ADVANCES IN NEUROLOGY
Volume 43

Advances in Neurology

Advances in Neurology

Volume 43

Myoclonus

Editors

Stanley Fahn, M.D.
H. Houston Merritt Professor
Department of Neurology
Columbia University
College of Physicians and Surgeons
New York, New York

C. David Marsden, M.D.
Department of Neurology
Institute of Psychiatry
London, England

Melvin H. Van Woert, M.D.
Professor
Department of Neurology
Mount Sinai School of Medicine
New York, New York

Raven Press ■ New York

Raven Press, 1140 Avenue of the Americas, New York, New York 10036

Made in the United States of America

Library of Congress Cataloging-in-Publication Data
Main entry under title:

Myoclonus.

    (Advances in neurology ; v. 43)
    Includes bibliographies and index.
    1. Myoclonus. I. Fahn, Stanley, 1933–
II. Marsden, C. David. III. Van Woert, Melvin H.
IV. Series. [DNLM: 1. Myoclonus. W1 AD684H v. 43 /
WE 550 M997]
RC321.A276 vol. 43   616.8 s   85-25798
[RC378]   [616.8]
ISBN 0-88167-122-3

Advances in Neurology Series

Preface

Myoclonus is a disorder that bridges the fields of epilepsy and involuntary movement disorders. Its varied etiologies, widespread sites of origin within the central nervous system, and multiple forms of clinical expression make it a highly complex disorder. Perhaps as a result of this complexity, no monograph has been available to summarize and distill what is known about myoclonus: This volume satisfies that need.

Beginning with a detailed discussion of the clinical aspects of myoclonus, subsequent sections review electrophysiological aspects, the role of the serotonin system, and animal models that can be used to study various aspects of the disorder.

This volume will facilitate a better understanding of myoclonus and will help clinicians in treating their myoclonic patients. Although current therapies for myoclonus can have dramatic effects, for many patients they provide only partial relief; disability remains. Because there is a need for further clinical and basic research, we feel that this volume will stimulate investigators to pursue their efforts to clarify the pathophysiology of the myoclonias and eventually to develop improved treatment.

STANLEY FAHN
C. DAVID MARSDEN
MELVIN H. VAN WOERT

Acknowledgement

The stimulus for organizing this volume came from the Myoclonus Research Fund, which together with the Department of Neurology of Columbia University College of Physicians and Surgeons cosponsored an international workshop on myoclonus at Arden House, New York. The bulk of financial support came from the Myoclonus Research Fund, with additional assistance from Abbott Pharmaceuticals, Sandoz Pharmaceuticals, and Hoffmann-La Roche. Much of the organizational work on arrangements for transportation and the amenities that make such a workshop run smoothly was handled by Mr. Norman Seiden, founder of the Myoclonus Research Fund, whose wife is a victim of anesthetic hypoxia-induced myoclonus. Mrs. Aida Malagold energetically and enthusiastically handled much of the correspondence. The staff at Arden House was most cooperative in making the facilities so accommodating and pleasant.

The organizers particularly thank the contributors and participants who took time from their busy schedules to meet, share information, and generate ideas on treatment and future research on myoclonus.

Contents

Clinical Aspects of Myoclonus

Electrophysiological Aspects of Myoclonus

Review of the Serotonin System

Animal Models of Myoclonus

Mechanism of Action of Antimyoclonic Drugs

Contributors

A

Aicardi, J., 11
Andermann, E., 87, 321
Andermann, F., 87, 321
Angel, A., 589
Artieda, J., 191
Azmitia, E. C., 407, 493

B

Baulac, M., 201
Boileau, J., 87
Bressman, S., 119, 287
Brin, M., 119
Brown, L. L., 519

C

Carmon, A., 545
Carpenter, S., 87
Carvey, P. M., 251, 509
Castaigne, P., 201
Chadwick, D., 183
Chapman, A. G., 661
Chung, E., 171, 565, 569, 653
Cirignotta, F., 295
Coccagna, G., 295
Côté, L., 309

D

De Léan, J., 215

E

Eisenberg, M., 119
*Escourolle, R., 201
Evron, S., 545

_____

*Deceased.

F

Fahn, S., 1, 119, 157, 197, 287,
    309, 645
Fuller, R. W., 469

G

Gannon, P., 407
Goetz, C. G., 251, 509
Goulon, M., 201

H

Hallett, M., 7, 183, 399
Halliday, A. M., 339
Hauw, J. J., 201
Hening, W., 309
Hopkins, L. C., 105

J

Jacobs, B. L., 481
Jenner, P., 183, 529, 553,
    577, 629

K

Kane, J. M., 231
Kinsbourne, M., 127
Klawans, H. L., 251, 509
Koskiniemi, M. L., 57

L

Lance, J. W., 33, 707
Lang, A. E., 191
Lapresle, J., 265
Leigh, N., 553
Lieberman, J. A., 231

xvii

Myoclonus

Advances in Neurology, Vol. 43: Myoclonus,
edited by S. Fahn et al. Raven Press,
New York © 1986.

Definition and Classification of Myoclonus

*Stanley Fahn, †C. David Marsden, and ‡Melvin H. Van Woert

*Department of Neurology, College of Physicians and Surgeons, Columbia University, New York, New York 10032; †Department of Neurology, Institute of Psychiatry, London SE5 8AF, United Kingdom; and ‡Department of Neurology, Mount Sinai School of Medicine, New York, New York 10029

The nosology and pathophysiology of myoclonus have been reviewed recently by Marsden et al. (14) and by Van Woert and Chung Hwang (19). These reviews offered a definition and classification of myoclonus, the basis of which is used here. New causes of myoclonus have been reported, some in this monograph, and we include this new information to update the etiologic classification of myoclonus.

DEFINITION

Myoclonus refers to sudden, brief, shocklike involuntary movements caused by muscular contractions (positive myoclonus) or inhibitions (negative myoclonus) arising from the central nervous system. This definition excludes the muscle twitches of fasiculations due to lesions of the lower motor neuron. However, it has become evident that phenomenologically similar muscle jerks may be produced by peripheral nerve or plexus lesions (see, for example, the report by Marsden et al., ref 16). The mechanism whereby such peripheral nerve lesions cause these jerks is not known, but it may be due to alteration of spinal motoneuron machinery.

The concept of negative myoclonus derives from the 1963 report of posthypoxic action myoclonus by Lance and Adams (11) who noted that some of the myoclonic jerking in this disorder is associated with electrical silent periods in muscle. The following year, Leavitt and Tyler (12) reported that asterixis may be associated with electrical silent periods in muscle. These observations, plus the physiologic studies by Marsden et al. (15), led to the concept of negative myoclonus. R. R. Young and B. T. Shahani *(this volume)* present a thorough analysis of asterixis as a form of negative myoclonus.

Myoclonus presents itself in various patterns. The myoclonic jerks can occur singly or repetitively. The amplitude of the jerks can range from small contractions not moving a joint to gross contractions moving limbs, head, or trunk. Single muscles or groups of muscles can be involved in a myoclonic jerk with a frequency rate that ranges from rare, isolated events to many contractions each minute. The distribution of myoclonus in the body can be focal (involving a single region), segmental (involving two or more contigious regions), or generalized (involving multiple regions of the body). Myoclonic jerks can occur bilaterally (symmetrical or asymmetrical) or unilaterally. A feature common and relatively distinct for myoclonus is synchrony; i.e., the simultaneous occurrence of muscle jerks, occurring within milliseconds of each other. Asynchronous jerking is also seen in patients with myoclonus.

Another feature relatively specific for myoclonus is that it is often stimulus-sensitive. For example, sudden and unexpected noise, light, visual threat, pin prick, or muscle stretch can trigger a myoclonic jerk. Some patients may be sensitive to ballistic movements (7), to sudden passive movements, or even to the command "try not to move" (5).

Activity can influence myoclonus. The jerks can be present with the patient at rest or it may arise during voluntary motor activity, especially when attempting to do a fine-motor task such as reaching for a target (action or intention myoclonus).

Myoclonus can vary from being very regular (rhythmic myoclonus) to irregular (arrhythmic myoclonus). Since rhythmic myoclonus tends to be persistent and uniform in its regularity, a third variety has been described, known as oscillatory myoclonus. This form is best described as jerky oscillations that often develop with a sudden stimulus or movement, last for a few seconds, and then fade away (6,17). More continuous irregular oscillatory myoclonus may also be seen (S. Bressman et al., *this volume*). Rhythmic myoclonus is usually associated with a lesion of brainstem or spinal cord, but it also has been observed in patients with no known cause and no other neurologic abnormality (S. Bressman and S. Fahn, *this volume*).

In classifying patients with myoclonus, the most important factor is the etiology, and this is discussed below. However, we believe it is also very helpful to classify patients according to certain aspects of the clinical phenomenology of the myoclonus, the most important of which are (a) distribution (focal, segmental, generalized); (b) regularity (arrhythmic, rhythmic, oscillatory); (c) synchronization (synchronous, asynchronous); (d) relation to motor activity (at rest, with action, intention); and (e) whether it is positive or negative myoclonus. These clinical features may eventually be found to be related to etiology, prognosis, severity, pharmacotherapy, or even surgical therapy. Moreover, when describing patients with myoclonus, indicating these clinical characteristics is useful in conveying a clear description of their neurological condition.

The differentiation of myoclonus from tics, chorea, dystonia, and tremor was made by Marsden et al. (14) in their review and does not require additional elaboration. However, it must be appreciated that myoclonic jerks are often seen in patients with, for example, Huntington's disease and various forms of dystonia. Furthermore, tics can sometimes be simple patterns of movements rather than complex, and they can resemble myoclonic jerks when they are of the "simple" pattern. The other typical abnormal movements identify these conditions as separate from the myoclonic disorders under discussion in this volume.

The disorder known as nocturnal myoclonus, originally described by Symonds (18), has been better characterized by using electrical recordings during the night. These involuntary movements of the legs are of fairly long duration (3), which precludes their being myoclonic jerks, as defined above. Since they recur repeatedly in periods of approximately 20 sec, the term periodic movements in sleep has been suggested (3). They often occur in patients who also have the restless-legs syndrome (2), and it seems more appropriate with our present state of knowledge to include them as part of the spectrum of the restless-legs syndrome. This is discussed in detail by E. Lugaresi et al. and by A. Walters et al., *this volume*.

CLASSIFICATION OF MYOCLONUS

Although myoclonus could be classified by pathophysiology, pharmacotherapy, or clinical phenomenology, the most important criterion is etiology because this allows extrapolation with regard to prognosis (1) and specific treatment. Marsden et al. (14) divided myoclonus into four major etiologic categories: physiologic, essential, epileptic, and symptomatic. We shall adopt this approach and update the listing by adding newly recognized causes of myoclonus and eliminate periodic movements in sleep as a form of myoclonus. Reference citations after an item listed denotes the additions made to this list.

I. Physiologic myoclonus (normal subjects)
   A. Sleep jerks (hypnic jerks)
   B. Anxiety-induced
   C. Exercise-induced
   D. Hiccough (singultus)
   E. Benign infantile myoclonus with feeding (13)
II. Essential myoclonus (no known cause and no other gross neurologic deficit)
   A. Hereditary (autosomal dominant)
   B. Sporadic
III. Epileptic myoclonus (seizures dominate and no encephalopathy, at least initially)
   A. Fragments of epilepsy
      Isolated epileptic myoclonic jerks
      Epilepsia partialis continua
      Idiopathic stimulus-sensitive myoclonus
      Photosensitive myoclonus
      Myoclonic absences in petit mal
   B. Childhood myoclonic epilepsies
      Infantile spasms
      Myoclonic astatic epilepsy (Lennox–Gastaut)
      Cryptogenic myoclonus epilepsy (Aicardi)
      Awakening myoclonus epilepsy of Janz (4,8,9)
   C. Benign familial myoclonic epilepsy (Rabot)
   D. Progressive myoclonus epilepsy: Baltic myoclonus (Unverricht–Lundborg)
IV. Symptomatic myoclonus (progressive or static encephalopathy dominates)
   A. Storage disease
      Lafora body disease
      Lipidoses, e.g., GM2 gangliosidosis, Tay–Sachs, Krabbe's
      Ceroid-lipofuscinosis (Batten)
      Sialidosis ("cherry-red spot")
   B. Spinocerebellar degeneration
      Ramsay Hunt syndrome
      Friedreich's ataxia
      Ataxia telangiectasia

C. Basal ganglia degenerations
    Wilson's disease
    Torsion dystonia
    Hallervorden–Spatz disease
    Progressive supranuclear palsy
    Huntington's disease
    Parkinson's disease

D. Dementias
    Creutzfeldt–Jakob disease
    Alzheimer's disease

E. Viral encephalopathies
    Subacute sclerosing panencephalitis
    Encephalitis lethargica
    Arbor virus encephalitis
    Herpes simplex encephalitis
    Postinfectious encephalitis

F. Metabolic
    Hepatic failure
    Renal failure
    Dialysis syndrome
    Hyponatremia
    Hypoglycemia
    Infantile myoclonic encephalopathy (polymyoclonus) ($\pm$ neuroblastoma)
    Nonketotic hyperglycemia
    Multiple carboxylase deficiency (S. Bressman et al., *this volume*)
    Biotin deficiency (S. Bressman et al., *this volume*)

G. Toxic encephalopathies
    Bismuth
    Heavy-metal poisons
    Methyl bromide, DDT
    Drugs, including levodopa (10)

H. Physical encephalopathies
    Posthypoxia (Lance–Adams)
    Post-traumatic
    Heat stroke
    Electric shock
    Decompression injury

I. Focal CNS damage
    Poststroke
    Postthalamotomy
    Tumor
    Trauma
    Olivodendate lesions (palatal myoclonus)

Most of the disorders listed are described in greater detail in this volume and in the reviews by Marsden et al. (14) and Van Woert and Chung Hwang (19) (see also Bressman et al., *this volume* and ref. 10). We added Parkinson's disease to the list of basal ganglia degenerations based on personal observations of patients with this disorder who have mild myoclonic jerks unrelated to medication. Levodopa-induced myoclonus due to toxicity with this drug in patients with parkinsonism has been recognized as well (10).

Segmental rhythmic myoclonus almost always indicates that this is a symptomatic form of myoclonus, and it has been reviewed by Marsden et al. (14). However, it can occasionally occur without a known cause, and in this situation it can be considered within the clinical spectrum of essential myoclonus (S. Bressman and S. Fahn, *this volume*).

Physiologic analysis of patients with myoclonus is leading to separate pathophysiologic groups, such as cortical reflex myoclonus and reticular reflex myoclonus. This is discussed in this volume. It is clearly known that posthypoxic action myoclonus can be associated with either of these two physiologic classification. Perhaps when other etiologies are similarly studied, some of them may also have disparate physiologic origins of the myoclonic jerking. We encourage such investigations and hope they will shed more light on this complex movement disorder.

REFERENCES

1. Aigner BR, Mulder DW. Myoclonus. Clinical significance and an approach to classification. *Arch Neurol* 1960;2:600–15.
2. Boghen D, Peyronnard JM. Myoclonus in familial restless legs syndrome. *Arch Neurol* 1976;33:368–70.
3. Coleman RM, Pollack CP, Weitzman ED. Periodic movements in sleep (nocturnal myoclonus): relation to sleep disorders. *Ann Neurol* 1980;8:416–21.
4. Delgado-Escueta AV, Enrile-Bascal F. Juvenile myoclonic epilepsy of Janz. *Neurology* 1984;34:285–94.
5. Fahn S. Atypical tremors, rare tremors, and unclassified tremors. In: Findley LJ, Capiledeo R, eds. *Movement disorders: tremor*. New York: Oxford University Press, 1984:431–43.
6. Fahn S, Singh N. An oscillating form of essential myoclonus. *Neurology* 1981;31(No. 4, Pt. 2):80.
7. Hallett M, Chadwick D, Marsden CD. Ballistic movement overflow myoclonus. A form of essential myoclonus. *Brain* 1977;100:299–312.
8. Janz D, Christian W. Impulsive petit mal. *Dtsch Z Nervenheilkunde* 1957;176:346–86.
9. Janz D, Mathes A. *Die Propulsiv Petit Mal Epilepsies*. New York: S. Karger, 1955.
10. Klawans HL, Goetz C, Bergen D. Levodopa-induced myoclonus. *Arch Neurol* 1975;32:331–4.
11. Lance JW, Adams RD. The syndrome of intention or action myoclonus as a sequel to hypoxic encephalopathy. *Brain* 1963;86:111–36.
12. Leavitt S, Tyler HR. Studies in asterixis. *Arch Neurol* 1964;10:360–8.
13. Lombroso CT, Fejerman N. Benign myoclonus of early infancy. *Ann Neurol* 1977;1:138–43.
14. Marsden CD, Hallett M, Fahn S. The nosology and pathophysiology of myoclonus. In: Marsden CD, Fahn S, eds. *Movement disorders*. London: Butterworth Scientific, 1982:196–248.
15. Marsden CD, Merton PA, Morton HB. Is the human stretch reflex cortical rather than spinal? *Lancet* 1973;1:759–61.
16. Marsden CD, Obeso JA, Traub MM, Rothwell JC, Kranz H, LaCruz F. Muscle spasms associated with Sudek's atrophy after injury. *Br Med J* 1984;1:173–6.
17. Obeso JA, Lang AE, Rothwell JC, Marsden CD. Postanoxic symptomatic oscillatory myoclonus. *Neurology* 1983;33:240–3.
18. Symonds CP. Nocturnal myoclonus. *J Neurol Neurosurg Psychiatry* 1953;16:166–71.
19. Van Woert MH, Chung Hwang E. Myoclonus. In: Vinken PJ, Bruyn GW, eds. *Handbook of clinical neurology*, vol. 38. Amsterdam; North-Holland Publishing Co., 1979:575–93.

Advances in Neurology, Vol. 43: Myoclonus,
edited by S. Fahn et al. Raven Press,
New York © 1986.

Early History of Myoclonus*

Mark Hallett

*Section of Neurology, Department of Medicine, Brigham and Women's Hospital and
Harvard Medical School, Boston, Massachusetts 02115*

On January 17, 1878, Professor Nikolaus Friedreich was called to do a consultation on Ludwig Beierlein in the Heidelberg Medical Clinic. This 50-year-old combmaker from Baden had been hospitalized for treatment of pneumonia. His doctors had noted the incidental problem of muscle jerks all over his body, which had affected him for the previous 5 years, and they wondered about the nature and significance of this disorder. The patient had suffered a fright at the onset of the muscle jerking, and no other history seemed relevant. There was no family history of neurological disease, his intelligence was normal, there was no epilepsy, and there was no other symptom or sign of neurological illness. The muscle jerking was not severe enough to disable him from practicing his trade.

In detail, there was multifocal jerking of all muscles in the body except those of the face. The frequency of jerking was 10 to 50 per minute. The jerks were often so small that joint movement did not occur. The movements were prominent at rest and disappeared with action; they could be induced by tactile or stretch stimuli.

Professor Friedreich was a well-known and respected physician with a good knowledge of neurology. He was Erb's mentor. For the previous 20 years he had been evaluating a family with ataxia and peripheral neuropathy with careful clinical and pathological studies. With the help of Schultze he had documented the pathology in the spinal cord. This illness is now known as Friedreich's ataxia.

The differential diagnosis available to Friedreich for this involuntary movement disorder was limited. There was epileptic clonus or clonic spasm, known since ancient times, which was a single jerk affecting part or all of the body in patients with epilepsy. Another described disorder was chorea, of which there were several subtypes. The term was originally used for the episodic dancing manias which affected entire communities in the middle ages; the best known of these was St. Vitus Dance. In 1686 Sydenham (19) borrowed the term to refer to the involuntary movements in patients with rheumatic fever. In 1846, Dubini (3) described patients with (presumably) only rapid movements and called this electric chorea. His patients were very ill, with an acute febrile illness which progressed to death in 90% of

*This chapter is a further analysis of material prepared for an earlier historical review which was part of a chapter by Marsden CD, Hallett M, Fahn S. The nosology and pathophysiology of myoclonus. In: Marsden CD, Fahn S, eds. Movement disorders. Butterworths International Medical Reviews, Neurology 2. London: Butterworth Scientific, 1982.

cases. The term electric chorea was subsequently used for an entirely different clinical picture by Henoch in 1861 and by Bergeron, reported by Berland in 1880 (1). Their patients were children about the age of puberty with multifocal muscle jerking and otherwise benign medical picture. At least for Bergeron's cases the disorder was self-limited. In 1872, Huntington (9) also used the term chorea to describe the involuntary movements in his patients with a hereditary disorder. Another entity, which Friedreich may not have known about, was convulsive tremor, originally described by Pritchard in 1822 (15) and revived by Hammond in 1867 (7). These patients had a dramatic disorder characterized by paroxysms of tremor and sweating with fever which lasted for a few minutes before completely disappearing. It was separated from epilepsy because consciousness was not impaired.

Clearly, none of the possibilities in the differential diagnostic list fit Ludwig Beierlein. A lesser man than Friedreich might have said that he did not know what this disorder was or that the disorder was closest to electric chorea, but that no cases had previously been described with adult onset. Friedreich, however, was confident that he was seeing a new disorder, and he thought it appropriate to describe and name it. In 1881 (4) he described the case in detail under the name of paramyoklonus multiplex. *Klonus* referred to a quick movement, but he used the modifier *myo* to clearly distinguish it from the epileptic disorder. *Para* indicated the symmetry, and *multiplex* indicated the involvement of multiple sites in the body.

Friedreich believed that the etiological factor in this case was the fright that Beierlein had experienced. In the discussion of his paper, Friedreich noted that fright was known to cause both chorea and epileptic convulsions. Moreover, in light of recent work, it was clear that fear was especially able to damage the spinal cord (and he quoted several references). In particular he mentioned nutritional disturbances and other organic changes. Therefore he believed that it was possible that paramyoklonus multiplex arose from a disorder in the spinal cord. We must remember that Friedreich had been studying the spinal cord carefully for the prior 20 years in relation to his cases of spinal ataxia. In this regard it would not have been surprising if he had given the name paramyeloklonus multiplex.

Unfortunately for Friedreich's theory, when Beierlein died 5 years later an autopsy by Schultze (limited to the spinal cord and muscles) failed to reveal any pathology. Nevertheless, the term became popular and was abbreviated to myoclonus.

Previously described phenomena were reclassified by many scholars as myoclonus. The electric choreas of Henoch and Bergeron were called myoclonus, but they probably fit better into the catetory of tic. It is notable in this regard that Gilles de la Tourette (5) described his cases 4 years after Friedreich and the publication that established tic as a distinct movement disorder was that of Meige and Feindel (13) in 1903. Hammond (6), in his textbook of neurology in 1892, claimed that his disorder of convulsive tremor was clearly "identical" to the case described by Friedreich. The case descriptions seem very different and looking back at Hammond's cases, it is difficult to know what to call them.

New phenomena were called myoclonus inappropriately. These include myoclonus fibrillaris multiplex of Kny (10) in 1888, fibrillary chorea of Morvan (14) in 1890, and myokymia of Schultze (17) in 1895. It is relevant to note that knowledge of the pathophysiology of the peripheral nervous system was also poor at that time. For example, it was not until 1938 that fibrillations and fasciculations were separated by Denny-Brown and Pennypacker (2).

Many new case reports of myoclonus appeared in the literature. Lowenfeld (11) described a case in 1883, proposing at that time to shorten the name to myoklonus. Seeligmüller (18) described a case in 1886, proposing to call the disorder myoclonie. Seeligmüller's patient was a 24-year-old man with jerks and vocalizations which were worse with anxiety and improved with galvanic current. This certainly would be classified as a tic today. In 1891 when Unverricht (20) reviewed the literature, he found 40 cases but thought that four-fifths were inappropriately designated. Unverricht also described patients for the first time with a familial disorder characterized by myoclonus, epilepsy, and mild progression.

In 1903, Lundborg (12) described additional patients with familial progressive myoclonic epilepsy and proposed a classification of the different cases of myoclonus, which remains a reasonable first approach. The first category is *symptomatic myoclonus*, which is myoclonus attributable to a definite disorder of the central nervous system (CNS). Dubini's cases were clear examples. The second category is *essential myoclonus*, which is myoclonus without any evident disorder of the CNS. Friedreich's case was the first described in this category. The third category was *familial myoclonic epilepsy*, of which there were two subtypes: nonprogressive, first described by Rabot (16) in 1899, and progressive, described by Unverricht and Lundborg.

Within 22 years, from Friedreich to Lundborg, myoclonus had come of age.

SUMMARY

The term myoclonus is a shortened form of the name *paramyoklonus multiplex* used by Nikolaus Friedreich to describe the involuntary movements of a patient whom today would be said to have a form of essential myoclonus. The details of this case and Friedreich's discussion of it have been reviewed. Other early cases and the initial classification scheme of H. Lundborg have been described.

REFERENCES

1. Bergeron, quoted by Berland (1880) on p. 1934 in Wilson SAK, *Neurology*, edited by Bruce AN, 2nd edition. Baltimore: Williams & Wilkins, 1955.
2. Denny-Brown D, Pennybacker JB. Fibrillations and fasiculations in voluntary muscle. *Brain*, 1938:61:311–34.
3. Dubini A. Primi cenni sulla corea electria. *Annals of the University of Medicine (Milano)* 1846:117:1–5, quoted in reference 18.
4. Friedreich N. Neuropathologische Beobachtung beim paramyokonus multiplex. *Virch Arch Pathol Anat Physiol Klin Med* 1881:86:421–34.
5. Gilles de la Tourette G. Étude sur une affection nerveuse caractérisée par de l'incoordination motrice accompagnée d'echolalie et de coprolalie. *Arch Neurol (Paris)* 1885:9:19–42, 159–200.

6. Hammond WA. *Diseases of the nervous system*. New York: Appleton, 1892.
7. Hammond WA. On convulsive tremor. *NY J Med* 1867:5:185–98.
8. Henoch (1861) quoted on p. 1933 in Wilson SAK, *Neurology*, edited by Bruce AN, 2nd edition. Baltimore: Williams & Wilkins, 1955.
9. Huntington G. On chorea. *Med Surg Reporter* 1872:26:317–21.
10. Kny E. Über ein dem Paramyoclonus Multiplex (Friedreich) nahestehendes Krankheitsbild. *Arch Psychiatr Nervenk* 1888:19:577–90.
11. Lowenfeld (1883), quoted in reference 18.
12. Lundborg H. *Die progressive Myoklonus-Epilepsie*. Uppsala: Almqvist and Wiksell, 1903.
13. Meige H, Feindel E. *Der Tic*. Berlin: Deuticke, 1903.
14. Morvan AM. De la chorée fibrillaire. *Gazette hebdomadaire de Medecine et de Chirurgie* 1890:27:173–176, 187–189, 200–202.
15. Pritchard (1822), quoted in reference 7.
16. Rabot L. *La Myoclonie Épileptique*. Thèse: Paris, 1899.
17. Schultze FR. Beiträge zur Muskelpathologie. Myokymie (Muskelwogen), besonder an den Unterestremitäten. *Deutsche Z Nervenheilkunde*, 1895:6:65–76, 167–168.
18. Seeligmüller A. Ein Fall von Paramyoklonus multiplex (Freidreich) (Myoclonia congenita). *Deutsche Med Wochenschift* 1886:12:405–408.
19. Sydenham T. Schedula monitoria de novae febris ingressu. Londini: G. Kettilby 1686.
20. Unverricht H. *Die Myoklonie*. Leipzig und Wien: Franz Deuticke, 1891.

Advances in Neurology, Vol. 43: Myoclonus,
edited by S. Fahn et al. Raven Press,
New York © 1986.

Myoclonic Epilepsies of Infancy and Childhood

Jean Aicardi

National Institute for Health and Medical Investigation, Hospital for Sick Children, 75743 Paris, France

All forms of myoclonus, whether massive or bilaterally symmetrical, segmental, or fragmentary (40), can occur with almost every type of epilepsy. It is customary, however, to use the term myoclonic epilepsy to designate those epilepsies characterized, exclusively or predominantly, by brief myoclonic, atonic, or tonic seizures (3) because they share several common clinical features: very frequent recurrence of fits of an apparently minor character, resistance to many conventional antiepileptic drugs, and frequent association with mental retardation. These resemblances are largely superficial, and a more precise analysis of the ictal and interictal manifestations by polygraphic and video monitoring shows that a number of these myoclonic phenomena consist of either a sudden loss of muscle tone (atonic seizures) or a brief increase in muscle tone (tonic seizures). The abruptness and brief duration of the ictal events explain why they are so commonly interpreted as myoclonias. Precise analysis permits us to distinguish true myoclonic seizures from pseudomyoclonic seizures. The former (81) are manifested in electromyographic records as short bursts of synchronized activity, which often involves at the same time agonist and antagonist muscles and are associated with fast (3 Hz or more), irregular spike–wave activity on the electroencephalogram (EEG) (Fig. 1). Pseudomyoclonic seizures of the tonic type appear on the electromyogram (EMG) as longer bursts of activity similar to voluntary muscle contraction. They are associated with a fast (10–20 Hz) rhythm or with a sudden flattening of the EEG tracings (Fig. 2) (44); atonic seizures are usually associated with spike–wave complexes with either a slow (>2.5 Hz) or a fast rhythm on the EEG, while the EMG of affected muscles shows suppression of the normal tonic activity (42,51). Some patients have only one seizure type, but several types may occur in the same patient and even in the same fit (e.g., a massive myoclonia may precede immediately loss of postural tone) (84). As a result, distinction of the various seizure mechanisms may be difficult, even when polygraphy is used.

This chapter reviews the various forms of epilepsy customarily referred to as myoclonic, irrespective of the neurophysiological mechanisms at play (2). However, epileptic syndromes featuring true or pseudomyoclonic seizures will be envisioned separately, when appropriate, since their outlook, treatment, and etiological factors are different.

11

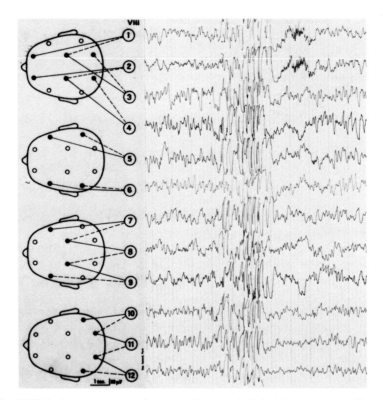

FIG. 1. EEG discharge accompanying a massive myoclonic jerk. Irregular polyspike–waves at 3 Hz.

In the International Classification of Epileptic Seizures (41), the vast majority of the seizures that constitute the myoclonic epilepsies are categorized, on clinical and EEG grounds, as generalized, under the headings of massive bilateral myoclonus, tonic or atonic seizures, and infantile spasms. However, in the 1981 revision of the classification (25), the latter are regarded as a syndrome rather than a seizure type. Localized forms of myoclonus may be associated with generalized myoclonias or represent the only or predominant myoclonic phenomenon in several epileptic syndromes. Erratic myoclonus, for instance, is often observed during the episodes of petit mal status or minor epileptic status (19,34) which may occur in the course of the Lennox–Gastaut syndrome or of certain true myoclonic epilepsies. Fragmentary or erratic myoclonus is also prominent in several disorders that belong to the group of the degenerative myoclonic epilepsies (Table 1) even though an epileptic mechanism is debatable in part of these cases (40). Localized epileptic myoclonus involving a fixed group of muscles is also a hallmark of epilepsia partialis continuans (85). In this syndrome, the myoclonus is associated with partial motor seizures starting in the area of the body which is the seat of the permanent myoclonias.

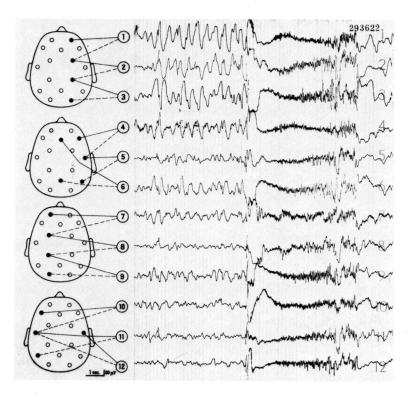

FIG. 2. EEG discharge accompanying a brief tonic seizure. Fast rhythm of 20 Hz with progressively increasing voltage.

This chapter is limited to the epilepsies with generalized myoclonus, which represent by far the most common types of myoclonic epilepsies. Approximately two-thirds of the myoclonic epilepsies occur during the first 5 years of life. A general classification of the disorders and syndromes associated with epileptic myoclonus is presented in Table 1, where they are divided into two groups: (a) those that are a symptom of a progressive, usually degenerative brain disorder (progressive myoclonic epilepsies), and (b) those in which myoclonic seizures are the major component of several epileptic syndromes not attributable to a known underlying progressive disease. The latter group in turn can be subdivided into the myoclonic epilepsies associated with a fixed encephalopathy manifested by neurological and/or mental signs predating the onset of the seizures (1,2,4,32), and the myoclonic epilepsies unassociated with any structural brain damage prior to the onset of fits. Proper assignment of a particular case to one or the other group may be difficult since apparent progression of the disorder is not infrequent in patients of the second group. This apparent progression can result from several mechanisms, such as drug toxicity, frequent seizures, and, especially, episodes of "petit mal status." During these episodes, erratic myoclonic jerks, mental deterio-

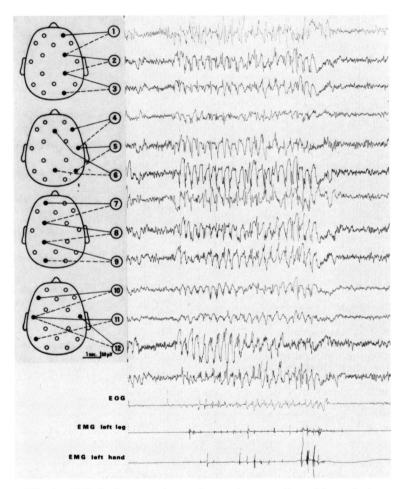

FIG. 3. EEG discharge accompanying an absence with eyelid myoclonias.

ration, obtundation, and ataxia (4,13,80) can mimic a degenerative disorder. The distinction between progressive and nonprogressive myoclonic epilepsies has obvious practical implications since the disorders of the first group have a dismal prognosis and are genetically transmitted. These progressive diseases are not discussed further in this chapter, which is limited to the study of the following: (a) infantile spasms and related syndromes, (b) Lennox–Gastaut syndrome and its variants, and (c) true myoclonic epilepsies of infancy, childhood, and adolescence. The former syndromes are mainly examples of pseudomyoclonic seizures.

INFANTILE SPASMS AND RELATED SYNDROMES

Infantile Spasms

Infantile spasms [also known as West's syndrome, flexor spasms, "propulsive petit mal," and Blitz–Nick–Salaam (BNS) krämpfe)] have been extensively reviewed

TABLE 1. *Classification of the myoclonic epilepsies of childhood*

Progressive myoclonic encephalopathies
  With demonstrated or probable metabolic disturbances
    Tay–Sachs disease
    juvenile Gaucher's disease
    ceroid-lipofuscinosis (Batten's disease)
    Lafora body disease
    sialosidosis and mucolipidosis
    nonketotic hyperglycinemia
  Genetic syndromes without known metabolic basis
    progressive degenerative myoclonic epilepsies (includes several types, including Baltic
      myoclonus and the Ramsay Hunt syndrome)
    infantile, nonspecific poliodystrophies (several types)
    juvenile neuroaxonal dystrophy
    Hallervorden–Spatz disease
    Huntington's chorea (myoclonic form)
    dominant myoclonus, ataxia, and hearing loss
    myoclonus associated with spinocerebellar degenerations
  Subacute sclerosing panencephalitis
Nonprogressive myoclonic encephalopathies
  of anoxic origin
  of other origins
Nonprogressive myoclonic epilepsies
  With mainly pseudomyoclonic seizures[a]
    infantile spasms (West's syndrome) and related syndromes
    Lennox–Gastaut syndrome
  With mainly true myoclonic seizures[a]
    cryptogenic myoclonic epilepsies (? several types)
    myoclonus associated with petit mal absences
    myoclonic absences
    eyelid myoclonia with absences
    myoclonic epilepsy of adolescence

[a]See text.

(5,23,43,58,61a,64,72,78) and are not dealt with in detail. The syndrome is observed exclusively during the first year of life, with a peak frequency between 4 and 9 months. In addition to the seizures, it comprises mental retardation or deterioration and a remarkable EEG abnormality known as hypsarrhythmia. The spasms consist of a sudden flexion of the head and limbs (34%), flexion of the trunk with extension of the upper and/or lower limbs (42%), and rarely, extension of the head, trunk, and limbs (23%). They supervene in clusters of several units or dozens, several seconds apart. They may be limited to a barely detectable head nod. Kellaway et al. (62) have shown by sophisticated polygraphic techniques that many of them go unrecognized, that their expression varies considerably in the same infant, and that isolated jerks are common in both sleep and wakefulness. Asymmetrical and even unilateral spasms may be observed, mainly in lesional cases (43,58). The usual EEG correlate of the spasms is a flattening of the tracing, temporarily suppressing the chaotic hypsarrhythmic pattern. A brief discharge of polyspike–waves may also be recorded (43,62). The interictal EEG pattern is devoid of background activity and entirely made of high-amplitude, asynchronous slow waves, haphazardly intermingled with sharp waves or spikes of multifocal origin.

The typical hypsarrhythmia may be absent in as many as 40% of the patients (58). A modified pattern with variable admixture of slow and sharp waves at times asymmetrical is then recorded. The contrast between a chaotic pattern while awake and one of synchronous polyspike–waves separated by low-amplitude tracing in sleep has a definite diagnostic value even when classic hypsarrhythmia is lacking (66). Sleep records should always be obtained, especially at the onset of the syndrome or following therapy, since they are modified earlier than waking ones.

Mental retardation may be obvious before onset of the spasms in symptomatic cases. In previously well infants, a definite behavioral regression is often observed. Regression may precede the spasms or be marked while these go unrecognized so that deterioration in an infant should lead one to suspect West's syndrome.

Infantile spasms are a syndrome with multiple causes (Table 2). The incidence of the syndrome is 0.25 to 0.35 per 1,000 live births (43,78). Boys are affected more often than girls (60%). Although the pathophysiology of the disorder is poorly understood, a diffuse cortical dysfunction seems likely, but no consistent neuro-

TABLE 2. *Main reported causes of West's syndrome[a]*

Neurocutaneous syndromes
tuberous sclerosis
neurofibromatosis
Sturge–Weber syndrome
incontinentia pigmenti
linear nevus sebaceus syndrome
Brain malformations
Aicardi's syndrome
lissencephaly–pachygyria syndrome
holoprosencephaly
agenesis of corpus callosum
heterotopias
micropolygyria
trisomy 21
Prenatal infections
cytomegalovirus
toxoplasmosis
rubella
Metabolic disorders
phenylketonuria
nonketotic hyperglycinemia
hyperornithinemia, hyperammonemia, and homocitrullinuria
Leigh's disease
soudanophilic leukodystrophy
neonatal hypoglycemia
Anoxic–ischemic perinatal encephalopathies
Postnatally acquired encephalopathies
CNS infections
acute dehydration
subdural hematoma and brain contusions
brain tumors (neurinoma, choroid plexus papilloma, sarcoma)

[a]Many of the listed disorders are also frequent causes of the Lennox–Gastaut syndrome.

pathological change has been found (15,43,61). The abnormalities of dendritic spines described by Huttenlocher (54) are of dubious specificity. Certain EEG and clinical characteristics of the spasms have suggested a brainstem origin, which is supported by the occurrence of spasms in anencephalic (31) and hydranencephalic (74) infants. In a majority (60–80%) of the cases, extensive brain lesions can be demonstrated. Prenatal causes are most common. Among the causes shown in Table 2, most are relatively nonspecific (e.g., perinatal anoxic–ischemic encephalopathy or cytomegalovirus infection) and are more often responsible for other epileptic or nonepileptic disturbances than for infantile spasms. Certain brain developmental defects and metabolic disorders have a more specific relationship with West's syndrome. Tuberous sclerosis may be responsible for 10 to up to 25% of the cases. It can be diagnosed early when achromic nevi are associated with the spasms (49). Subependymal calcifications can be demonstrated on computerized tomography (CT) scan as early as 3 to 5 months of age (47). The lissencephaly syndrome (50) and the syndrome of agenesis of the corpus callosum with lacunae of the retinal pigment epithelium, subependymal heterotopias, and vertebrocostal abnormalities in girls (Aicardi's syndrome) (7) are less common but are recognizable clinically and by CT scan.

Phenylketonuria and nonketotic hyperglycinemia are the only metabolic disorders significantly associated with West's syndrome. Brain damage of unknown origin is commonly shown by CT scan (47). Atrophic changes are of significance only if obtained before the start of hormonal therapy since brain shrinkage is commonly observed during such treatment (70).

In 20 to 30% of the patients, there is no obvious cause nor evidence of brain damage prior to the spasms. These cryptogenic cases have a much better prognosis. Cases occurring after diphtheria–tetanus–pertussis (DTP) immunization are probably only coincidental (73). Genetic factors are found only in a small minority of the patients.

Whatever the cause of the syndrome, the spasms and the hypsarrhythmic EEG pattern tend to disappear spontaneously before 3 years of age. Other seizures, especially those that constitute the Lennox–Gastaut syndrome, follow the spasms in about one-half the cases (43,59). Mental retardation, often associated with psychiatric disturbances (79), persists in about 90% of the patients.

The treatment of West's syndrome is still the subject of much controversy, which revolves about the value, indications, and modalities of hormonal therapy (52,64,65,82). Adrenocorticotropic hormone (ACTH) or corticosteroids are effective in stopping the fits in 50 to 70% of the cases. Long-term effects on mental development are much less impressive. The proportion of mentally normal children averages 35 to 40% in cryptogenic cases, whereas prognosis is uniformly poor in symptomatic cases. Some workers have claimed more favorable results with the use of very high dose (80–120 U i.v.) and prolonged therapy with ACTH or with a combined ACTH–corticosteroid regimen (65). The lack of uniform criteria for selection of patients and evaluation of the results, as well as the variety of regimens used, precludes any comparison between different series and any definitive conclusion regarding the most effective schedules (64). Recent trials of ACTH fragments without corticotropic activity have not been encouraging (88). The importance for the prognosis of such factors as age of onset, cause, and association with other types of seizures has been emphasized and these factors should be taken into account when studying the effects of therapy. Pending such an evaluation, hormonal therapy of all cases of West's syndrome not obviously symptomatic seems indicated. An early onset of treatment may improve the outlook (65,78). In symptomatic cases or in failures of hormonal therapy, sodium valproate (9) or the benzodiazepines (20,86) may provide favorable results.

Syndromes Related to Infantile Spasms: Early Infantile Epileptic Encephalopathy, Early Myoclonic Epileptic Encephalopathy, and Myoclonic Encephalopathy of the Newborn

Although infantile spasms may evolve as early as the first weeks of life, in this age range (until approximately 3 months) they tend to be less typical and to be associated with other types of fits.

The EEG pattern of typical hypsarrhythmia is virtually never seen before age 3 months. Various types of paroxysmal patterns are then observed. The most remarkable is made of complex paroxysmal bursts of irregular slow and sharp waves separated by intervals of low-voltage, almost inactive record (suppression–burst activity). Ohtahara (76) has proposed to place these early atypical cases in a separate category under the name of *early infantile epileptic encephalopathy*. This would represent a third type of age-dependent epileptic encephalopathy, together with West's and Lennox–Gastaut syndromes. The syndrome appears to be due to early and extensive brain insults, especially brain malformations. Aicardi's syndrome may be considered a subtype of early infantile epileptic encephalopathy in which the paroxysmal bursts occur independently over the two hemispheres (7,39). Early infantile epileptic encephalopathy tends to evolve into West's syndrome at about 4 to 6 months of age. However, infantile spasms do not follow in every case, and the nature and extent of brain damage, as well as the age of emergence, may be responsible for the peculiar clinical picture.

The suppression–burst pattern may also be found in newborns or in very young infants presenting clinically with erratic myoclonus, partial seizures, and severe neurological deterioration. Flexor spasms often supervene after a few weeks, whereas the erratic myoclonus tends to disappear. This picture is seen in nonketotic hyperglycinemia (26) and in the rare cases of D-glyceric acidemia (18). An identical picture, with a severe progressive course, may also occur in infants without known metabolic disturbances. Such cases, variably termed myoclonic encephalopathy of newborns (8) or early myoclonic epileptic encephalopathy (22,28), probably form a heterogeneous group. Familial cases are on record (8,28) and suggest the possibility of an undetermined metabolic disorder. A neuropathological picture of nonspecific poliodystrophy has been found in a few cases (8).

A syndrome of *benign myoclonus of infancy* has been reported (68). This syndrome comprises repetitive flexor spasms which closely resemble infantile spasms but without EEG abnormalities or mental dysfunction. In contradistinction to West's syndrome, benign myoclonus of infancy runs a benign, self-limited course and is probably related to tics rather than epilepsy.

THE LENNOX–GASTAUT SYNDROME: CHILDHOOD EPILEPTIC ENCEPHALOPATHY WITH SLOW SPIKE–WAVES

The term Lennox–Gastaut syndrome, as used in this chapter, refers to a form of severe epilepsy of childhood, characterized clinically by frequently repeated seizures of several types, often responsible for multiple falls, and electrically by an interictal pattern of diffuse slow spike–wave complexes at a rhythm of less than 2.5 Hz. This EEG pattern was initially described as petit mal variant (48). Other workers use the term in a broader or different sense. Some include under this heading all the clinical correlates of the diffuse slow spike–wave EEG pattern (17,71). Others base their description mainly on a clinical picture dominated by atonic seizures and massive myoclonias, regardless of the associated EEG pattern, which may be of the fast as well as of the slow spike–wave type. The latter use the descriptive term of myoclonic–astatic petit mal (33,35,63), which is often wrongly considered synonymous with that of the Lennox syndrome. These differences in criteria and definition have been responsible for an enormous nosological confusion. This is understandable because it is difficult to fix the limits of any specific syndrome within the large group of the severe epilepsies of early childhood with multiform, brief seizures, poor response to therapy, and frequent mental retardation. This group is certainly too heterogeneous to be regarded as a single entity, but subdivision into separate syndromes is bound to be arbitrary since many transitional cases occur.

The seizures of the Lennox–Gastaut syndrome, as defined in this chapter, are always of multiple types. The main types include the following: tonic fits involving mainly the axial muscles with frequent extension to the upper limbs and respiratory arrest, associated with a discharge of 10 to 15-Hz rhythm on the EEG (11,12,45); atonic seizures and atypical absences, variably associated with more or less rhythmical slow spike–waves or with a fast, 10-Hz rhythm (11,45); massive true myoclonias with irregular discharges of spike–wave complexes, usually at a rhythm of 2.5 Hz or more (24,45). Tonic and or atonic seizures (i.e., pseudomyoclonic) occur in more than 80% of the cases, whereas true myoclonias supervene in 10 to 30% (24,45). Whatever their type, the seizures are mainly brief (lasting less than 5–10 sec) and often produce falls in the standing child, either by throwing the patient out of balance (tonic and myoclonic attacks) or by inducing a sudden loss of muscle tone. The typical child experiences multiple daily falls, during which injuries to the teeth, nose, forehead, or occiput may be incurred; thus wearing a protective helmet is necessary. In milder fits, the head may nod and the knees sag although the child does not fall. Atypical absences marked by a brief period of immobility with a stare and at times palpebral jerks or a slow and saccading dropping forward of the head are also common, especially when the onset of the syndrome is relatively late, after 3 to 4 years of age (24). The tonic attacks are especially common during sleep even though they may be barely noticeable. The concomitant 10-Hz discharge on the EEG—the so-called grand mal discharge—is one of the most valuable EEG features of the Lennox–Gastaut syndrome (11,75). Seizures are also apt to be more frequent on awakening. Episodes of obtundation or blurring of consciousness, interspersed with atonic head nods, fluttering of eyelids, or slight erratic myoclonias of the face or segments of limbs, occur in 30 to 40% of patients (11,24,45). These episodes, variably termed petit mal status, epileptic stupor, absence status, and minor epileptic status (19,34,46), may last from minutes to hours or even days and weeks, at times in a subtle, almost unrecognizable form. Ataxia of a pseudocere-bellar type is common during some episodes of status (4,13,24) and may wrongly suggest the diagnosis of a progressive central nervous system (CNS) disorder. Episodes of tonic status, which may be life-threatening, occur in some patients and may be precipitated by the administration of benzodiazepines (16,83). In virtually all patients, good periods alternate with bad ones, with parallel fluctuations in intellectual performance (12,46). Other types of seizures (generalized tonic–clonic, unilateral, partial motor) are often associated with the tonic, atonic, and myoclonic fits which constitute the central ictal pattern of the Lennox–Gastaut syndrome.

The interictal EEG pattern features bilateral, synchronous, slow spike–wave complexes at 1 to 2.5 Hz, but spike–waves at a faster rhythm are quite common (17,46). The complexes occur in bursts lasting from seconds to minutes. They may be almost continuous during the bad periods and tend to become less regular to the point of resembling the hypsarrhythmic pattern (12). Complete symmetry is rather unusual, and some unilateral preponderance is the rule; however, the abnor-malities often shift from one side to the other, even during the same recording session (2). The paroxysms are little sensitive to hyperventilation and to intermittent photic stimulation but are strongly activated by sleep, during which runs of 10-Hz rhythm are common. The background activity is almost always abnormal, slow, and/or asymmetrical (17). Other abnormalities, whether generalized (3-Hz spike–waves), focal, or multifocal, are frequently associated with the characteristic pat-tern.

Mental retardation, of a severe degree in half the cases, is present before onset of the seizures in 20 to 60% of the patients (secondary cases), and in up to 75 to 95% after a few years (2,24,46). It is often accompanied by disturbances of behavior and personality. There is usually no obvious loss of previously acquired skills and no new neurological signs, except during episodes of status. This is important in differentiating the Lennox–Gastaut syndrome from the degenerative myoclonic epilepsies.

The incidence of the Lennox–Gastaut syndrome has been variously estimated from 3.0 to 10.7% of the epilepsies of childhood (21,46). The syndrome has its peak incidence between 2 and 8 years of age. It is often preceded by other seizure types, especially by infantile spasms. The same insults that produce the latter can be responsible for the Lennox–Gastaut syndrome, which may also result from a number of acquired brain lesions, such as trauma, infections, and prolonged convulsive seizures (2). A family history of convulsive disorders is present in 2.5 to 50% of the cases (2). Such large discrepancies probably result from the different definitions of the syndrome. No cause is found in 20 to 40% of the cases (primary cases).

The Lennox–Gastaut syndrome is one of the severest forms of childhood epilepsy. Only few patients are ultimately able to live independent lives because of mental retardation and/or neurological deficits. Approximately 80% of the patients will continue to have seizures. Even with the restricted definition used in this chapter, however, the syndrome is heterogeneous, which is reflected in the course. Chevrie and Aicardi (24), in a study of 80 patients with Lennox–Gastaut syndrome, found that tonic fits were prominent in cases of early onset, which were associated with a more severe outcome than cases of relatively late onset, in which myoclonic seizures and atypical absences were the predominant fits. Blume et al. (17) and Markand (71) came to similar conclusions. Beaumanoir (11), in a series of 103 cases, distinguished a typical or complete form, in which tonic fits, frequent petit mal or tonic statuses, and discharges of 10-Hz rhythm during sleep were all combined; and atypical or incomplete forms, in which certain seizure types (especially tonic fits and statuses) and the fast rhythms during sleep were lacking. After a mean follow-up of 21 years, the patients in the first group continued to exhibit the unchanged picture of the Lennox–Gastaut syndrome. In the second group, after a mean follow-up of 22.4 years, a majority of the patients presented either with partial seizures (mainly complex partial) or with multifocal or secondary generalized epilepsies and no longer had the characteristic seizures of the Lennox–Gastaut syndrome. In the latter group, the Lennox–Gastaut syndrome seemed to represent only a temporary and age-related modality of expression of several different forms of epilepsy. Frontal partial lesions may be particularly apt to produce a picture of the Lennox–Gastaut syndrome (2,10).

Treatment of the Lennox–Gastaut syndrome is disappointing. The benzodiazepines (86) and sodium valproate (60), or a combination of both, are partly and often temporarily effective. A ketogenic diet is favored by several workers (53). Either ACTH or steroids may be used to tide some patient over difficult periods, but their long-term use should be avoided. Overtreatment is a major hazard in such resistant epilepsies. Evidence has shown that limitation of the number of drugs utilized may not only improve the state of vigilance but also decrease the frequency of fits (87).

TRUE MYOCLONIC EPILEPSIES OF INFANCY, CHILDHOOD, AND ADOLESCENCE

During the past few years, the distinction made in this chapter between true and pseudomyoclonic seizures has gained increasing acceptance (1,4,37). As a result, the epileptic syndromes formerly grouped under the general heading of "myoclonic epilepsies" tend to be divided into those with mainly pseudomyoclonic seizures (West's and Lennox–Gastaut syndromes) and those in which true myoclonias represent the main seizure phenomenon. Such a distinction is of more than academic interest since true myoclonic epilepsies are associated with a different outlook and therapy than pseudomyoclonic ones (67). However, the distinction between true and pseudomyoclonic seizures is often difficult to draw in practice: (a) proper classification of such brief epileptic events may require the use of prolonged polygraphic recordings, which are not always available to establish their real nature; and (b) pure myoclonic seizures are uncommonly the sole type of ictal phenomena and other fits are frequently associated, especially atonic and tonic ones, so that assignment of a particular case to one or the other group may depend on the predominance rather than the exclusiveness of one type. Moreover, the epilepsies with true myoclonic seizures do not constitute a homogeneous group.

These difficulties explain why classification of the true myoclonic epilepsies remains so controversial. Jeavons (56) recognized three forms (myoclonic epilepsy of childhood, myoclonic epilepsy of adolescence, and eyelid myoclonias with absences), in addition to West's syndrome and the Lennox–Gastaut syndrome, which he terms "myoclonic-astatic epilepsy." He did not separate true from pseudomyoclonic seizures. Lombroso and Erba (67) clearly made this distinction. They recognized among patients with true myoclonic seizures a subgroup of children 5 years or older in whom myoclonias are part of other patterns of primary generalized epilepsy; a subgroup with earlier onset with frequent myoclonic status, and often with lesional causes; and a third and smaller subgroup of infants and young children without mental or neurological compromise and who rarely develop myoclonic status. The same authors distinguished in the large group of pseudomyoclonic seizures, a rare subgroup of children with purely atonic seizures and a common one featuring both tonic and atonic fits, which corresponds to the Lennox–Gastaut syndrome. Dravet et al. (37) divided their 142 patients into no less than seven categories (excluding the Lennox–Gastaut and West's syndromes) of which the main ones were myoclonic absences (24 patients), the myoclonic variant of the Lennox–Gastaut syndrome (14 patients), severe myoclonic epilepsy of infants (42 patients), and benign infantile myoclonic epilepsy (10 patients). They left 34 cases unclassified. Aicardi and Chevrie (1,2,4) separated cryptogenic myoclonic epilepsy of infancy and childhood from the myoclonic epilepsy associated with fixed encephalopathy, the myoclonic variant of the Lennox–Gastaut syndrome, myoclonic epilepsy of adolescence, and myoclonic petit mal. The nosological problem is further complicated by the use of the same terms (e.g., myoclonic–astatic epilepsy) to designate different, although overlapping syndromes and by the idiosyncratic terminology employed by each author.

In this section, myoclonic epilepsy of childhood is described under two headings: myoclonic epilepsy of infancy and early childhood, and myoclonic epilepsy of later childhood and adolescence.

Myoclonic Epilepsy of Infancy and Early Childhood

The myoclonic epilepsies of infancy and early childhood pose the most difficult problems in diagnosis and classification because they are often confused with the

Lennox–Gastaut syndrome, with which they share a number of common features (2,38). However, at least part of the myoclonic epilepsies of early childhood have a less gloomy outlook than the classic Lennox–Gastaut syndrome, and this different prognosis justifies their individualization. Two main subgroups can be recognized.

Symptomatic Myoclonic Epilepsies

Symptomatic myoclonic epilepsies have their onset between a few months and 3 to 4 years of age in patients who already exhibited definite psychomotor retardation and/or symptoms and signs of chronic organic brain damage, such as cerebral palsy. In the series of Aicardi and Chevrie, the mean age of onset of myoclonic seizures was 22 months; the youngest infant was only 4 months old at the time of the first fit. Neuroradiological evidence of diffuse brain atrophy is often present. The myoclonias may be the only seizure type or they may be associated with clonic or tonic–clonic generalized or partial seizures. Myoclonic status is a prominent feature in some patients (29). Absences and tonic seizures are not observed. Symptomatic myoclonic epilepsies accounted for 21 of 145 patients with myoclonic epilepsy in the series of Aicardi (1) but only for 10 of 142 in that of Dravet et al. (37). Mental prognosis is uniformly poor but the myoclonus can be controlled in some patients with benzodiazepine or valproate therapy.

Cryptogenic Myoclonic Epilepsy

Cryptogenic myoclonic epilepsy comprises those cases in which there is no evidence of previous brain damage. Genetic factors seem to play an important role, as epileptic seizures in relatives were noted in 26% (27,37) to 38% (3) of the patients. The age of onset ranges between 6 months and 5 years. The myoclonic seizures are often preceded by other fits, especially febrile convulsions. Other types of attacks are commonly associated with the myoclonias. These are mainly generalized tonic–clonic seizures and occasionally unilateral convulsions. Very brief absences are apt to accompany the myoclonic seizures and may become more prominent with the passing of time. The lack of tonic seizures is important for distinguishing cryptogenic myoclonic epilepsy from the Lennox–Gastaut syndrome (3). The occurrence of brief, nocturnal tonic attacks can be excluded only by prolonged monitoring, especially by all-night recordings. The incidence of early cryptogenic myoclonic epilepsy is impossible to evaluate as the syndrome is not separated from other types of myoclonic epilepsies by many workers. Pazzaglia et al. (77) give a figure of 1.4% of childhood epilepsies. Aicardi and Chevrie (1,4) had 35 patients with cryptogenic myoclonic epilepsy among 145 patients with different forms of epileptic myoclonus. However, some of these patients belonged to the myoclonic epilepsies of later childhood, with an onset after the age of 5 years.

The course of early cryptogenic myoclonic epilepsy is difficult to predict. Of the 55 patients studied by Aicardi (3), 27 had been seizure-free for a minimum of 1 year after a mean follow-up of 6 years 3 months. Twenty children had an IQ of 80 or more; 35 had some degree of mental impairment, but only six had an IQ of less than 50. Those children who had had no seizure prior to the onset of myoclonias had a significantly better outlook than the remainder of the patients. Conversely, a suspect mental development before onset was significantly linked to both the persistence of seizures and mental subnormality. Jeavons (57) found that the mental outlook was favorable in the group of true myoclonic epilepsy of childhood but that seizures recurred when treatment was discontinued in most cases. Lombroso and Erba (67) also regard cryptogenic myoclonic epilepsy as a relatively benign form of epilepsy, at least when it is compared with the Lennox–Gastaut syndrome. The group, however, is probably heterogeneous (4,37). Some workers (27,37), divide cryptogenic myoclonic epilepsy into benign (36) and severe (27,37) forms. According to these authors, the benign type has an early onset, before 2 years of age, and myoclonias represent the only seizure type, except for occasional febrile convulsions. The severe form usually starts during the first 9 months of life with generalized or unilateral convulsive seizures, often but not always triggered by fever. The convulsions are often long-lasting and frequently recurring. Myoclonias appear most commonly during the second part of the second year of life. They are associated with the persistence of convulsive fits and with partial complex and atypical seizures. Erratic myoclonus with pseudocerebellar ataxia may occur. The outlook is poor, both for seizures and for mental development, which stops progressing during the second year of life. According to Dravet et al. (37), this severe form of infantile myoclonic epilepsy corresponds in part to the centrencephalic myoclonic–astatic petit mal of Doose and Kruse (33,35,63) and to some cases of cryptogenic myoclonic epilepsy (2,4) and of true myoclonic epilepsy (56). Although both benign and severe forms of cryptogenic myoclonic epilepsy undoubtedly exist, such a sharp distinction is not always possible. In fact, 1 of the 7 patients with benign myoclonic epilepsy reported by Dravet and Bureau (36) had an IQ of 50 at the age of 13 years and only 3 had completely normal levels. Intermediate types between benign and malignant forms are also encountered.

Intermediate Forms Between True Myoclonic Epilepsy and the Lennox–Gastaut Syndrome

Some patients with early myoclonic epilepsy have pseudomyoclonic (tonic and/or atonic) seizures in association with true myoclonic ones. The proportions of each seizure type may vary in different patients thus realizing a full spectrum of epilepsies, from the purely myoclonic ones to the typical Lennox–Gastaut syndrome. From an EEG point of view the frequent coexistence of slow (<2.5 Hz) and fast (>2.5 Hz) spike–wave complexes has long been recognized in the Lennox–Gastaut syndrome (17,24,45,75). Conversely, slow spike-wave complexes can be the ictal EEG concomitant of typical myoclonic jerks (2,4). The epilepsies in which true myoclonic seizures constitute the predominant ictal manifestation but are associated with some pseudomyoclonic seizures are called the myoclonic variant of the Lennox–Gastaut syndrome by several workers (4,37,38). The prognosis for these epilepsies seems to be less unfavorable than that of the pure atonic–tonic form of the Lennox–Gastaut syndrome. In the above-mentioned series of Chevrie and Aicardi (24), 14 patients were categorized in the myoclonic variant. The mean age of onset for these patients was 35.8 months, as compared to 24.8 months in the remainder of the series. Only three (21%) were retarded, as opposed to 68% of the remaining patients. When the mental outcome of 14 patients with the myoclonic variant of the Lennox–Gastaut syndrome was compared with that of 35 patients with true cryptogenic myoclonic epilepsy, no difference was found, the proportions of severe mental retardation being 18 and 21%, respectively. On the other hand, the rate of severe mental retardation was much higher (62%) in the predominantly tonic–atonic type of the Lennox–Gastaut syndrome (J. Aicardi, *unpublished results*). These differences in outcome appear to be related to the presence and extent of brain damage, which is much less frequent in the myoclonic variant than in the classic Lennox–Gastaut syndrome (24).

Myoclonic and Atonic Phenomena in the Course of Certain Partial Epilepsies of Childhood

The occurrence of myoclonic and/or atonic seizures has been reported in the course of an atypical variant of benign partial epilepsy of childhood (6). These patients had occasional focal nocturnal seizures reminiscent of those of rolandic epilepsy and focal spikes in their waking EEGs. Myoclonic–atonic seizures producing repeated daily falls occurred in clusters usually lasting a few weeks. The EEG concomitants of these myoclonic seizures were brief bursts of fast spike–wave activity. The sleep tracings displayed an intense, continuous slow spike–wave activity, especially during the periods when myoclonic fits were occurring. Despite the frightening clinical and EEG manifestations, the course seemed to be benign. These cases should be distinguished from the Lennox–Gastaut syndrome for which they are regularly mistaken if grave errors in prognosis and treatment are to be avoided.

Myoclonic Epilepsy of Later Childhood and Adolescence

The myoclonic epilepsies of later childhood and adolescence are often part of other patterns of primary generalized epilepsies, such as absences or grand mal. Their etiology is usually idiopathic, with strong genetic predisposition; there is a relative lack of neurodevelopmental deficits (67).

Myoclonus Associated with Absences

Eyelid myoclonus is a common accompaniment of many petit mal absences. Uncommonly, massive myoclonic jerks are a prominent manifestation of some epilepsies of the petit mal group. Two subgroups can be recognized: In some patients, brief, massive jerks alternate with classic absences. The jerks are associated with bursts of 3-Hz irregular, arrhythmical spike–waves usually lasting less than 3 sec, whereas the absences are associated with longer (5 sec or more), more rhythmical discharges. In most cases, however, these discharges are somewhat less regular than those of pure absence epilepsy, the spike–wave complexes varying in duration and amplitude. In 31 such cases (1), the mean age of onset was 4.5 years. The outcome was more favorable than that of cryptogenic myoclonic epilepsy but less so than in pure absences without myoclonic jerks. In many patients, the myoclonic component tended to decrease over the years, but generalized tonic–clonic seizures frequently supervened. In other cases, the myoclonic jerks are an integral part of the absences. These myoclonic absences (84) are characterized by rhythmic jerks which occur approximately three times per second and are generalized but usually predominant in the proximal muscles of the upper limbs. When the lower limbs are severely affected, the patient may fall to the ground. The EEG discharge which accompanies myoclonic absences is indistinguishable from that normally observed in classic petit mal. Myoclonic absences occur many times daily and are resistant to therapy. In one study (69), 12 of 14 patients had an IQ below 80, 2 of them below 50, and in 2 patients atypical absences and/or tonic seizures developed after several years.

Eyelid Myoclonia with Absences

Jeavons (57) has described as eyelid myoclonia with absences, a type of photosensitive epilepsy characterized by marked jerking of the eyelids with upward deviation of the eyes, the attacks following eye closure. The patients also have typical electroclinical absences. Affected children are often thought to have habit spasms or tics. Jeavons emphasizes the severity of the eyelid jerking in these patients compared to the slight flicker of eyelids that may occur with other absences. The EEG pattern associated with eyelid jerks is of irregular 3-Hz spike–wave complexes. All patients are photosensitive. Attacks tend to be worse in bright light, and self-induction of seizures by slowly blinking or by watching a television screen (30) is common. Control of eyelid jerking is often difficult, and this type of epilepsy tends to persist into adult life.

In a number of children with photosensitive epilepsy, especially in self-induced cases, eyelid jerking may not be the only or even the predominant myoclonic phenomenon, and massive myoclonic jerks are also observed.

Myoclonic Epilepsy of Adolescence

This form usually appears after the age of 9 years and is more common in girls. It is marked by sudden jerks which involve mainly the arms bilaterally and symmetrically and are accompanied on the EEG by a polyspike–wave complex. The jerks may be isolated or occur several times in succession. In contrast with myoclonic absences, there is no loss of awareness. According to Janz (55), who has described in detail this type of epilepsy as "impulsive petit mal," the myoclonic jerks are associated with major tonic–clonic seizures in 90% of the cases but they often antedate the grand mal fits by several years and many cases with isolated jerks probably go unreported. The myoclonic jerks are most common after waking. Major attacks often occur during sleep, or they may be preceded by a succession of myoclonic jerks. At least half the patients show a paroxysmal EEG response to photostimulation. Complete control of the seizures is usually achieved but withdrawal of therapy is often followed by recurrence of the fits.

Treatment of the True Myoclonic Epilepsies

The myoclonic epilepsies are often resistant to many conventional antiepileptic drugs. The benzodiazepines (20,86) and sodium valproate or valproic acid (32,60) are usually the most effective agents. Some patients respond to ethosuximide or to a combination of ethosuximide and valproate (32). The ketogenic diet is advised in resistant cases by several authors. Jeavons et al. (60) has extensively discussed the therapy of the various types of myoclonic epilepsy.

CONCLUSION

This review of recent work in the field of the myoclonic epilepsies has shown the increasing complexity of the problem. The description of a number of new types or syndromes, most of which are based only on anecdotal evidence, makes the field a nosological jungle. The situation is rendered even worse by the lack of any standardized terminology, and some agreement on the use of the terms employed is highly desirable. The distinction between true and pseudomyoclonic seizures, on a neurophysiological basis, has helped to clarify the problem, especially with reference to the Lennox–Gastaut syndrome, which most recent works tend to separate from the true myoclonic epilepsies. In the latter group, however, a considerable degree of confusion still exists. The sharp distinctions between the proposed syndromes are blurred in actuality by the existence of a large number of unclassifiable and transitional forms, which makes it very difficult to determine prognosis in a particular patient. The classification presented in this chapter is obviously tentative and, at best, provisional. Further studies of large series of cases selected on predetermined criteria to constitute recognizable and relatively homogeneous groups and prospectively followed are clearly necessary.

SUMMARY

This chapter has reviewed the multiple types of childhood epilepsies customarily referred to as "myoclonic epilepsies" and has made an attempt at classification. A distinction was made on a clinical neurophysiological basis between true myoclonic and pseudomyoclonic seizures that include brief tonic and atonic attacks. The epilepsies characterized mainly by pseudomyoclonic seizures include infantile spasms (West's syndrome) and the Lennox–Gastaut syndrome. The epilepsies manifested principally by true myoclonic seizures comprise two subgroups: a symptomatic type, in which myoclonias are the result of fixed diffuse brain damage; and several cryptogenic forms. The latter may be divided, according to age of onset and clinical features, into several myoclonic syndromes: cryptogenic myoclonic epilepsy of infancy and early childhood, myoclonic epilepsy of childhood with absences, and myoclonic epilepsy of adolescence. Many intermediate and atypical forms exist; thus the proposed classification is only tentative.

ACKNOWLEDGMENT

We thank Dr. J. Misès and Dr. J. J. Chevrie for their help in the preparation of this manuscript and Miss B. Tricot for excellent secretarial assistance.

REFERENCES

1. Aicardi J. Myoclonic epilepsies. *Res. Clin. forums* 1980;2:47–55.
2. Aicardi J. Course and prognosis of certain childhood epilepsies with predominantly myoclonic seizures. In: Wada J, Penry JK, eds. *Advances in epileptology: The Xth epilepsy international symposium*. New York: Raven Press, 1980:159–63.
3. Aicardi J. Childhood epilepsies with brief myoclonic–atonic or tonic seizures. In: Laidlaw J, Richens A, eds. *A textbook of epilepsy*. Edinburgh: Churchill Livingstone, 1982:88–96.
4. Aicardi J, Chevrie JJ. Myoclonic epilepsies of childhood. *Neuropaediatrie* 1971;3:177–90.
5. Aicardi J, Chevrie JJ. Les spasmes infantiles. *Arch Fr. Pediatr* 1978;25:1015–23.
6. Aicardi J, Chevrie JJ. Atypical benign partial epilepsy. *Dev Med Child Neurol* 1982;24:281–92.
7. Aicardi J, Chevrie JJ, Rousselie F. Le syndrome spasmes en flexion, agénésie calleuse, lacunes choriorétiniennes. *Arch Fr. Pediatr* 1969;26:1103–20.
8. Aicardi J, Goutières F. Encéphalopathie myoclonique néonatale. *Rev EEG Neurophysiol* 1978;8:99–101.
9. Bachman DS. Use of valproic acid in treatment of infantile spasms. *Arch Neurol* 1982;33:49–52.
10. Bancaud J, Talairach J, Geier S, Scarabin JM. *EEG et SEEG dans les tumeurs cérébrales et l'épilepsie*. Paris: Edifor, 1973:266–75.
11. Beaumanoir A. Les limites nosologiques du syndrome de Lennox–Gastaut. *Rev EEG Neurophysiol* 1981;11:468–73.
12. Beaumanoir-Roger A, Guediche A. Syndromes de West et de Lennox, étude comparative. *Pediatr Fortbildungkurse Prax* 1972;26:57–80.
13. Bennett HS, Selman JE, Rapin I, Rose A. Nonconvulsive epileptiform activity appearing as ataxia. *Am J Dis Child* 1982;136:30–2.
14. Bentson J, Reza M, Winter J, Wilson G. Steroids and apparent cerebral atrophy on computed tomography scans. *J Comput Assist Tomogr* 1978;2:16–23.
15. Bignami A, Zappella M, Benedetti P. Infantile spasms with hypsarrhythmia. A pathological study. *Helv Paediatr Acta* 1964;19:326–42.
16. Bittencourt PRM, Richens A. Anticonvulsant-induced status epilepticus in Lennox–Gastaut syndrome. *Epilepsia* 1981;22:129–34.
17. Blume WT, David RB, Gomez MR. Generalized sharp and slow–wave complexes. Associated clinical features and long-term follow up. *Brain* 1973;96:289–306.
18. Brandt NJ, Rasmussen K, Brandt S, Schonheyder R. D-glyceric acidemia with hyperglucinemia. A new inborn error of metabolism. *Brit Med J* 1974;4:334–6.
19. Brett EM. Minor epileptic status. *J Neurol Sci* 1966;3:52.
20. Browne TR, Penry JK. Benzodiazepines in the treatment of epilepsy: a review. *Epilepsia* 1973;14:277–310.
21. Cavazzuti GB. Epidemiology of different types of epilepsy in school age children of Modena, Italy. *Epilepsia* 1980;21:57–62.
22. Cavazzuti GB, Nalin A, Ferrari F, Mordini B. Encefalopatie miocloniche nel primo anno di vita. *Riv Ital Ellettroencefal Neurofisiol Clin* 1979;2:253–61.
23. Charlton MH. *Myoclonic seizures*. Amsterdam: Excerpta Medica, 1975.
24. Chevrie JJ, Aicardi J. Childhood epileptic encephalopathy with slow spike–wave. A statistical study of 80 cases. *Epilepsia* 1972;13:259–71.
25. Commission of Classification and Terminology of the International League against Epilepsy.

Proposal for revised clinical and electroencephalographic classification of epileptic seizures. *Epilepsia* 1981;22:489–501.

26. Dalla Bernardina B, Aicardi J, Goutières F, Plouin P. Glycine encephalopathy. *Neuropaediatrie* 1979;10:209–25.
27. Dalla Bernardina B, Capovilla G, Colamaria V, Bondavalli S, Bureau M. Epilepsie myoclonique grave de la lère année (severe infant myoclonic epilepsy). *Rev EEG Neurophysiol* 1982;12:21–5.
28. Dalla Bernardina B, Dulac O, Bureau M, Dravet C, Del Zotti F, Roger J. Encéphalopathie myoclonique précoce avec épilepsie (early myoclonic epileptic encephalopathy). *Rev EEG Neurophysiol* 1982;12:8–14.
29. Dalla Bernardina B, Trevisan C, Bondavalli S, Colamaria V, Roger J, Bureau M, Dravet C. Une forme particulière d'épilepsie myoclonique chez des enfants porteurs d'encéphalopathie fixée. *Boll Lega It Contra Epil* 1980;29/30:183–8.
30. Darby CE, De Korte RA, Binnie CD, Wilkins AJ. The self-induction of epileptic seizures by eye closure. *Epilepsia* 1980;21:31–42.
31. De Ajuriaguerra J, Thomas A. Etude anatomoclinique de l'anencéphalie. In: Gruner J, Feld J, eds. Malformations congénitales du cerveau. Paris: Masson, 1959:207–67.
32. De Vivo DC. Myoclonic seizures. In: Morselli CE, Pippenger CE, Peñry JK, eds. *Antiepileptic drug therapy in pediatrics*. New York: Raven Press, 1983:137–43.
33. Doose J. Das akinetische Petit Mal. I. Das klinische und elektroencephalographische Bild der akinetischen Anfälle. *Arch Psychiatr Neurol* 1946;205:625–36.
34. Doose H. Non convulsive status epilepticus in childhood: clinical aspects and classification. In: Delgado-Escueta AV, Wasterlain CG, Treiman DM, Porter RJ, eds. *Advances in neurology, Vol. 34, status epilepticus*. New York: Raven Press, 1983:83–92.
35. Doose H, Gerken H, Leonhardt R, Völzke E, Völz C. Centrencephalic myoclonic-astatic Petit Mal. Clinical and genetic investigations. *Neuropaediatrie* 1970;2:59–78.
36. Dravet C, Bureau M. L'épilepsie myoclonique bénigne du nourrisson. *Rev EEG Neurophysiol* 1981;11:438–44.
37. Dravet C, Roger J, Bureau M, Dalla Bernardina B. Myoclonic epilepsies in childhood. In: Akimoto H, Kazamatsuri H, Seino M, Ward A eds. *Advances in epileptology: XIIIth epilepsy international symposium*. New York: Raven Press, 1982:135–40.
38. Erba G, Lombroso CT. La sindrome de Lennox-Gastaut. *Prospet Paediatr* 1973;3:145–65.
39. Fariello RG, Chun RW, Doro JM, Buncic JR, Prichard JS. EEG recognition of Aicardi's syndrome. *Arch Neurol* 1977;34:563–6.
40. Gastaut H, Séméiologie des myoclonies et nosologie analytique des syndromes myocloniques. *Rev Neurol* 1968;119:1–30.
41. Gastaut H. Clinical and electroencephalographic classification of epileptic seizures. *Epilepsia* 1970;11:102–13.
42. Gastaut H, Broughton R, Roger J, Tassinari CA. Generalized nonconvulsive seizures without local onset. In: Vinken PJ, Bruyn GW, eds. *Handbook of clinical neurology. The epilepsies*. Amsterdam: North-Holland, 1974:vol. 15;130–45.
43. Gastaut H, Soulayrol R, Roger J, Pinsard N, eds. *L'encéphalopathie myoclonique infantile avec hypsarythmie (syndrome de West)*. Paris: Masson, 1964.
44. Gastaut H, Roger J, Ouachi S, Timsit M, Broughton R. An electroclinical study of generalized epileptic seizures of tonic expression. *Epilepsia* 1963;4:15–44.
45. Gastaut H, Roger J, Soulayrol R, Tassinari CA, Regis H, Dravet C. Childhood epileptic encephalopathy with diffuse spike-waves (otherwise known as "Petit Mal Variant") or the Lennox syndrome. *Epilepsia* 1966;7:139–79.
46. Gastaut H, Dravet C, Loubier D, Giove C, Viani F, Gastaut JA, Gastaut JL. Evolution clinique et prognostic du syndrome de Lennox-Gastaut. In: Lugaresi E, Pazzaglia P, Tassinari CA. *Evolution and prognosis of epilepsies*. Bologna: Aulo Gaggi, 1973:133–54.
47. Gastaut H, Gastaut JL, Regis H, Bernard R, Pinsard N, Saint Jean M, Roger J, Dravet C. Computerized tomography in the study of West's syndrome. *Dev Med Child Neurol* 1978;20:21–7.
48. Gibbs FA, Gibbs EL. *Atlas of electroencephalography 1952 Vol. II, Epilespy*, 2nd ed. Reading: Addison-Wesley.
49. Gold AP, Freeman JM. Depigmented nevi: the earliest sign of tuberous sclerosis. *Pediatrics* 1965;55:1003–5.

50. Hakamada S, Watanabe K, Hara K, Miyazaki S. The evolution of electroencephalographic features in lissencephaly syndrome. *Brain Dev* 1979;1:277–83.
51. Hakamada S, Watanabe K, Hara K, Miyazaki S. Brief atonia associated with electroencephalographic paroxysm in an infant with infantile spasms. *Epilepsia* 1981;22:285–8.
52. Hrachovy RA, Frost JD, Kellaway P, Zion T. A controlled study of ACTH therapy in infantile spasms. *Epilepsia* 1980;21:631–6.
53. Huttenlocher PR. Ketonemia and seizures: metabolic and anticonvulsant effect of two ketogenic diets in childhood epilepsy. *Pediatr Res* 1976;10:536–40.
54. Huttenlocher PR. Dendritic development in neocortex of children with mental defect and infantile spasms. *Neurology (Minneap)* 1974;24:203–10.
55. Janz D. The natural history of primary generalized epilepsies with sporadic myoclonias of the "Impulsive Petit Mal" type. In: Lugaresi E, Pazzaglia P, Tassinari CA, eds. *Evolution and prognosis of epilepsies*. Bologna: Aulo Gaggi, 1973:55–61.
56. Jeavons PM. Nosological problems of myoclonic epilepsies in childhood and adolescence. *Dev Med Child Neurol* 1977;19:3–8.
57. Jeavons PM. Myoclonic epilepsies: therapy and prognosis. In: Akimoto H, Kazamatsuri H, Seino M, Ward A, eds. *Advances in epileptology. XIIIth Epilepsy international symposium*. Raven Press: New York, 1982:141–4.
58. Jeavons PM, Bower BD. *Infantile spasms. A review of the literature and a study of 112 cases.* London: Heinemann, 1964.
59. Jeavons PM, Bower BD, Dimitrakoudi M. Long-term prognosis of 150 cases of "West syndrome." *Epilepsia* 1973;14:153–64.
60. Jeavons PM, Clark JE, Maheshwari MC. Treatment of generalized epilepsies of childhood and adolescence with sodium valproate ("Epilim"). *Dev Med Child Neurol* 1977;19:9–25.
61. Jellinger K. Neuropathological aspects of hypsarrhythmia. *Neuropaediatrie* 1970;1:277–94.
61a. Kellaway P, Frost JD, Hrachovy RA. Infantile spasms. In: Morselli PL, Pippenger CE, Penry JK, eds. *Antiepileptic drug therapy in pediatrics*. New York: Raven Press, 1983:115–36.
62. Kellaway P, Hrachovy RA, Frost JD, Zion T. Precise characterization and quantification of infantile spasms. *Ann Neurol* 1979;6:214–8.
63. Kruse R. *Das myoklonisch-astatische Petit Mal*. Berlin: Springer, 1968.
64. Lacy J, Penry JK. *Infantile spasms*. New York: Raven Press, 1976.
65. Lerman P, Kivity S. The efficacy of corticotropin in primary infantile spasms. *J Pediatr* 1982;101:294–6.
66. Lombroso CT. A prospective study of infantile spasms: clinical and therapeutic correlations. *Epilepsia* 1983;24:135–58.
67. Lombroso C, Erba G. Myoclonic seizures: considerations in toxonomy. In: Akimoto H, Kazamatsuri H, Seino M, Ward A. eds. *Advances in epileptology: XIIIth Epilepsy international symposium*. New York: Raven Press, 1982:129–34.
68. Lombroso CT, Fejerman N. Benign myoclonus of early infancy. *Ann Neurol* 1977;1:38–43.
69. Lugaresi E, Pazzaglia P, Franck L, Roger J, Bureau-Paillas M, Ambrosetto G, and Tassinari CA. Evolution and prognosis of primary generalized epilepsies of the Petit Mal absence type. In: Lugaresi E, Pazzaglia P, Tassinari CA eds. *Evolution and prognosis of epilepsies*. Bologna: Aulo Gaggi, 1973:3–22.
70. Lyen KR, Holland IM, Lyen YC. Reversible cerebral atrophy in infantile spasms caused by corticotrophin. *Lancet* 1979;2:37–8.
71. Markand ON. Slow spike-wave activity in EEG and associated clinical features: often called "Lennox" or "Lennox-Gastaut" syndrome. *Neurology*, 1977;27:746–57.
72. Matsumoto A, Watanabe K, Negoro T, Iwase K, Hara K, Miyazaki S. Infantile spasms: etiological factors, clinical aspects and long-term prognosis in 200 cases. *Eur J Pediatr* 1981;135:239–44.
73. Melchior JC. Infantile spasms and early immunization against whooping cough. *Arch Dis Child* 1977;52:134–7.
74. Neville BGR. The origin of infantile spasms: evidence from a case of hydranencephaly. *Dev Med Child Neurol* 1972;14:644–56.
75. Niedermayer E. The Lennox–Gastaut syndrome: a severe type of childhood epilepsy. *Deutsch Z Nervenheilk* 1969;195:263–82.
76. Ohtahara S. Clinico-electrical delineation of epileptic encephalopathies in childhood. *Asian Med J* 1978;21:7–17.

77. Pazzaglia P, Franck L, Lugaresi E. Le epilessie generalizzate: problemi prognostici e di delimitazione nosografica. *Riv Neurol* 1971;41:1–17.
78. Riikonen R. A long-term follow-up study of 214 children with the syndrome of infantile spasms. *Neuropediatrics* 1982;13:14–23.
79. Riikonen R, Amnell G. Psychiatric disorders in children with earlier infantile spasms. *Dev Med Child Neurol* 1981;23:747–60.
80. Roger J, Lob H, Tassinari CA. Status epilepticus. In: Vinken PJ, Bruyn GW, eds. *Handbook of clinical neurology*, vol 15, the epilepsies. Amsterdam: North-Holland, 1974:145–88.
81. Shibasaki Y, Kuroiwa Y. Electroencephalographic correlates of myoclonus. *Electroencephalogr Clin Neurophysiol* 1975;39:455–63.
82. Singer WD, Rabe EF, Haller JS. The effect of ACTH therapy upon infantile spasms. *J Pediatr* 1980;96:485–9.
83. Tassinari CA, Dravet C, Roger J, Cano JP, Gastaut H. Tonic status epilepticus precipitated by intravenous benzodiazepine in five patients with Lennox–Gastaut syndrome. *Epilepsia* 1972;13:421–35.
84. Tassinari CA, Lyagoubi S, Santos V, Gambarelli F, Roger J, Dravet C, Gastaut H. Etude des décharges de pointe-ondes chez l'homme. Les aspects cliniques et électroencéphalographiques des absences myocloniques. *Rev Neurol* 1969;121:379–83.
85. Thomas J, Reggan J, Klass D. Epilepsia partialis continua. A review of 32 cases. *Arch Neurol* 1977;34:266–75.
86. Vassella F, Pavlincova E, Schneider HJ, Rudin HJ, Karbowski K. Treatment of infantile spasms and the Lennox–Gastaut syndrome with clonazepam (Rivotril). *Epilepsia* 1973;14:165–75.
87. Viani F, Avanzini G, Baruzzi A, Bordo B, Bossi L, Canger R, Porro G, Riboldi A, Sofficutini ME, Zanogi P, Morselli PL. Long-term monitoring of antiepileptic drugs in patients with the Lennox–Gastaut syndrome. In: Penry JK ed. *Epilepsy. The VIIIth international symposium.* New York: Raven Press, 1977:131–8.
88. Willig RP, Lagenstein I. Use of ACTH fragments in children with infantile spasms. *Neuropediatrics* 1982;13:55–8.

Advances in Neurology, Vol. 43: Myoclonus,
edited by S. Fahn et al. Raven Press,
New York © 1986.

Action Myoclonus, Ramsay Hunt Syndrome, and Other Cerebellar Myoclonic Syndromes

James W. Lance

Department of Neurology, The Prince Henry Hospital, School of Medicine, University of New South Wales, Sydney, New South Wales 2036, Australia

This chapter examines the concept of action myoclonus, the clinical conditions that may give rise to it, its specificity as a symptom or physical sign, and its association with cerebellar and other neurological disorders.

The term *action myoclonia* was introduced by Wohlfart and Höök (111) when they reported 10 patients with myoclonus epilepsy whose muscular jerking was initiated by movement, attempts at movement, and even intention to move. They also included three cases of Wilson's disease with involuntary movements (resembling myoclonus in at least one instance) brought about by movement and worsened by tests of coordination. The same phenomenon, observed as a sequel to hypoxic encephalopathy, was called "intention or action myoclonus" by Lance and Adams (62) who described "an arrhythmic fine or coarse jerking of a muscle or group of muscles in disorderly fashion, excited mainly by muscular activity, particularly when a conscious attempt at precision was required, worsened by emotional arousal, suppressed by barbiturates, and superimposed on a mild cerebellar ataxia."

Myoclonus is commonly precipitated by movement, regardless of the underlying cause of the disorder, a fact that is often obscured in the depths of lengthy case histories. The jerks of essential myoclonus or epileptic myoclonus usually follow attempted movement or assumption of a posture. The myoclonus associated with infections, toxins, metabolic changes, and diffuse degenerative cerebral diseases may be triggered by movement; it is also sensitive to a variety of afferent stimuli (muscle stretch, touch, and any form of startle). When neurological signs are present in such patients, cerebellar disturbance is most often encountered, and signs of basal ganglia or pyramidal disease and mental impairment are not uncommon (2,13).

Muscular twitchings and spasms, usually insufficient to move the limbs, present at rest and ceasing on movement were designated "paramyoclonus multiplex" by Friedreich in 1881 [cited by Aigner and Mulder (2), Bradshaw (13), Halliday (43), and Bonduelle (10)]. Myoclonus at rest, abolished by action, was also observed in three generations by Lindemulder (68). With the exception of this disorder and the rhythmic posturing of advanced subacute sclerosing panencephalitis (SSPE) and related conditions, most forms of myoclonus seem to be aggravated by movement.

Even in SSPE, a phase of action myoclonus may be observed in the early stages of the disease (61) (Table 1).

CONDITIONS IN WHICH ACTION MYOCLONUS HAS BEEN OBSERVED

Nonprogressive Myoclonus

It is possible that essential myoclonus is simply a variety of idiopathic epilepsy, since an isolated fit may appear in an otherwise impeccable history of "essential myoclonus" (61). Limb movement induces jerking in both instances (101). Myoclonus ceases with sleep but may be induced by shifting position or turning in bed (18).

Progressive Myoclonic Epilepsy

In 1891 and 1895, Unverricht reported two families in which half the children of one sibship of ten, and three of five in the other developed action myoclonus and epilepsy of increasing severity between the ages of 9 and 15 years. One patient had optic atrophy. Since Lundborg collected 50 similar cases in 30 families, which he published in 1903, the condition was subsequently known as Unverricht–Lundborg disease (43). Clinical and histological studies have made it clear that there are at least three forms of progressive myoclonic epilepsy (PME) (Table 2).

TABLE 1. *Causes of action myoclonus*

Nonprogressive myoclonus
  idiopathic epilepsy
  essential myoclonus
Progressive myoclonic epilepsy
  Lafora body disease
  lipidosis
  system degenerations
Metabolic disturbances
  anoxia
  uremia
Infections
  encephalitis: SSPE, rubella
  postencephalitic
Intoxications
  methyl bromide
  piperazine
Paraneoplastic cerebellar degeneration
  leukemia
  neuroblastomas
Focal cerebral lesions
  infarction
  multiple sclerosis

TABLE 2. *Progressive myoclonic epilepsy*

Lafora body disease
Cerebral storage disease
juvenile cerebroretinal degenerations
late-onset form (Kufs')
cherry-red-spot myoclonus syndrome
normal appearance
gargoyle facies
familial renal insufficiency with
action myoclonus
System degenerations
cerebellar
basal ganglia
spinal atrophy

Lafora Body Disease

In 1911, Lafora and Glueck found intraneuronal inclusion bodies in the brain of a 17-year-old boy who died after 2 years of illness characterized by myoclonus, epilepsy, and dementia (43). The amyloid substance of the inclusion bodies was shown to be an acid mucopolysaccharide by Harriman and Millar (45), who found inclusion bodies in heart and liver as well as in brain. The condition can thus be diagnosed by liver biopsy (77) and by muscle biopsy as well. These deposits are an unusual glucose polymer (4).

Halliday (43) summarized the data of 34 autopsied cases of Lafora body disease, with the age of onset varying from 5 to 20 years (mean, 14.3 years) and the age of death from 16 to 24 years (mean, 20 years). Diebold (24) recognized a form of later onset (17–33 years) in which the age of death varied from 42 to 65 years. The myoclonus of Lafora body disease is most pronounced on movement (45,100). The condition is inherited as an autosomal recessive.

Cerebral Storage Diseases
Cerebroretinal degeneration (amaurotic family idiocy; lipofuscinosis)

The late infantile form of cerebral lipidosis associated with myoclonus differs from the infantile variety (Tay–Sachs disease) because the retinal lesion involves rods and cones as well as ganglion cells. Macular lesions may appear as yellowish gray areas of degeneration in contrast to the cherry-red spots of Tay–Sachs disease. Juvenile lipidosis has been subdivided into categories on the grounds of age of onset, rapidity of progression, and severity of visual disturbance, myoclonus, dementia, and dystonia (1). Cerebral lipidosis as a cause of PME was emphasized by Watson and Denny Brown (109), who described one family with proven lipidosis in which myoclonus was precipitated by slight active or passive movements of the limbs.

Cerebral lipidosis of late onset (Kufs' disease)

Pallis et al. (80) reported the adult onset of cerebral lipidosis with cerebellar disturbance and action myoclonus starting at the age of 49 years and progressing to death 6 years later. Neurons and glial cells were found to be distended with lipofuscin. Pallis and his colleagues reviewed ten other adult cases of cerebral lipidosis, six of whom had cerebellar disturbance, but only one was recorded as having myoclonus.

Cherry-red-spot myoclonus syndrome

Action myoclonus is also a feature of another storage disease in which lipofuscin accumulates in neurons and hepatocytes, whereas a substance resembling muco-polysaccharide is found in Kupffer cells and hepatocytes (81). Sialic acid-containing oligosaccharides are excreted in the urine (52,81) and can be demonstrated in the viscera (84). Visual disturbance usually starts in childhood with the appearance of a cherry-red spot at the macula. Facial appearance is normal, unlike the "gargoyle facies" of other mucopolysaccharidoses and sialidoses, and there are no bony deformities. Myoclonus develops in early teenage years and is precipitated by passive movement, voluntary movement, or the thought of movement. The three patients (two of them sisters) described by Rapin and her collaborators (81) showed only mild signs of cerebellar disturbance, unlike the brothers with gross ataxia described by Itoyama et al. (52).

A variation on this theme is characterized by a gargoyle-like physical appearance, cherry-red spot at the macula, cerebellar ataxia, pyramidal signs, bony deformities, and vacuolated lymphocytes, with a deficiency of β-galactosidase in liver and brain (99).

Familial renal insufficiency with action myoclonus

Andermann et al. (3) described the familial occurrence of action myoclonus with renal failure as an autosomal recessive disorder. Nonneuronal accumulation of lipopigment was found in the cerebral cortex.

System Degenerations

Cerebellar disease

The association of myoclonus with hereditary cerebellar ataxia was recorded in 1913 by Boschi (11) who considered this to be a form of Unverricht's disease and remarked that myoclonus was provoked by movement. The family history of Bos-chi's case was interesting because one brother's illness resembled Friedreich's ataxia, whereas the other had a purely cerebellar degeneration. The link between cerebellar disorders and myoclonus is usually attributed to Ramsay Hunt (49) as a syndrome which bears his name. Hunt described two siblings who became ataxic in childhood or adolescence and developed myoclonus at the ages of 21 and 24 years, respectively. Tendon jerks were absent in both, and one sibling had loss of joint-position sense and a "tendency to pes cavus." Autopsy on the other sibling showed the spinal changes of Friedreich's ataxia without involvement of the corti-cospinal tracts but with degeneration of the dentate nucleus and its projections.

Hunt also described four other patients who developed myoclonus between the ages of 7 and 19 years, with the concomitant or later onset of cerebellar signs. None had a family history of a similar disorder. Many such patients have subsequently been reported, some with spinal cord changes resembling Friedreich's ataxia, again without pyramidal degeneration (9,17). One patient with typical Friedreich's ataxia developed continuous myoclonus, which finally caused her death (113). Action myoclonus was observed "to some extent." Autopsy disclosed atrophy of the dentate nucleus and superior cerebellar peduncle and loss of Purkinje cells as well as the spinal cord and peripheral nerve changes of Friedreich's ataxia (113). The most commonly reported pathological change is degeneration of the olivodentatorubral system (9,43). However, in some cases of Ramsay Hunt syndrome, the dentate nucleus may be spared (13,101); in others, the most outstanding feature has been the loss of Purkinje cells (58).

In 1960, I reported a family of six siblings from a marriage between first cousins once removed (78). Four of the children were subject to tonic–clonic seizures and myoclonus aggravated by movement, but only three of them showed signs of cerebellar impairment. An autopsy subsequently performed on one of the members of this family showed neuronal atrophy and fallout of Purkinje cells and cells in the dentate nucleus and inferior olives, which were stuffed with material positive to the periodic acid Schiff (PAS) technique. Marked neuronal loss was observed in the substantia nigra, but diencephalic nuclei were unaffected. Nucleus gracilis and cuneatus were remarkable for the presence of gigantic neurons containing vacuoles and large cytoplasmic inclusions that were not typical Lafora bodies. In this and most families reported, the disorder was transmitted by a recessive gene, but autosomal dominant transmission has also been described (59,70), with nerve deafness being an additional feature in the family described by May and White (70).

Families with cerebellar disturbance and action myoclonus without any other form of epilepsy have been described by Gilbert et al. (34) and by Jacobs (53) as an autosomal dominant trait (although the latter family of four affected siblings with no antecedents suggests recessive inheritance).

Koskiniemi et al. (58) reported a large series of 93 patients with progressive myoclonic epilepsy from Finland. This condition has subsequently been called *Baltic myoclonus* because of the prevalence in Finland and because Unverricht and Lundborg reported cases from Estonia and eastern Sweden (27). In Koskiniemi's series, myoclonus and tonic–clonic seizures started in childhood, followed by cerebellar disturbance, with the illness running a total course of approximately 10 years. Intellect was preserved, but signs of spasticity developed in 28% of cases. In the one patient with complete autopsy findings, there was a diffuse loss of Purkinje cells with relative preservation of the dentate nucleus. Neuronal degeneration was noted in the medial thalamic nuclei, which is of interest since experimental lesions in this area may induce myoclonus (72). There were no Lafora bodies or other inclusion material in brain or viscera. The condition appears to have autosomal recessive inheritance in most cases but "two of the parents had had attacks of unconsciousness and one jerks (58)."

To further complicate the issue, Smith et al. (91) reported a family in which a mother and three of her five children suffered from myoclonic epilepsy: The mother and son were ataxic, another son had additional features of Friedreich's ataxia, including extensor plantar responses, and a daughter had peroneal muscular atrophy (Charcot–Marie–Tooth disease) as well as myoclonus and ataxia. Two unrelated patients with Friedreich's ataxia, myoclonus, and muscular wasting were found to have a mitochondrial myopathy by Fukuhara et al. (31). Optic atrophy was present in one patient: Inheritance was autosomal dominant in both cases. The association of myoclonic epilepsy, ataxia, and mitochondrial myopathy has been reported briefly before by Tsairis et al. (105) in a family with dominant inheritance in which nerve deafness was also a symptom. Nerve deafness and mitochondrial myopathy were also features of patients with myoclonic epilepsy and ataxia reported by Fitzsimons et al. (30) and by Morgan-Hughes et al. (73). Biochemical studies in the latter patient demonstrated a defect in the mitochondrial respiratory chain caused by cytochrome-b deficiency (73). Another patient showed the combination of action myoclonus, ataxia, mitochondrial myopathy, and distal muscle weakness of neurogenic origin (29). A sporadic case of a boy with nerve deafness, action myoclonus, and muscular weakness without definite signs of cerebellar disturbance was reported by Lance and Evans (65), and in this case the weakness was caused by spinal muscular atrophy. Autopsy disclosed no significant changes in Purkinje cells and dentate nucleus with marked loss of motor neurons in cranial nerve nuclei and anterior horns of spinal cord. It is of interest that Koskiniemi et al. (58) reported muscular atrophy and weakness in the later stages of Baltic myoclonus, but the spinal cord was not examined at autopsy.

It thus appears that the common denominators of Ramsay Hunt syndrome are cerebellar disturbance and myoclonus and that the term embraces the following combinations of various system degenerations.

1. *Cerebellar signs and myoclonus without tonic–clonic seizures:* sporadic or familial (autosomal dominant or recessive), associated with neurogenic weakness in one sporadic case (29) and mitochondrial myopathy in two (29,73). Two of the 93 cases with PME reported by Koskiniemi (58) did not have major seizures.

2. *Cerebellar signs; myoclonus and tonic–clonic seizures;* sporadic or familial *(autosomal dominant or recessive)*. Patients in this category have also been reported to suffer from nerve deafness (30,70,105) and mitochondrial myopathy (30,105). One sporadic case (65) and one family (54) with action myoclonus, epilepsy, and spinal muscular atrophy *without* signs of cerebellar disease have also been described. Most of these mixed-system disorders are dominantly inherited (Table 3). Baltic myoclonus (Unverricht–Lundborg disease), which is usually inherited as a recessive gene, is included in this category, although spasticity was found in 28% of patients with this condition and a Babinski response in 4% (58).

TABLE 3. *System degenerations reported in PME*

Investigator	Ref. no.	Ataxia	Myoclonus	Epilepsy	Deafness	Spinal atrophy	Myopathy	Inheritance[a]	Generations	Special feature reported
						System degeneration				
Hunt (1921)	49	×	×	×				R		
Noad and Lance (1960)	78	×	×	×				R		Retardation
Gilbert et al. (1963)	34	×	×					D	4	
Jacobs (1965)	53	×	×					R(?)		
May and White (1968)	70	×	×	×	×			D	4	
Tsairis et al. (1973)	105	×	×	×	×		×	D	2	
Koskiniemi et al. (1974)	58	×	×	×		×(?)		R		Distal atrophy, spasticity 28%
Jankovic and Rivera (1979)	54		×	×		×		D	4	
Fukuhara et al. (1980)	31	×	×	×			×	D	2	Friedreich's ataxia
Fitzsimons et al. (1981)	30	×	×	×	×		×	D	2	Hypothalamic disorder
Morgan-Hughes et al. (1982)	73	×	×			×	×	S		Dementia; retinal degeneration
Feit et al. (1983)	29	×	×			×(?)	×	S		Distal atrophy Hypoventilation
Lance and Evans (1983)	65		×	×	×	×		R(?)		Finnish ancestry

[a]D, autosomal dominant inheritance; R, recessive inheritance; S, sporadic.

3. *Friedreich's ataxia with myoclonus (autosomal dominant or recessive).* One member of a reported family (91) had peroneal muscular atrophy and myoclonus. Other patients with Friedreich's ataxia and myoclonus have had optic atrophy and mitochondrial myopathy (31).

Basal ganglia disease

Hereditary dentatorubral–pallidoluysian atrophy. Naito and Oyanagi (74) described five different families with myoclonus, major epileptic seizures, cerebellar ataxia, choreoathetosis, and dementia. Some patients presented in childhood with epilepsy and dementia, whereas ataxia was the first symptom when the onset was in adult life. The myoclonus was stimulus-sensitive, but induction by movement was not specifically mentioned. Degenerative changes, without inclusion bodies, were found in the globus pallidus, subthalamic nucleus, and the fasciculus and ansa lenticularis, as well as in the dentatorubral pathway. The condition was transmitted as an autosomal dominant gene.

Atypical progressive supranuclear palsy. Action myoclonus of face and limbs was one of the early symptoms of a 58-year-old woman who developed a progressive pseudobulbar palsy with limitation of upward gaze and, later, of all eye movements (60). Neuronal loss and gliosis involved the deep layers of the cortex, midbrain, tegmentum, superior colliculus, periaqueductal gray matter, oculomotor nucleus, and dentate nucleus.

Wilson's disease. Action myoclonus was first noted in Wilson's disease by Wohlfart and Höök (111).

Other basal ganglia disorders. Typical action myoclonus has been reported in the rigid form of Huntington's disease (35). Myoclonic jerking has sometimes been observed in other basal ganglia disorders, such as Parkinson's disease, dystonia musculorum deformans, and Hallervorden–Spatz disease (69).

Spinal muscular atrophy

In 1938, Döring (25) reported the onset of action myoclonus at the same time as amyotrophic lateral sclerosis in a 68-year-old man. Jankovic and Rivera (54) described a family in which four generations were afflicted with distal spinal muscular atrophy, three members of which were also subject to myoclonus on maintaining a posture or voluntary movement. Apart from degeneration of motor neurons in brainstem and spinal cord, histological examination disclosed slight demyelination of the posterior columns and posterior spinocerebellar tracts. No details were given of some "degenerative changes in the basal ganglia and frontal cortex." A sporadic case of action myoclonus with spinal muscular atrophy (65) has been mentioned earlier.

Alzheimer's disease

Myoclonus has been reported in Alzheimer's disease (69) and was present at rest; there is no mention of it being aggravated by movement. (Variations on the theme of Ramsay Hunt syndrome are summarized in Table 4.)

Metabolic Disturbances

Anoxia

In discussing the effect of hypoxia, Courville (20) commented in 1939 that "muscular twitching of the extremities . . . at times assumed the proportions of true convulsive movements."

TABLE 4. *Progressive myoclonic epilepsy (systems degeneration type)*

Cerebellar
  Cerebellar ataxia
    No seizures: may be associated with neurogenic atrophy, myopathy
    Seizures: Ramsay Hunt syndrome; Baltic myoclonus,
      may be associated with optic atrophy, nerve deafness, spasticity, neurogenic atrophy,
      myopathy
   Friedreich's ataxia: seizures; may be associated with optic atrophy, myopathy
  Basal ganglia
  Spinal atrophy: may be associated with nerve deafness

In 1952, Gastaut and Rémond (33) listed anoxia as a cause of myoclonus without citing references. Hassler (46) used the term *anoxic myoclonus* for those patients who suffered cerebral damage in infancy, presumably at the time of birth. Aigner and Mulder (2) noted that two of 94 patients dated the onset of myoclonus from an operation, and at least one of these had experienced an episode of hypoxia during anesthesia (D. W. Mulder, *personal communication*). Swanson et al. (100), in their survey of 67 patients with myoclonus, included two cases that followed cardiac arrest. In 1963, Lance and Adams (62) analyzed the movement disorder in four patients with posthypoxic myoclonus resulting from respiratory obstruction or cardiac arrest. They pointed out that the disorder was precipitated particularly by voluntary movement, more so if coordination was required, but that passive movement and, in some cases, touch, tendon tap, pinprick, and sound were effective stimuli. Since then there have been many studies of posthypoxic action myoclonus (14,39,66,67,76,88). Fahn (28) recently reviewed 59 reported posthypoxic cases, as well as other causes of action myoclonus in a comprehensive article on the subject. Although some cases respond to therapy with serotonin precursors, only minor changes could be detected in the lower midbrain in the region corresponding to nucleus raphe dorsalis by de Léan and his colleagues (ref. 82 and *this volume*) and in two of the three posthypoxic patients with action myoclonus by Hauw et al. *(this volume)*. Histological examination of one previously reported case (14) showed neuronal loss and glial proliferation in the thalamus, subthalamic nucleus, and pons with some Purkinje cell loss, but the dentate nucleus was spared.

Uremia

Action myoclonus has been reported in renal failure (15,84,112), and I have observed this myself on a number of occasions. Uremic patients may also be susceptible to sound and muscle stretch, which provoke myoclonus.

Infections

Subacute sclerosing panencephalitis (SSPE) may be associated with action myoclonus in its early stages, before the characteristic bilateral rhythmic movements of this condition becomes apparent (61). I have also seen a syndrome of action myoclonus appear 2 weeks after an apparent encephalitic illness and resolve completely over a period of 7 weeks (61). Baringer et al. (6) described oscillopsia and action myoclonus of the trunk muscles in eight patients as a sequel to respiratory and gastrointestinal infections, with gradual recovery during 6 to 8 weeks. Incoordination, ataxia, and asymmetric myoclonic jerks have been reported with a chronic rubella encephalitis resembling SSPE (110), although whether the jerks were precipitated by movement was not stated.

Trauma

Action myoclonus has been reported as the result of head injury (41) and heat stroke (69).

Intoxications

Action myoclonus may be a sequel of methyl bromide poisoning (14) and may be limited to one limb (61). Castaigne and his colleagues (14) also refer to piperazine intoxication as a cause of action myoclonus. A generalized action myoclonus followed 1 hr after a patient was given 20 mg of the monoamine oxidase inhibitor tranylcypramine with 2 g of L-tryptophan orally and subsided within 24 hr (5).

Paraneoplastic Cerebellar Degeneration

A 23-year-old man with acute lymphocytic leukemia developed intention tremor and dysarthria followed by action myoclonus (79). He died approximately 10 days later, and histological examination showed a marked loss of Purkinje cells with neuronal degeneration in part of the dentate nucleus and substantia nigra. Although there was lymphoblastic infiltration of the leptomeninges and perivascular spaces, no neuronal changes were found in other parts of the brain.

Neuroblastoma may be associated with opsoclonus, ataxia, and myoclonus (87), although whether the latter is exacerbated by movement is uncertain. Abnormalities in an autopsied case were limited to the cerebellum, with loss of Purkinje cells, gliosis, and demyelination in the hilum of the dentate nucleus (114).

Focal Cerebral Lesions

Action or intention myoclonus may be restricted to a particular part of the body in patients with localized cerebral abnormalities. Shibasaki et al. (89) described a patient with action myoclonus involving the left arm and leg associated with independent left and right frontotemporal spike discharges in the electroencephalogram (EEG). An arteriovenous malformation had been removed from the left frontal pole 11 years previously, but the source of the left action myoclonus was undetermined. A 69-year-old patient with right-sided action myoclonus following a presumed left hemisphere infarction was reported by Sutton and Mayer (98). Her EEG showed paroxysmal spikes and polyspikes in the left centrotemporal region.

Severe action myoclonus (made worse by intentioned movement) has been described in multiple sclerosis and attributed to bilateral degeneration of the red nucleus (46,47). Bauer (7) also refers to "action myoclonia" in multiple sclerosis that may completely disable patients in whom other functions are well preserved.

DIFFERENTIATION AMONG THE VARIOUS FORMS OF ACTION MYOCLONUS

Clinical Features

From personal experience and cases recorded in the literature, it does not seem possible to distinguish on clinical grounds among the action myoclonus of any of the syndromes described above when the patient is examined at the height of the

nts, cortical evoked responses are increased in amplitude (21), especially
eriod of myoclonic activity (44,90). The myoclonic jerk itself is usually
ocklike muscular contraction of the type classified by Halliday (43) as
 although slower bilateral rhythmic contractions of the extrapyramidal
supervene as the patient's condition deteriorates.
nd Adams (62) reported EEG abnormalities in three of four patients
ypoxic myoclonus. Spikes or runs of spikes, often increasing in amplitude
ner of the "augmenting" and "recruiting" responses described by Demp-
rison (23), arose from the area overlying the sensorimotor cortex, being
n the side contralateral to myoclonic jerking. The latent interval for
jerks from the initial positive deflection of the cortical spike was 7 msec
l muscles, 12 msec for biceps, 16 msec for wrist extensors, and 32 msec
eps. The myoclonic jerk was propagated down the paravertebral muscles
ies indicating a spinal cord efferent conduction velocity of 30 to 40 m/
al spikes were followed by slow waves, which corresponded to silent
corded simultaneously in all muscle groups lasting up to 340 msec,
ch the limb fell lifelessly downward. This phenomenon appears to be
of the akinetic attacks that frequently accompany myoclonus. Between
jerks, muscle potentials were often grouped at 22 to 24 every second,
responding rhythm sometimes appearing on the EEG. A similar fast
ed to muscle activity in a patient with posthypoxic myoclonus has been
 Kelly et al. (56).
d Adams (62) proposed that action myoclonus might be caused by
s and repetitive discharges of the thalamocortical pathways; however,
t al. (67) made stereotaxic recordings from the ventrolateral thalamus,
a, and internal capsule to compare with cortical and muscular activity
 with posthypoxic action myoclonus and could not confirm this hypoth-
tency from cortical spike to jerk in facial muscles was 10 to 15 msec
 muscles 20 to 40 msec, whereas activity in the ventrolateral nucleus
 cortical spike at about the same latency. Stimulation and then destruc-
ventrolateral nucleus had no effect on myoclonus. On the other hand,
erks could be evoked by electrical stimulation of the motor cortex or
sule. Thus, in this instance, the cortex and descending motor pathways
e hyperexcitable in response to normal afferent volleys. This type of
vas termed *cortical reflex myoclonus* by Hallett et al. (41) who consid-
tion myoclonus is an "abnormal response to feedback during an on-
nent" (40).
l reflex myoclonus, myoclonic activity is preceded by a cortical spike
 recorded on the EEG, either directly or by back-averaging from the
e (41,90), and bursts of impulses are propagated downward from the
cles innervated by cranial nerves are thus activated from above down-
nasseter before facial muscles, the difference in latency between the
venth cranial nerve muscles being 3 to 8 msec. The latencies from
es to limb muscles in these studies were similar to those reported by

illness. Accompanying physical signs may certainly be of assistance in patients with cerebral lipidosis when there are characteristic macular changes in the fundi and in those patients in whom action myoclonus complicates basal ganglia disorders, such as Wilson's disease or progressive supranuclear palsy.

Most patients have signs of cerebellar degeneration that often parallel the severity of myoclonus, but this is not always the case. Approximately 25% of reported cases have signs of an upper motor neuron lesion or extrapyramidal rigidity, in addition to cerebellar disturbance. A considerable number of cases of PME have clinical signs of Friedreich's ataxia (or part thereof, such as pes cavus), but the corticospinal tracts are often spared.

The age and mode of onset, as well as the natural history of the disease, form the basis of the clinical diagnosis in most instances. For example, an episode of hypoxia, uremia, encephalitis, or methyl bromide poisoning provides an acute identifiable onset for the syndrome, which may be completely or partly reversible with the passage of time.

In contrast, the onset in childhood or adolescence of myoclonus in conjunction with increasing cerebellar or other neurological deficit justifies the term *progressive myoclonic epilepsy* (PME). The problem then remains to determine the variety of PME, although treatment remains symptomatic rather than curative in the present state of knowledge. The natural history is of some assistance. Lafora body disease usually appears in the second decade of life (mean, 14 years) and commonly leads to death within 10 years, the mean expectation of life being 6 years (43,45). Most cases of cerebral lipidosis causing PME manifest themselves in the first decade of life (although adult cases have been reported), have a variable life-span (1–23 years), and are commonly accompanied by dementia and dystonic postures in the later stages. Patients with the various forms of lipidosis develop myoclonus only in a minority of cases (43,80). Progressive myoclonic epilepsy of the Unverricht–Lundborg or Ramsay Hunt type has its onset at the end of the first decade or early in the second decade of life and may run a course of 20 years or more, depending on the nature and severity of the underlying system degeneration. On clinical grounds, it is not possible to discern any difference between the patients designated as having Unverricht–Lundborg disease and those with Ramsay Hunt syndrome. The symptoms and signs accompanying PME depend on the regions of the nervous system affected. Cerebellar disturbance is the most common abnormality, but degeneration of pyramidal and extrapyramidal pathways, posterior columns, and spinocerebellar tracts are not unusual, whereas anterior horn cells and muscle fibers have been involved in some cases. Nerve deafness has been associated with Ramsay Hunt syndrome (30,70,105), and one patient who suffered from spinal muscular atrophy (65). Mitochondrial myopathy has been associated with Ramsay Hunt syndrome in patients *with* (30,31,105) and *without* (29,73) major seizures. One patient with mitochondrial myopathy had the clinical features of Friedreich's ataxia and optic atrophy (31). It is thus difficult, and probably artificial, to draw lines of distinction among the many combinations of system degenerations that may accompany action myoclonus.

Pathological Changes of PME

Lafora bodies (amyloid bodies) show the staining reactions of an acid muco-polysaccharide. They have been found at autopsy in a patient suffering from epilepsy without myoclonus, although the patient's brother had the complete syndrome of PME (Buduls and Vilde, 1938, quoted in ref. 45). Nevertheless, their demonstration consistently in a subgroup of cases of PME suggests a disorder of carbohydrate metabolism with deposition in the cortex, basal ganglia (particularly substantia nigra), cerebellar cortex, dentate nucleus, olives, brainstem reticular formation, and viscera such as heart and liver.

Lipofuscin is not found in the normal infantile or adult human brain (80) but is present in the dentate nuclei of children with metachromatic leukodystrophy and Tay–Sachs disease, in cortical neurons in juvenile amaurotic idiocy, and in adult cerebral lipidosis. The lipid deposition in juvenile amaurotic idiocy affects cerebral and cerebellar cortex, basal ganglia, dentate nucleus, and olives.

Most of the system degenerations are also accompanied by evidence of diffuse neuronal disease (Table 5). The autopsy described by Ramsay Hunt in one of his patients with Friedreich's ataxia and myoclonus did not disclose evidence of corticospinal tract degeneration (which in fact excludes the diagnosis of Friedreich's ataxia) but did show atrophy of the dentate nucleus. In addition to atrophy of the dentate nucleus, degeneration of the posterior columns or nucleus gracilis and cuneatus and of the spinocerebellar tracts (but without corticospinal tract involvement) has been noted in other typical cases of Ramsay Hunt syndrome with cerebellar signs and action myoclonus (9,17). In most reports, degeneration of the cerebellar cortex, fallout of Purkinje cells, and atrophy of the dentate nucleus and

TABLE 5. *Sites of pathological disturbance reported*
in action myoclonus

Site of pathology	PME			Other	
	Lafora	Lipid	System	Anoxic	Neoplastic
Cortex	×	×	×		
Thalamus	×	×	×	×	
Basal ganglia	×	×	×	×	×
Cerebellum					
cortex	×	×	×	×	×
dentate	×	×	×		×
Brainstem					
reticular	×	×		×	
cranial nerve nuclei		×	×		
gracile, cuneate	×		×		
Cord					
sensory tracts			×		
motor neurons	×	×	×		
Dorsal root ganglia	×	×	×		
Muscle	×		×		
Viscera	×	×			

its projections have been the cardinal features, wi... also prominent (106).

There have been two reports of PME in wh... detected on histological examination: one autop... 47-year-old patient with a 20-year history (101)... on a 54-year-old woman with a 3-year history (13... a full autopsy on one patient in whom diffuse l... striking feature, with only a few atrophic or deg... in the dentate nucleus and medial thalamic nucle... of four other patients confirmed a patchy or alm... the dentate nuclei (and other structures examin... nigra, and striatum) appearing unremarkable. I... Hunt syndrome cannot be defined by structura... there is any abnormality, some changes will us... cells of the cerebellar cortex, the dentate nuclei...

Another system degeneration has been desc... system was affected as well as the dentatoru... progressive supranuclear palsy, midbrain gliosis... tion to dentate atrophy (60). In other instance... cranial motor nuclei and anterior horn cells of...

Pathological Changes in Other Cau...

Castaigne et al. (14) described the histologic... who had suffered posthypoxic myoclonus aft... cerebral white matter were intact, but marked... in the subthalamic nucleus and the ventrolater... nuclei of the thalamus. Neuronal lesions in cau... larly the large cells. Degenerative changes were... tegmentum, and some Purkinje cells of the cer... superior cerebellar peduncle were entirely no... Another patient who died with posthypoxic... showed minor changes in the vicinity of the n... nucleus) and adjacent midbrain gray matter b... De Léan et al., *this volume*).

The report by Oka et al. (79) is of unusual... action myoclonus developed as a complicatio... Purkinje cells with some neuronal degeneration... nigra were found at autopsy.

Physiological Studies of A...

The EEG of patients with PME of any var... spike or polyspike discharges and commonl... wave complexes on a background of mild slo...

some pat... during a... a brief, s... pyramida... type may...

Lance... with post... in the ma... sey and N... maximal... myocloni... for occipi... for quadri... with late... sec. Corti... periods re... during wh... the cause... myoclonic... with a co... rhythm li... observed...

Lance... synchrono... Lhermitte... basal gang... in a patien... esis. The... and in foo... *followed* th... tion of the... myoclonic... internal ca... appear to... myoclonus... ered that... going mov...

In cortic... that may b... muscle spi... cortex. Mu... ward; i.e.,... fifth and s... cortical sp...

illness. Accompanying physical signs may certainly be of assistance in patients with cerebral lipidosis when there are characteristic macular changes in the fundi and in those patients in whom action myoclonus complicates basal ganglia disorders, such as Wilson's disease or progressive supranuclear palsy.

Most patients have signs of cerebellar degeneration that often parallel the severity of myoclonus, but this is not always the case. Approximately 25% of reported cases have signs of an upper motor neuron lesion or extrapyramidal rigidity, in addition to cerebellar disturbance. A considerable number of cases of PME have clinical signs of Friedreich's ataxia (or part thereof, such as pes cavus), but the corticospinal tracts are often spared.

The age and mode of onset, as well as the natural history of the disease, form the basis of the clinical diagnosis in most instances. For example, an episode of hypoxia, uremia, encephalitis, or methyl bromide poisoning provides an acute identifiable onset for the syndrome, which may be completely or partly reversible with the passage of time.

In contrast, the onset in childhood or adolescence of myoclonus in conjunction with increasing cerebellar or other neurological deficit justifies the term *progressive myoclonic epilepsy* (PME). The problem then remains to determine the variety of PME, although treatment remains symptomatic rather than curative in the present state of knowledge. The natural history is of some assistance. Lafora body disease usually appears in the second decade of life (mean, 14 years) and commonly leads to death within 10 years, the mean expectation of life being 6 years (43,45). Most cases of cerebral lipidosis causing PME manifest themselves in the first decade of life (although adult cases have been reported), have a variable life-span (1–23 years), and are commonly accompanied by dementia and dystonic postures in the later stages. Patients with the various forms of lipidosis develop myoclonus only in a minority of cases (43,80). Progressive myoclonic epilepsy of the Unverricht–Lundborg or Ramsay Hunt type has its onset at the end of the first decade or early in the second decade of life and may run a course of 20 years or more, depending on the nature and severity of the underlying system degeneration. On clinical grounds, it is not possible to discern any difference between the patients designated as having Unverricht–Lundborg disease and those with Ramsay Hunt syndrome. The symptoms and signs accompanying PME depend on the regions of the nervous system affected. Cerebellar disturbance is the most common abnormality, but degeneration of pyramidal and extrapyramidal pathways, posterior columns, and spinocerebellar tracts are not unusual, whereas anterior horn cells and muscle fibers have been involved in some cases. Nerve deafness has been associated with Ramsay Hunt syndrome (30,70,105), and one patient who suffered from spinal muscular atrophy (65). Mitochondrial myopathy has been associated with Ramsay Hunt syndrome in patients *with* (30,31,105) and *without* (29,73) major seizures. One patient with mitochondrial myopathy had the clinical features of Friedreich's ataxia and optic atrophy (31). It is thus difficult, and probably artificial, to draw lines of distinction among the many combinations of system degenerations that may accompany action myoclonus.

Pathological Changes of PME

Lafora bodies (amyloid bodies) show the staining reactions of an acid mucopolysaccharide. They have been found at autopsy in a patient suffering from epilepsy without myoclonus, although the patient's brother had the complete syndrome of PME (Buduls and Vilde, 1938, quoted in ref. 45). Nevertheless, their demonstration consistently in a subgroup of cases of PME suggests a disorder of carbohydrate metabolism with deposition in the cortex, basal ganglia (particularly substantia nigra), cerebellar cortex, dentate nucleus, olives, brainstem reticular formation, and viscera such as heart and liver.

Lipofuscin is not found in the normal infantile or adult human brain (80) but is present in the dentate nuclei of children with metachromatic leukodystrophy and Tay–Sachs disease, in cortical neurons in juvenile amaurotic idiocy, and in adult cerebral lipidosis. The lipid deposition in juvenile amaurotic idiocy affects cerebral and cerebellar cortex, basal ganglia, dentate nucleus, and olives.

Most of the system degenerations are also accompanied by evidence of diffuse neuronal disease (Table 5). The autopsy described by Ramsay Hunt in one of his patients with Friedreich's ataxia and myoclonus did not disclose evidence of corticospinal tract degeneration (which in fact excludes the diagnosis of Friedreich's ataxia) but did show atrophy of the dentate nucleus. In addition to atrophy of the dentate nucleus, degeneration of the posterior columns or nucleus gracilis and cuneatus and of the spinocerebellar tracts (but without corticospinal tract involvement) has been noted in other typical cases of Ramsay Hunt syndrome with cerebellar signs and action myoclonus (9,17). In most reports, degeneration of the cerebellar cortex, fallout of Purkinje cells, and atrophy of the dentate nucleus and

TABLE 5. *Sites of pathological disturbance reported in action myoclonus*

	PME			Other	
Site of pathology	Lafora	Lipid	System	Anoxic	Neoplastic
Cortex	×	×	×		
Thalamus	×	×	×	×	
Basal ganglia	×	×	×	×	×
Cerebellum					
cortex	×	×	×	×	×
dentate	×	×	×		×
Brainstem					
reticular	×	×		×	
cranial nerve nuclei		×	×		
gracile, cuneate	×		×		
Cord					
sensory tracts			×		
motor neurons	×	×	×		
Dorsal root ganglia	×	×	×		
Muscle	×		×		
Viscera	×	×			

its projections have been the cardinal features, with changes in the substantia nigra also prominent (106).

There have been two reports of PME in which no cerebral abnormality was detected on histological examination: one autopsy by Dr. J. G. Greenfield, on a 47-year-old patient with a 20-year history (101) and another by Dr. W. G. P. Mair on a 54-year-old woman with a 3-year history (13). Koskiniemi et al. (58) reported a full autopsy on one patient in whom diffuse loss of Purkinje cells was the most striking feature, with only a few atrophic or degenerating nerve cells being found in the dentate nucleus and medial thalamic nuclei. Limited histological examination of four other patients confirmed a patchy or almost total loss of Purkinje cells with the dentate nuclei (and other structures examined, such as the olives, substantia nigra, and striatum) appearing unremarkable. It is thus apparent that the Ramsay Hunt syndrome cannot be defined by structural changes found at autopsy but, if there is any abnormality, some changes will usually be apparent in the Purkinje cells of the cerebellar cortex, the dentate nuclei, or both sites.

Another system degeneration has been described in which the pallidoluysian system was affected as well as the dentatorubral system (74). In one case of progressive supranuclear palsy, midbrain gliosis was a prominent feature, in addition to dentate atrophy (60). In other instances, the emphasis was on changes in cranial motor nuclei and anterior horn cells of the spinal cord (54,65).

Pathological Changes in Other Causes of Action Myoclonus

Castaigne et al. (14) described the histological findings in an 80-year-old woman who had suffered posthypoxic myoclonus after cardiac arrest. The cortex and cerebral white matter were intact, but marked degeneration and gliosis were seen in the subthalamic nucleus and the ventrolateral, ventromedial, and parafascicular nuclei of the thalamus. Neuronal lesions in caudate and putamen affected particularly the large cells. Degenerative changes were observed in the colliculi, the pontine tegmentum, and some Purkinje cells of the cerebellum, but the dentate nucleus and superior cerebellar peduncle were entirely normal (see also Hauw, *this volume*). Another patient who died with posthypoxic myoclonus at the age of 74 years showed minor changes in the vicinity of the nucleus raphe dorsalis (a serotonergic nucleus) and adjacent midbrain gray matter but little else of note (ref. 82 and J. De Léan et al., *this volume*).

The report by Oka et al. (79) is of unusual interest in that intention tremor and action myoclonus developed as a complication of acute leukemia. Marked loss of Purkinje cells with some neuronal degeneration in the dentate nucleus and substantia nigra were found at autopsy.

Physiological Studies of Action Myoclonus

The EEG of patients with PME of any variety usually shows episodic bilateral spike or polyspike discharges and commonly atypical spike–wave or polyspike–wave complexes on a background of mild slow-wave abnormalities (33,42,106). In some patients, cortical evoked responses are increased in amplitude (21), especially during a period of myoclonic activity (44,90). The myoclonic jerk itself is usually a brief, shocklike muscular contraction of the type classified by Halliday (43) as pyramidal, although slower bilateral rhythmic contractions of the extrapyramidal type may supervene as the patient's condition deteriorates.

Lance and Adams (62) reported EEG abnormalities in three of four patients with posthypoxic myoclonus. Spikes or runs of spikes, often increasing in amplitude in the manner of the "augmenting" and "recruiting" responses described by Dempsey and Morison (23), arose from the area overlying the sensorimotor cortex, being maximal on the side contralateral to myoclonic jerking. The latent interval for myoclonic jerks from the initial positive deflection of the cortical spike was 7 msec for occipital muscles, 12 msec for biceps, 16 msec for wrist extensors, and 32 msec for quadriceps. The myoclonic jerk was propagated down the paravertebral muscles with latencies indicating a spinal cord efferent conduction velocity of 30 to 40 m/sec. Cortical spikes were followed by slow waves, which corresponded to silent periods recorded simultaneously in all muscle groups lasting up to 340 msec, during which the limb fell lifelessly downward. This phenomenon appears to be the cause of the akinetic attacks that frequently accompany myoclonus. Between myoclonic jerks, muscle potentials were often grouped at 22 to 24 every second, with a corresponding rhythm sometimes appearing on the EEG. A similar fast rhythm linked to muscle activity in a patient with posthypoxic myoclonus has been observed by Kelly et al. (56).

Lance and Adams (62) proposed that action myoclonus might be caused by synchronous and repetitive discharges of the thalamocortical pathways; however, Lhermitte et al. (67) made stereotaxic recordings from the ventrolateral thalamus, basal ganglia, and internal capsule to compare with cortical and muscular activity in a patient with posthypoxic action myoclonus and could not confirm this hypothesis. The latency from cortical spike to jerk in facial muscles was 10 to 15 msec and in foot muscles 20 to 40 msec, whereas activity in the ventrolateral nucleus *followed* the cortical spike at about the same latency. Stimulation and then destruction of the ventrolateral nucleus had no effect on myoclonus. On the other hand, myoclonic jerks could be evoked by electrical stimulation of the motor cortex or internal capsule. Thus, in this instance, the cortex and descending motor pathways appear to be hyperexcitable in response to normal afferent volleys. This type of myoclonus was termed *cortical reflex myoclonus* by Hallett et al. (41) who considered that action myoclonus is an "abnormal response to feedback during an ongoing movement" (40).

In cortical reflex myoclonus, myoclonic activity is preceded by a cortical spike that may be recorded on the EEG, either directly or by back-averaging from the muscle spike (41,90), and bursts of impulses are propagated downward from the cortex. Muscles innervated by cranial nerves are thus activated from above downward; i.e., masseter before facial muscles, the difference in latency between the fifth and seventh cranial nerve muscles being 3 to 8 msec. The latencies from cortical spikes to limb muscles in these studies were similar to those reported by

Lance and Adams (62) and compatible with those elicited by direct cortical stimulation (41,67). Dawson (21) and Halliday (44) have shown that sensory evoked responses are increased in myoclonic states, and this augmented cortical response is probably identical with the spike–wave recorded in myoclonus. One site of signal amplification in action myoclonus thus appears to be the sensorimotor cortex, which could account for the sensitivity of many patients to afferent stimulation, including muscle stretch, because there is ample physiological evidence for the projection of muscle afferents to the cerebral cortex (32,95). Action myoclonus may be limited to one part of the body if that part is selectively stimulated or can be restricted to one part of the body as the result of a focal cortical lesion (98). The effective stimulus may be touch or pressure rather than muscle stretch (97). Conversely, generalized myoclonic jerks may be elicited by stimulation of a specific area of the body (76), which suggests the possibility of amplification of the signal at a subcortical level with resulting bilateral spread of synchronized and often repetitive motor activity.

The term *reticular reflex myoclonus* was introduced by Hallett et al. (39) after studying a patient with posthypoxic action myoclonus who was also sensitive to sensory stimuli, such as noise or tendon tap. Myoclonic jerks were recorded in facial musculature before the masseter muscle, suggesting that the motor disturbance was ascending through the brainstem. Most remarkable of all, the sternomastoid muscle, innervated from the cervical cord through the spinal accessory nerve, was involved in myoclonic contraction from 7 to 16 msec before the cranial musculature. The authors refer to the "11th nerve nucleus" being activated 4 msec before the cervical cord, but the relevant part of the eleventh nerve nucleus is of course in the spinal cord, in the segments immediately rostral to the motor neurons supplying the biceps muscle. One can only conclude that the generator of the myoclonic jerk was in the caudal part of the medulla or upper cervical cord and propagated upward and downward from this site. Cortical spikes in this form of myoclonus are not time-locked to myoclonic jerks as they are in cortical reflex myoclonus.

Clinical observations concur with the concept of hyperactivity of both cortex and reticular formation in action myoclonus. A small movement of one limb or a sensory stimulus applied to a limb may lead to jerking of that limb (cortical reflex myoclonus). As movements or sensory stimuli are increased, the resulting myoclonic jerks may overflow to the opposite side of the body, spread from upper to lower limb, and involve all the body musculature (reticular reflex myoclonus). It is clear that the origin of action myoclonus lies in the withdrawal of a diffusely distributed inhibitory or modulating system rather than in damage to some discrete locus in the nervous system.

MECHANISM OF ACTION MYOCLONUS

Action myoclonus is an augmented, synchronized, and irradiated motor response to attempted voluntary movement. Some cases may react to specific afferent stimulation as well. A subclinical muscle contraction may be detected in normal subjects in response to auditory, photic, or somatosensory stimulation by computer-averaged electromyography (8). Stimulus-sensitive myoclonus could be an exaggeration of this normal reflex response. What modulating system or systems must be withdrawn to permit such excessive and misplaced enthusiasm on the part of the central nervous system?

Damage to the medial nuclei of the thalamus in monkeys can cause spontaneous myoclonus, but this is not aggravated by movement (72). It is possible that a lesion of the medial thalamic nuclei may underlie focal myoclonus in some cases of localized cerebral damage or may play a part in other forms of action myoclonus, since degeneration of medial thalamic nuclei was reported in Unverricht–Lundborg disease (Baltic myoclonus) by Koskiniemi et al. (58) and in posthypoxic myoclonus by Castaigne et al. (14). The most consistent pathological change noted at autopsy in patients with action myoclonus has been degeneration of Purkinje cells or dentate nuclei. Purkinje cell output inhibits the deep cerebellar nuclei, which in turn have an excitatory action on their target nuclei, including the brainstem reticular formation (26). Removal of Purkinje cell inhibition would therefore increase the excitability of the reticular formation to sensory input.

Purkinje cell loss is not uncommon in patients suffering from forms of epilepsy other than myoclonus (69), although the association with myoclonus (48) has aroused most interest. The changes are unlikely to be caused solely by hypoxia during epileptic fits, since they have been found in a biopsy specimen from an epileptic patient without a history of major seizures (86), and the possibility that loss of Purkinje cells is related to phenytoin medication (27) cannot be excluded at present. Degeneration of the cerebellar cortex and dentate nucleus is likely to be an adjuvant factor rather than a primary cause of myoclonus because of the capricious nature of the involvement of these structures in autopsied cases and because of the lack of correlation between cerebellar signs and severity of myoclonus.

The findings that the main metabolite of serotonin, 5 hydroxyindoleacetic acid (5-HIAA), was present in abnormally low concentrations in the cerebrospinal fluid of some patients with posthypoxic myoclonus (16,38,82,108) led to successful treatment with serotonin precursors in combination with decarboxylase or monoamine oxidase inhibitors. Serotonergic systems are concentrated in the median raphe nuclei of the brainstem and generally have a central inhibitory action, for example, on pain mechanisms. Minor changes have been found in an area corresponding to the nucleus raphe dorsalis and adjacent gray matter in autopsied cases of posthypoxic myoclonus, but the disorder nevertheless appears to be one of serotonergic transmission without any convincing structural basis.

Contrary to what one would expect from the clinical data, experimental myoclonus has been produced by the administration of the serotonin precursor 5-hydroxytryptophan (5-HTP) to immature guinea pigs (57). Moreover, myoclonus was consistently induced by 5-HTP in rats pretreated with desmethylimipramine intraperitoneally (to protect noradrenergic neurons) and dihydroxytryptamine intracisternally (to destroy other amine-containing neurons) by Stewart et al. (96). Myoclonus in the pretreated rats was attributed to supersensitivity of postsynaptic serotonin receptors because it was partially blocked by methysergide and a centrally active dose of decarboxylase inhibitor but was potentiated by a monoamine oxidase inhibitor. Autoradiographic analysis after [^{14}C]deoxyglucose given to guinea pigs with 5-HTP-induced myoclonus showed that glucose metabolism was increased in ventral and ventral anterior thalamic nuclei but diminished in the cerebral cortex (104). This form of experimental myoclonus in guinea pigs was suppressed by the daily administration of cortisol for 2 weeks (75). The injection into rats of *p*-chloroamphetamine, which releases serotonin from nerve terminals, also produces a myoclonic syndrome (36).

In contrast to the implications of these experiments and more in line with clinical observations, myoclonus resulting from the intragastric administration of *p,p'*-DDT in mice and rats was reduced by L-5-HTP (as well as by a serotonin agonist and a serotonin-releasing agent) and was enhanced by the serotonin-blocking agent meth-ysergide (50). Cerebral content of 5-HIAA was increased, suggesting increased serotonin turnover. Possibly, *p,p'*-DDT inhibits serotonin release, thus causing a feedback enhancement of serotonin synthesis.

Focal myoclonus has been caused in rats by a combination of cortical damage and the injection of picrotoxin or allylglycine into the caudate nucleus. Such myoclonus was abolished by the injection of γ-aminobutyric acid (GABA) or the destruction of globus pallidus (102).

Do these experimental models help us to understand action myoclonus in humans? Clearly, inhibitory areas or systems have been put out of action in the various forms of focal or generalized neuronal disease that underlie action myoclonus in humans. There is sound evidence for the involvement of serotonergic pathways in humans, but animal studies thus far obfuscate rather than elucidate the mechanism. Whether GABA pathways are also compromised remains speculative.

Finally, why is movement, particularly precise or coordinated movement, such a potent trigger for myoclonus? Action myoclonus may be initiated by a corollary discharge from motor cortex or reticular formation, the general concept of which was presented by McCloskey (71). Alternatively or additionally, it may be provoked by projections of muscle afferents to the motor cortex (32,95) as an abnormal response to feedback while a movement is in progress, as suggested by Hallett et al. (41).

Treatment of Action Myoclonus

Action myoclonus may be reduced appreciably in some cases by conventional anticonvulsants, such as phenytoin and primidone (78), or by barbiturates (62,85). Phenytoin may have adverse long-term effects in PME (27). Lance (61) evaluated the medications available at that time in the management of 46 patients in whom myoclonus was the presenting symptom or one of the main complaints. He concluded that nitrazepam was the most useful (preventing myoclonic attacks in nine of the 25 patients in whom it was used and improving another six patients), whereas diazepam was less effective, although some patients responded satisfactorily (see also refs. 85 and 88).

An important advance was made with the discovery that 5-HTP almost completely relieved posthypoxic action myoclonus and L-DOPA with a monoamine oxidase inhibitor caused some improvement, whereas agents that blocked noradrenergic and serotonergic transmission aggravated myoclonus (66). These results have been amply confirmed (16,22,38,107). It is now apparent that doses of L-5-HTP of the order of 1,000 mg daily, with or without a decarboxylase inhibitor, improve most but not all patients with posthypoxic myoclonus and some patients with other varieties of PME (29,37,103,108). The high incidence of nausea, vomiting, and diarrhea and affective disturbances (mania, depression) as side effects of 5-HTP therapy limit its application.

When clonazepam, a successor to diazepam and nitrazepam in the benzodiazepine series, became available, it was found to be effective in posthypoxic encephalopathy (12), as well as in some patients with action myoclonus from other causes (35). The introduction of sodium valproate provided another effective treatment for posthypoxic myoclonus (83,93), as well as for PME (63,92). Lance and Anthony (64) compared the action of clonazepam and sodium valproate in 60 epileptic patients, 17 of whom suffered from myoclonus, and concluded that both drugs were effective in the majority of patients but that some responded unpredictably to one rather than the other. Hormonal influences may alter responses to medication: estrogen therapy improved one posthypoxic patient reported by Fahn (28). Iivanainen and Himberg (51) have recently recorded their experiences in Finland with 26 patients suffering from PME, of whom all but one improved conspicuously after their conventional drug regimen was changed to a combination of clonazepam, sodium valproate, and phenobarbital.

Kelly et al. (55) divided myoclonic patients into two groups: "epileptic" if they were also subject to nonmyoclonic seizures or had spike or spike–wave discharges in their EEGs, and "nonepileptic" if they had not. The former group responded better to anticonvulsants than the latter. Unfortunately, not all patients with epileptic myoclonus can be controlled satisfactorily, even with the newer anticonvulsants. It remains to be proven whether clonazepam and sodium valproate owe their efficacy to actions on serotonin and GABA mechanisms, respectively.

The action myoclonus of multiple sclerosis has been relieved by stereotaxic destruction of the zona incerta immediately below the thalamus (47), and Jacobs (53) reported that two of his family with action myoclonus improved after thalamotomy. Stereotaxic destruction of the ventrolateral thalamic nucleus has not reduced posthypoxic action myoclonus (29,67), but improvement has been reported with chronic cerebellar stimulation (19).

It can be seen that the understanding and treatment of action myoclonus has made great advances over the past 20 years, and this gives rise to cautious optimism for the future.

SUMMARY

Action myoclonus, reviewed in this chapter, is the term applied to arrhythmic muscular jerking induced by voluntary movement. It is made worse by attempts at precise or coordinated movement (intention myoclonus) and may also be provoked by certain sensory stimuli. The effective stimuli for action myoclonus is probably feedback from muscle afferents, although it may be initiated by corollary discharge from motor cortex to reticular formation before or at the onset of voluntary movement.

The condition is usually associated with diffuse neuronal disease such as post-hypoxic encephalopathy, uremia, and the various forms of PME, although action myoclonus may be limited to one limb in some cases of focal cerebral damage. It is caused by hyperexcitability of the sensorimotor cortex (cortical reflex myoclonus) or reticular formation (reticular reflex myoclonus), or both. No consistent pathological change has been reported in autopsied cases of action myoclonus. The underlying disorder appears to be a loss of inhibitory mechanisms involving serotonin and possibly GABA as transmitter agents.

The term PME is used for the association of myoclonus with degenerative changes in the nervous system which are commonly diffuse but may predominate in certain systems. There may or may not be associated tonic–clonic seizures, other manifestations of epilepsy, or dementia. Those cases of PME associated with Lafora inclusion bodies and cerebral storage diseases can be distinguished from the system degenerations. Systems which may be involved in the latter group include cerebellodentatorubral, pyramidal, extrapyramidal, optic, auditory, posterior columns and gracile and cuneate nuclei, spinocerebellar pathways, motor neurons of cranial nerves and anterior horns, and muscle fibers. Confronted with this diversity of pathological change, it seems unnecessary to make any clinical distinction between Ramsay Hunt syndrome and Unverricht–Lundborg syndrome (Baltic myoclonus) because cerebellar signs are found in patients described under both headings. Additional systems may be involved in individuals or families who are otherwise typical. All three names could well be joined in an eponymous title (Unverricht–Lundborg–Hunt disease) or the condition simply known as the systems degeneration type of PME, as Halliday (43) suggested. The cause of the condition (or spectrum of conditions) is at present unknown.

Action myoclonus usually responds to sodium valproate or clonazepam, and some individuals, particularly those with posthypoxic myoclonus, improve with the administration of serotonin precursors.

REFERENCES

1. Adams R, Victor M. *Principles of neurology*. Second ed. New York: McGraw Hill, 1981:692–3.
2. Aigner BR, Mulder DW. Myoclonus. Clinical significance and an approach to classification. *Arch Neurol* 1960;2:600–15.
3. Andermann F, Carpenter S, Wolfe LS, Andermann E, Patry G, Boileau J, Nelson R, Warren Y, Barcelo R. Myoclonus epilepsy and renal failure: a new syndrome (abstr.). *Neurology* 1981;31(2):68.
4. Austin J, Sakai M. Disorders of glycogen and related macromolecules in the nervous system. In: Vinken PJ, Bruyn GW, eds. Handbook of clinical neurology, vol. 27. Amsterdam: North-Holland, 1976:169–219.
5. Baloh RW, Dietz, J, Spooner JW. Myoclonus and ocular oscillations induced by L-tryptophan. *Ann Neurol* 1982;11:95–7.

6. Baringer JR, Sweeney VP, Winkler GF. An acute syndrome of ocular oscillations and truncal myoclonus. *Brain* 1968;91:473–80.

7. Bauer HJ. Problems of symptomatic therapy in multiple sclerosis. *Neurology* 1978;28(2):8–20.

8. Bickford RG, Jacobson JL, Cody DTR. Nature of average evoked potentials to sound and other stimuli in man. *Ann NY Acad Sci* 1964;112:204–23.

9. Bird TD, Shaw CM. Progressive myoclonus and epilepsy with dentatorubral degeneration: a clinicopathological study of the Ramsay Hunt syndrome. *J Neurol Neurosurg Psychiatry* 1978;41:140–9.

10. Bonduelle M. The myoclonias. In: Vinken PJ, Bruyn GW, eds. Handbook of clinical neurology, vol 6. Amsterdam: North-Holland, 1968:761–81.

11. Boschi G. Ataxie héréditaire avec paramyoclonus multiplex type Unverricht. *J Neurol* 1913;18:141–50.

12. Boudouresques J, Roger J, Khalil R, Vigouroux RA, Gosset A, Pellister JF, Tassinari CA. A propos de 2 observations du syndrome de Lance and Adams. Effet thérapeutique du Ro-05-4023. *Rev Neurol* 1971;15:306–7.

13. Bradshaw J. A study of myoclonus. *Brain* 1954;77:138–57.

14. Castaigne P, Cambier, J, Escourolle R. Les myoclonies d'intention et d'action. *Rev Neurol* 1968;119:107–20.

15. Chadwick D, French AT. Uraemic myoclonus: an example of reticular reflex myoclonus? *J Neurol Neurosurg Psychiatry* 1979;42:52–5.

16. Chadwick D, Hallett M, Harris R, Jenner P, Reynolds EH, Marsden CD. Clinical, biochemical and physiological factors distinguishing myoclonus responsive to 5-hydroxytryptophan, tryptophan plus a monoamine oxidase inhibitor and clonazepam. *Brain* 1977;100:455–87.

17. Christophe J, Gruner J. La dyssynergie cérébelleuse myoclonique de Ramsay Hunt. Étude anatomique d'un cas. *Rev Neurol* 1956;95:297–309.

18. Clark LP. A case of myoclonia occurring only after rest or sleep. *JAMA* 1912;58:1666–8.

19. Cooper IS, Amin I, Riklan M, Waltz JM, Poon TP. Chronic cerebellar stimulation in epilepsy. Clinical and anatomical studies. *Arch Neurol* 1976;33:559–70.

20. Courville CB. *Untoward effects of nitrous oxide Anesthesia.* Mountain View, California: Pacific Press, 1939.

21. Dawson GD. Investigations on a patient subject to myoclonic seizures after sensory stimulation. *J Neurol Neurosurg Psychiatry* 1947;10:141–62.

22. De Léan, J, Richardson JC, Hornykiewicz O. Beneficial effects of serotonin precursors in postanoxic action myoclonus. *Neurology* 1976;26:863–8.

23. Dempsey EW, Morison PS. The electrical activity of a thalamocortical relay system. *Am J Physiol* 1943;138:283–96.

24. Diebold K. Vier Erbtypen oder Krankheitsformen der progressiven Myoklonus epilepsien. *Arch Psychiatr Nervenkrankh* 1972;215:362–75.

25. Döring G. Myoklonus Syndrom bei Amyotrophischer Lateralsklerose. *Deutsche Z Nervenheilk* 1938;147:26–35.

26. Eccles JC, Ito M, Szentágothai J. *The cerebellum as a neuronal machine.* New York: Springer, 1967:227–99.

27. Eldridge R, Iivanainen M, Stern R, Koerber T. Baltic myoclonus epilepsy: a treatable, inherited disorder distinct from Lafora disease *(abstr.)*. *Neurology* 1981;31(2):67–8.

28. Fahn S. Posthypoxic action myoclonus: review of the literature and report of two new cases with response to valproate and estrogen. *Adv Neurol* 1979;26:49–84.

29. Feit H, Kirkpatrick J, Van Woert MH, Pandian G. Myoclonus, ataxia and hypoventilation: response to L-5-hydroxytryptophan. *Neurology* 1983;33:109–12.

30. Fitzsimons RB, Clifton-Bligh P, Wolfenden WH. Mitochondrial myopathy and lactic acidaemia with myoclonic epilepsy, ataxia and hypothalamic infertility: a variant of Ramsay-Hunt syndrome? *J Neurol Neurosurg Psychiatry* 1981;44:79–82.

31. Fukuhara N, Tokiguchi S, Shirakawa K, Tsubaki T. Myoclonus epilepsy associated with ragged-red fibres (mitochondrial abnormalities): disease entity or a syndrome? *J Neurol Sci* 1980;47:117–33.

32. Gandevia S, Burke D, McKeon B. The relationship between the size of a muscle afferent volley and the cerebral potential it produces. *J Neurol Neurosurg Psychiatry* 1982;45:705–10.

33. Gastaut H, Rémond A. Étude électroencéphalographique des myoclonies. *Rev Neurol* 1952;85:596–609.

34. Gilbert GJ, McEntee WJ, Glaser GH. Familial myoclonus and ataxia. Pathophysiologic implications. *Neurology* 1963;13:365–72.
35. Goldberg MA, Dorman JD. Intention myoclonus: successful treatment with clonazepam. *Neurology* 1976;26:24–6.
36. Growdon JH. Postural changes, tremor, and myoclonus in the rat immediately following injections of p-chloroamphetamine. *Neurology* 1977;27:1074–7.
37. Growdon JH, Young RR, Shahani BT. L-5-hydroxytryptophan in treatment of several different syndromes in which myoclonus is prominent. *Neurology* 1976;26:1135–40.
38. Guilleminault C, Tharp BR, Cousin D. HVA and 5HIAA CSF measurements and 5HTP trials in some patients with involuntary movements. *J Neurol Sci* 1973;18:435–41.
39. Hallett M, Chadwick D, Adam J, Marsden CD. Reticular reflex myoclonus: a physiological type of human post-hypoxic myoclonus. *J Neurol Neurosurg Psychiatry* 1977;40:253–64.
40. Hallett M, Chadwick D, Marsden CD. Ballistic movement overflow myoclonus. A form of essential myoclonus. *Brain* 1977;100:299–312.
41. Hallett M, Chadwick D, Marsden CD. Cortical reflex myoclonus. *Neurology* 1979;29:1107–25.
42. Halliday AM. The electrophysiological study of myoclonus in man. *Brain* 1967;90:241–84.
43. Halliday AM. The clinical incidence of myoclonus. In: Williams D, ed. *Modern trends in neurology*, vol. 4. London: Butterworths, 1967:69–105.
44. Halliday AM. Cerebral evoked potentials in familial progressive myoclonic epilepsy. *J Coll Phys Lond* 1967;1:123–34.
45. Harriman DGF, Millar JHD. Progressive familial myoclonic epilepsy in three families: its clinical features and pathological basis. *Brain* 1955;78:325–49.
46. Hassler R. Myoclonies extrapyramidales traitées par coagulation stéréotaxique de la voie dentato-thalamique et leur mécanisme physiopathologique. *Rev Neurol* 1968;119:409–18.
47. Hassler R, Bronisch F, Mundinger F, Riechert T. Intention myoclonus of multiple sclerosis, its patho-anatomical basis and its stereotactic relief. *Neurochirurgie* 1975;18:90–106.
48. Hodskins MB, Yakovlev PI. Anatomicoclinical observation on myoclonus in epileptics and on related symptom complexes. *Am J Psychiatry* 1930;86:827–48.
49. Hunt JR. Dyssynergia cerebellaris myoclonica—primary atrophy of the dentate system: a contribution to the pathology and symptomatology of the cerebellum. *Brain* 1921;44:490–538.
50. Hwang EC, Van Woert MH. p,p'-DDT-induced neurotoxic syndrome: experimental myoclonus. *Neurology* 1978;28:1020–5.
51. Iivanainen M, Himberg J-J. Valproate and clonazepam in the treatment of severe progressive myoclonic epilepsy. *Arch Neurol* 1982;39:236–8.
52. Itoyama Y, Goto I, Kuroiwa Y, Takeichi M, Kawabuchi M, Tanaka Y. Familial juvenile neuronal storage disease. New disease or variant of juvenile lipidosis? *Arch Neurol* 1978;35:792–800.
53. Jacobs H. Myoclonus and ataxia occurring in a family. *J Neurol Neurosurg Psychiatry* 1965;28:272–5.
54. Jankovic J, Rivera VM. Hereditary myoclonus and progressive distal muscular atrophy. *Ann Neurol* 1979;6:227–31.
55. Kelly JJ, Sharbrough FW, Daube JR. A clinical and electrophysiological evaluation of myoclonus. *Neurology* 1981;31:581–9.
56. Kelly JJ, Sharbrough FW, Westmoreland BF. Movement-activated central fast rhythms: an EEG finding in action myoclonus. *Neurology* 1978;28:1037–40.
57. Klawans HL Jr, Groetz C, Weiner WJ. 5-Hydroxytryptophan-induced myoclonus in guinea pigs and the possible role of serotonin in infantile myoclonus. *Neurology* 1973;23:1234–40.
58. Koskiniemi M, Donner M, Majuri H, Haltia M, Norio R. Progressive myoclonus epilepsy. A clinical and histopathological study. *Acta Neurol Scand* 1974;50:307–32.
59. Kreindler A, Crighel I, Poilici I. Clinical and electroencephalographic investigations in myoclonic cerebellar dyssynergia. *J Neurol Neurosurg Psychiatry* 1959;22:232–7.
60. Kurihara T, Landau WM, Torack RM. Progressive supranuclear palsy with action myoclonus, seizures. *Neurology* 1974;24:219–23.
61. Lance JW. Myoclonic jerks and falls: aetiology, classification and treatment. *Med J Aust* 1968;1:113–20.
62. Lance JW, Adams RD. The syndrome of intention or action myoclonus as a sequel to hypoxic encephalopathy. *Brain* 1963;86:111–36.
63. Lance JW, Anthony M. The anticonvulsant action of sodium valproate (Epilim) in 100 patients with various forms of epilepsy. *Med J Aust* 1977;1:911–5.

64. Lance JW, Anthony M. Sodium valproate and clonazepam in the treatment of intractable epilepsy. *Arch Neurol* 1977;34:14–7.
65. Lance JW, Evans WA. Progressive myoclonic epilepsy nerve deafness and spinal muscular atrophy. *Clin Exp Neurol*, 1984;20:141–51.
66. Lhermitte F, Marteau R, Degos C-F. Analyse pharmacologique d'un nouveau cas de myoclonies d'intention et d'action post-anoxiques. *Rev Neurol* 1972;126:107–14.
67. Lhermitte F, Talairach J, Buser P, Gautier J-C, Bancaud J, Gras R, Truelle J-L. Myoclonies d'intention et d'action post-anoxiques. Étude stéréotaxique et destruction du noyau ventral latéral du thalamus. *Rev Neurol* 1971;124:5–20.
68. Lindemulder FG. Familial myoclonia occurring in three successive generations. *J Nerv Ment Dis* 1933;77:489–91.
69. Marsden CD, Hallett M, Fahn S. The nosology and pathophysiology of myoclonus. In: Marsden CD, Fahn S, eds. *Movement disorders*. London: Butterworths, 1981:196–248.
70. May DL, White HH. Familial myoclonus, cerebellar ataxia and deafness. Specific genetically-determined disease. *Arch Neurol* 1968;19:331–8.
71. McCloskey DI. Corollary discharges: motor commands and perception. In: Brooks VB, ed. *Handbook of physiology—the nervous system II*. Bethesda: American Physiological Society, 1982;1415–47.
72. Milhorat TH. Experimental myoclonus of thalamic origin. *Arch Neurol* 1967;17:365–78.
73. Morgan-Hughes JA, Hayes DJ, Clark JB, Landon DN, Swash M, Stark RJ, Rudge P. Mitochondrial encephalomyopathies. Biochemical studies in two cases revealing defects in the respiratory chain. *Brain* 1982;105:553–82.
74. Naito H, Oyanagi S. Familial myoclonus epilepsy and choreoathetosis: hereditary dentatorubral–pallidoluysian atrophy. *Neurology* 1982;32:798–807.
75. Nausieda PA, Weiner WJ, Carvey PM, Braun A. The effect of chronic corticosteroid administration on an animal model of myoclonus (abstr.). *Ann Neurol* 1981;10:94.
76. Niedermeyer E, Bauer G, Burnite R, Reichenbach D. Selective stimulus-sensitive myoclonus in acute cerebral anoxia. *Arch Neurol* 1977;34:365–8.
77. Nishimura RN, Ishak KG, Reddick R, Porter, R, James S, Barranger JA. Lafora disease: diagnosis by liver biopsy. *Ann Neurol*. 1980;8:409–15.
78. Noad KB, Lance JW. Familial myoclonic epilepsy and its association with cerebellar disturbance. *Brain* 1960;83:618–30.
79. Oka H, Matsushima M, Ando K, Hoshizaki H. Intention myoclonus in acute leukaemia. *Brain* 1972;95:395–8.
80. Pallis CA, Duckett S, Pearse AGE. Diffuse lipofuscinosis of the central nervous system. *Neurology* 1967;17:381–94.
81. Rapin I, Goldfischer S, Katzman R, Engel J, O'Brien JS. The cherry-red-spot-myoclonus syndrome. *Ann Neurol* 1978;3:234–42.
82. Richardson JC, Rewcastle NB, de Léan J. Hypoxic myoclonus: clinical and pathological observations. In: Rose FC, ed. *Physiological aspects of clinical neurology*. Oxford: Blackwell, 1977:231–45.
83. Rollinson RD, Gilligan BS. Postanoxic action myoclonus (Lance–Adams syndrome) responding to valproate. *Arch Neurol* 1979;36:44–5.
84. Rose AL, O'Brien J, Bhutt K, Nicastri A. Cherry-red-spot-myoclonus syndrome (Sialidosis Type 1): report of another family and characterization of storage material in the viscera (abstr.). *Ann Neurol* 1981;10:294.
85. Rosen AD, Berenyi KJ, Laurenceau V. Intention myoclonus—diazepam and phenobarbital treatment. *JAMA* 1969;209:772–3.
86. Salcman M, Defendini R, Correll J, Gilman S. Neuropathological changes in cerebellar biopsies of epileptic patients. *Ann Neurol* 1978;3:10–9.
87. Senelick RC, Bray PF, Lahey ME, Van Dyk HJL, Johnson DG. Neuroblastoma and myoclonic encephalopathy. *Pediatr Surg* 1973;8:623–32.
88. Sherwin I, Redmon W. Successful treatment in action myoclonus. *Neurology* 1969;19:846–50.
89. Shibasaki H, Logothetis JA, Torres F. Intention myoclonus: a case report. *Neurology* 1971;21:655–8.
90. Shibasaki H, Yamashita Y, Kuroiwa Y. Electroencephalographic studies of myoclonus. *Brain* 1978;101:447–60.
91. Smith NJ, Espir MLE, Matthews WB. Familial myoclonic epilepsy with ataxia and neuropathy

with additional features of Friedreich's ataxia and peroneal muscular atrophy. *Brain* 1978;101:461–72.

92. Somerville ER, Olanow W. Valproic acid. Treatment of myoclonus in dyssynergia cerebellaris myoclonica. *Arch Neurol* 1982;39:527–8.
93. Sotaniemi K. Valproic acid in the treatment of nonepileptic myoclonus. Report of three cases. *Arch Neurol* 1982;39:448–9.
94. Stark RJ. Reversible myoclonus with uraemia. *Br Med J* 1981;1:1119–20.
95. Starr A, McKeon B, Skuse NF, Burke D. Cerebral potentials evoked by muscle stretch in man. *Brain* 1981;104:149–66.
96. Stewart RM, Growdon JH, Cancian D, Baldessarini RJ. Myoclonus after 5-hydroxytryptophan in rats with lesions of indoleamine neurons in the central nervous system. *Neurology* 1976;26:690–2.
97. Sutton GG. Receptors in focal reflex myoclonus. *J Neurol Neurosurg Psychiatry* 1975;38:505–7.
98. Sutton GG, Mayer RF. Focal reflex myoclonus. *J Neurol Neurosurg Psychiatry* 1974;37:207–17.
99. Suzuki Y, Nakamura N, Shimada Y, Yotsumoto H, Endo H, Nagashima K. Macular cherry-red spots and β-galactosidase deficiency in an adult. *Arch Neurol* 1977;34:157–61.
100. Swanson PD, Luttrell CN, Magladery JW. Myoclonus—a report of 67 cases and review of the literature. *Medicine* 1962;41:339–56.
101. Symonds C. Myoclonus. *Med J Aust* 1954;1:765–8.
102. Tarsy D, Pycock CJ, Meldrum BS, Marsden CD. Focal contralateral myoclonus produced by inhibition of GABA action in the caudate nucleus of rats. *Brain* 1978;101:143–62.
103. Thal LJ, Sharpless NS, Wolfson L, Katzman R. Treatment of myoclonus with L-5-hydroxytryptophan and carbidopa: clinical, electrophysiological, and biochemical investigations. *Ann Neurol* 1980;7:570–6.
104. Thal LJ, Wolfson LI. Functional anatomy of L-5-hydroxytryptophan-induced myoclonus in the guinea pig. *Neurology* 1981;31:955–60.
105. Tsairis P, Engel WK, Kark P. Familial myoclonic epilepsy syndrome associated with skeletal muscle mitochondrial abnormalities (abstr.). *Neurology* 1973;23:408.
106. Van Bogaert L, Radermecker J, Titeca J. Les syndromes myocloniques. *Folia Psychiatr Neurol Neurochirurg Neerl* 1950;53:650–90.
107. Van Woert MH, Sethy VH. Therapy of intention myoclonus with L-5-hydroxytryptophan and a peripheral decarboxylase inhibitor, MK486. *Neurology* 1975;25:135–40.
108. Van Woert MH, Rosenbaum D, Howieson J, Bowers MB. Long-term treatment of myoclonus and other neurologic disorders with L-5-hydroxytryptophan and carbidopa. *N Engl J Med* 1977;296:70–5.
109. Watson CW, Denny-Brown D. Myoclonus epilepsy as a symptom of diffuse neuronal disease. *Arch Neurol Psychiatry* 1953;70:151–68.
110. Weil ML, Itabashi HH, Cremer NE, Oshiro LS, Lennette EH, Carnay L. Chronic progressive panencephalitis due to rubella virus simulating subacute sclerosing panencephalitis. *N Engl J Med* 1975;292:994–8.
111. Wohlfart G, Höök O. A clinical analysis of myoclonic epilepsy (Unverricht-Lundborg), myoclonic cerebellar dyssynergy (Hunt) and hepatolenticular degeneration (Wilson). *Acta Psychiatr Neurol Scand* 1951;26:219–45.
112. Wolf P, Becker H. Aktionmyoklonus bei akuter Dekompensation einer chronischen Niereninsuffizienz. *J Neurol* 1974;207:247–52.
113. Ziegler DK, Van Speybroech NW, Seitz EF. Myoclonic epilepsia partialis continua and Friedreich ataxia. *Arch Neurol* 1974;31:308–11.
114. Ziter FM, Bray PF, Cancilla PA. Neuropathologic findings in a patient with neuroblastoma and myoclonic encephalopathy. *Arch Neurol* 1979;36:51.

Advances in Neurology, Vol. 43: Myoclonus,
edited by S. Fahn et al. Raven Press,
New York © 1986.

Baltic Myoclonus

M. L. Koskiniemi

*Department of Neurology and Children's Hospital, University of Helsinki,
00290 Helsinki 29, Finland*

Progressive myoclonus epilepsy (PME) as an entity was first described by Unverricht in 1891 (22). Since then this syndrome has been reported from different parts of the world. Subsequent cases have been more heterogeneous (5,6,19,21). Many subgroups have been described (2,6,24). The most well-known form has become PME with intranuclear inclusion bodies, described by Lafora in 1911 (16). However, no histopathological knowledge exists in Unverricht's patients. On closer examination, the clinical pictures of Unverricht's and Lafora's patients are different. Finnish PME patients closely mimic Unverricht's patients; only degenerative alterations have been found in neurons (4,11). Swedish PME patients are clinically similar to these cases (18). In other parts of the world, the Lafora type of PME is more frequent. Therefore, cases without inclusion bodies could be called Unverricht–Lundborg's syndrome or Baltic/Nordic PME.

DIAGNOSTIC CRITERIA

The diagnosis of PME without Lafora bodies is based on the following criteria, of which at least three are needed in addition to stimulus-sensitive myoclonic jerks: (a) age at onset, 6 to 15 years, (b) grand mal seizures, (c) characteristic electroencephalogram (EEG), and (d) progressive course (11).

CLINICAL FEATURES

The early development of these children is normal (11). They usually attend school at the same age (7 years) as healthy children. The first symptom suggesting the PME syndrome—stimulus-sensitive myoclonic jerks or grand mal seizures—appears at the age of 6 to 15 years. The other follows some months or years later. In a few patients, fatigue, clumsiness of the legs, syncopal attacks, or blinking may be noted earlier.

Myoclonic jerks mostly appear in the morning on awakening or when tired. All stimuli, either external or from the patient himself, increase the involuntary jerks. These affect gait, speech, swallowing, and every aspect of the patient's daily life. Infectious diseases are common. In the later stages of the disease, some patients have urinary and fecal incontinence. Over a course of approximately 5 years, myoclonic jerks, in particular, incapacitate the patient. Support in walking is needed by the age of 18 years, on average. Some years later the patients often are confined to bed. The mean age at death has been 24 years, or approximately 14 years after the appearance of the first symptoms. The age at death and the duration of the illness appear to be increasing. The most common cause of death has been pneumonia. Some patients have committed suicide.

On neurological and physical examination, myoclonic jerks, ataxia, and intention tremor are the most prominent features 1 to 3 years after the onset of the disease. In some patients, however, no abnormal signs are detected for years. Later, gait and speech disorders and emotional lability are present. Growth in height and weight continue normally, although later many patients lose weight and a few may gain much weight. A raised arterial blood pressure is found in some. Neuroophthalmological examination reveals a decrease in visual acuity in a few far-advanced cases. The optic discs occasionally may be pale.

The skull is thicker than average on X-ray. Osteoporosis of the vertebrae sometimes is seen. Pneumoencephalographic examination has not shown cerebral or cerebellar atrophy. Computed tomography of the head is normal.

Therapy is symptomatic. Hitherto, diphenylhydantoin medication was usual, but this caused acne, gingival hypertrophy, and/or hirsutism, and may have contributed to loss of Purkinje cells (1). The combination of sodium valproate and clonazepam is currently the most effective treatment in doses of 400 to 2,000 and 0.5 to 8 mg/day, respectively. Phenobarbital may be combined at night in order to prevent symptoms in the early morning hours. During the initial years, sodium valproate alone has been sufficient; it has stabilized both the clinical symptoms as well as the EEG paroxysms, particularly the sensitivity to stimuli.

PSYCHOLOGICAL FEATURES

The patients' intelligence is relatively unimpaired (7,11). The mean WAIS intelligence quotient at the onset of the disease is 92, representing the low normal range. The level diminishes about 10 points in 10 years (Figs. 1 and 2). Among verbal subtests, performance on "similarities" and "information" is preserved best. Diminished performance is most obvious in tests of "arithmetic" and "digit span." The mental deficits found may depend, to a large extent, on the patients' poor physical condition, difficulty in speech, and the triggering of myoclonus by stimuli so characteristic of the syndrome. The patients have little contact outside home and many have to interrupt school because of physical incapacity. Rapid dementia is never seen. Bedridden patients often are alert, following events with their eyes; although unable to speak, they may respond with appropriate facial expressions.

Depression is common. Some patients have inappropriate laughter and visual or auditory hallucinations. Many are infantile and emotionally immature. Lability of mood is conspicuous and has a marked impact on the physical condition.

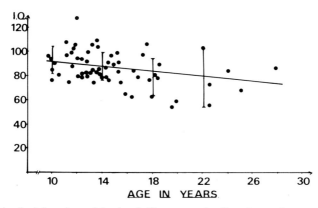

FIG. 1. IQ (ordinate) and age (abscissa). The regression line shows changes as the patients aged. The correlation between age and IQ was − 0.36 (*p*<0.001). *Small dots*, mean; *vertical bars*, SD.

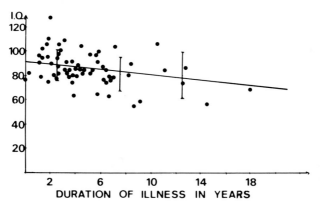

FIG. 2. IQ (ordinate) and duration of the disease (abscissa). The regression line shows the change with time from onset. The estimated IQ when the illness became manifest was 92; the IQ diminished about 10 points in 10 years. The correlation between IQ and duration was − 0.37 (*p*<0.001). *Small dots*, mean; *vertical bars*, SD.

ELECTROENCEPHALOGRAM

The EEG is abnormal from the beginning of the disease in PME patients without Lafora bodies (14). Irregular theta activity is dominant. Alpha activity is sparse initially and usually decreases further, while the amount of beta activity increases.

Generalized spike–wave paroxysms, ranging in amplitude from 250 to 500 μV, and in frequency from 3 to 5 Hz, are seen in the early stages of the disease, even 3 years before the first symptoms are manifest. Polyspike–wave paroxysms appear in half of the patients (Figs. 3 and 4).

The sensitivity to photic stimulation is distinct from about 4 Hz of flash. Paroxysmal activity increases and, if photic stimulation is continued, a generalized seizure may result.

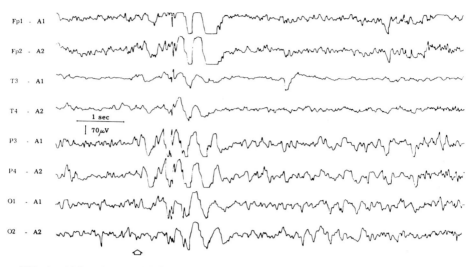

FIG. 3. Male, 13 years old, ill for 4 years. Spike–wave paroxysms immediately after a sudden noise.

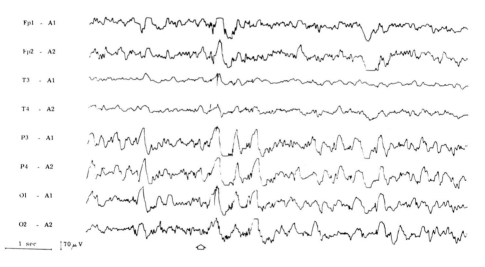

FIG. 4. Male, 13 years old, ill for 4 years. Spike–wave paroxysms after a tactile stimulation.

The EEG abnormality is most prominent 3 to 8 years after the first symptoms of PME. Later, the activity stabilizes. Anticonvulsant medication appears to be associated with an increase in beta activity. Clonazepam has the strongest effect, producing high beta activity. Sodium valproate diminishes the sensitivity to photic stimulation.

In the EEGs of the parents, a slight episodic slowing is seen in some recordings. Normal siblings more than 15 years of age usually have a normal EEG. Every sibling less than 15 years of age shows some kind of abnormality in their EEG, either an increased amount of slow activity or even spike–wave paroxysms.

BIOCHEMICAL ALTERATIONS

Routine laboratory examinations on blood and serum are normal. Urinalysis usually is normal, but PME patients are prone to urinary infections. Total protein concentration and cell count show no marked abnormalities in the cerebrospinal fluid (CSF) (8).

The most obvious finding is increased excretion of indican, originally reported by Unverricht (8,23). During therapy with sodium valproate, the excretion decreases (10). The concentration of plasma tryptophan is lower in PME patients without Lafora bodies than in controls (9). After oral L-tryptophan administration, the level remains lower than in controls.

The concentration of 5-hydroxyindoleacetic acid (5-HIAA) and vanillic mandelic acid in the CSF have been reported to be low (17). Using reverse phase liquid chromatography with electrochemical detection, no consistent differences in CSF indole levels have been noted between PME patients and controls (13,15). Oral L-tryptophan administration increases levels of tryptophan and 5-HIAA in the CSF.

HISTOPATHOLOGICAL FINDINGS

A diffuse loss of Purkinje cells has been the only consistent neuropathological finding (4,11). The dentate nucleus is relatively well preserved, with only a few atrophic or degenerating nerve cells. Except for some neuronal degeneration in the medial thalamic nuclei, no other certain neuropathological alterations have been described. No Lafora bodies have been found. The liver, cardiac muscle, and other viscera do not contain deposits characteristic to the Lafora body type of PME syndrome. Sural nerve specimens have been normal. Some nerve fibers may display a wallerian type of degeneration.

GENETICS

Autosomal recessive transmission is evident in PME patients without Lafora bodies. The 107 Finnish patients described by Norio and Koskiniemi (20) belonged to 74 families. Of the 68 marriages (six illegitimate), 15 (22%) were consanguinous. The proportion of affected sibs was 0.260. Sex distribution was equal.

The incidence is estimated to exceed 1:20,000. The disease occurs in all parts of Finland, but the geographical distribution is uneven, the majority of the patients coming from the southeastern parts of the country. This is accentuated by the distribution of birth places of the grandparents (Fig. 5). No clear heterozygous manifestations are seen.

CONCLUSIONS

The PME syndrome without Lafora bodies is most frequent in Finland, as are many rare hereditary diseases (3). Finnish PME patients mimic closely Unverricht's

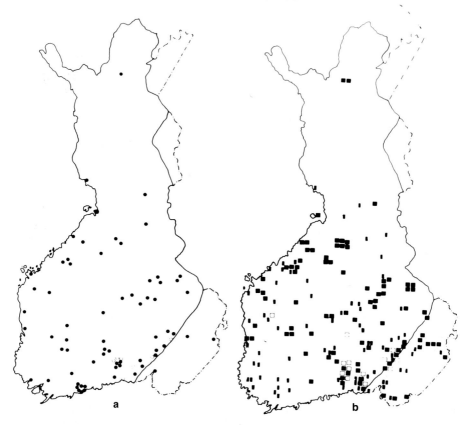

FIG. 5. Birth places of **(a)** the patients (one dot/sibship) and **(b)** the grandparents. In **b**, the whole square indicates that both maternal or both paternal grandparents were born in the same locality (established locality for a recessive PME gene), the half square indicates the birth place of one grandparent, if his/her wife/husband was not born in the same locality (uncertain locality for a PME gene). *Solid symbols*, basic series; *open symbols*, families found during the study. *Broken line*, eastern boundary of Finland before the Second World War.

"original" PME patients as well as Lundborg's Swedish patients, in whom no histopathological data are available. In Finnish patients only degenerative histopathological alterations have been seen. The clinical features of these three series from neighboring countries are similar. The age at onset and the mild mental alterations are characteristic. These patients could be defined as single-entity, Baltic or Nordic PME. Criteria set for Lafora's disease are sufficient to distinguish it from the PME syndrome without inclusion bodies (6,16,21).

The etiology and pathogenesis of Baltic PME is unknown. The clinical picture suggests a deficient inhibitory neuronal transmission allowing overflow of stimuli. The level of the possible defect is obscure and only vague suggestions are available. Tryptophan metabolism has been investigated, and the role of 5-hydroxytryptamine as a transmitter is well known. Both its metabolites and precursors have been measured, but the data so far are fragmentary (13,15,17). On the other hand, tryptophan administration has transiently benefited PME patients (12). As a whole, it appears that PME without Lafora bodies belongs to a larger spectrum of diseases characterized by myoclonic jerks, which have a common biochemical background.

SUMMARY

It has been found that PME without Lafora bodies is more common in Finland than elsewhere. The incidence is 1:20,000. The mode of inheritance is autosomal recessive.

At first the children are healthy. Stimulus-sensitive myoclonic jerks and grand mal seizures appear at the age of 6 to 15 years. The EEG shows a generalized disturbance with spike–wave or polyspike–wave paroxysms which increase during photic stimulation. Myoclonic jerks incapacitate the patient. Within 5 years after the onset of the first symptoms, many patients have a disorder of gait and may become confined to bed. Sodium valproate alone or combined with clonazepam is the most effective therapy. However, the course of the disease is progressive. The mean age at death has been 24 years but appears to be increasing.

The etiology and pathogenesis of PME without Lafora bodies are unknown. Increased excretion of indican has been noted, suggesting deficient intestinal absorption of L-tryptophan. A loss of Purkinje cells is the most prominent neuropathological feature. No inclusion bodies are present.

Finnish PME patients are similar to the patients described by Unverricht from Estonia and by Lundborg from Sweden. Neuropathological data from these patients are not available. Clinically, these patients could form an entity with Finnish patients defined as a Baltic or Nordic type of PME. The gene is enriched in Finland, but elsewhere it is rare.

REFERENCES

1. Dam M. The density and ultrastructure of the Purkinje cells following diphenylhydantoin treatment in animals and man. *Acta Neurol Scand* 1972;48(suppl 49):1–65.
2. Diebold K. Vier Erbtypen oder Krankheitsformen der progressiven Myoklonusepilepsien. *Arch Psychiatr Nervenkr* 1972;215:362–75.
3. Eriksson AW, ed. *Population structure and genetic disorders*. London: Academic Press, 1980.
4. Haltia M, Kristensson K, Sourander P. Neuropathological studies in three Scandinavian cases of progressive myoclonus epilepsy. *Acta Neurol Scand* 1968;45:63–77.
5. Harenko A, Toivakka EI. Myoclonus epilepsy (Unverricht–Lundborg) in Finland. *Acta Neurol Scand* 1961;37:282–96.
6. Van Heycop Ten Ham MW, De Jager H. Progressive myoclonus epilepsy with Lafora bodies. Clinicalpathological features. *Epilepsia* 1963;4:95–119.
7. Koskiniemi M. Psychological findings in progressive myoclonus epilepsy without Lafora bodies. *Epilepsia* 1974;15:537–45.
8. Koskiniemi M. Findings in routine laboratory examinations in progressive myoclonus epilepsy. *Acta Neurol Scand* 1975;51:12–20.
9. Koskiniemi M-L. Deficient intestinal absorption of L-tryptophan in progressive myoclonus epilepsy without Lafora bodies. *J Neurol Sci* 1980;47:1–6.
10. Koskiniemi M, Palo J. Urinary excretion of indican in progressive myoclonus epilepsy without Lafora bodies—the effect of sodium valproate. *J Neurol Sci* 1978;39:235–9.

11. Koskiniemi M, Donner M, Majuri H, Haltia M, Norio R. Progressive myoclonus epilepsy—a clinical and histopathological study. *Acta Neurol Scand* 1974;50:307–32.
12. Koskiniemi M, Hyyppä M, Sainio K, Salmi T, Sarna S, Uotila L. Transient effect of L-tryptophan in progressive myoclonus epilepsy without Lafora bodies: clinical and electrophysiological study. *Epilepsia* 1980;21:351–7.
13. Koskiniemi M-L, Laakso J, Kuurne T, Laipio M-L, Härkönen M. Indole levels in human lumbar and ventricular cerebrospinal fluid and effect of L-tryptophan administration. *Acta Neurol Scand* 1985;71:127–32.
14. Koskiniemi M, Toivakka E, Donner M. Progressive myoclonus epilepsy. Electroencephalographical findings. *Acta Neurol Scand* 1974;50:333–59.
15. Laakso JT, Koskiniemi M-L, Wahlroos Ö, Härkönen M. Simultaneous determination of tryptophan and its 5-hydroxy metabolites in human cerebrospinal fluid by reversed phase liquid chromatography with electrochemical detection. *Scand J Clin Lab Invest* 1983;43:463–72.
16. Lafora GR. Über das Vorkommen amyloider Körperchen im inneren der Ganglienzellen. *Virchows Arch (Pathol Anat)* 1911;205:295.
17. Leino E, MacDonald E, Airaksinen MM, Riekkinen PJ. Homovanillic acid and 5-hydroxyindoleacetic acid levels in cerebrospinal fluid of patients with progressive myoclonus epilepsy. *Acta Neurol Scand* 1980;62:41–54.
18. Lundborg H. Der Erbgang der progressiven Myoklonus-epilepsie. *Z Gesamte Neurol Psychiatr* 1912;9:353–8.
19. Matthews WB, Howell DA, Stevens DL. Progressive myoclonus epilepsy without Lafora bodies. *J Neurol Neurosurg Psychiatry* 1969;32:116–22.
20. Norio R, Koskiniemi M-L. Progressive myoclonus epilepsy: genetic and nosological aspects with special reference to 107 Finnish patients. *Clin Genet* 1979;15:382–98.
21. Schwarz GA, Yanoff M. Lafora's disease. Distinct clinicopathologic form of Unverricht's syndrome. *Arch Neurol* 1965;12:172–88.
22. Unverricht H. *Die Myoclonie*. Leipzig, Wien: Franz Deuticke, 1891:128.
23. Unverricht H. Über familiare Myoclonie. *Dtsch Z Nervenheilk* 1895;7:32–67.
24. Vogel F, Häfner H, Diebold K. Zur Genetik der progressiven Myoklonus-epilepsien. *Humangenetik* 1965;1:437–75.

Advances in Neurology, Vol. 43: Myoclonus,
edited by S. Fahn et al. Raven Press,
New York © 1986.

Myoclonus in Neuronal Storage and Lafora Diseases

Isabelle Rapin

*Saul R. Korey Department of Neurology and Rose F. Kennedy Center for Research in
Mental Retardation and Human Development, Albert Einstein College of Medicine,
Bronx, New York 10461*

Myoclonus is a prominent feature of a number of genetic-metabolic diseases and often provides an important clue to clinical diagnosis. The character of the myoclonus differs in different diseases, presumably because its mechanism differs depending on the population of neurons and neurotransmitters selectively affected by the metabolic error. Detailed study of the myoclonus of different diseases may thus provide information on its pathogenesis and deserves to be pursued in more detail than has typically been done.

This chapter focuses on the following conditions: the sphingolipidoses, sialidoses, ceroid-lipofuscinoses, and progressive myoclonus epilepsy of the Lafora type. It concentrates on patients in whom a definitive diagnosis was made by enzymatic assay or pathologic examination, or both. The glycogenoses, mucopolysaccharidoses, mucolipidoses, and leukodystrophies are not considered because myoclonus is not one of their typical features.

THE SPHINGOLIPIDOSES

Among the disorders of sphingolipid metabolism, only two are characterized by prominent myoclonus: infantile GM_2 gangliosidosis and juvenile neuropathic Gaucher's disease (glucocerebroside storage disease). Infants with Krabbe's disease, one of the leukodystrophies, are usually sensitive to many stimuli, but these evoke fretful crying rather than myoclonus. One patient suffering from a variant of Niemann–Pick type C is said to have had prominent myoclonus (28).

Infantile GM_2 Gangliosidosis: Tay–Sachs Disease

Classic Tay–Sachs disease is attributable to hexosaminidase A deficiency. Sandhoff's disease, where both hexosaminidases A and B are deficient, has a phenotype virtually identical to Tay–Sachs disease, including the typical startle reaction to sound. Myoclonus is not as characteristic of other variants of GM_2 or GM_1 gangliosidosis.

Startling is a normal stereotyped response to sudden sound and other unexpected stimuli that habituates with repetition (31). It is mediated entirely at brainstem levels, by activity in the nucleus gigantocellularis of the medullary reticular formation (20). Landis and Hunt (31) distinguish it from the Moro response, whose effective trigger is sudden extension of the neck.

An exaggerated startle response to sound is the presenting symptom of infants with Tay–Sachs disease and is recognized from birth by mothers in their second affected infant. There is controversy in the literature as to whether the exaggerated startle to sound of Tay–Sachs infants should be considered a myoclonic response. Gastaut (14) classifies it among the intermittent bilateral generalized myoclonic jerks of long duration (greater than 250 msec) that are rarely associated with a corresponding electroencephalographic (EEG) discharge. It was present by 2 months of age in 14 of 17 infants studied by Schneck and co-workers (51). Even though it is often called hyperacusis, it does not denote increased auditory sensitivity (58). It consists of tonic extension, adduction and elevation of the arms, clenching of the hands, flexion or extension of the legs, a startled facial expression, and a sharp cry. A brief metallic bang elicits it more reliably than a hand clap or a pure tone (51). Pure tones are most effective when their frequency lies between 700 and 2,100 Hz and their intensity above 90 dB, although Tanaka and colleagues (58) elicited startles at intensities as low as 30 dB. The amplitude of the response decreases rapidly with repeated stimulation. M. Cox and I have found that, after complete habituation, the refractory period before it resumes full amplitude is extremely long, of the order of 100 sec. (This was strikingly different from the myoclonus to sound regularly elicited in an infant with bilateral cortical damage secondary to neonatal meningitis in whom myoclonus to sound hardly habituated at all.) The exaggerated myoclonus to sound in Tay–Sachs disease is inhibited by heavy sedation and anticonvulsant drugs and does not have an EEG correlate (42).

After age 18 months, the increased startle to sound is often followed by focal or generalized clonic movements and, occasionally, by a generalized seizure. With repetitive noise at intervals of at least 15 sec, Schneck and colleagues (51) were able to drive a clonic reaction of the hands that persisted long after the extensor response had habituated. In older infants, they duplicated the startle response to sound by sustained or repetitive dorsiflexion of the foot. In the very advanced stages of the illness, M. Cox and I observed that the startle response to sound becomes difficult or impossible to elicit.

Morrell and Torres (36) report that by 21 months the infant they studied had developed spontaneous segmental and generalized myoclonic twitches that could be triggered by sensory stimuli in any modality, i.e., light, sound, touch, tap, pinprick; although they stated that these stimuli evoked giant potentials in the appropriate cortical sensory area, other investigators do not mention this finding (6,42,66). Pampiglione and co-workers (43) and Schneck (50) report that the EEG is essentially normal until about 1 year, when it deteriorates with loss of rhythmicity and photic driving; it becomes disorganized, slower, and higher voltage, with irregular sharp waves and random spikes. After 2 years the EEG becomes flatter and even slower. Prolonged tonic responses to noise or pain no longer have an EEG correlate, whereas focal seizures are still accompanied by runs of sharp waves or low-voltage spikes. The electroretinogram (ERG) remains normal until very late in the illness; visual evoked responses (VER) become simplified and lower voltage and are no longer elicited after 18 months (6,65).

The pathology in Tay–Sachs disease is diffuse. Storage involves the cortex, brainstem, cerebellum, and spinal cord. Neuronal dropout and gliosis are severe in late stages of the illness. Some types of neurons (e.g., cortical pyramids) develop meganeurites and aberrant dendrites, whereas others (e.g., stellate interneurons) do not (44). One can surmise that it will be difficult to unravel the anatomic substrates of the changing myoclonic features of this illness.

In summary (Table 1), the increased startle or diffuse reflex myoclonic jerk to sound characteristic of the early stages of Tay–Sachs disease is without overt EEG correlate; present from birth, it is superseded at 18 to 24 months by segmental and diffuse myoclonus and by prolonged tonic seizures, both spontaneous and stimulus driven. The spikes and sharp waves of the EEG in the second year are replaced by a flattened, featureless, slow EEG by the third.

Juvenile Neuropathic Gaucher's Disease

Infantile neuropathic Gaucher's disease (type II) affects the brainstem predominantly; it is associated with organomegaly, opisthotonos, spasticity, and dysphagia, and leads to death before age 2 years. The EEG is normal, and myoclonus does not seem to occur. Classic juvenile Gaucher's disease (type I) does not affect the brain, although a few patients are reported to have had an abnormal EEG (37). There are a heterogeneous group of patients with enzymatically, biochemically, and/or pathologically proven Gaucher's disease who do not fit either of these classic types and who have been collectively labeled type III. Many of them had myoclonus and a disorder of horizontal eye movements as prominent symptoms (4,18,26,37,63). It involved saccadic horizontal eye movements selectively with preservation of smooth pursuit, opticokinetic, doll's eyes, and vertical movements.

These patients have an abnormal EEG, and they usually suffer seizures, cerebellar deficits, and some degree of dementia. In several families (18,26,63) severe intention myoclonus, photosensitivity, and, in some, touch myoclonus were important features. Although myoclonus was not mentioned in other reports, patients were said to have jerky movements (23) or asterixis (35). Myoclonus eventually becomes

TABLE 1. *Tay–Sachs disease*

Startle to sound	Segmental and generalized myoclonus
Onset at birth	Onset after 1 year
No EEG correlate	Spontaneous
Long duration (>250 msec)	Stimulus driven
Rapid habituation	Precedes seizures
Long refractory period (seconds)	ERG: N − VER ↓
VER and SER (?): Normal	

so severe as to disable the patients completely and render them anarthric. The EEG characteristically shows runs of 6- to 10-Hz multiple spike-and-sharp-wave complexes, predominantly posteriorly or multifocally, against a normal or slow background (37). Photic stimulation at 6 to 10 Hz produces a photomyoclonic response. Spontaneous spike-and-wave complexes are enhanced by drowsiness. In a single patient who is presumed to have suffered from this variant of Gaucher's disease, Halliday and Halliday (20) noted relatively normal VER and markedly enlarged somatosensory evoked responses (SER).

The disease is compatible with survival to mid-adulthood in some patients or has led to death in less than a decade in others. There is no detailed report of an autopsy in this variant. One of the patients of Grover et al. (18) who underwent appendiceal and cortical biopsy at ages 6 and 8 years had no neuronal storage in either site and had only one Gaucher cell in her bone marrow.

In summary (Table 2), a heterogeneous group of patients with β-glucocerebrosidase deficiency developed a disorder of horizontal eye movements, cerebellar signs, dementia, and devastating spontaneous, intention, and photosensitive myoclonus, with 6- to 10-Hz multiple spike–waves predominating in posterior derivations. Evoked response studies in a single patient showed larger SER than VER. The pathology of this form of Gaucher's disease is not yet known.

THE SIALIDOSES

Since 1977–1978, when deficiency of α-2-6 sialidase (neuraminidase) was described by O'Brien (38,39) and Thomas and co-workers (60) in patients with the cherry-red-spot myoclonus syndrome [sialidosis type I of Lowden and O'Brien (33)], a number of clinical and, presumably, genetic variants of sialidosis have come to be recognized (2). Myoclonus is an important feature of most variants, although it was not described in severe infantile nephrosialidosis with chondrodystrophy, dementia, and early death (34). Myoclonus is prominent in other variants, notably in the one or more juvenile and adult variants, seemingly most common in Japan, with mild chondrodystrophy, angiokeratoma, mild to moderate dementia, and associated partial deficiency of β-galactosidase–sialidosis type II of Lowden and O'Brien (33) or galactosialidosis (29), and in the chronic cherry-red-spot myoclonus syndrome variant of juvenile or young adult onset that lacks de-

TABLE 2. *Juvenile neuropathic*
Gaucher's disease

↓ Horizontal eye movements
Severe myoclonus
   spontaneous
   photosensitive
   intention
6 to 10 Hz occipital spike–wave
SER >> VER
Dementia, cerebellar signs

---

mentia or systemic signs (45). Cherry-red spots at the macula are present, at least at some stage of the disease, in virtually all patients with sialidosis. More severely impaired vision than can be accounted for by punctate opacities of the lens and, in some variants, of the cornea may be due to degeneration of the occipital cortex, recently documented in an adult with galactosialidosis (29). The ERGs are normal. Most of the patients have cerebellar signs, including, in some, nystagmus, although evaluation of cerebellar function is complicated by severe intention myoclonus. Most patients have mild signs of corticospinal involvement with hyperreflexia without frank spasticity. Some variants have signs of a neuropathy or evidence of anterior horn cell degeneration.

The neurophysiologic aspects of the cherry-red-spot myoclonus variant of sialidosis have been studied in detail by Engel and co-workers (11). Some of their findings are duplicated in other, less detailed reports (15,21,60). Myoclonus is often the presenting sign of the illness and eventually dominates the clinical picture. It occurs spontaneously but is characteristically precipitated by voluntary movement or even the thought of movement, or less effectively by touch. It seems to be evoked by sensory feedback since it was abolished in the legs of one of Engel's patients by light epidural anesthesia that did not preclude movement. Myoclonus to touch habituates rapidly. In most patients myoclonus is not evoked by light or by sound unless it triggers a startle response. Engel argues that the myoclonus of sialidosis is not true action myoclonus, in the sense of Lance and Adams (30), because the jerk induced by movement is massive and bilateral rather than restricted to the moved limb and because passive movement is as effective a trigger as voluntary movement. Myoclonus was enhanced by eye closure, premenstrually, and with emotional tension in Engel's patients and was decreased by concentration and α-blocking; it was made worse by cigarette smoking in Thomas and co-workers' patient (61) who reported that orgasm caused the myoclonus to abate for several hours.

Engel and co-workers (11) described two separate types of myoclonus in their patients: massive myoclonic jerks and facial myoclonus (Table 3). The massive myoclonic jerks were bilaterally synchronous, intermittent, brief, and stimulus sensitive. Agonist and antagonist muscles were both involved. The patients exhibited

TABLE 3. *Sialidosis (cherry-red-spot myoclonus syndrome)*

Massive myoclonus	Facial myoclonus
Spontaneous	Spontaneous
Reflex	Stimulus-insensitive
Voluntary movement	
Passive movement	
Thought of movement	
Touch	
Decreases in slow-wave sleep	Persists in slow-wave sleep
Small vertex positive spikes	No EEG correlate

paroxysmal inspiration, often with vocalization, elevation of the eyes, extension of the neck, abduction of the shoulder, elevation of the arm, flexion of the elbow, extension of the wrist, and flexion of the hip. Mild jerks involved only neck extension and eye elevation. Jerks occurred approximately 20 times per minute, and patients rarely went for more than 2 min without a jerk. Occasionally, repeated jerks culminated in a myoclonic status lasting several minutes and, exceptionally, in a generalized seizure with loss of consciousness.

Facial myoclonus was spontaneous and not stimulus sensitive. It was restricted to the lower face and mouth and interfered with speech. It was intermittent, irregular, and often asymmetric. It occurred independently of the massive myoclonus. It did not resemble palatal myoclonus that was reported in one patient with galactosialidosis (24).

The background EEG of these patients was low voltage and fast. This was also true of two patients with the mucolipidosis I variant of sialidosis (10), whereas some patients with sialidosis associated with dementia had slow background EEGs (15,21,60). The facial myoclonus had no EEG correlate (Fig. 1). The massive myoclonus was associated with trains of small vertex positive spikes that were regularly obliterated by the muscle artifacts caused by the myoclonus. The trains of spikes were 20 to 100 μV in amplitude and occurred in runs of 10 to 20/sec, terminating by a slow wave of 0.5 to 1 sec. Each spike preceded a muscle potential by 15 msec for neck, 20 msec for arm, and 30 msec for leg muscles. Occasionally, one or more spikes in the train occurred before any muscle activity was recorded. Franceschetti and co-workers (13) confirmed these findings with the backward

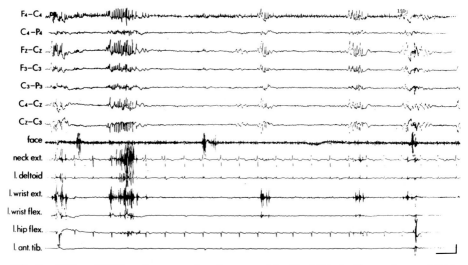

FIG. 1. EEG and EMG surface recordings from an adult with sialidosis. The background EEG is low voltage and fast. Frequent runs of vertex positive spikes are associated and often precede massive myoclonic jerks (this time relationship was more clearly shown at higher paper speeds). Note the lack of EEG correlate of the facial myoclonus and its independence from the massive body jerks. Calibration, 100 μV, 1 sec. (Reproduced with permission from Engel et al., ref. 11.)

averaging technique; they recorded a 30-msec spike occurring 5 to 15 times per second over the contralateral sensorimotor cortex 17 msec before the electromyogram (EMG) discharge in the arm.

These two types of myoclonus were differentially affected by slow-wave sleep [rapid eye movement (REM) sleep was not identified with certainty in these patients or in those of Hambert and Petersen (21)]. The facial myoclonus persisted unchanged throughout sleep, whereas the massive myoclonus abated progressively in sleep phases I and II and disappeared in phases III and IV. There was a dissociation between myoclonus and spikes in deep sleep: runs of spikes superimposed on slow waves occupied virtually 100% of the EEG record, whereas small muscle twitches replaced the massive jerks of the waking state.

As noted earlier, the patients had loss of vision. The ERG in Engel's patient 1 was normal, but the VER had decreased in amplitude (Table 4), suggesting cortical visual loss in these patients as well as in galactosialidosis (47). Late cortical auditory evoked responses (AER) were normal. In contrast, SER to median nerve stimulation recorded from parietal electrodes were polyphasic, greatly enhanced in amplitude, and bilaterally symmetric in distribution. Positive peaks occurred at approximately 25, 65 to 72, and 105 to 120 msec at an amplitude of up to 100 μV (Fig. 2). Since myoclonic jerks in the arm produced by median nerve stimulation had a latency of 90 msec and since vertex positive spikes preceded spontaneous arm myoclonus by 20 msec, it was concluded that the 65- to 72-msec component of the SER and the vertex positive spikes shared a common neuronal mechanism. The later positive peak might be the response evoked by the myoclonic jerk since, when median nerve

TABLE 4. *Sialidosis (cherry-red-spot myoclonus syndrome)*

Evoked responses	Finding
ERG	Normal
AER	Normal
VER	Amplitude decreased
SER	Giant, symmetric bilateral
	Polyphasic
	+ Peaks at 25, 65–72, 105–120 msec

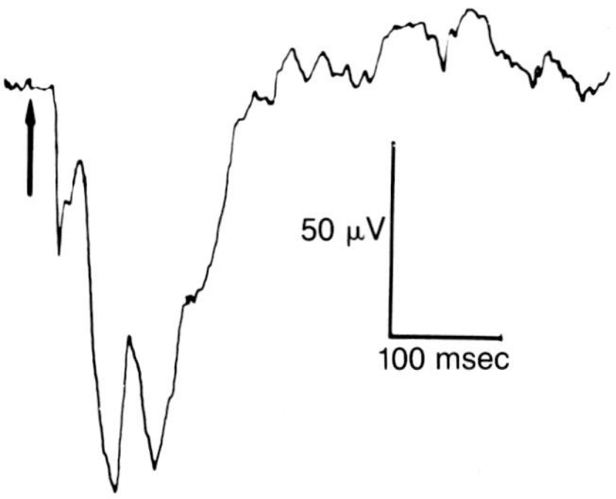

FIG. 2. SER recorded from left parietal to left frontal derivation following 30 shocks to the right median nerve at the wrist in an adult with sialidosis. Compare the response with that in late infantile ceroid-lipofuscinosis (Fig. 3). Analysis time, 500 msec; calibration, 50 μV, 100 msec. Positivity at the active electrode is down. (Reproduced with permission from Engel et al., ref. 11.)

50 μV

100 msec

stimulation was below threshold for producing a direct motor response, the SER consisted of a single positive spike with onset at 24 msec and peak at 75 msec; the early positive response could not be clearly identified. These findings differ from those of Halliday and Halliday (20) in adult patients with "progressive myoclonic epilepsy." These investigators recorded an enlarged positive peak 32 msec after digital nerve stimulation that was enlarged only if the patient had a myoclonic response to stimulation; the patients did not have the later 65- to 72-msec positive peak of the patients with sialidosis.

The patients' generalized seizures were well controlled with standard anticonvulsants; the drugs had no effect on the myoclonus, which was resistant to all drugs tried. 5-Hydroxytrytophan (5-HTP) with carbidopa in high dose reduced the myoclonus, the EEG paroxysms, and the amplitude of the SER but did not produce meaningful functional improvement (11,45,59). A manic state was precipitated by 5-HTP in one patient who went into a severe depression lasting several weeks upon withdrawal. Intravenous diazepam abolished the myoclonus transiently; clonazepam was not effective; in one patient, valproic acid has a persistent although modest effect on the massive myoclonic jerks.

Several patients with galactosialidosis (sialidosis type II) have come to postmortem examination (27,47,56,62). Distension of neurons by lipofuscin granules and membranous and lamellar inclusions was widespread. In general the lateral geniculate bodies, brainstem nuclei, dentate nuclei, and Purkinje cells were more affected that the cortex, although complete loss of neurons was noted in the calcarine cortex of one patient (47). A frontalcortical biopsy at age 10 years in case 1 of Rapin et al. (45) and Engel et al. (11) revealed lipofuscin, lysosome-like, and membranovesicular bodies in cortical neurons (16).

In summary, spontaneous and intention myoclonus is a characteristic feature of sialidosis of most types. In the cherry-red-spot myoclonus syndrome, it is of two kinds: massive bilaterally symmetric myoclonic jerks that are sensitive to somatosensory stimulation, suppressed in slow-wave sleep, and preceded by vertex positive spikes; and facial myoclonus that is irregular, asymmetric, stimulus insensitive, does not change during slow-wave sleep, and does not have an EEG correlate. Massive myoclonus is precipitated by active and passive movement, the thought of movement, and touch, but not by light or sound. Giant SER with bilateral distribution and late large positive peaks at 65 to 72 and 105 to 120 msec seem characteristic of this illness. Diazepam, 5-HTP, and valproic acid decrease the myoclonus somewhat but without satisfactory control.

THE CEROID-LIPOFUSCINOSES (BATTEN DISEASE)

This group of illnesses is characterized by retinal degeneration, dementia, seizures, myoclonus, and a variety of motor deficits. The biochemistry of these cerebromacular degenerations is not understood, and enzymatic deficiencies have yet to be described. Three well-defined autosomal recessive syndromes of childhood are easily recognized on the basis of their clinical features and pathology: infantile, late infantile, and juvenile variants (Table 5). Other childhood cases that defy classification are not discussed here.

Adult variants, often called Kufs' disease even though it is clear that they are heterogeneous, usually do not have retinal degeneration. Some patients have myoclonus. Prominent intention myoclonus and truncal and facial myoclonus of a type reminiscent of the myoclonus of sialidosis were present in an adult with a 6-year dementing illness (40). The patient's myoclonus was a wild jerking made worse by voluntary movement and flashing lights. The EEG was slow, with giant SER and photomyoclonic responses. Lipofuscin granules were present throughout the nervous system; storage was mild in the cortex and severe in the inferior olive. There was dropout of Purkinje cells and dentate nucleus cells. Two siblings with seizures but no myoclonus had normal brainstem AER and VER but had giant multiphasic late SER (65). Fine and co-workers (12) reviewed the literature on Kufs' disease and described a patient who did not become demented. He had severe muscle wasting, ataxia, "intermittent coarse rhythmical tremors" of the forearms and hands, and irregular perioral and periorbital tremors with dysarthria. His EEG was dysrhythmic. He had profound cerebellar atrophy with severe loss of granular cells and diffuse lipofuscinosis of the brain and cord, including brainstem nuclei and Purkinje cell dendrites. Boehme and colleagues (3) classified as Kufs' disease a family with dominant inheritance. Eleven members over four generations died in mid-adult life after a decade or less of progressive dementia, cerebellar deficit with nystagmus, myoclonus (spontaneous and movement induced), and frequent seizures. Their EEGs were slow with runs of 4- to 7-Hz slow waves preceded by high-voltage spikes and atypical spike–wave complexes. They too had diffuse lipofuscinosis and cerebellar atrophy at postmortem examination. There was severe dropout of Purkinje cells and cells of the substantia nigra where remaining neurons contained "myoclonus bodies of the protein type." Storage in the thalamus, brainstem, and pons was striking. The nosologic classification of this family is especially problematic.

Infantile "Finnish" Variant of Ceroid-Lipofuscinosis

Santavuori and colleagues (49) described 40 children with this illness, which is relatively frequent in Finland but has also been seen elsewhere, including the United

TABLE 5. *Ceroid lipofuscinosis (Batten disease)*

Parameter	Infantile	Late infantile	Juvenile	Adult
Age (years)				
at onset	8–18 months	2½–4	5–7	Variable
at death	5–10	6–10	15–25	+10
Blind	Yes	Yes	Yes	No
Seizures	Variable	Frequent	Delayed	Variable
First sign	Regression	Seizures	Visual loss	Ataxia, myoclonus

States. Hagberg and colleagues (19,57) reported an increase in monoenoic fatty acids and a decrease in fatty acids of the linolenic series in the brains and viscera of three children with this illness. Other chemical changes reflected neuronal devastation, which is virtually complete in the cortex and cerebellum (both Purkinje and granular cells) and very severe in the basal ganglia, thalamus, substantia nigra, pontine, dentate, and inferior olivary nuclei. The white matter is poorly myelinated and atrophic. Brain weight is typically less than 500 g at age 5 to 10 years. There is a marked increase of autofluorescent lipofuscin-like granules in remaining neurons, glial cells, and proliferated macrophages. The stored material appears finely granular by electron microscopy.

Clinically, the infants present between 8 and 18 months with progressive loss of motor milestones, hypotonia, ataxia, dementia, and impaired vision with diffuse pallor of the retina. Some but not all develop generalized seizures. Myoclonic jerks start between 18 and 24 months; they involve the limbs first, the face and trunk later. The children characteristically develop transient "knitting" (myoclonic?) movements of the hands between the ages of 2 and 3 years. After 3 to 4 years, the children are in a permanently decorticate state, in which any form of stimulation (no details provided) precipitates myoclonic jerks (Table 6). In the early stages of the illness, the EEG is relatively high voltage and slow, with irregular spike–wave complexes. By 18 to 24 months of age, normal background rhythms disappear; the EEG flattens, becomes featureless, and eventually isoelectric, usually between 3 and 4 years (48). Photosensitivity is not present, and photic driving disappears before 2 years of age when the ERG becomes extinguished and the infants blind. Physiologic studies of the myoclonus and of evoked responses were not encountered.

In summary, this illness presents by 12 to 18 months of age and devastates the brain and cerebellum by 3 to 4 years of age. The cortex and cerebellum become essentially aneuronal. Myoclonus appears by 2 years and by 3 years is severe and stimulus sensitive. Electrophysiologic correlates, if any, of this myoclonus are not described.

Late Infantile Ceroid-Lipofuscinosis (Jansky–Bielchowsky Disease)

This variant of the disease usually starts with a seizure somewhere between 2½ and 4 years (41). In addition to generalized seizures, children may develop atypical

TABLE 6. *Ceroid lipofuscinosis (Batten disease)*

	Infantile	Late infantile	Juvenile	Adult
Myoclonus				
Onset	18–24 months	3–4 years	Late	Early
Spontaneous	+ + +	+ + + (Late)	+	+ + +
Induced	All stimuli	Light (slow)	?	Movement
Induced		(Other stimuli)		(Light)
Evoked		Giant VER		Giant SER
responses		(+ SER)		(+ VER)

absences and akinetic spells. These are followed within a few months by myoclonus that is at first segmental, asymmetric, and spontaneous and that interrupts movement; it eventually precludes ambulation and hand use and, late in the course, produces virtually continuous small amplitude tremulousness present as long as the child is awake (status myoclonicus). At times myoclonic jerks culminate in a generalized seizure. Intellectual deterioration is an early sign followed by loss of central vision with a granular, mahogany appearance of the macula (not a cherry-red spot), and optic atrophy. The children become spastic and survive for a few years in a decorticate state. Age at death is usually 6 to 10 years.

Postmortem examination shows severe loss of cortical and cerebellar neurons. The brain is atrophic, weighing 500 to 800 g. In the cerebellum, there is almost total dropout of Purkinje and granular cells with severe gliosis of the molecular layer. Neuronal dropout is severe but less so in the cerebral cortex and still less in the basal ganglia and brainstem structures. Remaining neurons are distended by autofluorescent pigmented inclusions that typically have the appearance of curvilinear membranes by electron microscopy. Similar inclusions are abundant in the viscera in this form of the illness (8). The chemistry of the disease is unknown except for increased excretion of dolichols in the urine.

The EEG is typically slow, high voltage, and disorganized in the early stages of the illness, with spikes, sharp waves, and polyphasic spikes first in a posterior distribution, later more diffusely (17,41,66). As the disease progresses, fast rhythms, including sleep spindles, disappear, and the record becomes flatter and slower. Myoclonic jerks sometimes but not always are preceded by a spike or spike–wave discharge. The characteristic feature of this illness is the response to slow photic stimulation: flicker rates below 3 Hz trigger the appearance of high-amplitude polyphasic spikes measuring 200 to 500 μV, usually in posterior derivations although at times more anteriorly as well, corresponding to the giant VER. The interspike interval is 250 to 450 msec, so that the spikes are not driven to higher rates when the flicker frequency is increased above 4 Hz. The spikes are frequently associated with a myoclonic jerk. Jerks may persist for several seconds after cessation of photic stimulation and occasionally culminate in a seizure. The discharges persist in sleep, even though the myoclonus subsides. The virtually constant myoclonic state characteristic of the late stages of the illness is not reflected by an increase in paroxysmal discharges in the EEG. Photic sensitivity persists to age 6 to 7 years, when vision deteriorates severely and the ERG becomes extinguished. At that stage, any stimulus will enhance the myoclonus.

The ERG is present but abnormal because of decreased amplitude, increased latency, and a polyphasic appearance (6,66). The VER consists of a high-amplitude surface positive wave with a peak latency of 40 to 50 msec followed by a negativity at 70 to 90 msec, another large positive wave at 120 to 130 msec, and a broad late negative component peaking at 230 to 300 msec. Amplitude is 8 to 10 times that of control subjects. The SER exhibit normal morphology and latency, but peak-to-peak amplitude is abnormally large (Fig. 3). These findings confirm Green's (17) report; he noted that, followed median nerve stimulation, enlarged sensory evoked

FIG. 3. SER recorded from the parietal hand area with ear reference following 50 shocks to the contralateral median nerve at the wrist in a 4½-year-old child with late infantile ceroid-lipofuscinosis. The child also had giant VER. Compare the response with that in sialidosis (Fig. 2). Analysis time, 500 msec; calibration, 100 μv, 50 msec. Positivity at active electrode is down. (Courtesy D. R. Giblin.)

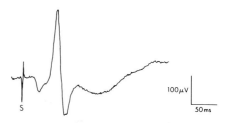

responses can often be seen contralaterally in the plain EEG. He noted that the response was larger when it was associated with a twitch than when it was not. Median nerve stimulation precipitated a focal seizure on the stimulated side in one of his patients.

In summary, this illness usually starts with seizures at 2½ to 4 years. Myoclonus, which appears in the ensuing months, is segmental and asymmetric, typically photosensitive, and sensitive to somatosensory stimulation as well. (Responses to sound have not been reported.) Myoclonus eventually becomes generalized and virtually continuous in the waking state. Although it abates during sleep, spike discharges persist in the EEG. Photomyoclonic responses with giant polyphasic occipital potentials at slow flicker rates are characteristic. Somatosensory potentials are also enlarged. Death occurs in a vegetative state at 6 to 10 years. Loss of cerebellar neurons and, to a lesser extent, cortical neurons and ubiquitous storage of autofluorescent material with curvilinear profiles are the pathologic features of the illness.

Juvenile Ceroid-Lipofuscinosis (Spielmeyer–Vogt–Sjögren Disease)

This is a relatively common illness that is widespread in its geographic distribution, although the largest series of patients have been reported from Sweden (54) and Denmark (32,55). The illness starts at early school age by loss of central vision and the retinal findings of macular degeneration with pigmentary degeneration of the retina. Visual loss progresses to blindness over the next several years. Neurologic symptoms are usually delayed by 2 or more years and consist of seizures and insidious intellectual decline. Most of the seizures are generalized, but other types occur, including complex partial and sporadic jerking. Many of the children can attend a school for the blind until their teens, when motor findings impede ambulation. The children develop the stooped posture and accelerated stuttering speech that are pathognomonic of the illness. Cerebellar and corticospinal findings are usually mild. The facies is masked, associated movements decrease, and tone increases. It is typically a severe motor apraxia that puts the patients into a wheelchair: they forget how to walk unless propelled forward or how to sit unless forced down. Seizures usually become more frequent, and spontaneous myoclonus of small amplitude involving the face and later the hands makes its appearance. In the late stages, intellectual and motor deterioration become severe; death usually supervenes in the late teens or early twenties. Psychotic episodes have occurred in several of my patients and are stressed by the Danish authors (32,55), who report the frequent occurrence of visual hallucinations in these blind adolescents.

The myoclonus of this illness is poorly described and often mistaken for a tremor of basal ganglia or cerebellar origin. In one patient with advanced disease, severe myoclonus of the legs lasting for 30 min or more often culminated in a generalized seizure. Myoclonus was induced by passive movement. The EEG background is slow and becomes disorganized; slow waves, sharp waves, spikes, and spike–wave complexes appear in random distribution or in bursts. Sleep activates paroxysmal EEG discharges (66). Green (17) recorded contralaterally enlarged SER upon median nerve stimulation in the plain EEG. The ERG is extinguished early in these patients, and photic driving produces neither behavioral nor EEG response. The averaging studies of d'Allest and co-workers (6) confirm the degradation of the VER. No report of averaged somatosensory stimulation was encountered.

There is only mild brain atrophy in this variant, although storage of autofluorescent material is widespread in neurons and glia. There may be some loss of granular cells in the cerebellum. Large inclusions may be seen in the substantia nigra, dentate nucleus, and inferior olive (68). The predominant ultrastructural appearance is that of fingerprint membranous profiles, although curvilinear, and typical lipofuscin inclusions are also seen. With the exception of urinary dolichol excretion, the chemistry of the illness is unknown.

In summary, myoclonus has not been well described in the juvenile variant. It may consist of sporadic jerks, small amplitude persistent facial myoclonus, or more violent myoclonus of the limbs culminating in a seizure. The electrophysiologic correlates of the myoclonus and its clinical characteristics remain to be studied.

LAFORA DISEASE

The literature on the progressive myoclonus epilepsies is plagued by lack of knowledge of their underlying metabolic defects. Some investigators have not clearly distinguished Lafora disease, the only one discussed here, from other variants, such as the Unverricht–Lundborg and Ramsay Hunt syndromes. From a clinical standpoint, Lafora disease is quite homogeneous (1,9,52,64); pathologically, abundant Lafora bodies occur in characteristic distribution in the brain, and polyglycan-like deposits are found in myocardium, skeletal muscle, and liver (5,22). The occasional presence of mature Lafora bodies, with their dark basophilic core and lighter periphery and their granular and fibrillar appearance by electron microscopy, in brains of patients with other conditions does not detract from the individuality of Lafora disease. Lafora bodies contain polysaccharides, mostly glucose, so that the disease has been tentatively classified among the autosomal recessive metabolic diseases of carbohydrate metabolism, even though its enzymatic basis is unknown.

The disease is one of adolescence. Most patients become ill between 10 and 18 years and die within less than a decade. The first sign is invariably a generalized seizure. The seizures are at first sporadic, but other seizure types, notably absences and drop attacks, supervene. Characteristically, the seizures are preceded by a visual aura of flashing or colored lights. The patients are photosensitive. Myoclonic jerks appear in the following months and are at first infrequent, sporadic, irregular, asymmetric, and of such small amplitude as not to move the limb. They are likely to involve the face and, occasionally, the extraocular muscles. The frequency of occurrence and severity of the myoclonus may fluctuate widely from day to day; it is enhanced by emotional tension. Prolonged episodes of myoclonus of increasing intensity often herald a generalized seizure. As the disease progresses, the myoclonus remains asymmetric and segmental but becomes almost constant and grossly incapacitating when it precludes ambulation, self-help, and speech.

Signs of an insidious and rather rapidly progressing dementia, often with apraxia, develop, usually within months to 1 or 2 years of the onset of seizures. The patient may evince behavioral difficulties, have periods of agitation, and suffer delusions of psychotic proportion. Motor findings are variable, relatively inconspicuous, and tend to occur late in the course of the illness; the most frequently mentioned include ataxia, hyperreflexia, and wasting. Vision usually deteriorates markedly despite normal fundi. The patients eventually become totally disabled and mute and expire after a variable period of vegetative existence.

The anatomic distribution of lesions was studied by de Ajuriaguerra and colleagues (7) and Seitelberger and co-workers (52). Areas with the greatest density of Lafora bodies are the substantia nigra, dentate nucleus, superior olive, pontine reticular nuclei, nonspecific thalamic nuclei, lateral geniculate body, globus pallidus, and sensorimotor cortex. Areas less severely affected include the cerebellar cortex, cerebral cortex, cingulate gyrus, other thalamic nuclei, hypothalamus, and retina (67). The red nucleus and subthalamic nucleus are relatively spared, and the inferior olive, caudate, and putamen are mildly affected. Cord involvement, rarely mentioned (64), was prominent in the brother of one of my patients. Neuronal dropout involves the granular and Purkinje cells of the cerebellum but is not a striking feature of this illness, which produces relatively little if any brain atrophy. Most Lafora bodies are found in the perikaryon of neurons but may be found in the neuropil. They are not membrane bound and do not represent storage in lysosomes.

The EEG becomes disorganized relatively early in the illness, with loss of α-rhythms, considerable amounts of 2.5- to 3.5-Hz slow waves, often in runs, and sporadic spikes and sharp waves. Trains of high voltage, usually bilaterally symmetric spike and polyspike–wave complexes, make their appearance, with a frontocentral preponderance. The EEG persists relatively unchanged until the terminal state of the illness. Although spikes may be temporally related to myoclonic jerks, the relationship is not obligatory (25,46,64). Photic stimulation, especially at high flash rates, induces multiple spike and spike–wave complexes and myoclonus and may precipitate seizures. There are variable reports of the effects of sound and touch on the myoclonus, but it appears that, in the majority of cases, they are ineffective. Myoclonus is enhanced, in some patients at least, by voluntary movement. Sleep regularly diminishes the amplitude and frequency of occurrence of the myoclonus without abolishing the spikes in the EEG (25). Shibasaki *(this volume)* recorded evoked potentials in one patient with this illness.

The early generalized seizures respond well to anticonvulsant medications. The myoclonus is difficult to treat, although some patients have obtained temporary benefit from drugs such as ethosuximide and clonazepam.

In summary, the myoclonus of Lafora disease is rarely an early sign of the illness and is preceded by seizures that characteristically have a visual aura (Table 7). The patients are photosensitive but usually not sensitive to sound or touch, although intention myoclonus is reported in advanced stages of the illness. The myoclonus is segmental and asymmetric, although severe bilateral myoclonus may lead to tonic and generalized seizures. It tends to vary strikingly from day to day. The EEG shows bilaterally symmetric spike, polyspike, and spike–wave complexes with a frontocentral preponderance. The patients become demented, often have psychotic episodes, become blind despite normal fundi, and are eventually totally incapacitated. Motor findings occur late and are variable. The disease occurs in adolescents and typically lasts 5 to 8 years. Its chemical basis is unknown.

COMMENT

Neurologists often rely on the presence of myoclonus and its particular characteristics for diagnosis in the individual patient. Yet we have no understanding of why myoclonus is an important feature of some illnesses—even dominating the clinical picture in the cherry-red-spot myoclonus variant of sialidosis or in the Ramsay Hunt syndrome—and why it does not occur in others with rather similar pathology.

In order to identify the missing enzymes, research on the storage diseases has tended to focus on biochemical analysis of the stored material and pathways of its synthesis and degradation. This type of endeavor, in which brain tissue is minced, homogenized, and chromatographed, is unlikely to shed light on a symptom arising from distorted communication between neuronal systems. Knowing that α-2-6-neuraminidase deficiency causes sialidosis—and we still are ignorant of how different mutations affecting a single enzyme molecule produce phenotypically distinct variants of sialidosis—sheds no light on why sialidosis almost invariably causes

TABLE 7. *Lafora disease*

Seizures with visual aura
Photosensitivity
Myoclonus
  Later
  Asymmetric, segmental
  Variable day to day
EEG: symmetric spike–wave
Dementia, psychosis
Visual loss with normal fundi
Motor signs late, variable

---

myoclonus. Answering that kind of question will require more than awareness that storage is ubiquitous with predilection for this or that nucleus; it will require detailed attention to quantitative aspects of both storage and cell loss in each nucleus. A start in that direction was provided by Tokuda et al. (62) and Koga et al. (27) for adult Japanese galactosialidosis and by de Ajuriaguerra et al. (7) and Seitelberger and colleagues (52) for Lafora disease. In addition to this microanatomic type of study, we must address the question at the level of cellular specificity: Why, in infantile gangliosidosis, do cortical pyramids develop meganeurites and grow aberrant dendrites on them when adjacent stellate cells do not (44)? Understanding an illness at the molecular level or even at the level of the gene will not exhaust what we need to know in order to understand its clinical manifestations.

Review of the myoclonus in the individual storage disorders considered here highlights remarkable differences among them, differences for which we have no explanation today (Table 8). For example, light flashes provoke a different reflex myoclonus in three of these diseases: late infantile ceroid-lipofuscinosis, juvenile Gaucher's disease, and Lafora disease. In Jansky–Bielchowsky disease, flashes lose their effectiveness for provoking giant VER and myoclonic jerks if their rate exceeds approximately 3 Hz (17,41), whereas in juvenile Gaucher's disease, the flash rate is 6 to 10 Hz (37), and in Lafora disease, fast rates seem most effective (46). The relative refractory period for the myoclonic jerks to sound of Tay–Sachs infants is of the order of many seconds, while the massive myoclonus to hand claps of an infant of the same age whose brain was devastated by neonatal meningitis did not habituate at all. What are the neurophysiologic mechanisms that underlie these gross differences? Why is it that movement is so much more potent a trigger of myoclonus than light or sound in sialidosis, the Ramsay Hunt syndrome, and adult ceroid-lipofuscinosis, and sound so selectively effective in young Tay–Sachs infants?

Before we can hope to answer these questions, we need much better descriptions of the myoclonus of each disease. We must record in detail characteristics of effective and ineffective sensory stimuli, such as intensity, rate of stimulation, and refractory period. We must map responses in the plain EEG as well as record averaged brainstem and cortical evoked response correlates of these stimuli. In

TABLE 8. *Differences among diseases*

Disease	Induced myoclonus				Evoked responses	
	Light	Sound	Proprioception	All	VER	SER
Tay–Sachs		+ + +		+ +	↓	
Juvenile Gaucher's	+ + +		+ +		↑	↑ ↑
Sialidosis			+ + +		↓	↑ ↑
Ceroid lipofuscinosis						
Infantile				+ + +	↓	↓
Late infantile	+ +			+ +	↑ ↑	↑
Juvenile					↓	
Adult	+		+ + +		↑	↑ ↑
Lafora	+ +					

order to dissect the relationship between potentials that precede jerks and potentials produced by jerks, we must perform forward and backward averaging studies triggered from the myoclonic jerks (13,53) and use stimuli at intensities that both trigger and do not trigger jerks. This type of study enabled Engel and co-workers (11) to show that the late positive component of the polyphasic giant SER of sialidosis probably represent feedback from the jerk, and that earlier components are closely related if not identical to the vertex positive spikes that precede spontaneous jerks.

The usefulness of several excellent physiologic studies carried out in patients with myoclonus is marred by lack of an exact diagnosis; "progressive myoclonus epilepsy" may mean Ramsay Hunt syndrome, Lafora disease, adult ceroid-lipofuscinosis (and that is not even a diagnosis!), sphingolipidosis of some type or other, or sialidosis. This lack is deplorable but understandable in the case of diseases for which enzymatic or pathologic diagnosis is unavailable: Patients are alive when studied, and postmortem tissue may not be available for years, if at all. By the time the patient's brain is studied, anatomic examination is unlikely to be carried out with the detail required to answer some of these physiologic questions, unless the clinician remains involved until it is time to guide the pathologist's inquiry.

Pharmacologic control of the myoclonus of storage diseases has been, in large part, a dismal failure. Part of the reason may be that therapeutic trials have rarely been systematic and their effects recorded in adequate detail (59). Yet such trials may provide a tantalizing clue for unraveling the pathogenesis of the myoclonus. For example, 5-HTP, a precursor of serotonin, was modestly successful in controlling the massive jerks of two patients with sialidosis. It is known that slow-wave sleep is at least partially under serotonergic control and that slow-wave sleep strongly inhibits the myoclonus of several of these diseases without abolishing the cortical spikes that accompany it in the waking state. These observations suggest the hypothesis that slow-wave sleep (and possibly serotonin) inhibits the spinal but not the cortical projections of the myoclonic-generating system in sialidosis. They also suggest that it does not inhibit the generator itself, any more than it inhibits the generator for the facial myoclonus that does not abate in sleep. Clues of this type must be exploited by measuring metabolites of serotonin and other neurotransmitters and neuromodulators in spinal fluid and other body fluids in living patients and with immunocytochemical approaches in their tissues after death.

If the enhanced startle response to sound of Tay–Sachs infants truly does not have an EEG correlate (it seems not to have been investigated with modern averaging techniques), does it share some pathways with the facial myoclonus of sialidosis, which also does not, despite their obvious differences? The nucleus gigantocellularis of the reticular formation has been implicated by Halliday and Halliday (20) both in the startle response as well as in the chronic myoclonus of the progressive myoclonic epilepsies that have both upstream and downstream projections. How are we to reconcile these discrepancies?

The type of question raised by this chapter requires a long-term and much more rigorous program of research than has been typical thus far. It requires clinicians, neurophysiologists, pharmacologists, neurochemists, and morphologists (pathologists-turned-anatomists) to join forces in order to exploit the experiments of nature provided by patients with these rare genetic diseases. The patients themselves and their families are often eager for investigators to carry out noninvasive studies of their symptoms, yet investigators have not always responded with adequately planned and systematic research and with the long-term commitment to follow the patients to diagnosis or demise. Finally, physiologists must join neuropathologists and neurochemists in investigations of existing and yet-to-be discovered animal models of these diseases. These will allow the performance of the more detailed experiments with more proximate answers forbidden by the sensitive care of human victims of these same mutations.

SUMMARY

Genetic storage diseases with prominent myoclonus include classic infantile Tay–Sachs disease and juvenile neuropathic Gaucher's disease among the sphingolipidoses, most of the variants of the sialidoses and ceroid-lipofuscinoses, and Lafora disease. The character of the myoclonus differs from disease to disease and often changes as the disease runs its course. For example, massive myoclonic jerks to sound with rapid habituation and a prolonged refractory period are characteristic of the early stages of Tay–Sachs disease; children with late infantile ceroid-lipofuscinosis are most sensitive to light flashes below 3 Hz, those with juvenile Gaucher's disease at 6 to 10 Hz, and those with Lafora disease at 15 to 20 Hz, whereas young adults with sialidosis are not sensitive to either light or sound but are highly sensitive to somatosensory stimulation and movement. Some patients with sialidosis were found to have two distinct types of myoclonus: (a) a stimulus-insensitive facial myoclonus without EEG correlate that persisted in slow-wave sleep and (b) stimulus-sensitive massive jerks associated with vertex positive EEG spikes on which sleep had the paradoxic effect of suppressing jerks while stimulating spikes. Systematic EEG and event-related potential studies, including backward averaging from jerks and detailed anatomic studies of postmortem specimens with modern histochemical techniques, may help illuminate these intriguing differences. New modalities are needed to treat the myoclonus of these diseases since it generally responds poorly to currently available pharmacologic agents.

ACKNOWLEDGMENT

This work was supported in part by grant NS 3356-23 from the National Institute of Neurologic Diseases, Communication Disorders and Stroke.

REFERENCES

1. Austin J, Sakai M. Lafora's myoclonus epilepsy. In: Vinken PJ, Bruyn, GW, eds. *Handbook of clinical neurology*, vol. 27. Amsterdam: North-Holland, 1976:171–95.
2. Beaudet AL. Sialidosis. In: Stanbury JB, Wyngaarden GB, Fredrickson DS, Goldstein JL, Brown MS, eds. *The metabolic basis of inherited disease*, 5th ed. New York: McGraw Hill, 1983:795–7.

3. Boehme DH, Cottrell JC, Leonberg SC, Zeman W. A dominant form of neuronal ceroid-lipofuscinosis. *Brain* 1971;94:745–60.
4. Brady RO, Pentchev PG, Gal AE, Hibbert SR, Dekaban AS. Replacement therapy for inherited enzyme deficiency: use of purified glucocerebrosidase in Gaucher's disease. *N Engl J Med* 1974;291:989–93.
5. Carpenter S, Karpati G, Andermann F, Jacob JC, and Andermann E. Lafora disease: peroxisomal storage in skeletal muscle. *Neurology* 1974;24:531–8.
6. d'Allest AM, Laget P, Raimbault J. Visual and somesthetic potentials in neurolipidosis. In: Courjon J, Mauguiere F, Revol M, eds. *Clinical applications of evoked potentials in neurology*. New York: Raven Press, 1982:397–407.
7. de Ajuriaguerra J, Sigwald J, Piot C. Myoclonie-épilepsie familiale de type Unverricht. Etude clinique, électroencéphalographique et anatomique. *Presse Med* 1954;62:1813–6.
8. de Baecque CM, Pollack MA, Suzuki K. Late infantile neuronal storage disease with curvilinear bodies. *Arch Pathol Lab Med* 1976;100:139–44.
9. de Barsy T, Myle C, Troch C, Mattley R, Martin JJ. La dyssynergie myoclonique (R. Hunt): affection autonome ou variante du type dégénératif de l'épilepsie-myoclonie progressive (Unverricht–Lundborg). Approche anatomoclinique. *J Neurol Sci* 1968;8:111–27.
10. Doose H, Spranger J, Warner M. EEG in mucolipidosis I. *Neuropaediatrie* 1975;6:98–101.
11. Engel J Jr, Rapin I, Giblin DR. Electrophysiological studies in two patients with cherry red spot-myoclonus syndrome. *Epilepsia* 1977;18:73–87.
12. Fine DI, Barron KD, Hirano A. Central nervous system lipidosis in an adult with atrophy of the cerebellar granular layer. A case report. *J Neuropathol Exp Neurol* 1960;19:355–69.
13. Franceschetti S, Uziel G, Di Donato S, Caimi L, Avanzini G. Cherry-red spot myoclonus syndrome and alpha-neuraminidase deficiency: neurophysiological, pharmacological and biochemical study in an adult. *J Neurol Neurosurg Psychiatry* 1980;43:934–40.
14. Gastaut H. Séméiologie des myoclonies. *Rev Neurol* 1968;119:1–30.
15. Goldstein ML, Kolodny EH, Gascon GG, Gilles FH. Macular cherry-red spot, myoclonic epilepsy, and neurovisceral storage in a 17-year-old girl. *Trans Am Neurol Assoc* 1974;99:110–2.
16. Gonatas NK, Terry RD, Winkler R, Korey SR, Gomez CJ, Stein A. A case of juvenile lipidosis: the significance of electronmicroscopic and biochemical observations of a cerebral biopsy. *J Neuropathol Exp Neurol* 1963;22:557–80.
17. Green JB. Neurophysiological studies in Batten's disease. *Dev Med Child Neurol* 1971;13:477–89.
18. Grover WD, Tucker SH, Wenger DA. Clinical variation in two related children with neuropathic Gaucher's disease. *Ann Neurol* 1978;3:281–3.
19. Hagberg B, Haltia M, Sourander P, Svennerholm L, Eeg-Olofsson O. Polyunsaturated fatty acid lipidosis: infantile form of so-called neuronal ceroid-lipofuscinosis. I. Clinical and morphological aspects. *Acta Paediatr Scand* 1974;63:753–63.
20. Halliday AM, Halliday E. Cerebral somatosensory and visual evoked potentials in different clinical forms of myoclonus. In: Desmedt JE, ed. *Clinical uses of cerebral, brain stem and spinal somatosensory potentials*, vol 7. Basel: Karger, 1980:292–310. (Progress in clinical neurophysiology.)
21. Hambert O, Petersen I. Clinical, electroencephalographical and neuropharmacological studies in syndromes of progressive myoclonus epilepsy. *Acta Neurol Scand* 1970;46:149–86.
22. Harriman DGF, Millar JHD, Stevenson AL. Progressive familial myoclonic epilepsy in three families: its clinical features and pathological basis. *Brain* 1955;78:325–49.
23. Herrlin K-M, Hillborg PO. Neurological signs in the juvenile form of Gaucher's disease. *Acta Paediatr* 1962;51:137–54.
24. Itoyama Y, Goto I, Kuroiwa Y, Takeichi M, Kawabuchi M, Tanaka Y. Familial juvenile neuronal storage disease: new disease or variant of juvenile lipidosis? *Arch Neurol* 1978;35:792–800.
25. Janeway R, Ravens JR, Pearce LA, Odor DL, Suzuki K. Progressive myoclonus epilepsy with Lafora inclusion bodies. I. Clinical, genetic, histopathologic, and biochemical aspects. *Arch Neurol* 1967;16:565–82.
26. King JO. Progressive myoclonic epilepsy due to Gaucher's disease in an adult. *J Neurol Neurosurg Psychiatry* 1975;38:849–54.
27. Koga M, Sato T, Ikuta F, Nakashima S, Kameyama K, Kojima K. An autopsy case of familial neurovisceral storage disease of late onset. *Folia Psychiatr Neurol Jpn* 1978;32:299–308.

28. Kunishita T, Taketomi T. Sphingomyelin storage in a patient with myoclonus epilepsy as a main clinical symptom—a variant of Niemann-Pick disease Type C? *Jpn J Exp Med* 1979;49:151–6.
29. Kuriyama M, Okada S, Tanaka Y, Umezaki H. Adult mucolipidosis with beta-galactosidase and neuraminidase deficiencies. *J Neurol Sci* 1980;46:245–54.
30. Lance JW, Adams RD. The syndrome of intention or action myoclonus as a sequel to hypoxic encephalopathy. *Brain* 1963;86:111–36.
31. Landis C, Hunt WA. *The Startle Pattern*. New York: Farrar and Rhinehart, 1939.
32. Lou HC, Kristensen K. A clinical and psychological investigation into juvenile amaurotic idiocy in Denmark. *Dev Med Child Neurol* 1973;15:313–23.
33. Lowden JA, O'Brien JS. Sialidosis: a review of human neuraminidase deficiency. *Am J Human Genet* 1979;31:1–18.
34. Maroteaux P, Humbel R, Strecker G, Michalski J-C, Mande R. Un nouveau type de sialidose avec atteinte rénale: la néphrosialidose. *Arch Franc Pediatr* 1978;35:819–29.
35. Miller JD, McCluer R, Kanfer JN. Gaucher's disease: neurologic disorder in adult siblings. *Ann Int Med* 1973;78:883–7.
36. Morrell F, Torres F. Electrophysiological analysis of a case of Tay–Sachs disease. *Brain* 1960;83:213–24.
37. Nishimura R, Omos-Lau N, Ajmone-Marsan C, Barranger JA. Electroencephalographic findings in Gaucher disease. *Neurology* 1980;30:152–9.
38. O'Brien JS. Neuraminidase deficiency in the cherry red spot-myoclonus syndrome. *Biochem Biophys Res Commun* 1977;79:1136–41.
39. O'Brien JS. The cherry red spot-myoclonus syndrome: a newly recognized inherited lysosomal storage disease due to acid neuraminidase deficiency. *Clin Genet* 1978;14:55–60.
40. Pallis CA, Duckett S, Pearse AGE. Diffuse lipofuscinosis of the central nervous system. *Neurology* 1967;17:381–394.
41. Pampiglione G, Harden A. Neurophysiological identification of a late infantile form of neuronal lipidosis. *J Neurol Neurosurg Psychiatry* 1973;36:68–74.
42. Pampiglione G, Lehovsky M. The evolution of EEG features in Tay-Sachs disease and amaurotic family idiocy in 24 children. In: Kellaway P, Petersen I, eds. *Clinical electroencephalography of children*. New York: Grune & Stratton, 1968:287–306.
43. Pampiglione G, Privett G, Harden A. Tay-Sachs disease: Neurophysiological studies in 20 children. *Dev Med Child Neurol* 1974;16:201–8.
44. Purpura DP, Suzuki K. Distortion of neuronal geometry and formation of aberrant synapses in neuronal storage disease. *Brain Res* 1976;116:1–21.
45. Rapin I, Goldfisher S, Katzman R, Engel J Jr, O'Brien JS. The cherry-red spot-myoclonus syndrome. *Ann Neurol* 1978;3:234–42.
46. Roger J, Gastaut H, Toga M, Soulayrol R, Riges H, Lob H, Tassinari A, Dubois D, Poinso Y, Mesdjian E. Epilepsie myoclonique progressive avec corps de Lafora (etude clinique, polygraphique et anatomique d'un cas). *Rev Neurol* 1965;112:50–61.
47. Sakuraba H, Suzuki Y, Akagi M, Sakai M, Amano N. Beta-galactosidase-neuraminidase deficiency (galactosialidosis): clinical, pathological, and enzymatic studies in a postmortem case. *Ann Neurol* 1983;13:497–503.
48. Santavuori P. EEG in the infantile type of so-called neuronal ceroid-lipofuscinosis. *Neuropaediatrie* 1973;4:375–87.
49. Santavuori P, Haltia M, Rapola J, Raitta C. Infantile type of so-called neuronal ceroid-lipofuscinosis. Part 1. A clinical study of 15 patients. *J Neurol Sci* 1973;18:257–67.
50. Schneck L. The early electroencephalographic and seizure characteristics of Tay-Sachs. *Acta Neurol Scand* 1965;41:163–71.
51. Schneck L, Maisel J, Volk BW. The startle response and serum enzyme profile in early detection of Tay-Sachs' disease. *J Pediatr* 1964;65:749–56.
52. Seitelberger F, Jacob H, Peiffer J, Colmant HJ. Die Myoklonuskörperkrankheit: Eine angeborene Störung des Kohlenhydratstoffwechsels. Klinishpathologische Studie an fünf Fällen. *Fortschr Neurol Psychiatr* 1964;32:305–45.
53. Shibasaki H, Yamashita Y, Kuroiwa Y. Electroencephalographic studies of myoclonus: myoclonus related cortical spikes and high amplitude somatosensory evoked potentials. *Brain* 1978;101:447–60.
54. Sjögren T. Die juvenile amaurotische Idiotie, klinische und erblichkeitsmedizinische Untersuchungen. *Hereditas* 1931;14:197–425.

55. Sorensen JB, Parnas P. A clinical study of 44 patients with juvenile amaurotic idiocy. *Acta Psychiatr Scand* 1979;59:449–61.
56. Suzuki Y, Nakamura N, Shimada Y, Yotsumoto H, Endo H, Nagashima K. Macular cherry-red spots and beta-galactosidase deficiency in an adult: an autopsy case with progressive cerebellar ataxia, myoclonus, thrombocytopathy, and accumulation of polysaccharide in the liver. *Arch Neurol* 1977;34:157–61.
57. Svennerholm L, Hagberg B, Haltia M, Sourander P, Vanier M-T. Polyunsaturated fatty acid lipidosis. II. Lipid biochemical studies. *Acta Pediatr Scand* 1975;64:489–96.
58. Tanaka Y, Taguchi K, Arayama T. Auditory responses in Tay-Sachs disease. *Pract Otorhinolaryngol* 1969;31:46–53.
59. Thal LJ, Sharpless NS, Wolfson L, Katzman R. Treatment of myoclonus with L-5-hydroxytryptophan and carbidopa: clinical, electrophysiological, and biochemical observations. *Ann Neurol* 1980;7:570–6.
60. Thomas GH, Tipton RE, Ch'ien LT, Reynolds LW, Miller CS. Sialidase (alpha-N-acetyl neuraminidase) deficiency: the enzyme defect in an adult with macular cherry-red spots and myoclonus without dementia. *Clin Genet* 1978;13:369–79.
61. Thomas PK, Abrams JD, Swallow D, Stewart G. Sialidosis type 1: cherry red spot-myoclonus syndrome with sialidase deficiency and altered electrophoretic mobilities of some enzymes known to be glycoproteins. I. Clinical findings. *J Neurol Neurosurg Psychiatry* 1979;42:873–880.
62. Tokuda Y, Harada K, Yamagami M, Shiradi H. An autopsy case of a late form of familial amaurotic idiocy in comparison to the clinical and pathological findings on the two siblings with the same disease. *Folia Psychiatr Neurol Jpn* 1967;69:401–28.
63. Tripp JH, Lake BD, Young E, Ngn J, Brett EM. Juvenile Gaucher's disease with horizontal gaze palsy in three siblings. *J Neurol Neurosurg Psychiatry* 1977;40:470–8.
64. Van Haycop Ten Ham MW, DeJager H. Progressive myoclonus epilepsy with Lafora bodies. Clinical–pathological features. *Epilepsia* 1963;4:95–119.
65. Vercruyssen A, Martin JJ, Ceurerick C, Jacobs K, Swerts L. Adult ceroid-lipofuscinosis: diagnostic value of biopsies and of neurophysiological investigations. *J Neurol Neurosurg Psychiatry* 1982;45:1056–9.
66. Westmoreland BF, Groover RV, Sharbrough FW. Electrographic findings in three types of cerebral macular degeneration. *Mayo Clin Proc* 1979;54:12–21.
67. Yanoff M, Schwarz GA. Lafora's disease—a distinct genetically determined form of Unverricht's syndrome. *J Genet Hum* 1965;14:235–44.
68. Zeman W. The neuronal ceroid-lipofuscinoses. In: Zimmerman HM, ed. *Progress in neuropathology*, vol III. Orlando: Grune and Stratton 1976:203–23.

Advances in Neurology, Vol. 43: Myoclonus,
edited by S. Fahn et al. Raven Press,
New York © 1986.

Action Myoclonus–Renal Failure Syndrome: A Previously Unrecognized Neurological Disorder Unmasked by Advances in Nephrology

Eva Andermann,[1,2] Frederick Andermann,[2] Stirling Carpenter,[1] Leonhard S. Wolfe,[1] Robert Nelson,[3] Georges Patry,[4] and Jean Boileau[5]

Montreal Neurological Hospital and Institute, Montreal, Canada

In recent years we have encountered a progressive neurological disease associated with renal failure in four young French Canadian patients. The neurological features are tremor of fingers and hands starting in the late teens, followed by action myoclonus, ataxia, dysarthria, and generalized tonic–clonic seizures. Proteinuria is noted at the same age as the initial neurological symptoms and proceeds to renal failure, requiring dialysis or transplantation.

The neurological syndrome is not considered to be merely the result of a metabolic encephalopathy due to the renal failure; rather, the primary disease process appears to involve both brain and kidneys. To our knowledge the syndrome has not been recognized previously.

CASE REPORTS

Patient 1

This 24-year-old woman, S.T., was the seventh of nine liveborn siblings (Fig. 1). She was born to apparently unrelated parents originating from small adjacent villages in the Beauce region of Québec (Figs. 1 and 2). There was no family history of renal or relevant neurological disease. She was born at term, weighing 8 lbs, walked at 10 months, and talked at 15 months. She had a concussion at age 6 years. At age 13 years, she developed pyelonephritis, for which she received a single injection of penicillin and was found to have albuminuria. She had enuresis to age 12 years.

[1]Department of Neurology and Neurosurgery, McGill University, Montreal, Canada.
[2]Centre for Human Genetics, McGill University, Montreal, Canada.
[3]University of Ottawa, Ottawa, Canada.
[4]Laval University, Canada.
[5]University of Montreal, Montreal, Canada.

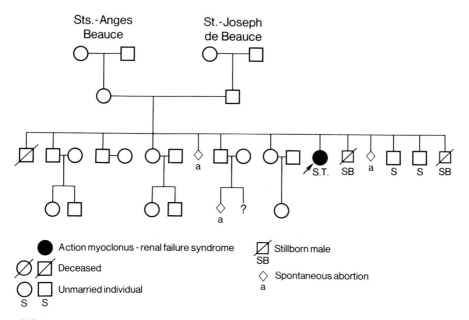

FIG. 1. Pedigree of family T. The grandparents were born in adjacent small communities.

At the age of 18 years, she noted fine shaking of the fingers bilaterally at rest. This was increased by delicate movement, such as writing. Jerking of the upper and then the lower extremities started at age 19 years. Her voice became tremulous, and she began to fall. She stopped working at age 20 years because of her neurological symptoms. At this age, urinalysis and renal function studies were normal.

At the age of 21 years, she developed infrequent generalized seizures. They started with a cry, generalized clonic jerking, and revulsion of the eyes, of which she was aware, followed by loss of consciousness and urinary incontinence. An electroencephalogram (EEG) showed irregular generalized spike–wave discharges increased by hyperventilation and intermittent photic stimulation.

At 22 years, she developed ankle swelling followed by generalized edema, insomnia, headache, nausea, and dyspnea. A renal biopsy showed chronic glomerulonephritis. Immunofluorescence revealed immunoglobulin M (IgM) and complement in the glomerular loops and in the mesangium. She was started on dialysis.

At 24 years of age, she was bedridden because of severe action myoclonus. At rest she had myoclonic jerks of the arms or legs, often proximal, asynchronous, and of variable severity. Movements of the limbs or talking greatly increased the amplitude and amount of myoclonus. Attempts at speaking induced violent myoclonus of the bulbar musculature. Intelligence and affect were normal. Muscle tone and power, reflexes, and sensation were normal. There was no clear tremor at this time. Cerebellar function could not be assessed because of the myoclonus.

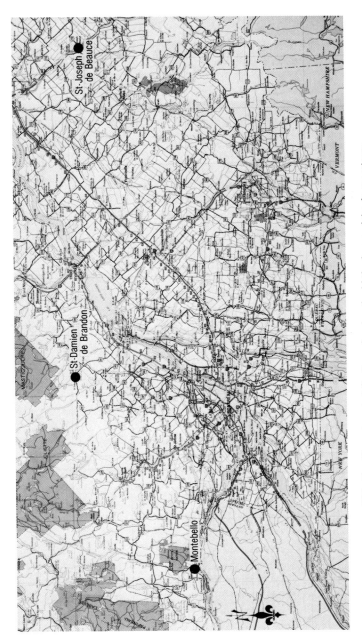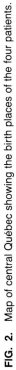

FIG. 2. Map of central Québec showing the birth places of the four patients.

The EEGs showed slow background activity at 6.5 to 7.5 Hz and rather infrequent, relatively low-voltage spike and spike–wave discharges, bilaterally synchronous and generalized or confined to the central vertex or both occipital regions. Some of the brief spike potentials would have been difficult to distinguish from muscle potentials except that they were seen at the vertex where there is no muscle artifact. The electromyogram (EMG) myoclonic potentials were sometimes associated with cerebral potentials and at other times occurred independently. Intermittent photic stimulation produced whole body myoclonus with multiple spikes in the EEG record associated with slow waves. The photosensitivity was greatly reduced for 20 min following subcutaneous administration of a subemetic dose of apomorphine; this also temporarily reduced spontaneous myoclonic activity and generalized epileptogenic discharge. There was some reduction of epileptic activity 2 hr after administration of a tryptophan loading dose. A computerized tomography (CT) scan showed mild dilatation of the third and lateral ventricles and slight prominence of the sulci, suggesting mild diffuse cerebral atrophy.

Total and free tryptophan were measured and found to be markedly reduced (50% of lower limit of normal). This was most likely due to the dialysis and was corrected by 4 g/day tryptophan supplements. There was, however, no clear reduction in myoclonus associated with increased tryptophan levels.

Valproic acid reduced the action myoclonus but had to be discontinued because it led to pancreatitis on three occasions. Only slight reduction in myoclonus resulted from administration of 6 mg clonazepam and 15 mg nitrazepam daily. On the other hand, the generalized seizures were easily controlled with 300 mg phenytoin/day.

No kidney of suitable tissue type was available for transplantation. The patient died at the age of 25 years of complications related to her dialysis.

Patient 2

A 34-year-old man, B.B., from St. Damien de Brandon in the Joliette region of Québec (Fig. 2) was the second of six siblings (Fig. 3). His parents were second-degree cousins. The oldest sister, who was severely retarded as a result of prematurity and perinatal anoxia, had several seizures. A younger brother died at 14 years of age due to suspected collagen vascular disease. The patient was hit with a hammer at the age of 12 years and had a subdural hematoma removed. He recovered over a period of 1 year, repeated seventh grade, and went to work on a farm at age 14 years.

He developed swelling of the legs at the age of 20 years. Because of renal failure he was dialyzed for 14 months and had a renal transplant at age 21. He developed unsteadiness of gait at age 20 and within a year started to have intention myoclonus manifest when he would pick up objects or make other purposeful movements. At 22 years of age, he developed generalized seizures that were infrequent and easily controlled with a low dose of phenytoin.

At age 34 years, the renal transplant was functioning well. The parents stated that the action myoclonus had increased over the last few years. He was confined

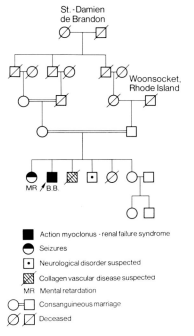

St.-Damien
de Brandon

Woonsocket,
Rhode Island

MR   B.B.

■ Action myoclonus - renal failure syndrome
◐ Seizures
⊡ Neurological disorder suspected
⊠ Collagen vascular disease suspected
MR Mental retardation
○─□ Consanguineous marriage
⌀ ⬚ Deceased

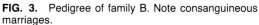

FIG. 3. Pedigree of family B. Note consanguineous marriages.

to a wheelchair and had to be strapped in because of the severity of the myoclonus. Power, tone, reflexes, and sensation appeared normal. No tremor was apparent, and coordination could not be tested because of the violence of the action myoclonus. His speech was dysarthric above and beyond the jerky interruptions related to the myoclonus of the bulbar musculature. Intelligence and affect were normal. He was living with a disabled young woman in an institution for the physically handicapped and was able to maneuver his electrical wheelchair.

Patient 3

Patient 3, V.P., was born at Montebello, in the Outaouais region of Québec, the ninth child of apparently unrelated parents (Figs. 2 and 4). He developed a tremor of his limbs at the age of 17 years. He lost his job as a waiter at a resort hotel because of the tremor, which was obvious when he was serving at table. He noticed that the tremor was relieved by alcohol. At the same age, he was found to have proteinuria. At the age of 20, his tremor involved in addition his head, legs, and voice. It was aggravated by intention and partially relieved by 40 mg propranolol/day. He startled excessively, perspired profusely, and was hyperreflexic throughout, with slight increase in tone in the lower extremities.

At the age of 21 years, he developed generalized seizures, and his EEG showed a generalized epileptic abnormality increased by hyperventilation. Cerebrospinal fluid (CSF) protein was 21 mg% and γ-globulin 11.8%. He had unsustained

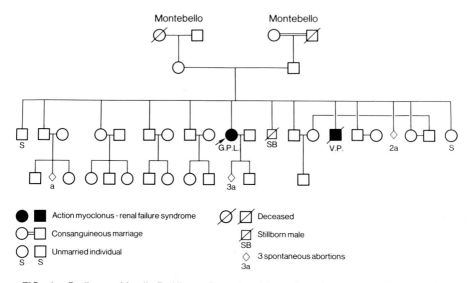

FIG. 4. Pedigree of family P. All grandparents originate from the same small community.

nystagmus, vertical ocular dysmetria, and loss of smooth pursuit movements. Later that year he developed myoclonic jerks of all extremities. He was unable to stand and could barely sit up in bed. He had unsustained patellar clonus and crossed adduction reflexes, but the plantar responses were flexor. He underwent renal transplantation at age 22 years.

At age 23, he was markedly dysarthric and had gross nystagmus on lateral gaze. He had a pronounced tremor of the tongue and violent intention myoclonus. Reflexes were brisk, and sensory examination was normal. A CT scan showed enlargement of lateral ventricles and cerebral sulci. Carbidopa (100 mg/day) and 300 mg hydroxytryptophan produced some transient improvement in the myoclonus. He was treated with valproic acid, clonazepam, carbamazepine, and phenobarbital. He died at 25 years of age due to complications related to rejection of his renal transplant. An autopsy was performed.

Patient 4

Patient 4, G.P.L., was a sister of V.P., the sixth child of the family (Fig. 4). At the age of 18 years, she was found to have proteinuria during an examination prior to tonsillectomy. During pregnancy at age 22, she developed a nephrotic syndrome. At age 23 years, she lost 7 g protein/day, and a biopsy showed membranous nephropathy. That year she developed action myoclonus and became unable to write. She also started to have generalized nocturnal seizures. An EEG showed only diffuse slowing of background. At age 24 years, she had a renal transplant with a rejection reaction 2 months later. She then was noted to have ataxia of gait.

At age 27, she had moderate dysarthria. With the arms held extended there was only mild tremulousness, but she had a very marked intention tremor on finger-to-nose test. Her gait was broad based and unsteady. Occasional myoclonic jerks of perioral muscles were seen, and she had marked intention myoclonus: if she were asked to pick up an object, her hand would suddenly start off in an oblique direction just before achieving her goal. She had no nystagmus. Cranial nerves were normal, as were her reflexes, sensation, and intelligence. An EEG showed a generalized photosensitive epileptogenic abnormality. A CT scan showed moderate cerebellar atrophy with widened sulci, an enlarged fourth ventricle, and a shrunken vermis. Cerebral hemispheres were slightly atrophic.

At the age of 29 years, she was confined to bed; opening of the eyes or attempts to speak or take an object produced violent myoclonic jerks, which were focal or generalized. There was a notable absence of horizontal nystagmus, although there were a few beats of rotatory nystagmus on upward gaze. Her speech was somewhat dysarthric, and she exhibited "scanning" but had no difficulty with repeated sounds. Although her speech was barely intelligible, her mentation was normal. The most striking finding was an intention tremor, present in all four extremities and disappearing at rest. There was a mild Holmes rebound phenomenon in both arms. She had great difficulty with heel-to-shin test. The intention myoclonus could be distinguished from the intention tremor in that at the end point of carrying out a specific movement, her arm suddenly jerked involuntarily; this seemed irrespective of the degree of intention tremor exhibited with the particular movement. She also had occasional spontaneous myoclonic jerks of her face, particularly around the mouth. Deep tendon reflexes were present, with some pendular features. Plantar responses were normal, and she had no sensory abnormalities. Brief improvement in myoclonus was produced by L-tryptophan with carbidopa, but diarrhea limited the dose to 400 mg/day. She died at the age of 29 years due to complications related to her renal transplant.

PATHOLOGICAL FINDINGS

The autopsy of patient 3, V.P., showed swelling of his grafted kidney, hemorrhagic cystitis and ureteritis, and marked atrophy of the patient's own kidneys, which each weighed 30 g. His brain was normal in size without convolutional atrophy. There was mild but definite dilatation of the lateral ventricles. The substantia nigra showed less black pigmentation than normal, as well as a spreading of brownish pigmentation along its lower border. The globus pallidus was not noticeably pigmented.

Microscopic examination showed no neuronal loss or significant gliosis. The only abnormality was the presence of pigment granules, which appeared to be in astrocytes and in certain cells in the meninges. The staining reactions of the pigment are indicated in Table 1. There appears to be a spectrum of reactions between the small granules and the large granules which were up to 10 μm in size. In the cortex, pigment was seen in the first two layers (Figs. 5 and 6). In the molecular layer, the granules were small, numerous, and clustered, whereas in the second cortical layer, they were considerably larger but fewer. Small pigment granules

TABLE 1. *Staining reactions of nonneuronal pigment*

Method	Reaction of small granules	Reaction of large granules
Unstained	Colorless to tan	Brown
Ultraviolet light	Lemon to bright cadmium yellow	Dark center, bright yellow periphery
Hematoxylin–eosin	Colorless to tan	Brown
Luxol fast blue-cresyl violet	Gray to black	Brown center, black periphery
Sudan black-B	Black	Golden brown
Iron	Negative	Negative

were numerous in the inner and outer parts of the globus pallidus and in the reticular part of the substantia nigra. Occasionally they appeared to be increased in number around vessels in this area. Numerous small pigment granules were seen in the hippocampus in glial cells in fields H2, H3, H4, and H5 and in the stratum lacunosum of all fields (Fig. 7). They were also seen in the molecular layer of the dentate gyrus. In the cerebellum they were prominent in the layer of the Bergmann glia (Fig. 8); here, as in the second layer of the cerebral cortex, there were granules up to 10 μm in size which were brown on unstained sections. Neurons contained

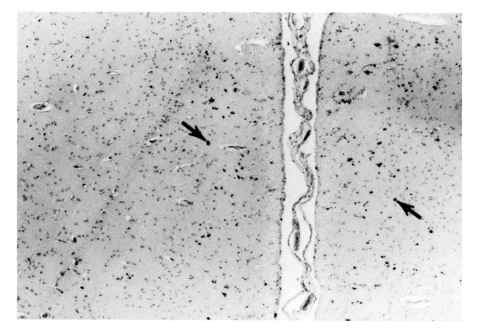

FIG. 5. This photomicrograph shows large and small pigment granules (some marked with arrows) in the outer two cortical layers of gyri at the base of the temporal lobe. Paraffin section, hematoxylin–eosin. ×50.

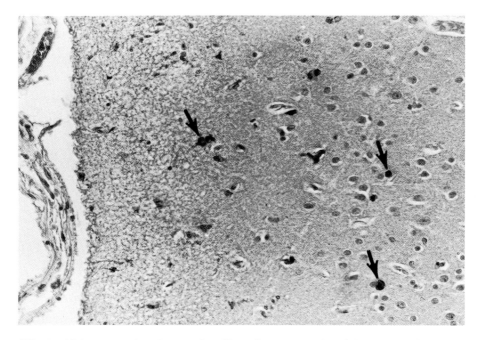

FIG. 6. Higher power view of an area from Fig. 5. *Arrows*, examples of pigment. Paraffin section, hematoxylin–eosin. × 220.

what appeared to be normal amounts of lipofuscin. This shared the quality of yellow autofluorescence with the extraneuronal pigment but differed from it by being consistently colorless on unstained sections and colorless by luxol fast blue-cresyl violet. Electron microscopy showed osmiophilic bodies, which were probably located in astrocytic processes. At high magnification, they were seen to contain tightly packed lamellae with a periodicity of 6 to 7 nm (Figs.9–11).

A muscle biopsy from the gastrocnemius of patient 1 showed mild denervation atrophy. Lipofuscin in muscle cells was unremarkable in amount and in ultrastructure. A biopsy of her sural nerve showed mild axonal degenerative neuropathy. A skin biopsy was within normal limits.

Renal biopsies from the four patients were reviewed. Interstitial fibrosis was seen in three. Sclerosis of a proportion of the glomeruli was seen in all, but no specific features could be found. There was no suggestion of storage.

BIOCHEMICAL FINDINGS

Thin-layer chromatography of the urine developed with orcinol and resorcinol reagents for neutral and sialyl oligosaccharides was normal for patients 1, 2, and 4 (S.T, B.B., and G.P.L.). The results of leukocyte and fibroblast α-neuraminidase and leukocyte β-galactosidase assayed with the synthetic 4-methylumbelliferyl substrates in patient 1 are shown in Table 2. It is clear that a diagnosis of mucolipidosis I (sialidosis type I) can be excluded.

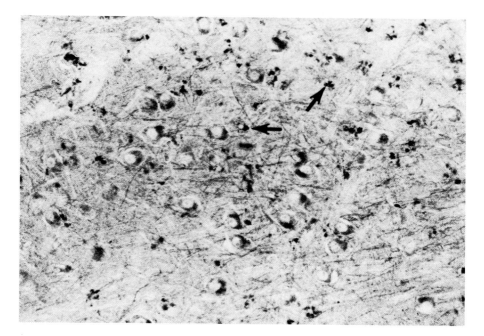

FIG. 7. In the endplate of the hippocampus, Sudan black-B stains small granules in astrocytes (some marked with arrows). The neurons contain normal amounts of lipopigment. Paraffin section. ×220.

DISCUSSION

These four patients, members of three sibships, had quite similar neurological abnormalities, considering that the initial neurological histories and examinations were performed by different neurologists, and that the families differed in their historic ability.

The first symptom was commonly a tremor of fingers and hands (Table 3), exacerbated by intention and responding partially to alcohol and propranolol. The description of this tremor is reminiscent of essential or familial tremor and also of involvement of the dentatorubral system. In patient B.B., the tremor was not a striking feature. Certainly it was not clearly apparent when he was older and when his action myoclonus was violent. In the early stages of the illness, it was not noted by himself or his family, and early medical observations were sketchy. In all patients, as in this man, the tremor was largely masked by the striking action myoclonus as the disease progressed, although it could still be demonstrated in patient G.P.L. at the age of 29 years.

Onset of action myoclonus ranged between the ages of 19 to 23 years; it involved bulbar as well as proximal and distal appendicular musculature. It was extremely severe in all patients, representing the most disabling symptom of the neurological disease. At least in one patient, the myoclonus was sensitive to light. It responded poorly or transiently to tryptophan in the three patients in whom this was tried.

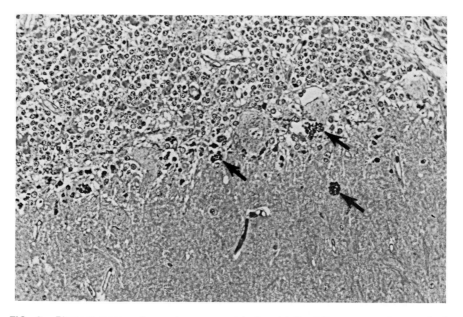

FIG. 8. Pigment masses *(arrows)* are present in the vicinity of Bergmann astrocytes in the cerebellar cortex. Epoxy resin section, paraphenylene diamine, phase optics. ×220.

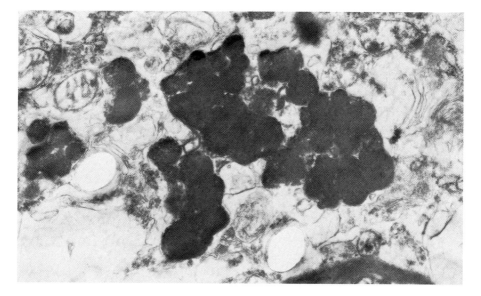

FIG. 9. This electron micrograph shows pigment granules from the vicinity of Bergmann astrocytes in the cerebellum. ×25,000.

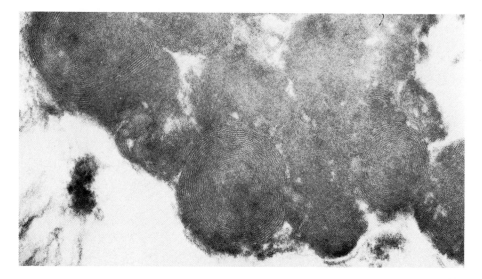

FIG. 10.   This electron micrograph shows at higher power that within the granules of Fig. 9 there are lamellar profiles. × 100,000.

The response to valproic acid and to clonazepam was also not striking. The myoclonic jerks were at times accompanied by a cerebral discharge, but at other times no clear EEG accompaniment was seen. This pattern was suggestive of a subcortical origin.

Generalized seizures started to occur between the ages of 21 and 23 years and were diurnal or nocturnal. They seemed to start with a generalized clonic phase with preserved consciousness and proceed to unconsciousness and urinary incontinence. This pattern is similar to that seen in some patients with other forms of

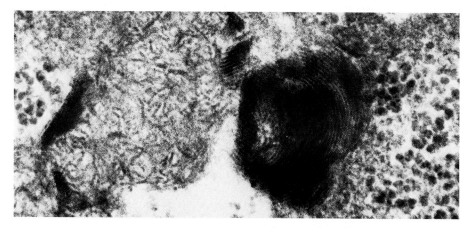

FIG. 11.   This electron micrograph shows, for contrast, the appearance of the fingerprint profiles (systems of paired parallel lines) which accumulate in juvenile Batten disease. × 100,000.

TABLE 2. *Biochemistry on patient S.T.*

Biochemistry[a]	nmole/mg Protein/hr
Leukocyte α-neuraminidase	
S.T.	1.12, 1.26, 2.95
Normals (5)	2.61 (1.00–4.50)
Leukocyte β-galactosidase	
S.T.	15.42
Normals	20.86 (15.00–24.00)
Fibroblast α-neuraminidase	
S.T.	122.0, 95.7
Controls	103.7, 105.8

[a]Urine sialyl oligosaccharides on patients S.T., B.B., and G.L. negative.

progressive myoclonus epilepsy (e.g., Baltic myoclonus) and is not unusual in patients with the myoclonic form of primary generalized corticoreticular epilepsy (Janz syndrome). The EEG and clinical findings suggested a secondary generalized corticoreticular epileptic disorder. The gradual buildup of myoclonus leading to a generalized seizure has not been well studied physiologically; the excessive artifact associated with such seizures would make such studies difficult. This pattern appears to be different, however, from the more common generalized tonic–clonic seizures.

The blockade of the photosensitivity in response to apomorphine (a dopamine agonist) suggested the presence of an abnormality in the dopaminergic system at the level of the striate cortex (9). At any rate, the seizures in this disease were not prolonged, and patients did not show a tendency to develop status epilepticus. The attacks were easily controlled with phenytoin or carbamazepine.

Ataxia and dysarthria appeared around the ages of 21 to 23 years. In one patient, these represented the earliest neurological symptoms, whereas in the others, they tended to occur later. The cerebellar abnormalities were not severe and did not represent the limiting factor in the patients' disability. They were overshadowed by the action myoclonus, which made it difficult to distinguish them and which represented the major functional disability. Pendular reflexes, abnormal rebound,

TABLE 3. *Age of onset: Action myoclonus–renal failure syndrome*

Symptom	Age (years)
Tremor of fingers and hands	17–18
Proteinuria	17–18
Action myoclonus	19–23
Renal failure	20–22
Ataxia and dysarthria	21–23
Infrequent generalized seizures	21–23

and nystagmus were found in some patients, confirming the clinical evidence for cerebellar involvement.

Remarkably, the patients remained normal in intelligence, judging by casual observation and the opinion of their families. Psychometric testing, however, has not been carried out late in the illness. Although hyperreflexia sometimes has been noted, there was no good evidence for a pyramidal syndrome in this disorder, and there were no extrapyramidal signs.

The neurological manifestations of renal failure are well known and have been described in detail by Tyler (13) and by Raskin and Fishman (11). The neuropathological findings have been reviewed by Olsen (8). The advent of dialysis and renal transplantation has led to more uremic patients being under careful medical scrutiny for longer periods of time, and new syndromes, such as dialysis dementia (1) and a progressive cerebellar syndrome resembling olivopontine cerebellar disease (6), have been described.

Abnormalities of movement are among the most common manifestations of renal failure. Tremor and tremulousness may be seen even in well-controlled patients but are more obvious as the sensorium becomes impaired. Asterixis involving the hands, legs, and head is associated with more severe uremia; according to Raskin and Fishman (11), myoclonus does not appear until stupor and coma have intervened. Myoclonus is multifocal and involves particularly the face and proximal upper limbs. The myoclonus may be so severe as to resemble multifocal seizures and may be incapacitating.

Focal and generalized seizures also occur with acute renal failure or as a terminal event. Between these clinical extremes, seizures may be associated with excessive dialysis and dialysis disequilibrium, or hypertensive encephalopathy, or they may be due to various drugs which are not readily excreted by the uremic patient.

The second hallmark of the disease described here is renal involvement. This begins with proteinuria at 17 to 18 years of age, proceeding to renal failure at 20 to 22 years. The proteinuria may be found when the first neurological manifestations occur, or even earlier. One patient developed renal failure when only minimal neurological symptoms were present. The others, however, had developed florid neurological disability by the time renal failure became apparent. The myoclonus and other neurological symptoms are unlike the myoclonus and other cerebral manifestations of uremic metabolic encephalopathy.

In this condition, the clinical manifestations appear to be due to independent or separate involvement of brain and kidney by one pathological process, which is probably an inherited metabolic defect. Transplanted kidneys have functioned for as long as 13 years in one patient without clinical evidence of being affected by the pathological process in the same way as the original organs. The neurological disease seemed to progress with time independently of the renal function and was not improved by dialysis or by renal transplantation. The condition has probably not been described before the advent of dialysis and renal transplantation because of its rapidly fatal course due to the renal failure.

Feinfeld et al. (2) have reported a case described by Rapin et al. (10) and diagnosed as having the cherry-red-spot myoclonus syndrome (sialidosis type I), who developed lupus nephritis at age 25 years. A patient of Dr. A. L. Rose (*personal communication*, 1983) with onset of myoclonus at age 10 years and bilateral cherry-red spots who developed renal involvement at age 13 was also diagnosed to have α-neuraminidase deficiency by J. S. O'Brien (*personal communication*, 1983). He and an older sister who had a similar syndrome died of renal failure. The normal α-neuraminidase levels in one of the patients in this report indicates that the disease reported here is different from sialidosis type I.

A search of the literature revealed one case similar to our patients, a girl reported by Horoupian and Ross (3) as suffering from the "pigment variant of neuronal ceroid-lipofuscinosis (Kufs' disease)." At 19 years of age, she had the onset of tremor, followed by action myoclonus seizures. She also developed dysarthria and ataxia. In the late stages of her illness, she was extremely photosensitive. She was said to be demented during her final admission, although she was capable of logical thinking in the last year of her life. At 21 years, she developed proteinuria. Kidney biopsy showed focal sclerosing glomerulonephritis and immune damage to the basement membrane with a rather smooth pattern. She died in renal failure at age 25 years. The findings of extraneuronal pigment in the brain closely resembled those in our case 3. On the other hand, dark pigmentation of the globus pallidus was visible on gross examination. Microscopically, there was felt to be an excess of intraneuronal periodic acid Schiff (PAS)-positive granules in thalamus and sub-thalamus. Dr. Ross informed us that the mother was French; whether or not she was from Québec is unclear, but there is a large French population in Manitoba originating from Québec. The father was born in the south of England. Horoupian and Ross (3) felt that their case belonged with those who had been reported to have the pigment variant of amaurotic idiocy. Those cases, however, have a different clinical picture, without myoclonus or renal failure (4,5,7,12,14), whereas our four cases as well as that of Horoupian and Ross appear to have a uniform and fairly closely age-related pattern of neurological and renal involvement. Furthermore, patients with the pigment variant of amaurotic family idiocy apparently show definite neuronal storage as well as the extraneuronal pigment which is generally similar to that in our cases and that of Horoupian and Ross (3).

A case of myoclonus epilepsy with atrophy of brainstem and Hallervorden–Spatz type of pathological change in the pallidum, substantia nigra, and dentate nucleus was reported by Yakovlev (14) in 1942. This patient developed seizures at age 17 years and died at age 30. There was no mention of renal failure. In addition to the iron deposits, this patient also had neuronal pigment storage and thus appears to have a different disorder.

Our patients appear pathologically distinct from other well-defined entities. They differ from those who have ceroid-lipofuscinosis (Batten–Kufs' disease) by lacking storage in neurons and visceral secretory cells and by having a different ultrastructural appearance of the stored material. They differ from Hallervorden–Spatz disease by lacking iron deposition in the basal ganglia and axonal dystrophy. They lack the storage in neurons and secretory cells that occurs in sialidosis, not to mention the specific enzyme defect. The pathogenesis of the extraneuronal pigment storage and of the glomerular damage in our cases remains unknown. The finding of HLA types A2 and B35 in two patients in different sibships may be of interest.

All our patients are French Canadian from the province of Québec. Although they appear to originate in different parts of the province (Fig. 2), common surnames may be found among ancestors of the three families, indicating a possible founder effect. Two of the families may be traced to "colons" bearing the same name but with different spelling (Poulain and Poulin), originating from Île de France and Normandie, adjacent French provinces, in the 17th century. The location of the communities of origin of the grandparents is compatible with the pattern of settlement and migration of the French Canadian population from the initially established communities in the vicinity of the city of Québec. The absence of affected cases in previous generations, the presence of two affected siblings in one family, and parental consanguinity in another all suggest autosomal recessive inheritance.

ACKNOWLEDGMENT

We thank Dr. Serge Jothy for reviewing the renal biopsies, and Ms. Geneviève Limoges for typing the manuscript.

REFERENCES

1. Alfrey AC, LeGendre GR, Kaehny WD. Dialysis encephalopathy syndrome (possible aluminum toxicity). *N Eng J Med* 1976;294:184–8.
2. Feinfeld DA, Scholnick HR, Janis R. Lupus nephritis in a neuronal storage disease. *Arch Intern Med* 1977;137:693–4.
3. Horoupian DS, Ross RT. Pigment variant of neuronal ceroid-lipofuscinosis (Kufs' disease). *Can J Neurol Sci* 1977;4:67–75.
4. Jakob H, Kolkmann FW. Zur Pigmentvariante der adulten Form der amaurotischen Idiotie (Kufs). *Acta Neuropathol (Berl)* 1973;26:225–36.
5. Jervis GA. Hallervorden–Spatz disease associated with atypical amaurotic idiocy. *J Neuropathol Exp Neurol* 1952;11:4–18.
6. Massry SG, Glassock RJ. *Textbook of nephrology*. Baltimore: Williams & Wilkins, 1983.
7. Moschel R. Amaurotische Idiotie mit einer besonderen Form von Pigmentablagerung. *Deutsche Ztschr Nervenh* 1954;172:102–10.
8. Olsen, S. The brain in uremia. *Acta Psychiatr Neurol Scand [Suppl]* 1961;36:156.
9. Quesney LF, Andermann F, Lal S, Prelevic S. Transient abolition of generalized photosensitive epileptic discharge in man by apomorphine, a dopamine receptor agonist. *Neurology* 1980;30:1169–74.
10. Rapin I, Goldfischer S, Katzman R, Engel J, O'Brien JS. The cherry-red spot-myoclonus syndrome. *Ann Neurol* 1978;3:234–42.
11. Raskin NH, Fishman RA. Neurological disorders in renal failure. *N Engl J Med* 1976;294:143–8; 204–10.
12. Seitelberger F, Simma K. On the pigment variant of amaurotic idiocy. In: Aronson SM, Volk BW, eds *Cerebral sphingolipidoses*. New York: McGraw-Hill, pp. 29–47.
13. Tyler HR. Neurological disorders in renal failure. *Am J Med* 1968;44:734–48.

14. Yakovlev PI. A case of myoclonus epilepsy with atrophy of brain-stem and Hallervorden-Spatz type of pathologic change in the pallidum, substantia nigra and dentate nucleus. *Trans Am Neurol Assoc* 1942;95–100.
15. Zeman W, Scarpelli DG. The non-specific lesions of Hallervorden–Spatz disease. A histochemical study. *J Neuropathol Exp Neurol* 1958;17:622–30.

Advances in Neurology, Vol. 43: Myoclonus,
edited by S. Fahn et al. Raven Press,
New York © 1986.

Myoclonus and Mitochondrial Myopathy

Linton C. Hopkins and Howard S. Rosing

Department of Neurology, Emory University School of Medicine, Atlanta, Georgia 30322

Mitochondrial myopathies are disorders in which the structure or function of muscle mitochondria is abnormal. When structure is affected, the dominant pathologic change in skeletal muscle is an increase in the number of mitochondria that usually have abnormal morphology. Typically, muscle fibers have a "ragged red" appearance when stained with the modified Gomori trichrome technique. They have been recognized since Luft et al. (27) described a patient with nonthyroid hypermetabolism who had abnormal muscle mitochondria. Although hypermetabolism due to mitochondrial myopathy is extremely rare, numerous reports of mitochondrial myopathy have appeared, most commonly associated with progressive external ophthalmoplegia. Observation of these patients and others without ophthalmoplegia indicates that central nervous system (CNS) dysfunction is commonly present in patients who have mitochondrial accumulation in skeletal muscle. More recently, it has been recognized that overt, sometimes fatal, brain disease may occur. Myoclonus has been described in some of these patients.

CNS DISEASE AND MITOCHONDRIAL MYOPATHY WITH MYOCLONUS

Myoclonus was reported in a patient with a structural abnormality of muscle mitochondria by Spiro et al. (42). Patient 2 was a 16-year-old boy who was considered to have slow intellectual development. At age 8 years, he developed decreased visual acuity. At age 11 years, he had a generalized motor seizure, which was followed by progressive gait ataxia, reduction in intellectual function, and slowly progressive weakness. Examination showed mental retardation, generalized proximal weakness, bilateral foot drop, severe ataxia, and many small-amplitude random asymmetric myoclonic jerks. He was areflexic and had bilateral extensor plantar responses and decreased joint position sense in the lower extremities. Muscle biopsy showed an increase in subsarcolemmal red staining material when stained with the modified Gomori trichrome technique; electron microscopy showed an increase in number of normal muscle mitochondria. Biochemical analysis of muscle showed loose coupling of oxidative phosphorylation and a reduction in the concentration of cytochrome b.

Autosomal dominant inheritance and variability of expression are indicated by the somewhat different clinical history of his father, who developed ataxia and dysarthria at age 33 years, followed by progressive weakness, cramps, and fasciculations but no myoclonus or seizures. His examination showed generalized ataxia and muscle weakness, fasciculations, slightly diminished proprioception in the legs, and extensor plantar responses. The father's muscle biopsy did not show subsarcolemmal red staining material on trichrome stain but did show an increase in number of normal muscle mitochondria on electron microscopy.

In 1973, Tsairis et al. (45) reported a family with an inherited disorder characterized by myoclonic epilepsy, ataxia, and diffuse weakness with associated sensorineural hearing loss but with sparing of intelligence. There was photic sensitivity on the electroencephalogram (EEG) with photic-induced myoclonic jerking in two family members who did not have ataxia or hearing loss. Marked mitochondrial accumulation was noted on both light and electron microscopy in all five patients. Muscle biochemical studies were not reported, but serum lactate and pyruvate were increased in three family members. Variability of clinical expression is illustrated again by this family, as the mother had weakness, EEG abnormalities, and photic-induced myoclonus but no ataxia or hearing loss. Two daughters had myoclonic epilepsy, ataxia, weakness, and hearing loss. A third daughter was clinically normal and had a normal EEG; like all the other affected family members, however, she had obvious mitochondrial myopathy on light and electron microscopy. Although reported as autosomal dominant, the pedigree is compatible with maternal inheritance.

Shapira et al. (40) reported two siblings with myoclonus and other seizure types. One patient's muscle biopsy had many ragged red fibers on light microscopy and large irregular mitochondria with paracrystallin bodies on ultrastructural study. The patient with documented mitochondrial myopathy, developed periodic headaches with hemianopia, progressive dementia, increasing focal myoclonic seizures, and deafness; she died at age 16 years. Her brother developed blindness with macular degeneration, right hemiparesis, and progressive dementia; he died at age 10 years with refractory generalized seizures. The pattern of inheritance is uncertain, but is also compatible with maternal inheritance. At 40 years of age, their mother had night blindness and diminishing peripheral vision but no myoclonus. She refused muscle biopsy. Biochemical abnormalities showed elevated serum and urine lactate and pyruvate, but respiratory chain biochemistry was not reported. Pathologic changes in the brain included mild cortical atrophy, focal zones of cortical softening which microscopically showed neuronal loss, microcyst formation, gliosis, and vascular proliferation. Except in these focal areas, cortex was normal, as were Sommer's sector of Ammon's horn and cerebellar Purkinje cells. Ferrocalcific deposits were present in the blood vessels of the globus pallidus and putamen, but there was no loss of neurons and no gliosis in these deep nuclei. Ultrastructural study of the brain was not reported.

Fukuhara et al. (14) reported two patients with early onset of myoclonus who had mental deterioration, intention tremor, ataxia, muscle atrophy, and foot deformities. Muscle biopsy showed ragged red fibers, which were shown to contain excess mitochondria by electron microscopy. One of the patients had elevated blood lactate and pyruvate. Either an autosomal dominant or maternal inheritance pattern is suggested as one patient's mother and brother had abnormal EEGs. The other patient's mother had died at age 33 years with a history of ataxia. Another brother had ataxia. Brain pathology was reported in one patient but may have been affected by numerous severe accidental head injuries sustained 1 year prior to death at age 22 years. The brain showed multiple minute infarcts in the thalamus, putamen, corpus callosum, and fornix. Neuronal degeneration and gliosis were present in the subthalamic nucleus, striatum, and globus pallidus. The red nucleus showed mild demyelination and axonal degeneration. Cerebellar Purkinje cells showed numerous axonal torpedoes and abnormal dendrites, and there was mild granular cell depopulation. The dentate nuclei showed marked loss and degeneration of neurons and profound fibrillary gliosis with accompanying atrophy of cerebellar peduncles. Severe gliosis was also present in the inferior olivary nuclei, and there was also degeneration of the posterior columns of the spinal cord and loss of neurons in cuneate and gracile nuclei. Ultrastructural studies of the brain were not reported.

Fitzsimons et al. (13) reported a single patient with mitochondrial myopathy with ragged red fibers and confirmatory electron microscopy who also had overt myoclonic epilepsy, cerebellar ataxia, and high tone hearing loss. Once again, maternal inheritance is by a mother and maternal aunt who had involuntary movements. The patient had proximal weakness, preservation of reflexes, normal creatine phosphokinase, and a reduced serum level of leutinizing hormone. There was no dementia.

Morgan-Hughes et al. (33) reported two patients with ragged red fiber myopathy confirmed as mitochondria with electron microscopy. One patient developed myoclonus at age 33 years, which was followed 10 years later by progressive ataxia, deafness, and dementia. Cytochrome b was reduced in her muscle.

Feit et al. (12) reported a patient with myoclonus and mitochondrial myopathy who had hypoventilation. Severe respiratory depression occurred on clonazepam.

Roger et al. (37) reported a single patient with mitochondrial myopathy who developed myoclonus at age 16 years. Sudden loss of visual acuity occurred at age 19 years.

Holliday et al. (19) have reported three patients, two with myoclonus, who had mitochondrial myopathy, progressive dementia, ataxia, and loss of vision and hearing. Severe periodic headaches occurred. Lactate and pyruvate were increased. The BAER were abnormal.

Riggs et al. (35) showed reduced succinate-cytochrome c reductase activity in two siblings who had developed ataxia at age 5 years. Intellectual impairment, myoclonus, rare seizures, and small stature were described. There were many ragged red fibers on muscle biopsy. Serum pyruvate and lactate were normal.

A patient with many similarities to the above group who also had a deficiency of cytochrome b and cytochrome c was reported by Prick et al. (34) as an example of progressive infantile poliodystrophy (Alper's disease). He was a 3-year-old boy who had severe psychomotor retardation, quadriparesis, ataxia, and myoclonus. Skeletal muscle pathology showed no ragged red fibers or abnormal mitochondria on electron microscopy, although lipid storage was present. Cardiac muscle showed abnormal mitochondrial accumulation. Two previous patients with progressive infantile poliodystrophy with myoclonus had been found to have giant neuronal mitochondria in brain by Suzuki and Rapin (44) and by Sandbank and Lerman (39).

Rosing et al. (38) reported a three-generation pedigree containing nine patients affected with mitochondrial myopathy. Three patients had myoclonus. Maternal inheritance and variability of clinical expression were emphasized. The most severely affected living patient had pes cavus deformity at birth and hearing loss in childhood but developed normally until age 14 years, when absence seizures began. Constant repetitive myoclonic jerks appeared and were accompanied by ataxia and dementia. Hyperactive reflexes, extensor plantar responses, severe bilateral sensorineural hearing loss, and chronic hypoventilation were other clinical features. Low-dose clonazepam was used to treat the myoclonus, but respiratory depression occurred, which required intubation. The myoclonus was later reduced but not obliterated by valproic acid.

Her mother and maternal grandmother were both aware of lifelong hearing loss but were not aware of any other difficulty yet both were found to have numerous ragged red fibers on muscle biopsy. One family member with myoclonus was observed over 20 years with minimal CNS deterioration. Two family members, a 16-year-old girl and her 14-year-old sister, were completely asymptomatic, without myoclonus, hearing loss, or ataxia; but they had many abnormal mitochondria-laden muscle fibers.

The EEG, visual evoked responses (VER), somatosensory evoked responses (SER), and brainstem auditory evoked responses (BAER) were performed on members of the family. Like Halliday and Halliday (18), the authors observed in the one patient with active myoclonus that large SER appeared only when accompanied by a clinical myoclonic jerk. However, an unexpected finding was that single evoked responses were uniformly high in amplitude in the least affected family members. Amplitude of photic driving was correspondingly high on EEG. These minimally affected patients never had myoclonus, ataxia, or dementia but were affected with mitochondrial myopathy and hearing loss. The evolution of the electrophysiologic findings from mildly affected to severely affected suggested that the evoked response amplitudes and EEG photic driving responses returned to the normal range as the disease progressed, while diffuse background slowing appeared on the EEG. The BAER were not obtainable in the severely affected patient but were normal in the others. Mitochondrial biochemistry has not been reported in this family, but serum lactate and pyruvate were elevated in two patients, and pyruvate alone was elevated in two other patients.

Nineteen patients have been reviewed who have both mitochondrial myopathy and frequent myoclonus. The majority of the patients had elevated lactate and pyruvate. Four have had measurements of enzymes in the respiratory chain. Two had deficiency of cytochrome b, and two had reduced succinate-cytochrome c reductase. One also had a slight reduction in cytochrome a (see Tables 1 and 2).

TABLE 1. *Myoclonus and mitochondrial myopathy: Clinical and EEG features*

Date	Number with myoclonus	Inheritance[a]	Dementia	Ataxia	Deafness	EEG (photic response)	Ref.
1970	1 of 2	AD	+	+	NR	NR	42
1973	2 of 5	AD or M	0	+	+	+	45
1975	2	AD or M	+	+	+(1)	+ (Photic NR)	40
1980	2	AD or M	+	+	0	+	14
1981	1	AD or M	0	+	+	+ (Photic NR)	13
1981	1	?	+	+	NR	+ (Photic NR)	34
1982	1 of 2	?	+	+	+	+ (Atypical spike–wave)	33
1982	1	?	0	+	NR	+	37
1983	2 of 3	?	+	+	+		19
1983	1	?	+	+	NR	+	12
1983	2	AR	+	NR	NR	Occipital spikes	35
1985	3 of 9	AD	0	+	+	+ (Photic NR)	38

[a]AD, autosomal dominant; AR, autosomal recessive; M, maternal; NR, not reported.

CNS DISEASE AND MITOCHONDRIAL MYOPATHY WITHOUT MYOCLONUS

The preceding discussion has been limited to those few patients with mitochondrial myopathy and CNS disease associated with myoclonus. However, more patients have been reported with mitochondrial myopathy and brain dysfunction who have not had myoclonus.

Hackett et al. (17) reported two patients with mitochondrial myopathy who had elevated serum lactate and pyruvate. One had deafness, and the other had focal motor and generalized seizures. One patient died of refractory lactic acidosis.

A patient reported by Crosby and Chou (7) as an example of Leigh's disease had mitochondrial myopathy, ataxia, extensor plantar responses, sensorineural hearing loss, nystagmus, and lethargy. The CNS pathology showed granular ependymitis; gray-brown discoloration of the globus pallidus, posterior hypothalmus, substantia nigra, and tegmentum of the midbrain, pons, and medulla; an arachnoid cyst in the inferior midline cerebellum; and pancerebellar atrophy, more severe in the anterior vermis. There was mild atrophy of the posterior lateral region of the spinal cord. Microscopically there was a severe symmetric spongiform encephalopathy with rarefaction of the neuropil and spongy or microcyst degeneration but relative preservation of neurons and axis cylinders. The cerebral white matter was involved in a patchy fashion. The change was most severe in globus pallidus, cerebellar white matter, and brainstem tegmentum but also involved substantia nigra, subthalamic nucleus, dorsal gray of the spinal cord, dorsal white matter of the spinal cord, optic radiations, and centrum semiovale. In addition, capillary proliferation and hyperplasia were superimposed and were most severe in periventricular hypothalamus, periaqueductal midbrain, and tegmentum of the medulla, particularly the medial region of the floor of the fourth ventricle. Except for Purkinje cells,

TABLE 2. Myoclonus and mitochondrial myopathy: Pathologic and biochemical features

Date	Number	Ragged red fibers	Electron microscopy[a]	Cytochrome b	Other	Serum lactate	Serum pyruvate	Ref.
		Pathology						
1970	1 of 2	+	+	↓	Cytochrome a ↓	NR	NR	42
1973	2 of 5	+	+	NR	NR	↑3/5	↑3/5	45
1975	2	+(1)	+	NR	NR	↓	↓	40
1980	2	+	+	NR	NR	↓	↓	14
1981	1	+	+	NR	NR	NR	NR	13
1981	1	(Heart)	− skeletal muscle	↓	Cytochrome c ↓	N	N	34
1982	1	+	+	↓	NAOH–CoQ ↓ (1)	↓	↓	33
1982	1	+	NR	NR	NR	↓	↓	37
1983	2 of 3	+	+	NR	NR	N	N	19
1983	2	+	+	Normal: cytochrome c oxidase NADH-cytochrome c reductase	Succinate: cytochrome c reductase ↓	N	N	35
1983	1	+	+	NR	NR	NR	NR	12
1985	3 of 9	+	+	NR	NR	↓	↑	38

[a]NR, not reported; N, normal.

which were abnormal, there were no definite abnormalities of neurons. Electron microscopic study of the brain was not reported.

A patient reported by McLeod et al. (30) had dementia, seizures, and ataxia. No CNS pathology was available.

Although CNS pathology was not reported in the cases reviewed by Bertorini et al. (3), computerized tomography (CT) scans were done on 13 patients with progressive external ophthalmoplegia associated with mitochondrial myopathy who had a high incidence of intellectual impairment and hearing loss. The CT showed diffuse attenuation of the white matter (leukoencephalopathy) in three patients and brainstem atrophy in one. One of the patients showed diffuse leukoencephalopathy in the cerebral hemispheres, cerebellum, and brainstem.

Askanas et al. (1) reported two patients with mitochondrial myopathy and seizures and very abnormal EEGs. The authors were able to reproduce the mitochondrial abnormality in the muscle in cultured muscle cells, suggesting that the defect producing the abnormal mitochondria was intrinsic. Lactic acidosis was present, but mitochondrial biochemistry was not reported.

The patient reported by Skoglund (41) had mitochondrial myopathy, lactic acidemia, hemianopia, and alexia. No CNS pathology was reported, but a CT scan showed lucencies in both parietal and occipital regions and increased density in the area of the basal ganglia bilaterally.

Markesbery (28) reported a patient with mitochondrial myopathy and lactic acidosis who had basal ganglia calcifications on CT scan in the presence of normal serum calcium and phosphorus. Basal ganglia calcifications had also been noted in other muscle mitochondrial disorders reported by Britton et al. (6), Hart et al. (22), and Shapira et al. (40).

Hart et al. (22) reported a dominantly inherited form of poliodystrophy (Alper's disease) associated with mitochondrial myopathy. The proband had mitochondrial myopathy, progressive dementia, absence spells, tonic spasms, progressive deterioration, and mild hearing loss. A CT scan showed dilated ventricles. His sister developed seizures at age 7 years and then homonymous hemianopia, numerous minor and major seizures, episodes of mutism, and episodes of total blindness. She developed permanent hemiplegia and died at 18 years of age. Muscle pathology was not obtained. The CNS pathology showed cortical atrophy with loss of neurons in cortex, gliosis, and spongy alteration of layers of the cerebral cortex. In addition, profound neuronal alterations were present in the basal ganglia and in the granular cell layer of the cerebellum but not in hippocampus. The basal ganglia contained granular basophilic deposits consistent with an iron mucopolysaccharide calcium complex, which were largely confined to blood vessels. Serum lactate and pyruvate were increased.

The type of mitochondrial myopathy with the largest number of patients, progressive external ophthalmoplegia, was extensively discussed by Berenberg et al. (2) with specific interest in the CNS manifestations. The authors reviewed 35 patients with progressive external ophthalmoplegia, atypical pigmentary degeneration of retina, and heart block. All patients had abnormal muscle mitochondria.

There was a high incidence of CNS abnormalities. Cerebellar signs occurred in 24 (69%), sensorineural hearing loss in 19 (54%), mental retardation in 14 (40%), and dysfunction of the vestibular system in 11 of 13 patients who were tested (85%). Of the 35 patients, 31 (89%) had either cerebellar signs, hearing loss, vestibular dysfunction, or impaired intellect.

Finally, Harden et al. (21) found CNS dysfunction in every case in an unselected series of patients with mitochondrial myopathy when specifically searched for with modern electroencephalography, electroretinography, and VER. Eight of 13 had progressive external ophthalmoplegia (10). Only two of their 13 patients had seizures that were both focal and grand mal, not myoclonic. However, four patients showed paroxysmal features during photic stimulation, which in one patient was associated with a single, whole-body jerk.

Like those with myoclonus, patients with mitochondrial myopathy and CNS disease without myoclonus have ataxia, deafness, dementia, and elevated lactate and pyruvate levels. Other features may include hemianopia and ophthalmoplegia, basal ganglia calcification, and CT signs of leukoencephalopathy. Two patients had diffuse spongiform encephalopathy.

RELATIONSHIP TO OTHER DISORDERS WITH MYOCLONUS

An etiologic classification of myoclonus by Marsden et al. (29) included four categories: (a) physiologic (normal subjects), (b) essential (no other deficit), (c) epileptic (seizures dominate but no encephalopathy), and (d) symptomatic (in which a progressive or static encephalopathy dominates). They recognized nine varieties of symptomatic myoclonus: (a) storage diseases (including Lafora body disease), (b) spinocerebellar degenerations (including the Ramsay Hunt syndrome), (c) basal ganglia degenerations, (d) dementias, (e) viral encephalopathies, (f) metabolic encephalopathies, (g) toxic encephalopathies, (h) physical encephalopathies, and (i) focal CNS damage. Myoclonus associated with mitochondrial myopathy does not conform to any one of these types of symptomatic myoclonus.

Patients with myoclonus and mitochondrial myopathy have not been shown to have storage disease. No material has been found comparable to a Lafora body, and there is no other evidence of storage material.

The Ramsay Hunt syndrome has been classified by Marsden et al. (29) under spinocerebellar degenerations. The Ramsay Hunt syndrome and Unverricht–Lundborg disease are recessively inherited disorders that have been referred to as degenerative types of myoclonic epilepsies by others. Myoclonus associated with mitochondrial myopathy usually follows either a maternal or autosomal dominant inheritance, but patients resemble those with degenerative myoclonic epilepsy. It is possible that those older series contained individual families who had mitochondrial myopathy, but muscle pathology was not reported. Because of the muscle mitochondrial abnormality and biochemical defects, patients with myoclonus associated with mitochondrial myopathy should not be classified under spinocerebellar degenerations.

Basal ganglia pathology has been reported in myoclonus with mitochondrial myopathy, but extensive cortical and cerebellar changes are present as well. Dementia occurs in severely affected patients, but less severely affected family members may not be demented. No viral encephalopathy has been found. Metabolic defects (reduced components of the respiratory chain and lactate acidemia) are common, but the syndrome does not fit well into the group of metabolic encephalopathies. No toxin has been discovered, nor has any physical brain injury been found. Finally, multifocal CNS damage has been reported, but the implications of the classification is that a single focal lesion may cause myoclonus. These patients are more complex.

Until more complete biochemical studies are available, myoclonus associated with mitochondrial myopathy should be listed separately in the symptomatic myoclonus category.

RELATIONSHIP TO KNOWN MITOCHONDRIAL MYOPATHIES

Mitochondrial myopathies have been reviewed by DiMauro (9). He identified 15 categories which he separated on the basis of biochemical features when known and on clinical grounds when biochemical data were lacking. Patients in seven of the 15 categories frequently have evidence of CNS involvement:

1. Pyruvate dehydrogenase complex deficiency (4,5,11,36,43): psychomotor retardation, microcephaly, ataxia, progressive encephalopathy;
2. Pyruvate carboxylase deficiency (8): psychomotor retardation, dystonia, seizures;
3. Subacute necrotizing encephalomyelopathy (Leigh's disease) (7,47): progressive encephalopathy with ataxia, ophthalmoplegia, respiratory disturbance; one patient had muscle cytochrome c oxidase deficiency;
4. Cytochrome b deficiency (32–34,42): one with myoclonus, ataxia, dementia, ophthalmoplegia; one without CNS signs;
5. Cerebrohepatorenal syndrome of Zellweger (16): nystagmus, hypotonia, CNS pathology;
6. Progressive external ophthalmoplegia (2,3): ataxia, hearing loss, mental retardation; and
7. Myopathy, growth retardation, lactic acidosis and cerebral disease (15,22, 31,40,41): includes patients with myoclonus.

DISCUSSION

It is clear that CNS disease exists in many patients who have mitochondrial myopathy, and that many have evidence of defective substrate utilization and energy production by mitochondria with elevation of serum lactate and pyruvate and deficiency of components of the respiratory chain. This suggests that mitochondrial proliferation is a secondary phenomenon, an effort to compensate for the inborn defect.

There is experimental evidence that muscle mitochondria do proliferate in response to metabolic stress. Experimental ischemia will produce mitochondrial alterations in muscle (20,23–25). In addition, Walter et al. (46) showed that abnormal muscle mitochondria will appear after experimental sciatic nerve stimulation, after uncoupling of oxidative phosphorylation, and after inhibition of membrane adenosine triphosphatase by ouabain.

Because most reports of mitochondrial myopathy have not included electron microscopy of brain tissue, it is not clear if the CNS manifestations are accompanied by the same type of change in mitochondria that is present in muscle. It is known, however, that CNS mitochondria will also proliferate in response to metabolic stress. Anoxia, hypoglycemia, puromycin injection, and viral infection have been associated with changes in brain mitochondria (44).

It is not clear why myoclonus occurs in some patients with mitochondrial myopathy and not in others. It is tempting to speculate that myoclonus and other epileptic phenomena indicate that the abnormality in those patients is particularly severe in neurons or at least in cerebral cortex as opposed to white matter. Two pathologic studies of those with myoclonus and one study of those without support this distinction. More nerve cell involvement was present in the patients with myoclonus (14,40). The white matter was more involved, and neurons were relatively spared in the patient with CNS disease who did not have myoclonus (7).

CONCLUSIONS

Encephalopathy may accompany mitochondrial myopathy, dominate the clinical picture, and be accompanied by myoclonus. In other patients, the encephalopathy may be so mild that it is not clinically apparent, and electrophysiologic studies may be required to demonstrate any CNS abnormality.

If a patient with unexplained myoclonus is found to have elevation of serum lactate and pyruvate, abnormal mitochondrial biochemistry should be suspected, and muscle biopsy for appropriate studies should be considered.

Mitochondrial disease may be maternally inherited. This type of inheritance is present if the pedigree shows that myoclonus or some other clinical feature, such as hearing loss, is transmitted by affected females to all her offspring of both sexes but not transmitted to any offspring by affected males.

Pathologic changes in the nervous system have a wide distribution in severely affected patients with mitochondrial myopathy and CNS disease. Multiple clinical manifestations appear, which reflect this widespread involvement.

It is not known if the neuronal changes in patients with myoclonus are accompanied by mitochondrial accumulation. Perhaps electron microscopic study of cerebral cortex and deep nuclei in those with myoclonus and those without will provide useful information.

SUMMARY

The CNS diseases that are associated with mitochondrial myopathy have been reviewed in this chapter. The disorders causing myoclonus have been compared to those in which myoclonus has been reported. Both groups have been associated with lactate and pyruvate accumulation, and both have a wide spectrum of clinical and pathologic findings.

Deficiency of components of the respiratory chain has been offered as an explanation for the mitochondrial accumulation in the muscles of these patients. Skeletal muscle respiratory-chain components may be deficient, and there is experimental evidence that indicates that mitochondria will proliferate in muscle and other tissues when vital nutrients are withheld.

There are two features of these patients that separate them from other patients with myoclonus. The first is the elevation of serum lactate and pyruvate due to deficient oxidative phosphorylation. The second is a pedigree that indicates maternal inheritance.

ACKNOWLEDGMENTS

The authors thank Drs. Robert F. Kibler, Douglas C. Wallace, and Charles M. Epstein for their assistance and advice. Also, we especially thank Mrs. Mary Ellen Skehan for her editorial assistance and for typing the manuscript.

REFERENCES

1. Askanas V, Engel WK, Britton DE, Adornato BT, Eiben RM. Reincarnation in cultured muscle of mitochondrial abnormalities. Two patients with epilepsy and lactic acidosis. *Arch Neurol* 1978; 35:801–9.
2. Berenberg RA, Pellock JM, DiMauro S, Schotland DL, Bonilla E, Eastwood A, Hayes A, Vicale CT, Behrens M, Schutorian A, Rowland LP. Lumping or splitting. "Ophthalmoplegia-plus" or Kearns-Sayre syndrome? *Ann Neurol* 1977; 1:37–54.
3. Bertorini T, Engel WK, DiChiro G, Dalakas M. Leukoencephalopathy in oculocraniosomatic neuromuscular disease with ragged red fibers (mitochondrial abnormalities). *Arch Neurol* 1978; 35:643–7.
4. Blass JP, Gibson GE, Kark RAP. Pyruvate dehydrogenase phosphatase deficiency: a cause of congenital chronic lactic acidosis in infancy. *Pediatr Res* 1975; 9:939.
5. Blass JP, Cederbaum SD, Gibson GE. Clinical and metabolic abnormalities accompanying deficiencies in pyruvate oxidation. In: Hommes FA, van der Berg CJ, eds. *Normal and pathological development of energy metabolism.* London: Wiley & Sons, 1975:193–210.
6. Britton DE, Pellock JM, Eiben RN. Acute hemiplegia of childhood, lactate pyruvate acidemia and mitochondrial disorder. *Ann Neurol* 1977; 22:265.
7. Crosby TW, Chou SM. "Ragged red" fibers in Leigh's disease. *Neurology* 1974; 24:49–54.
8. DeVivo DC, Haymond MW, Leckie MP, Bussmann YL, McDouglas DB, Pagliara AS. The clinical and biochemical implications of pyruvate carboxylase deficiency. *J Clin Endocrinol Metab* 1977; 45:1281–96.
9. DiMauro S. Metabolic myopathies. In: Vinken PJ, Byrun GW, eds. *Handbook of clinical neurology.* Amsterdam: Elsevier North-Holland, 1979; 41:175–234.
10. Egger J, Lake BD, Wilson J. Mitochondrial cytopathy. A multisystem disorder with ragged red fibers on muscle biopsy. *Arch Dis Child* 1981; 56:741–52.
11. Farrell DF, Clark AF, Scott CR, Wennberg RP. Absence of pyruvate decarboxylase activity in man: a cause of congenital lactic acidosis. *Science* 1975; 187:1082–4.
12. Feit H, Kirkpatrick J, VanWoert MH, Pandian G. Myoclonus, ataxia and hypoventilation: response to L-5 hydroxytryptophane. *Neurology* 1983; 33:109–12.
13. Fitzsimons RB, Clifton-Bligh P, Wolfenden WH. Mitochondrial myopathy and lactate acidemia with myoclonic epilepsy, ataxia and hypothalamic infertility: a variant of Ramsay-Hunt syndrome? *J Neurol Neurosurg Psychiatry* 1981; 44:79–82.
14. Fukuhara N, Tokiguchi S, Shirakawa K, Tsubaki T. Myoclonus epilepsy associated with ragged

red fibers (mitochondrial abnormalities): disease entity or a syndrome? *J Neurol Sci* 1980; 47:117–33.

15. Gardner-Medwin D, Dale G, Parkin JM. Lactic acidosis and mitochondrial myopathy and recurrent coma. *Internat Congr Child Neurol Toronto 1st.* 1975:47(Abstr).

16. Goldfischer S, Moore CL, Johnson AB, Spiro AJ, Valsamis MP, Wisniewski HK, Ritch RH, Norton WT, Rapin I, Gartner LM. Peroxisomal and mitochondrial defects in the cerebro-hepatorenal syndrome. *Science* 1973; 182:62–4.

17. Hackett TN, Bray PF, Ziter FA, Nyhan WL, Creer KM. A metabolic myopathy associated with chronic lactic acidemia, growth failure, and nerve deafness. *J Pediatr* 1973; 83:426–31.

18. Halliday AM, Halliday E. Cerebral somatosensory and visual evoked potentials in different clinical forms of myoclonus. In: Desmedt JE, ed. *Clinical uses of cerebral brainstem and spinal somatosensory evoked potentials.* Basal: Karger, 1980:292–310. (Progress in clinical neurophysiology, vol. 7.)

19. Holliday PR, Climie ARW, Gilgroy J, Mahmud MZ. Mitochondrial myopathy and encephalopathy: three cases-a deficiency of NAOH–CoQ dehydrogenase? *Neurology* 1983;33:1619–22.

20. Hanzlikova V, Schiaffino S. Mitochondrial changes in ischemic skeletal muscle. *J Ultrastruct Res* 1977; 60:121–33.

21. Harden A, Pampiglione G, Battaglia A. "Mitochondrial myopathy" or mitochondrial disease? EEG, ERG, VEP studies in 13 children. *J Neurol Neurosurg Psychiatry* 1982; 45:627–32.

22. Hart ZH, Chang CH, Perrin EVD, Neerunjuin JS, Ayyar R. Familial poliodystrophy, mitochondrial myopathy and lactate acidemia. *Arch Neurol* 1977; 34:180–5.

23. Heffner RR, Barron SA. The early effects of ischemia upon skeletal muscle mitochondria. *J Neurol Sci* 1978; 38:295–315.

24. Karpati G, Carpenter S, Melmed C, Eisen AA. Experimental ischemic myopathy. *J Neurol Sci* 1974; 23:129–61.

25. Kelts KA, Kaiser KK. Experimental ischemic myopathy. *J Neurol Sci* 1979; 40:23–7.

26. Koenigsberger MR, Pellock JM, DiMauro S, Eastwood AB. Juvenile mitochondrial myopathy, short stature, and lactic acidosis: a clinical ultrastructural and biochemical study. *Nat Meet Child Neurol Soc Monterey, 5th. 1976* (Abstr.).

27. Luft R, Ikkos D, Palmieri G, Eruster, Afzelius B. A case of severe hypermetabolism of nonthyroid origin with a defect in the maintenance of mitochondrial respiratory control: a correlated clinical, biochemical, and morphological study. *J Clin Invest* 1962; 41:1776–804.

28. Markesbery WR. Lactic acidemia, mitochondrial myopathy and basal ganglia calcification. *Neurology* 1979; 29:1057–61.

29. Marsden CD, Hallett M, Fahn S. The nosology and pathophysiology of myoclonus. In: *Movement disorders.* London: Butterworth, 1982:196–248.

30. McLeod JG, Baker WC, Shorey CD, Kerr CB. Mitochondrial myopathy with multisystem abnormalities and normal ocular movements. *J Neurol Sci* 1975; 24:39–52.

31. Monnens LF, Gabreels F, Willems J. A metabolic myopathy associated with chronic lactic acidemia, growth failure, and nerve deafness. *J Pediatr* 1975; 86:983.

32. Morgan-Hughes JA, Darveniza P, Kahn SN, Landon DN, Sherratt RM, Land JM, Clark JB. A mitochondrial myopathy characterized by a deficiency in reducible cytochrome b. *Brain* 1977; 100:617–40.

33. Morgan-Hughes JA, Hayes DJ, Clark JB, Landon DN, Swash M, Stark RJ, Rudge P. Mitochondrial encephalomyopathies, biochemical studies in two cases revealing defects in the respiratory chain. *Brain* 1982; 105:553–82.

34. Prick MJJ, Gabreels FJM, Renier WO, Trijbels JMF, Sengers RCA, Slooff JL. Progressive infantile poliodystrophy. *Arch Neurol* 1981; 38:767–72.

35. Riggs JE, Schochet DD, Fakadej AV, Papadimitrious A, DiMauro S, Crosby TW, Gutman L, Moxley RT. Mitochondrial encephalomyopathy with decreased succinate cytochrome c reductase activity. *Neurology* 1984;34:48–53.

36. Robinson BH, Sherwood WG. Pyruvate dehydrogenase phosphatase deficiency: a cause of congenital chronic lactic acidosis in infancy. *Pediatr Res* 1975; 9:935–9.

37. Roger J, Pellissier JF, Dravet C, Bureau-Paillas M, Arnoux M, Larrieu JL. Degenerescence spinocerebelleuse-atrophie optique-epilepsie-myoclonus-myopathic mitochondriale. Cent. Saint-Paul, 13009 Marseille, France. *Rev Neurol (Paris)* 1982; 138/3:187–200.

38. Rosing HS, Hopkins LC, Wallace DC, Epstein CM, Weidenheim K. Maternally inherited mitochondrial myopathy and myoclonic epilepsy. *Ann Neurol* 1984;17:228–37.

39. Sandbank U, Lerman P. Progressive cerebral poliodystrophy—Alper's disease. *J Neurol Neurosurg Psychiatry* 1972; 35:749–55.
40. Shapira Y, Cederbaum SD, Cancilla PA, Nielsen D, Lippe BM. Familial poliodystrophy, mitochondrial myopathy and lactate acidemia. *Neurology* 1975; 23:614–21.
41. Skoglund RR. Reversible alexia, mitochondrial myopathy and lactic acidemia. *Neurology* 1979; 29:717–20.
42. Spiro AJ, Moore SL, Prineas JW, Strasberg PM, Rapin I. A cytochrome related inherited disorder of the nervous system and muscle. *Arch Neurol* 1970; 23:103–12.
43. Stromme JH, Borud O, Moe P. Fatal lactic acidosis in a newborn attributable to a congenital defect of pyruvate dehydrogenase. *Pediatr Res* 1976; 10:60–6.
44. Suzuki K, Rapin I. Giant neuronal mitochondria in an infant with microcephaly and seizure disorder. *Arch Neurol* 1969; 220:62–72.
45. Tsairis P, Engel WK, Kark P. Familial myoclonic epilepsy syndrome associated with skeletal muscle mitochondrial abnormalities. *Neurology* 1973; 23:409 (Abstr.).
46. Walter GF, Brucher JM, Tassin S, Bergmans J. Experimental changes in muscle mitochondria induced by electric stimulation and inhibition of energy metabolism. In: Busch HFM, Jennenkens FGI, Scholte HR, eds. *Mitochondria and muscular diseases.* Beetsterzwaag, The Netherlands: Mefar BV, 1981:107–11.
47. Williems JL, Mommens LAM, Trijbels JMF, Veerkamp JH, Meyer AEFH, Van Dam K, Van Haelst U. Leigh's encephalomyelopathy in a patient with cytochrome c oxidase deficiency in muscle tissue. *Pediatrics* 1977; 60:850–7.

Advances in Neurology, Vol. 43: Myoclonus,
edited by S. Fahn et al. Raven Press,
New York © 1986.

Biotin-Responsive Encephalopathy with Myoclonus, Ataxia, and Seizures

Susan Bressman, Stanley Fahn, Max Eisenberg, Mitchell Brin, and
William Maltese

*Departments of Neurology and Biochemistry, and Division of Pediatric Neurology,
Columbia University, College of Physicians and Surgeons, and The Neurological Institute
of New York, New York, New York 10032*

Biotin, a water-soluble vitamin, serves in man as a coenzyme in four carboxylation reactions: pyruvate (PC), propionyl-CoA (PCC), methylcrotonyl-CoA (MCC), and acetyl-CoA (ACC) carboxylase (Figs. 1 and 2) (1,2). Biotin is covalently bound to the various apocarboxylases to form holoenzyme in a two-step reaction activated by holocarboxylase synthetase:

$$(A) \quad d\text{-biotin} + ATP \overset{Mg^{2+}}{\rightleftharpoons} d\text{-biotinyl-5'-AMP} + PP_i$$

$$(B) \quad d\text{-biotinyl-5'-AMP} + apocarboxylase \rightarrow holocarboxylase + AMP$$

$$Net: \quad d\text{-biotin} + ATP + apocarboxylase \overset{Mg^{2+}}{\rightarrow} holocarboxylase + AMP + PP_i$$

It is thought to be recycled for reutilization by the enzyme biotinidase, which cleaves biotin from the ϵ-amino group of lysine, through which biotin is covalently bound to the carboxylases (3). The absorption in man of biotin has not been fully established, but dietary sources as well as gut bacterial synthesis appear to contribute to nutritional requirements (1,2).

Recent reports (2,4–6) have drawn attention to the clinical significance of biotin dependence and deficiency in human disease and the use of biotin as a therapeutic agent. In particular, there has been elucidation of the clinical and biochemical findings in infants and young children with biotin-responsive multiple carboxylase deficiencies (MCD).

Two major subtypes of MCD have been proposed (2,10,12). The first, a neonatal form, generally appears in the first days to first weeks of life in the form of lethargy, vomiting, and metabolic acidosis. The biotin-dependent carboxylase activities are diminished in both fresh leukocytes and fibroblasts grown in biotin-deficient media; plasma biotin levels are normal. The primary enzymatic defect is an abnormality of holocarboxylase synthetase (2,7–9).

The second form, known as late-onset or juvenile MCD, generally appears in the first months of life; clinical features include skin rash, alopecia, seizures,

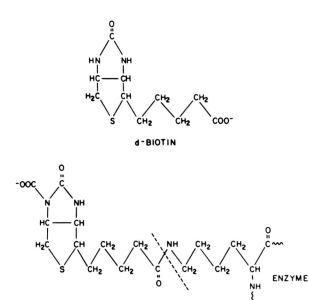

d-BIOTIN

N-CARBOXYBIOTIN   LYSYL RESIDUE

FIG. 1. The structure of *d*-biotin and *N*-carboxybiotin covalently attached to the ε-lysine residue of a carboxylase enzyme (2).

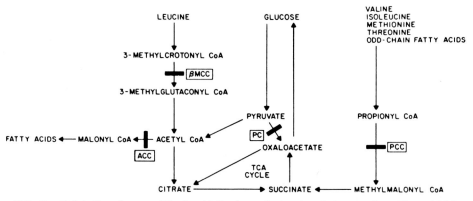

FIG. 2. Metabolic pathways of the four biotin-dependent carboxylation reactions. Sites of PCC, PC, BMCC, and ACC are indicated by black bars (2).

myoclonus, ataxia, immunologic disturbances, and hearing loss (2,10). Ketoacidosis and organic aciduria are frequently but not uniformly present (11). Carboxylase activities in fresh leukocytes are often diminished. Fibroblasts, however, display the same carboxylase activities as controls regardless of the biotin concentration of the culture medium. Biotin levels are low or normal (10–13). Recent studies suggest that the primary enzyme defect in many of these patients is a deficiency of biotinidase (14–17).

Although there is considerable variation in the clinical and biochemical expressions in reported cases of biotin-responsive MCD, all were symptomatic by 24 months (11,14). In contrast to these inborn errors of metabolism, acquired deficiencies have been reported in adults and children. Causes for such acquired deficiency include ingestion of avidin (contained in raw egg whites), which binds biotin (18), and parenteral alimentation lacking biotin in patients with intestinal abnormalities that presumably result in impaired microbial biosynthesis and/or absorption of biotin (19). Symptoms include skin rash, hair loss, pallor, lethargy, hallucinations, headache, hyperesthesias, anorexia, and vomiting.

We present a young woman with adult-onset myoclonus, ataxia, hearing loss, seizures, hemianopia, and hemiparesis who had a low plasma level of biotin despite a normal diet and apparent normal absorption and who responded to pharmacologic dosages of biotin.

CASE REPORT

The patient is a 30-year-old right-handed woman. Her parents are unrelated, and there is no family history of neurologic disease. Her diet and development were normal, and she was always considered an excellent athlete and student. She had occasional problems hearing as an adolescent, but these were not evaluated. In her early twenties, she experienced intermittent unsteadiness and in gym class was forbidden to climb ropes. Nevertheless, she became a superb rock climber.

At age 23, during her training to become a physical therapist, a routine physical examination was normal. At age 24, her colleagues told her she was having occasional jerking movements of her trunk. She became aware of increased hearing difficulty, and became unsteady while walking. One year later, seizures began and were difficult to control. Clonazepam, phenytoin, phenobarbital, carbamazepine, and valproate were given for seizures and myoclonus but were ineffective or toxic. Some caused attacks of bronchospasm and skin rash, although these also occurred spontaneously. At age 25, a sustained right hemiparesis developed after a right focal seizure. Several weeks later, serial examinations revealed an evolving left hemianopia. A trial of 5-hydroxytryptophan and carbidopa reduced the myoclonus but had no effect on other symptoms.

In February 1983 at the age of 28, she was admitted to the hospital. Mentation was normal. A homonymous left hemianopia was present. There was ocular dysmetria, jerky pursuit, fixation instability, and slowing of saccades. There was a moderately severe sensorineural hearing loss with 48% speech discrimination on the left and a profound hearing loss with 44% speech discrimination on the right. She used sign language and lip-reading to communicate. The limbs were hypotonic, and a right hemiparesis was present. There was marked limb and gait ataxia. Low-amplitude spontaneous and action multifocal myoclonus were present. There were hyperreflexia with sustained ankle clonus and bilateral Babinski signs.

Laboratory studies that were normal included computed tomography (CT) scan; cerebrospinal fluid (CSF) protein, glucose, cell count, γ-globulin and oligoclonal bands; nerve-conduction velocities; electromyogram (EMG); muscle, nerve, and rectal biopsies; arterial pH, lactate and ammonia; and plasma amino acids. The electroencephalogram (EEG) was mildly and diffusely slow. Serum IgG was depressed at 479 mg/dl.

Since we were aware that the juvenile MCD syndrome resembled our patient clinically, a plasma biotin level was obtained. It was found to be undetectable as measured by an auxanographic procedure using a biotin auxotroph of *E. coli* (controls, 290–500 pg/ml). Pyruvate carboxylase activity in fresh leukocytes was undetectable as well. All four biotin-dependent carboxylase enzyme activities, however, were the same as in control skin fibroblasts grown in biotin-enriched and -deficient media. The organic acids 3-hydroxyisovaleric and 3-hydroxypropionic were elevated in urine. Both clinical and laboratory findings suggested biotin-dependent carboxylase deficiencies, and she was treated with pharmacologic dosages of oral biotin varying from 3 to 20 mg/day. After 48 h, there was marked improvement. After 4 days, myoclonus, ataxia, hemianopia, and hemiparesis resolved. Hearing on the left and eye movements were entirely normal. A moderate right hearing loss remained, and reflexes were brisk. Plasma biotin level determined on day 4, ½ hour after an oral dose of 1.5 mg (25μ/kg) of biotin, was markedly elevated at >5,000 pg/ml. Pyruvate carboxylase activity in fresh leukocytes was the same as controls, and urinary organic acids were now normal.

The patient did well for 2 months and then had partial recurrence of symptoms despite increasing biotin dosages to 75 mg/day and elevated plasma biotin levels. There was return of moderate gait and mild limb ataxia, ankle and wrist clonus, and Babinski signs. Episodic respiratory insufficiency also occurred. This was secondary to upper and lower airway and laryngeal dyscoordination, as well as to bronchospasm. The latter responded partially to steroids and bronchodilators.

During the summer of 1983, while the patient remained on steroids, biotin was discontinued. After 2 months, there was respiratory and to a lesser extent neurological deterioration. Biotin level was normal and propionyl CoA and β-methyl-crotonyl CoA carboxylase (BMCC) activities in fresh leukocytes did not change significantly during this period off biotin. However, activities of PCC were <25% of controls and BMCC activities were <40% of controls before, during, and at the conclusion of the trial off biotin. There was no organic aciduria 2 months after discontinuation of biotin.

Biotin was restarted at 300 mg, and peak plasma level exceeded that in the control subject (Fig. 3), suggesting adequate absorption. There was clinical improvement after reinstitution of biotin. Subsequently, during the past year, neurological deterioration has consistently occurred after discontinuation of biotin. A tracheostomy was performed for respiratory insufficiency, and the respiratory status has remained stable despite tapering of the steroids. Furthermore, a recent episode of headache, nausea, and vomiting was followed by left hemiparesis and confusion. The hemiparesis resolved over days with reinstitution of biotin 3.0 mg/day. An MRI scan was performed at the time and was entirely normal. The patient's biotindase activity in serum was assessed colorimetrically in two different labora-

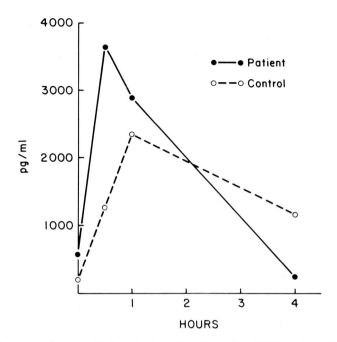

FIG. 3. Response of plasma biotin to the ingestion of 5 µg/kg of biotin in the patient (●) and in a normal control (○).

tories by measuring *p*-aminobenzoate liberation from *N*-biotinyl-*p*-aminobenzoate. It was found to be normal.

DISCUSSION

Our patient has adult-onset encephalopathy with myoclonus, ataxia, fluctuating hemiparesis, hearing loss, hemianopia, and seizures. Her initial response to pharmacologic dosages of biotin was dramatic with near resolution of all symptoms. Subsequently, there has been partial recurrence of symptoms, although seizures have not recurred; vision is normal, and hearing loss and myoclonus remain markedly improved on biotin. Her initial laboratory findings of (a) low plasma biotin, (b) low leukocyte pyruvate carboxylase activity, (c) organic aciduria, and (d) fibroblast carboxylase activities similar to normal controls, suggested late-onset MCD. Many of these patients have a deficiency of biotinidase, which is not present in our patient. Also, she appears to have normal absorption of biotin. We have not, however, studied renal excretion of biotin, which has been reported to be abnormal in children with late-onset MCD (6,17).

Further investigations are necessary to delineate the metabolic defect in this patient. She does not appear to fit either subcategory of MCD. Carboxylase activities of fibroblasts grown in biotin-deficient media were the same as controls, excluding infantile-onset holocarboxylase synthetase deficiency; further, biotinidase activity was normal, thus excluding what appears to be the major cause of late-onset MCD. Possible alternative explanations include the presence of some other deficiency state that results in abnormal carboxylation and partial response to biotin, or the presence of a competitor or inhibitor of biotin. Indeed, a recent paper (20) reported the successful treatment of myoclonus with biotin in chronically hemodialyzed patients. The authors propose a circulating inhibitor (possibly a metal) of the biotin-dependent carboxylases in uremia.

There are many patients with unexplained myoclonic syndromes with ataxia and seizures. A subset of these patients may, like our patient, improve with biotin therapy. We therefore advocate that these patients be evaluated for biotin-dependent carboxylase deficiencies and possible therapy with biotin.

SUMMARY

Prominent neurological abnormalities, including myoclonus, seizures, ataxia, and hearing loss, have been noted in juvenile-onset biotin-responsive MCD. The underlying defect in many of these patients, who generally present in the first year of life, appears to be a deficiency of biotinidase. We have presented a young woman with adult-onset myoclonus, ataxia, hearing loss, seizures, hemianopia, and hemiparesis who responded to pharmacologic dosages of biotin. Although she displayed many of the clinical and biochemical features of juvenile-onset MCD, she did not have a biotinidase deficiency, and the underlying defect remains to be determined. Because of her response to biotin, we have advocated that other patients with unexplained myoclonus syndromes be evaluated for biotin-dependent carboxylase deficiencies and undergo a therapeutic trial with biotin.

REFERENCES

1. Roth KS. Biotin in clinical medicine—a review. *Am J Clin Nutr* 1981;34:1967–74.
2. Wolf B, Feldman GL. The biotin-dependent carboxylase deficiencies. *Am J Hum Genet* 1982;34(5):699–716.
3. Koivvsalo M, Pispa J. Biotinidase activity in animal tissues. *Acta Physiol Scand* 1963;58:13–19.
4. Sander JE, Malamud N, Cowan MJ, Packman S, Amman AJ, Wara DW. Intermittent ataxia and immunodeficiency with multiple carboxylase deficiencies: a biotin-responsive disorder. *Ann Neurol* 1980;8(5):544–7.
5. Munnich A, Saudubray JM, Cotisson A, Coude FX, Ogier H, Charpentier C, Marsac C, Carre G, Bourgeay-Causse M, Frezal J. The biotin-dependent multiple carboxylase deficiency presenting as a congenital lacticacidosis. *Eur J Pediatr* 1981;137(2):203–6.
6. Thoene JG, Lemons R, Baker H. Impaired intestinal absorption of biotin in juvenile multiple carboxylase deficiency. *N Engl J Med* 1983;308(11):639–42.
7. Saunders ME, Sherwood WG, Duthie M, Surh L, Gravel RA. Evidence for a defect of holocarboxylase synthetase activity in cultured lymphoblasts from a patient with biotin-responsive multiple carboxylase deficiency. *Am J Hum Genet* 1982;34(4):590–601.
8. Burri BJ, Sweetman L, Nyhan WL. Mutant holocarboxylase synthetase; evidence for the enzyme defect in early infantile biotin-responsive multiple carboxylase deficiency. *J Clin Invest* 1981;68(6):1491–5.
9. Roth KJ, Yang W, Foreman JW, Rothman R, Segal S. Holocarboxylase synthetase deficiency. A biotin-responsive organic acidemia. *J Pediatr* 1980;96:845–9.
10. Thoene J, Baker H, Yoshino M, Sweetman L. Biotin-responsive carboxylase deficiency associated with subnormal plasma and urinary biotin. *N Engl J Med* 1981;304:817–20.

11. Swick HM, Kien CL. Biotin deficiency with neurologic and cutaneous manifestations but without organic aciduria. *J Pediatr* 1983;103(2):265–7.

12. Packman S, Caswell NM, Baker H. Biochemical evidence for diverse etiologies in biotin-responsive multiple carboxylase deficiency. *Biochem Genet* 1982;20(1-2):17–28.

13. Packman S, Sweetman L, Yoshino M, Baker H, Cowan M. Biotin-responsive multiple carboxylase deficiency of infantile onset. *J Pediatr* 1981;99:421–3.

14. Wolf B, Grier RE, Allen RJ, Goodman SL, Kien CL, Parker WD, Howell DM, Hurst DL. Phenotypic variation in biotinidase deficiency. *J Pediatr* 1983;103(2):233–7.

15. Wolf B, Grier RE, Allen RJ, Goodman SL, Kien CL. Biotinidase deficiency: the enzymatic defect in late-onset multiple carboxylase deficiency. *Clin Chem Acta* 1983;131(3):273–81.

16. Thoene J, Wolf B. Biotinidase deficiency in juvenile multiple carboxylase deficiency. *Lancet* 1983;2(8346):398.

17. Baumgartner ER, Suormala T, Wick H, Bonjour JP. Biotin-responsive multiple carboxylase deficiency: deficient biotinidase activity associated with renal loss of biotin. *J Inherited Metab Dis* 1984;6(Suppl 2):123–5.

18. Sweetman L, Surh L, Baker H, Peterson RM, Nyhan WL. The clinical and metabolic abnormalities in a boy with dietary deficiency of biotin. *Pediatrics* 1981;68(4):553–8.

19. Mock DM, Delorimer AA, Leibman WM, Sweetman L, Baker H. Biotin deficiency, an unusual complication of parenteral alimentation. *N Engl J Med* 1981;304(14):820–3.

20. Yatzidis H, Koutsicos D, Agroyannis B, Papastephanidis C, Francos-Plemenos M, Delatola Z. Biotin in the management of uremic neurologic disorders. *Nephron* 1984;36(3):183–6.

Advances in Neurology, Vol. 43: Myoclonus,
edited by S. Fahn et al. Raven Press,
New York © 1986.

Myoclonic Encephalopathy of Infants

*Ira Lott and †Marcel Kinsbourne

*University of California at Irvine Medical Center, Irvine California 92717; and †Eunice
Kennedy Shriver Center and Harvard Medical School, Boston, Massachusetts 02115

Rare neurological syndromes occasionally generate an interest that is out of proportion to their frequency of occurrence because of the basic neurobiological questions that are raised by studies of their pathogenesis. Such is the case in the "dancing-eyes–dancing-feet" syndrome of myoclonic encephalopathy of infants, which highlights the relationships among myoclonus, oncology, and neuroimmunology.

INDEX REPORT

In 1962, Kinsbourne (23) reported six cases with a unique form of myoclonic encephalopathy. The ages of the three male and three female infants ranged from 6 to 18 months at the time of onset of their symptoms. Previous developmental status was normal except for one case whose maturation was slightly delayed. Each infant developed an involuntary movement disorder with intense and continual shocklike muscular contractions that reached maximal intensity within 1 week. The movements were irregular in timing and in their wide distribution across the musculature, were of variable amplitude, and were asymmetrical. They were increased by startle, continuously present at rest, and abolished only by deep sleep. Although not temporally related to the somatic myoclonus, abnormal eye movements were equally prominent. The term *dancing eyes* was coined to describe rapid and irregular conjugate ocular movements that showed by cine recording up to eight displacements or rotations every second. The eye movements were noted in every direction of gaze and seemed to be exacerbated by the same stimuli as the body myoclonus. There were no other neurological abnormalities identified. There was neither cerebellar ataxia nor mental clouding. Typically, the disorder reached its height within 48 hr of a nonspecific respiratory or gastrointestinal infection. Electroencephalograms, performed in each case, were normal. An air encephalogram and cerebral cortical biopsy performed in one individual were negative. The course did not appear to be progressive but was prolonged and fluctuated over a period of years.

This initial report described a remarkable response to steroids, wherein the somatic and ocular movement abnormalities remitted completely when the children were given adrenocorticotropic hormone (ACTH) or prednisolone. In some cases, improvement was sustained for many months after the steroids were discontinued.

In other instances this led to relapse, and it was necessary to reinstitute the regimen for several years before remission became permanent. In general, 5 to 20 mg of prednisolone or 20 to 40 units of ACTH were required daily for therapeutic benefit. The dose could usually be titrated down to a stable level below which myoclonus would begin to intrude.

SUBSEQUENT CLINICAL OBSERVATIONS

More than 100 cases have been recorded since the original report (5). Reference has been made to this disorder under several names, including Kinsbourne's syndrome (19), infantile polymyoclonia (14), and syndrome of rapid irregular movements of eyes and limbs in childhood (35). As additional cases have accumulated, the symptomatology originally reported has been confirmed. Myoclonus continues to be the essential ingredient of the disorder. We have, however, seen one case in which the myoclonus was punctuated by periods of choreoathetosis. Classification of the eye-movement abnormality has been the subject of considerable interest. The fact that the ocular dance is rapid, irregular, conjugate, and present in all planes distinguishes it from the rhythmicity of nystagmus or the rotatory movements of Pelizaeus–Merzbacher disease. According to Smith and Walsh (45), the term *opsoclonus* was first coined by Orzechowski in 1913 to describe an eye condition in nonepidemic encephalitis, associated with somatic myoclonus and characterized by continuous, rapid, variable conjugate eye movements. The plane was mainly horizontal with some deviation into the vertical and diagonal directions. The deviation was maximal at the beginning of a voluntary eye movement. Orzechowski considered these movements to be the ocular equivalent of myoclonus. Cogan (10) distinguished opsoclonus from both ocular dysmetria and flutter. He described ocular dysmetria as an intention tremor at the globe and flutter as spontaneous periodic horizontal movements of the eyeballs. Moreover, Dyken and Kolar (14) reported a spectrum of eye-movement abnormalities in their cases of infantile polymyoclonia, with opsoclonus seen early in the disorder, and movements resembling flutter noted as the somatic myoclonus lessened in severity. Perhaps opsoclonus differs from dysmetria only in the degree of severity.

The onset of the myoclonus is typically acute, although at times the disorder reaches its peak over up to 7 days. Subsequently, the course varies from apparently complete recovery after 3 months to several years of persistence of the full-blown syndrome. The latter is the more frequent picture. Occasionally, incomplete spontaneous recovery is followed by relapse. Relapses are common in relation to infection as well as to the discontinuation of steroid therapy, when effective. Cases of either type respond to corticosteroid therapy, and it is not clear whether ACTH or cortisone is the more effective. After the myoclonic state is over, more than half the children turn out to be in some permanent fashion developmentally handicapped: half the cases mentally retarded, in most instances dysarthric, sometimes with selective educational difficulty or attention deficit. Somewhat less serious sequelae are recorded for the type associated with neuroblastoma, but they still occur with significant frequency.

In the very early acute phase, irritability, vomiting, and head tilt may raise suspicion of a posterior fossa tumor, but by far the most relevant differential diagnosis is with respect to acute cerebellar ataxia. In this condition, as in the myoclonic state, the child, if old enough to have been previously ambulatory, is ataxic, and intentional movement is prejudiced by what appears to be a tremor. Neck muscles are affected by titubation; however, the dense myoclonus may suffice to account for these manifestations in the myoclonic encephalopathy cases without the need to posit cerebellar ataxia as an independent but associated phenomenon.

Opsoclonus may be observed in brainstem or cerebellar outflow (dentatothalamocortical connections) dysfunction or in both in association with benign encephalitis (11). It has also been reported in adults with pathologically demonstrated cerebellar disease in association with carcinoma of the uterus, breast (15), and lung (39). The characteristics of the changes in cerebellum and dentate nucleus have been reviewed by Ellenberger and Nelsky (16). One should distinguish opsoclonus from ocular bobbing, which may sometimes be seen in palatal myoclonus (21). The chaotic irregularity of the involuntary eye movements distinguishes them from the phasic nystagmus of some cases of acute cerebellar ataxia [which can also be associated with myoclonus (24)], the opsoclonia found on occasion in nonepidemic encephalitis (33), polioencephalitis (28), and the "cog-wheel" rotatory nystagmus of the Pelizaeus–Merzbacher syndrome. The irregularity and distribution of the involuntary movements, which affect the limbs, eyes, and axial musculature, differentiate the condition from spasmus nutans (34).

ELECTRODIAGNOSTIC STUDIES

Pampiglione and Maria (35) applied electrodiagnostic criteria to 16 children with the syndrome of rapid, irregular movements of eyes and limbs, six of whom had been described by Kinsbourne (23) in his original report. Detailed electroencephalographic (EEG) studies showed nonrhythmic discharges consisting of single or multiple spikes corresponding to the involuntary movements. There was an irregular grouping of the muscle action potentials in the agonist, but not in the antagonist, muscles. Of interest was the absence of any spikes or complex waveforms on the EEG at the time of multiple EMG discharges. Variations in the electro-oculogram were related to the displacement of the eyeballs in either the horizontal or the vertical plane. Most of the wild movements of the globes tended to occur in symmetrical bursts regardless of the amplitude of the excursion. No classical rhythmical nystagmus was observed, but there were occasional brief episodes of less irregular rapid components occurring at 5 to 12 Hz. The authors were of the opinion that this constellation of electrodiagnostic signs differed from the findings in myoclonic epilepsy, cerebellar ataxia, tremor, and choreic syndromes.

SUBSEQUENT COURSE

Although dramatic improvement with steroids is common, subsequent cases have indicated a variable prognosis for this form of the syndrome. In a long-term follow-up study of 26 children with myoclonic encephalopathy of infants, 16 were judged to have significant neurological sequelae despite a marked initial improvement in 22 of 24 cases (29). The deficits have included severe mental retardation, other types of educational handicaps, ataxia, tremor, and clumsiness. Personal experience includes a teenage girl whose visuomotor incoordination was ameliorated when cortiosteroids were again given. Case 3 of Kinsbourne's (1982) series, now aged 22 years and long remitted, has come under the care of Dr. Charles Barlow, having developed an unexplained ataxic syndrome (without myoclonus) after a nonspecific infection. Raised serum pyruvate and lactate levels were the only biochemical abnormalities found. Case 3 had intellectual function generally within the normal range, but exhibited disinhibited behavior patterns suggestive of frontal lobe dysfunction. Brain electrical activity mapping (Dr. F. Duffy) indicated bilaterally abnormal frontotemporal function.

ASSOCIATION WITH NEUROBLASTOMA

In 1968, Solomon and Chutorian (46) described two cases of biopsy-proved neuroblastoma with opsoclonus and irregular limb movements. The myoclonic state was the first sign of disease. This association proved to be more than coincidental. By 1976, 28 cases could be summarized (1). Thoracic localization was disproportionately represented in the opsomyoclonus group with neuroblastoma (49%), and eight of the patients for whom histopathological data were available showed evidence of ganglioneuroblastoma, a tumor of favorable prognosis (4). Indeed, the prognosis for the opsoclonus–neuroblastoma group as a whole seems to reflect a survival rate of 90% compared to a 2-year survival rate of 30 to 40% for an age-matched population with neuroblastoma alone (9,25). When patients were staged according to the extent of disease, 71% of the opsoclonus–myoclonus patients were classified in the prognostically favorable stage I, II, or IVS categories, compared with only 33% of the overall neuroblastoma group. However, even with advanced disease (stages III and IV), where survival of the overall group was less than 33%, 71% of the opsomyoclonus patients were long-term survivors. The good prognosis of the opsomyoclonus group is not because the neurologic symptomatology expedites early diagnosis, because, as Altman and Baehner (1) argue, there is no evidence that the neurologic signs actually coincided with the onset of the malignancy. Moreover, there was not a disproportionate number of children under 1 year of age, as might be expected in the early diagnosis of a tumor of presumptive embryonal origin. Nickerson and Hutter (32) have also indicated that neurological symptomatology may be independent of tumor activity, with signs and symptoms occurring months before a tumor is found (43). The tumor is usually found within 3 months of symptom onset (58% of cases). Reflecting the predominantly thoracic location of the tumor, plain X-ray of the chest is the most commonly effective diagnostic maneuver, and films of the abdomen reveal most of the remaining cases. Urinary catecholamine levels are rarely diagnostic.

Like the idiopathic type, this variant shows response to steroids. According to recent reviews (5,32), many (but not all) children respond to ACTH or orally administered steroids. A comparable incidence of favorable response (approximately 60%) is seen in groups with and without neuroblastoma (36). An initial improvement after the use of steroids did not appear to be a reliable indicator of the eventual outcome.

The response of the opsomyoclonus to tumor resection has also been variable. The neurological symptoms may improve dramatically (3,12,30,32,41,42) but may recur at a later time (1,3,7,31,32,43). The long-term outlook with respect to residual deficits is only a little improved by tumor resection (5) and does not substantially differ from that of the ideopathic type. The movement disorder may resolve spontaneously months or years after the tumor has been resected. In one instance, the tumor did recur without renewed opsomyoclonus (6). In two reported cases, the encephalopathy began well after the neuroblastoma had been removed, at intervals of 15 and 19 months, respectively (13,40).

A comparison of myoclonic encephalopathy of infants with and without neuroblastoma is presented in Table 1, based on a review of the literature to date.

PATHOGENESIS

Neuropathological studies of myoclonic encephalopathy of infants have not clarified the pathogenesis of this disorder. Kinsbourne's (23) first case (1962) had a negative frontal cortical biopsy, and reported autopsy examinations were either normal (27,51) or remarkable only for mild demyelination around the dentate nucleus (6). Case 5 of Kinsbourne's (1982) series died at age 33 months. Her brain exhibited no more than perivascular lymphocytic aggregations scattered in the

TABLE 1. *Clinical findings in myoclonic encephalopathy of infants[a]*

	Isolated cases	Cases with neuroblastoma	Total cases
Sex			
Male	25	25	50
Female	30	35	65
Age (years)			
1	15	15	30
1–2	26	32	58
2–3	8	10	18
3	8	5	13
Opsoclonus	56	57	113
Myoclonus	47	51	98
Ataxia	49	62	111
ACTH treatment			
improved	11	12	23
no change	0	2	2
regressed	7	4	11
Spontaneous improvement	8	9	17

[a]Modified and updated from Pinsard et al. (36); includes refs 2,8,17,18,20, 22,26,32,37,38,44,48,49,51.

brainstem. She had been successfully treated with ACTH, but at the time of her death she was still subject to relapse as soon as it was discontinued.

The anatomic locus of opsoclonus (separate from infantile polymyoclonia) has been theorized to be in the mesencephalon by Orzechowski (33) and Atkins and Bender, but this formulation has been disputed by Cogan (10). In a 61-year-old man that he had examined, the autopsy revealed an encephalitis with perivascular lymphocytic infiltration in the hypothalamus, midbrain, and pons. Another adult patient reported by Ross and Zeman (39) showed a mild diffuse Purkinje cell loss and an even milder loss of olivary cells. These studies suggest that opsomyoclonus does not correspond to any clear pattern of anatomic damage visible at the level of the light microscope.

Speculation about an immune disorder involving brainstem structures has gained ascendency in recent years. Based on the dramatic responses of his original cases to ACTH and corticosteroids, Kinsbourne (23) suggested that an autoimmune process might be responsible for the exacerbations of the illness. Two of Kinsbourne's patients (cases 2 and 5) had hypergammaglobulinemia; another (case 4) showed complement-fixation tests, suggesting recent infection with lymphocytic choriomeningitis virus; and another (case 3) had the onset of myoclonus after an immunization. The three patients reported by Dyken and Kolar (14) had cerebrospinal fluid plasmacytosis and abnormalities in IgG immunoglobulins. The presence of abnormalities in spinal fluid immunoelectrophoresis 2 and 4 years after the onset of the disease was considered to support the concept of an autoimmune process. More recently, it has been shown that leukocytes from children with proven neuroblastomas are inhibited by tumor extracts in a capillary migration test (47). Five children with opsoclonus but without proven neuroblastoma showed the same inhibition of leukocyte migration, whereas children with other cerebellar syndromes did not. Stephenson et al. (47) have suggested that the neuroblastoma and cerebellum are "joint targets of an immunological attack" (explaining the relatively good prognosis for neuroblastoma when present). Neuroblastoma in the children with opsoclonus but no demonstrated tumor might have had the tumor at a microscopic level (*in situ*). The "dancing-eyes" syndrome may be useful as a model of natural tumor regression. The postulate of an immunologic factor operating on a subcellular structure in this disorder is compatible with the absence of any significant gross neuropathological changes.

Thus, the pathophysiology of myoclonic encephalopathy remains a matter for conjecture. With reference to certain adult cases of opsoclonus, Zee and Robinson (50) have suggested that this is a release phenomenon: Saccadic burst cells are released from their inhibition by pontine "pause" cells. This suggestion raises the more general issue that myoclonus of any kind can be due in principle either to pathologically increased excitation or to pathological release from inhibition. Which of these alternatives better describes the situation in myoclonic encephalopathy of infants is not known.

As pointed out by Bray et al. (6), the association between the neuroblastoma and opsoclonus may be explained along three possible lines. In the first instance, a neurotropic virus could infect both neural crest structures and cerebellar nuclei around the dentate, causing malignant transformation in the former and encephalopathic dysfunction in the latter. Second, opsoclonus may be a remote effect of cancer in which excessive quantities of a metabolite toxic to the cerebellum and its connections are liberated by the neuroblastoma. Third, antibody to neuroblastoma antigen may cross-react with a common antigen in the cerebellar cells and thereby create damage. An additional possibility is that a congenital defect in midline cerebellar structures predisposes toward opsoclonus in some children with neuroblastoma.

Coxsackie B3 virus has recently been cultured from the stool of two children, following acute onset of opsomyoclonus, and from the cerebrospinal fluid of one of them (26). Admittedly, the syndrome deviated from typical myoclonic encephalopathy of infants in that it was relatively short lived, and the ages of onset (3 years, 7 months and 3 years, 11 months) were somewhat greater than usual. Nevertheless, the clear view is that viruses can leave opsomyoclonus by direct attack on relevant brain structures.

If myoclonic encephalopathy represents an immune reaction, we note that ACTH and corticosteroid, although effectively subduing the reaction against the brain, do not appear to compromise the hypothesized defense against neuroblastoma. There is no evidence that the rate of growth of neuroblastoma increases under steroid therapy.

RELATIVE INCIDENCE OF THE TWO VARIANTS

The relative probability of the two outcomes remains perplexingly uncertain. Were one simply to count published cases, one would assume a tumor discovery rate of nearly 50% (2,18); but to do so ignores an obvious publication bias in favor of cases associated with neuroblastoma. These cases raise issues of investigative technique (especially imaging) and surgical intervention and outcome that are quite suitable for airing in the medical literature, whereas there is less known about, and therefore to be said about, the idiopathic cases. Also, some series are based on secondary sources (such as Farrelly et al.'s tumor registry) that simply exclude the other type of case from attention. Only those series that features unselected, consecutive cases of myoclonic encephalopathy of infants can be used as a basis for relative incidence estimates. These give a surprisingly consistent picture that is grossly at variance with the literature-based impression that neoplasia is a relatively frequent associate of the syndrome.

The original series of six cases were all children who had been or were subsequently followed over a number of years (23). Indeed, case 3, currently 25 years old, still shows no trace of a neoplasm. Case 5 died at age 33 months, and autopsy by Dr. Barbara Ockenden revealed no tumor. Of the six cases of Pinsard et al. (36), only one had neuroblastoma, whereas none of Boltshauser et al.'s (5) seven personal cases had neoplasms. More surprising yet, neuroblastoma was found in none of the 16 cases followed over the long term by Marshall et al. (29).

Would the latest in diagnostic technology have revealed more tumors? Farrelly et al.'s enthusiasm for whole-body computed tomography notwithstanding, we note that five of the six cases so diagnosed in their series were also found to be identifiable by a combination of more conventional methods. One cannot dismiss these experiences as due to inadequate investigation. Most of the children were followed well beyond 1969, when Solomon and Chutorian (46) first drew attention to the relationship between myoclonic encephalopathy and neoplasm. Also, failure to declare itself over, sometimes, many years of follow-up is inconsistent with the natural history of progressive neuroblastoma. It is not inconsistent, however, with neuroblastoma that regresses or remains microscopic.

This train of thought leads one to the main missing datum—the natural history of the neoplasm to whose early identification the syndrome was a clue. Note the surely not fortuitous tendency of myoclonic encephalopathy to occur before the neoplasm becomes symptomatic.

One can hardly fault the universal practice of excising or otherwise treating the neoplasm when discovered. After all, there are a few cases on record in which the neuroblastoma progressed, metastasized, and caused death (27). Nevertheless, it is quite possible that untreated, many such tumors might regress—an outcome not unknown in neuroblastoma and consistent with its notably favorable prognosis (1).

Returning to the issue of relative incidence, we are compelled to conclude that if idiopathic and neuroblastoma-related myoclonic encephalopathy are distinct conditions, the latter is relatively uncommon and certainly represents far fewer than 50% of all cases. If both represent a reaction against neuroblastoma formation, this defense appears to be sufficiently effective, in most cases, to contain the neuroblastoma to an extent that renders it undiagnosable by existing investigative techniques.

REFERENCES

1. Altman AJ, Baehner RL. Favorable prognosis for survival in children with coincident opsomyoclonus and neuroblastoma. *Cancer* 1976; 37:846–52.
2. Baker ME, Kirks DR, Korobkin M, Bowie JD, Filston HC. The association of neuroblastoma and myoclonic encephalopathy: An imaging approach. *Ped Radiol (In press.)*
3. Berg BO, Ablin AR, Wang W, Skoglund R. Encephalopathy associated with occult neuroblastoma. *J Neurosurg* 1974; 41:567–72.
4. Bill AH, Morgan A. Evidence for immune reactions to neuroblastoma and future possibilities for investigation. *J Pediatr Surg* 1970; 5:111–6.
5. Bolthauser E, Deonna TH, Hirt HR. Myoclonic encephalopathy of infants or "dancing eyes syndrome" *Helv Pediatr Acta* 1979; 34:119–33.
6. Bray PF, Ziter FA, Lahey ME, Myers GG. The coincidence of neuroblastoma and acute cerebellar encephalopathy. *J Pediatr* 1969; 75:983–90.
7. Brissaud HE, Beauvais P. Opsoclonus and neuroblastoma. *N Eng J Med* 1969; 280:1242.
8. Burrows FA, Seeman RG. Ketamine and myoclonic encephalopathy of infants (Kinsbourne syndrome). *Anesthesia and Analgesia* 1982; 61:873–5.
9. Clatworthy HW. The treatment of neuroblastoma. *Cancer* 1968; 3:146–50.
10. Cogan DG. Ocular dysmetria: Flutter-like oscillations of the eyes and opsoclonus. *Arch Ophthalmol* 1954; 51:318–35.
11. Cogan DG. Opsoclonus, body tremulousness and benign encephalitis. *Arch Ophthalmol* 1968; 79:545–51.

12. Davidson M, Tolentino Y, Sapir S. Opsoclonus and neuroblastoma. *N Eng J Med* 1968; 279:948.
13. Delalieux C, Ebinger G, Maurus R, Sliwowski H. Myoclonic encephalopathy and neuroblastoma. *N Eng J Med* 1975; 292:46–7.
14. Dyken P, Kolar O. Dancing eyes, dancing feet: Infantile polymyoclonia. *Brain* 1968; 91:305–20.
15. Ellenberger C Jr, Campa JF, Netsky MG. Opsoclonus and parenchymatous degeneration of the cerebellum. *Neurology (Minneap.)* 1968; 18:1041–6.
16. Ellenberger C Jr, Welch KWA, Netskey MG. Anatomic basis and diagnostic value of opsoclonus. *Arch Ophthalmol* 1970; 83:307–10.
17. Evans RW. Opsoclonus in a confirmed case of St. Louis encephalitis. *J Neurol Neurosurg Psychiatry* 1982; 45:660–1.
18. Farrelly C, Daneman A, Chan HSL, Martin DJ. Occult neuroblastoma presenting with opsomyoclonus. *Am J Radiol* 1984; 142 (Apr):807–10.
19. Ford FR. Myoclonic encephalopathy of infants (Kinsbourne). The dancing eyes syndrome. In: *Diseases of the nervous system in infancy, childhood, and adolescence*, 5th ed. Springfield: Thomas, 1966:301–3.
20. Gumbinas M, Gratz ES, Johnston GS, Schwartz AD. Positive gallium scan in the syndrome of opsoclonus–myoclonus treated with adrenocorticotropic hormone. *Cancer* 1984; 54:815–6.
21. Haymaker W, Kuhlenbeck H. Disorders of the brainstem and its cranial nerves. In: Baker AB, Baker LH, eds. *Clinical Neurology*. New York: Harper and Row, 1971.
22. Kinast M, Levin HS, Rothner DA, Evenberg G, Wacksman J, Judge J. Cerebellar ataxia, opsoclonus, and occult neural crest tumor, *Am J Dis Child* 1980; 134:1057–9.
23. Kinsbourne M. Myoclonic encephalopathy of infants. *J Neurol Neurosurg Psychiatry* 1962; 25:271–9.
24. Klingman WD, Hodges RG. Acute ataxia of unknown origins in children. *J Pediatr* 1944; 24:536–43.
25. Koop CE, Johnson DG. Neuroblastoma: An assessment of therapy in reference to staging. *J Pediatr Surg* 1971; 6:595–600.
26. Kuban KC, Ephros MA, Freeman RL, Laffell LB, Bresnan MJ. Syndrome of opsoclonus–myoclonus caused by Coxsackie B3 infection. *Ann Neurol* 1983; 13:69–71.
27. Lemerle J, Lemerle M, Aicardi J, Messica C, Schweisguth O. Report of three cases of the association of an oculocerebello–myoclonic syndrome with a neuroblastoma. *Arch Fr Pediatr* 1969; 26:547–8.
28. Marmion DE, Sandilands J. Opsoclonia—A rare ocular sign in polioencephalitis. *Lancet* 1947;2:508.
29. Marshall PC, Brett EM, Wilson J. Myoclonic encephalopathy of Childhood (the dancing eyes syndrome): A long-term follow-up study. *Neurology* 1978; 28:348.
30. Martin ES, Griffith JF. Myoclonic encephalopathy and neuroblastoma. *Am J Dis Child* 1971; 122:257–8.
31. Moe PG, Nellhaus G. Infantile polymyoclonia–opsoclonus syndrome and neural crest tumors. *Neurology* 1970; 20:756–64.
32. Nickerson BG, Hutter JJ. Opsomyoclonus and neuroblastoma: Response to ACTH. *Clin Pediatr (Phila)* 1979; 18 (July):446–8.
33. Orzechowski C. De l'ataxie des yeux: Remarques sur l'ataxie des yeux dite myoclonique (opsoclonie, opsochorie). *JPsychiatr Neurol* 1927; 35:1–18.
34. Osterberg G. On spasmus nutans. *Acta Ophthalmol (Copenh)* 1937; 15:457.
35. Pampiglione G, Maria M. Syndrome of rapid irregular movements of eyes and limbs in childhood. *Br Med J (Clin Res)* 1972; 1:469–73.
36. Pinsard N, Pons-Cerdan C, Mancini J, Livet MO, Bernard R. Le syndrome ataxie–opsoclonies–myoclonies. *Sem Hop Paris* 1981; 57:488–94.
37. Rivner MH, Jay WM, Green JB, Dyken PR. Opsoclonus in hemophilus influenzae meningitis. *Neurology* 1982; 32:661–3.
38. Rosenberg N. Hearing loss as an initial symptom of the opsoclonus–myoclonus syndrome. *Arch Neourol.* 1984;41(Sep):998–9.
39. Ross AT, Zeman W. Opsoclonus, occult carcinoma, and chemical pathology in dentate nuclei. *Arch Neurol* 1967; 17:546–51.
40. Rupprecht L, Mortier W. Cerebellare Bewegungsstorung und Neuroblastoma. *Monatschr Kinderheilkd* 1975; 123:392–3.
41. Sandok BA, Kranz H. Opsoclonus as the initial manifestations of occult neuroblastoma. *Arch Ophthalmol* 1971; 86:235–6.

42. Savino PJ, Glaser JS. Opsoclonus, pattern of regression in a child with neuroblastoma. *Br J Ophthalmol* 1975; 59:696–8.
43. Senelick RC, Bray PF, Lahey ME, Van Dyk HHL, Johnson DG. Neuroblastoma and myoclonic encephalopathy: Two cases and a review of the literature. *J Pediatr Surg* 1973; 8:623–32.
44. Sheinman BD, Gawler J. Opsoclonus and polymyoclonia complicating oat-cell carcinoma of the bronchus. *Postgrad Med J* 1982; 58:704–5.
45. Smith JL, Walsh FB. Opsoclonus–ataxic conjugate movements of the eyes. *Arch Ophthalmol* 1960; 64:108–14.
46. Solomon GE, Chutorian AM. Opsoclonus and occult neuroblastoma. *N Eng J Med* 1968; 279:475–7.
47. Stephenson JBP, Graham-Pole J, Ogg L, Cochran AJ. Reactivity to neuroblastoma extracts in childhood cerebellar encephalopathy ("dancing eyes" syndrome) *Lancet* 1976; II:975–6.
48. Tal Y, Jaffe M, Sharf B, Amin N. Steroid-dependent state in a child with opsoclonus. *Pediatr* 1983; 103:420–1.
49. Willis J, Collada M, Robertson H. Cerebellar lesion in myoclonic encephalopathy of infants. *Arch Neurol* 1983; 40:818–9.
50. Zee DS, and Robinson DA. A hypothetical explanation of saccadic oscillations. *Ann Neurol* 1979; 5:405–14.
51. Ziter FA, Bray PF, Cancilla PA. Neuropathologic findings in a patient with neuroblastoma and myoclonic encephalopathy. *Arch Neurol* 1979; 36:51.

Advances in Neurology, Vol. 43: Myoclonus,
edited by S. Fahn et al. Raven Press,
New York © 1986.

Asterixis: One Type of Negative Myoclonus

Robert R. Young and Bhagwan T. Shahani

*Clinical Neurophysiology Laboratory and Movement Disorder Clinic, Department of
Neurology, Harvard Medical School, Massachusetts General Hospital,
Boston, Massachusetts 02114*

In 1949, Adams and Foley (1), in their description of the neurologic abnormalities seen with hepatic encephalopathy, emphasized an "*almost* rhythmical" tremor which is seen only during active maintenance of a posture and is accompanied by "occasional bursts of exacerbation and acceleration." In their subsequent paper in 1953 (2), they demonstrated that the bilateral jerky, twitching movements seen with this "flapping tremor" are asynchronous on the two sides and are caused by intermittent pauses in ongoing electromyographic (EMG) activity rather than by short periods of excessive muscle contraction, as had previously been supposed. To differentiate these jerky movements from the tremor itself, they coined the term *asterixis* to describe the lapses of posture. They and others (8) soon recognized that asterixis occurs not only with liver disease but also as a symptom of uremia, pulmonary failure with hypercarbia, drug intoxications of various kinds (including sedatives and tranquilizers), electrolyte imbalance, and other types of metabolic encephalopathy (Table 1). Asterixis seemed invariably to be accompanied by tremor and a reduced state of alertness or clouding of consciousness. Because of the supposed nonspecific nature of the numerous metabolic abnormalities that result in asterixis (Table 1) and the nonspecific alterations in mental state that seemed to be its inevitable accompaniment, asterixis initially was felt to reflect an equally nonspecific, generalized (that is, nonfocal) abnormality of the motor system—a concept which, as unfolds below, has subsequently been revised (21b,28,39,41).

In 1964, Leavitt and Tyler (15) reported that much of the tremulousness seen with asterixis also is due to short pauses in voluntary EMG activity. They noted that these pauses are briefer and less profound (i.e., complete EMG silence is not always present) and do not occur simultaneously in all muscles within the limb. This is in contrast to those longer, more generalized pauses seen with the larger lapses of posture called asterixis. This tremulousness (which they termed *metabolic tremor*) appeared to them to be "a manifestation of the same phenomena that underlie asterixis," and they thought it was best considered a less intense variety of asterixis rather than yet another type of abnormal movement. They too invariably found an abnormal mental status and a diffusely slow electroencephalogram (EEG) in patients with asterixis and considered asterixis to be a result of diffuse, widespread derangement of central nervous system (CNS) function. They did, however, mention "extremely rare" patients with asterixis due to thalamic or parietal disorders

137

TABLE 1. *Complex toxic–metabolic encephalopathies that include asterixis[a]*

Chronic pulmonary disease with CO_2 narcosis; ?Effects of hypoxia, acidosis, and elevated
    intracranial pressure worse with narcotics or pulmonary infection
Portal–systemic encephalopathy
    ?Role of hyperammonemia, increase in neutral amino acids in brain, decreased branched
    chain amino acids in blood
    Worse with thiazide diuretics, NH_4Cl loading, increased dietary protein, blood in
    gastrointestinal tract, infection, abnormal electrolyte levels, including hypokalemia,
    narcotics, sedatives, tranquilizers
Seen with NH_4Cl loading and alkalosis with normal liver and portal–systemic circulation
Uremic encephalopathy
Chronic hemodialysis with dialysis dementia: worse with benzodiazepines
Toxicity of sepsis: ?role of increased levels of neutral amino acids in plasma and brain
Anticonvulsant therapy: phenytoin, primidone, valproate, carbamazepine, bromides
Convulsants: metrizamide
Delerium tremens and fat embolism syndrome
Abnormal electrolyte levels: hypokalemia, hyponatremia/hypoosmolar state,
    hyperparathyroidism/hypercalcemia, magnesium deficiency, lithium toxicity
Steatorrhea–malabsorption syndromes
    Idiopathic or Whipple's disease
    ?Role of abnormal electrolyte levels
Salicylate toxicity
Cardiac failure
Hyperviscosity syndrome–polycythemia
Toxic encephalopathy in elderly Parkinson patients on levodopa

---

[a]The factors responsible for asterixis are not clear.

which had produced severe sensory loss, particularly severe loss of joint position sense, an abnormality they felt correlated best with the presence of asterixis. Tyler and Leavitt (34) postulated a "high-level defect in the continuous integration of joint position and other sensory information as important in the production of asterixis."

In 1973 (39), we described unilateral asterixis, produced by certain focal CNS lesions enumerated below, in patients without abnormalities of joint position sensation, without loss of strength or dexterity, and without any alteration in mental status. Asterixis was thereby demonstrated to be a symptom or sign in its own right, dissociable from stupor and other complex symptoms of diffuse CNS origin. That paper (39) also first reported the association of asterixis with anticonvulsant medication.

Although asterixis can arise from a small focal lesion within specific areas of the motor system, most commonly it is seen as part of a metabolic encephalopathy where, we suppose, the neurochemical abnormality disrupts normal function in the same specific areas of the motor system. For example, Glantz et al. (12) reported bilateral asterixis in a small fraction of their elderly patients with Parkinson's disease whose toxic psychosis cleared as levodopa therapy was reduced. They suggested that asterixis may be due to involvement of dopaminergic or serotonergic systems. Although the anatomic, physiologic, and biochemical derangements necessary for production of any type of asterixis are still poorly understood, it seems to be a disorder of those neural mechanisms that are involved with sustained or tonic muscle contractions.

We have also stressed the similarities between asterixis and myoclonus and, as developed in more detail below, have suggested that asterixis is one type of negative myoclonus (28,29). We used the term *negative myoclonus* (29) to emphasize the EMG silent periods that are responsible for the abnormal movements, even though the latter (e.g., asterixis) look myoclonic.

OBSERVATIONS AND GENERALIZATIONS

In our laboratory, we have studied more than 70 patients with various types of asterixis and have arrived at several generalizations which we propose, hoping other investigators will either confirm or refute them, thereby advancing our knowledge of this interesting phenomenon. Certain of these generalizations have evolved from, or at least are in agreement with, reports in the literature (21a). Although it is likely that all types of asterixis may not represent one and the same disorder (i.e., they all may not operate through the same mechanism), we will, for purposes of simplicity, assume until proven otherwise that asterixis, whether bilateral or unilateral, is one pathophysiologic entity.

Asterixis is easily recognized clinically when a gross, arrhythmic, involuntary, very brief lapse of posture occurs at a joint during tonic contraction. This is illustrated in Fig. 1, where the voluntarily outstretched, extended, pronated hand is passively flexed at the wrist by gravity during the period of EMG silence (Fig. 2), and is then quickly jerked back to its original position. In the absence of such gross lapses, when only a tremor is present, asterixis is more difficult to recognize unless one is particularly sensitive to any irregularity of the tremor. Under these circumstances, surface EMG recordings are necessary because only they can clearly demonstrate the brief, irregular silent periods (Fig. 3) that may occur in any one muscle as often as 5 or 6 times each second or as rarely as several times a minute. These lapses in posture/brief cessations of tonic muscle contraction have been seen in each skeletal muscle we have studied: orbicularis oculi, neck flexors, finger or wrist flexors or extensors, hip extensors, and so on.

Although asterixis most often occurs in the presence of typical toxic–metabolic encephalopathies, it may also be seen during the recovery phase following general anesthesia, with sedative medications, and as a result of chronic administration of various anticonvulsant drugs ["anticonvulsant asterixis" including "phenytoin flap" (20,39)] (see Table 1). It can also be seen in perfectly normal people who are simply drowsy. A sudden lapse in head posture with unsuspected jerking of the head back to its normal position is familiar to all of us who have been drowsy while sitting upright during a lecture, for example. Typical asterixis of the forearms is also a common experience for those who have been reading when drowsy and are surprised to be alerted by the sudden drift down and jerking back up of the hands and arms. Thus there appears to be a close relationship between asterixis and various disorders of alertness. As a complement to lists such as Table 1, it

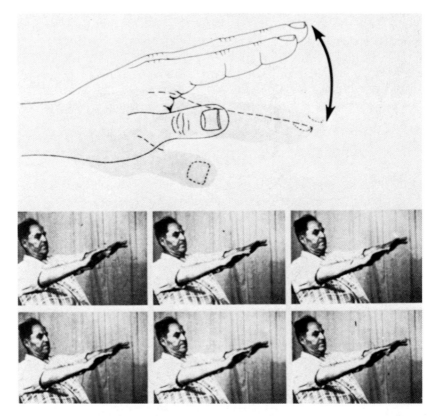

FIG. 1. Asterixis is most often demonstrated clinically by asking the patient to hold out his hands. As depicted in the bottom series of frames approximately 85 msec apart from a movie (to be read horizontally beginning at the upper left and proceeding to the lower right), the patient's right hand flexes suddenly at the wrist and then returns to the original posture. This movement is illustrated in the drawing. (Reprinted with permission from Shahani and Young, ref. 28.)

would be interesting to know if any toxic–metabolic encephalopathies are *not* associated with asterixis.

Asterixis either does not appear, or is difficult to recognize, during the course of a quick, phasic movement, although it can occasionally be recorded during the course of tonic contraction even if a slow change in posture (i.e., a slow, ramp movement) is permitted. With quicker movements, after a new position of the limb is reached, an interval of several seconds or more occurs before asterixis is seen. Our hypothesis is that asterixis is a disorder of those CNS mechanisms/programs responsible for the maintenance of posture (or slow, unidirectional movements) as distinct from those concerned with movement itself (28). It remains to be seen if this dichotomy can usefully be expressed in terms such as ballistic versus nonballistic muscular contraction. Asterixis can interrupt a grasp reflex and a "supporting reaction," such as when an arm is stiffly extended to keep a person who is tilted

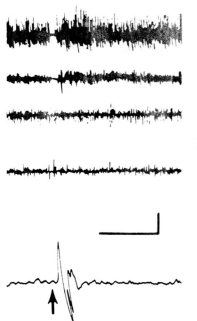

FIG. 2. Top four traces are surface EMG recorded from extensors and flexors of the wrist and elbow (from top down). The bottom trace is from an accelerometer on the hand. The silent period begins at the arrow, and the movement of asterixis begins shortly after with acceleration of the hand downward followed by deceleration and then acceleration back upward. Time calibration, 1 sec. (Reprinted with permission from Shahani and Young, ref. 28.)

from falling over when seated or standing. The following question remains unanswered: Is asterixis present only with voluntarily mediated drive on the spinal motor neuron pool (including "voluntary" postures), or can it occur during various types of involuntary (for example, dystonic) muscle contraction?

Because asterixis is most apt to occur when movement has not recently occurred at the joint involved, as was first pointed out by Leavitt and Tyler (15), we use the following stratagem to provide a clinical answer to the question of whether or not

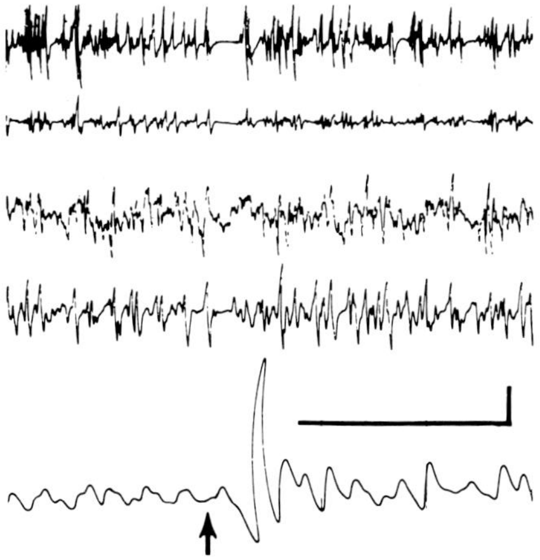

FIG. 3. The traces here are the same as in Fig. 2. Asterixis of the usual type (following the arrow) is often accompanied by shorter EMG pauses which produce a tremulous movement of the hand, as shown by the accelerometer trace. Time calibration, 1 sec. (Reprinted with permission from Young and Shahani, ref. 40.)

a patient has asterixis: We require simple dorsiflexion of the index finger for 30 sec with the patient watching the finger carefully to minimize movements there.

Asterixis is completely involuntary; the patient has no warning it will occur, is surprised to see it happen because he thinks he is contracting his muscles as steadily as ever, and is unable to prevent its occurrence except perhaps indirectly by moving the limb. Since, in physiologic terms, asterixis is the absence of EMG activity, it cannot be produced or recognized without background EMG contraction and therefore falls into the category of "action tremors" or "action myoclonus." The latter term refers to myoclonic movements that are worse during activity, perhaps, in part at least, because action requires background muscle contraction, in the midst of which asterixis or negative myoclonus can appear. The EMG silence underlying asterixis typically varies in length from 50 to 100 msec in facial muscles and 50 to 200 msec in limb muscles. On occasions, periods of EMG silence lasting 300 to 500 msec may be seen, but under those circumstances it is often difficult to be certain that a lapse of attention or momentary decrease in voluntary effort has not occurred. These EMG silent periods tend to occur synchronously in muscles throughout one limb but are not of equal magnitude throughout; any single flapping movement usually occurs at only one joint. Furthermore, although asterixis of the common sort occurs bilaterally, the jerky movements and silent periods are not bilaterally synchronous except in the face (Fig. 4). Further studies are needed to evaluate the degree of bilateral synchrony in other axial muscles which, like the face, have a high degree of bilateral cerebral cortical representation. On the other hand, focal CNS lesions can produce asterixis affecting only one side of the face (9).

ANTICONVULSANT ASTERIXIS INCLUDING PHENYTOIN FLAP

The situation regarding anticonvulsant medications and asterixis is not a simple one. As noted below, unilateral asterixis has been seen in patients who have been taking phenytoin (DPH) and whose DPH blood levels are well within the therapeutic range (i.e., not excessive), providing those patients also have a lesion within the contralateral cerebral hemisphere. This latter lesion may not be symptomatic otherwise. Attention may be drawn to a cerebral lesion by virtue of the unilateral asterixis produced by anticonvulsant therapy, or the lesion may have been symptomatic earlier (as in the acute phase following a thalamotomy) but no longer productive of any neurologic sign or symptom unless the patient is given an anticonvulsant. In the presence of an appropriate CNS lesion, modest doses of anticonvulsants (e.g., a single 50-mg i.v. dose of DPH) produce asterixis and do so very quickly, especially if the medication is given parenterally.

The general physician responsible for the first patient in whom we recognized unilateral asterixis obtained a history, several weeks after an acute paralysis of the patient's left leg due to a right anterior cerebral artery occlusion, of episodic jerking movements which had, shortly after the ictus, involved her left arm (39). Her arm was neurologically normal at the time of examination and, in retrospect, the jerking

A

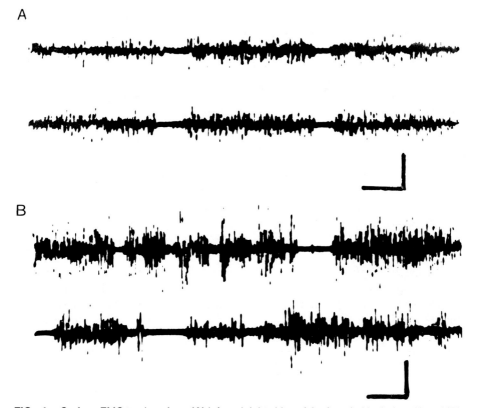

B

FIG. 4. Surface EMG tracings from **(A)** left and right sides of the face (orbicularis coli) and **(B)** left and right arms (extensors of the wrist). Time calibrations, 250 msec.

movements probably represented unilateral asterixis which had subsequently subsided. She was started on DPH because her physician thought the abnormal movements might have been focal seizures. DPH therapy produced renewed jerking of the left arm which, when she was seen by us, was obviously unilateral asterixis. By that time, DPH therapy had been supplemented with phenobarbital because the jerky movements had become more frequent. On several other occasions, physicians have mistaken unilateral asterixis for focal seizures and/or positive myoclonus; usually such patients were already receiving phenytoin, and its failure to stop the abnormal movements resulted in a neurologic consultation.

Higher doses of DPH (resulting in serum levels greater than the therapeutic range) produce a toxic–metabolic encephalopathy with decreased alertness, mental slowing, and loss of spontaneity. This can also be associated with typical metabolic asterixis of the usual bilateral type (20). We have seen the same syndrome in patients with excessive levels of primidone, and it has been reported to accompany intoxication with bromides (8), an anticonvulsant no longer in use. In these settings, the bilateral asterixis disappears as anticonvulsant concentrations are reduced to

TABLE 2. *Anatomic lesions that have produced asterixis*

Asterixis	No. of patients	Ref.
Unilateral		
Infarct or ischemia	12[a,b]	8, 9 (*12, 17*)[c], 11, 13, 17 (*1, 2*), 26 (*1, 2*), 33, 38, 39
Thalamotomy	9[b]	39, 41
Intracerebral hemorrhage	8	9 (*10, 11*), 11, 13 (*1, 2*), 17 (*3*), 26, (*3–5*)
Glioblastoma	6[a]	8, 9 (*8, 13*), 24
Abscess or granuloma	2[b]	9 (*7*), 13 (*3*)
Metastasis	3	9 (*5, 6*), 26 (*6*)
Subdural hematoma	1	35
Focal encephalitis	1[b]	39
Bilateral		
Infarcts	3[b]	5, 32, 39
Bilateral metastases	1[b]	39
Subdural empyema	1	23
Subdural hematoma	1	25
Intraventricular hemorrhage with hydrocephalus	1[b]	37

[a]Unilateral asterixis appeared as first sign of glioblastoma (one patient) or impending carotid occlusion (three patients).
[b]Asterixis seen only during receipt of phenytoin (seven patients).
[c]Numbers in italics refer to case numbers within the cited reference.

more normal levels and an anatomic lesion of the CNS is not discovered. Sodium valproate is reported to have caused asterixis in two patients with blood levels within the therapeutic range, but both were also receiving three other anticonvulsants, including phenytoin and primidone (21d).

Whatever mechanisms eventually are shown to underlie unilateral asterixis and its exacerbation by anticonvulsants, one should remember that some lesion, even asymptomatic and perhaps functional as well as structural is presumably required for the production of asterixis by compounds such as phenytoin, for example. Anticonvulsant asterixis of the bilateral variety (requiring excessive levels of medication) may also be conditioned by the patient's prior neurologic (and neurotherapeutic) history. Recognition of the syndrome of anticonvulsant asterixis may lead to reductions in dosage of that medication (or exceptionally, its complete withdrawal) but, if the asterixis is unilateral, it should strongly suggest the presence of a lesion within the CNS structures outlined below, a lesion that might otherwise not be clinically evident.

UNILATERAL ASTERIXIS AND ASTERIXIS
CAUSED BY FOCAL LESIONS

Although generalized or bilateral asterixis is most common, several interesting points emerge from analysis of the unilateral asterixis that has been seen as a result of different types of lesions affecting the CNS (Table 2). As noted above, we first observed typical asterixis (28,39) in only one arm (which was neither weak nor insensitive) in a patient following an anterior cerebral artery occlusion with infarction of the medial aspect of the contralateral hemisphere. This stroke produced paralysis of the patient's leg on the same side as the arm with asterixis. Subsequently, we have seen patients with metastatic deposits within the medial frontal or parietal regions, who had unilateral (or, with biparietal metastases, bilateral) asterixis. Embolic infarcts of the parietal area or posterior medial surface of the hemisphere, focal encephalitis, and thalamotomies have also produced unilateral asterixis in our patients. We have seen asterixis as an accompaniment of cerebral vasospasm following a subarachnoid hemorrhage in the absence of a demonstrable infarct. Others (8,9,11) have reported unilateral asterixis in the phase immediately prior to a cerebral infarction caused by carotid occlusion; that is, asterixis was the only sign of cerebral ischemia, i.e., a prodromal symptom for hemiparesis which appeared as the ischemic region enlarged. In one patient (9), it was the first sign of a cerebral tumor. As shown in Table 2, in nine patients (four unilateral), asterixis was seen only when phenytoin was given in the presence of a focal CNS lesion. In addition, there have been reports of infarcts (9,13,21b,26,33), hemorrhages (9,10,13,19,21b,26), or tumors (6,9,21b,24,26) within the thalamus and/or adjacent internal capsule, midbrain, or parietal cortex causing unilateral asterixis (see Tables 2 and 3).

As emphasized by Goldblatt and Griggs (13) and Osawa (21b), a hemiparesis is quite compatible with the presence of asterixis; that is, hemiparesis does not diminish the likelihood of its appearance as it does for most other movement disorders. Asterixis, of course, cannot be seen in the presence of a complete hemiplegia. Are there lesions which, short of producing complete paralysis, eliminate asterixis? Such a lesion would be demonstrable in a patient with a metabolic encephalopathy who would otherwise have bilateral asterixis. It would also be a unique example of unilateral asterixis where the CNS lesion was ipsilateral.

More than 74 patients have been reported with asterixis caused by anatomic (as opposed to biochemical) lesions which are more or less focal (Table 2); in seven, asterixis was bilateral. The location of most of these lesions is poorly defined. Often the lesion was "localized" only by clinical criteria. This was particularly the case for putative midbrain lesions (9), the locations of which were inferred from neuroophthalmic signs. In only 56 of these 74 were any reasonably objective criteria given for localization of the lesions (Table 3). Apart from nine patients with thalamotomy, only 35 others of the 56 had very well-localized lesions. Only one of these had autopsy confirmation (medial frontal infarction). In the other 34, lesions were localized by computerized tomography (CT) scan: one, with bilateral asterixis, had an infarct in the rostral midbrain tegmentum; the other nine (unilateral asterixis) had infarcts involving the internal capsule (genu and anterior portion of posterior limb) and adjacent thalamus or thalamic hemorrhages with more or less compression of (or extension into) adjacent capsule or midbrain. In the absence of a detailed postmortem anatomic evaluation, CT scan localization is not sufficiently precise for one to be certain which of these structures (i.e., internal capsule or

TABLE 3. *Localization of single lesions that have produced asterixis*

Asterixis	No. of patients	Ref.
Unilateral		
Thalamus	15[a]	6, 10, 13, 26 (*3, 4, 5*),[c] 39, 41
Parietal lobe	7	9 (*5–8, 10, 12*), 39
Internal capsule	6[b]	9 (*13, 16*), 17, 26, (*2*), 29, 38
Medial frontal cortex	3	26 (*1*), 33, 39
Bilateral: rostral midbrain tegmentum	1	5

[a]Nine were stereotactic thalamotomies (39,41).
[b]Without postmortem anatomic evidence, it is possible that these lesions produce asterixis by involving the thalamus or that thalamotomies produce asterixis by involving the internal capsule.
[c]Numbers in italics refer to case numbers within the cited references.

adjacent thalamus) must be involved, with a minimal lesion, for asterixis to result. The most discrete lesions producing asterixis are tiny (0.1 cc) ventrolateral thalamotomies (41) (Fig. 5) placed by neurosurgeons for the treatment of tremor or rigidity. Providing the lesion is within the ventrolateral thalamus (and not in globus pallidus), such stereotactic operations, inevitably produce asterixis acutely perhaps by affecting descending motor fibers in the adjacent internal capsule. However, it disappears after several days or weeks, as it does following the other nonprogressive focal lesions listed above. When, as time passes following one of these lesions, unilateral asterixis has disappeared, it can quickly be brought out again by the administration of DPH, even intravenous infusion of as little as 50 mg. When the latter technique is employed, asterixis reappears within a few minutes and lasts approximately 30 min.

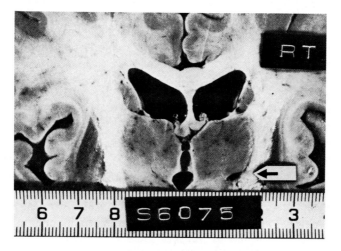

FIG. 5. Coronal section of the human brain in which a stereotactically placed lesion is visible in the ventrolateral area of the right thalamus *(arrow)* (20a).

Careful neuropathologic studies of brains from patients with typical unilateral asterixis are now underway (36), but precise anatomic details of those lesions are not yet available. Nevertheless, asterixis is not attributable to nonspecific hemispheral disease since the vast majority of patients with cerebral lesions do not have it. Our speculation is that lesions affecting structures either near the supplementary motor area or in the posterior parietal cortex or circuitry within the ventrolateral thalamus (all three areas perhaps being part of one motor subsystem) produce asterixis.

MECHANISMS UNDERLYING ASTERIXIS

Mechanisms responsible for EMG pauses, the larger ones of which are associated with asterixis, are still unclear. A number of interesting preliminary observations have been made which bear on the possible cerebral structures involved and various clinical settings (see Tables 2 and 3), apart from metabolic encephalopathies, in which asterixis is seen. As outlined above, damage to specific circuitry in the basal thalamus (including possibly the rostral midbrain), mesial hemisphere, or parietal cortex can produce asterixis, whereas cerebral lesions in other locations certainly do not. Apart from these few precisely localized lesions on the one hand and metabolic encephalopathies on the other, what other circumstances are associated with asterixis?

During seizures, asterixis of a localized or generalized sort can be recorded. This is particularly true of the "drop attacks" or "myoclonic jerks" seen with petit mal seizures, but patients with focal seizures, including epilepsia partialis continua, also have a mixture of excessive EMG bursts and, at other times, unexpected brief pauses in otherwise ongoing EMG contraction. Marsden et al. (16) report that transcutaneous electrical stimulation of human motor cortex (18) produces either electrically induced twitches of the appropriate body part or, if stimulus parameters are changed slightly, electrically induced brief silent periods in voluntarily contracting muscles, which are then associated with postural lapses. Their conclusion is that "activity in the motor cortex may either cause muscle contraction or asterixis." Whereas it is often possible to record from the scalp (sometimes even without averaging EEG activity) "spontaneous" electrocortical events which precede EMG bursts responsible for myoclonic jerks (16,40), we have not been able, using backward averaging [see Shibasaki et al. (30) and *this volume* for a similar technique], to recognize electrocerebral activity (or EEG silent periods) preceding the movements of asterixis. Electrical stimulation within the human internal capsule has also been reported (22) to produce either short-latency EMG activation or 50- to 200-msec periods of EMG silence during voluntary or postural contraction. This suppression of ongoing EMG activity sometimes followed an electrically induced burst of EMG, but very often, particularly with stimulation near the capsular–thalamic boundary, only a brief period of EMG inactivity was produced, "not preceded by any motor response" (22).

In patients with posthypoxic intention myoclonus, jerky irregularities of movement are produced by both bursts of excessive myoclonic EMG activity and aste-

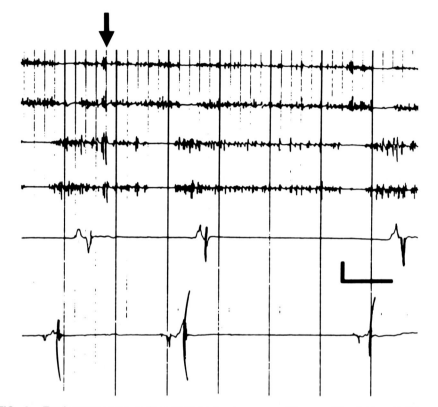

FIG. 6. Top four traces are surface EMG from extensors and flexors of the right and left knees (from top down) of a patient with posthypoxic intention myoclonus. The bottom two traces are from accelerometers on the right and left foot, respectively. Note the movements of asterixis-negative myoclonus which follow EMG silent periods and occur asynchronously on the two sides. Note also the synchronous EMG burst seen in all four muscles *(arrow)*, which represent positive myoclonus. Time calibration, 500 msec. (Reprinted with permission from Young and Shahani, ref. 40.)

rixis-like silent periods in ongoing EMG (Fig. 6) (14,40). It is impossible to tell clinically whether individual jerky movements in posthypoxic patients (or in those with similar-appearing progressive but nonhypoxic myoclonic syndromes) are due to excessive or insufficient EMG activity; only careful EMG recordings can make that differentiation.

In their original description of the syndrome, Lance and Adams (14) suggested that the silent periods in EMG activity seen in patients with posthypoxic intention myoclonus are not likely to be due entirely to refractoriness of the motor neuron pool following its synchronous activation by a preceding EMG twitch. This postdischarge inactivity may account for some of the silent periods in such patients but probably is not an important cause of asterixis-like EMG pauses in general. These pauses do not always (or even usually) follow a myoclonic EMG burst; single unit recordings show sudden lapses in the repetitive firing of single motor unit potentials which do not usually follow a burst of EMG or any other increase in activity (Fig. 7). Second, after a true proprioceptive- or exteroceptive-induced silent period (electrical stimulation of a mixed or sensory nerve during voluntary contraction) (27), as motor neurons resume their discharges, they tend to fire synchronously so that EMG bursts can be seen for a few cycles after the silent period—something not usually evident with asterixis (Fig. 2). Since asterixis is present in facial muscles, such as orbicularis oculi, which do not contain muscle spindles, function of the stretch reflex arc (and group IA afferents) appears not to be necessary for the production of these silent periods. During a proprioceptive silent period produced by unloading muscle spindles, one usually finds stretch reflex EMG activity in antagonist muscles; such antagonist EMG activity is not seen during asterixis. Third, silent periods which are due to (i.e., follow upon) synchronous motor unit discharge do not completely unfuse a prior tetanic contraction of the muscle and therefore do not produce very dramatic postural lapses. Therefore, we are reluctant to explain either the silent period seen with asterixis of the usual sort or the asterixis-like silent periods of various myoclonic or epileptic patients simply in terms of synchronized refractory periods within the motor neuron pool. When discussing silent periods in general, it should be noted that proprioceptive- or exteroceptive-induced silent periods, like asterixis, tend to be shorter or absent during the course of a brisk movement.

ASTERIXIS AS ONE TYPE OF MYOCLONUS

Does asterixis have any relationship to myoclonus? We suggest that asterixis and similar brief involuntary silent periods during ongoing EMG activity (such as during the accompanying tremor) produce movements that appear to be just as myoclonic as those produced by the equally brief involuntary bursts of EMG activity seen with other types of myoclonus when muscles are either at rest or contracting. Unfortunately, the presence of phenomena responsible for these pauses in EMG activity cannot be demonstrated in humans except against the background of more-or-less continuous EMG discharge. Myoclonic jerks of the classic type—that is, those produced by brief involuntary EMG bursts—are, if one applies Jacksonian terminology to EMG phenomena, a positive symptom/sign or, at least, can be said to be due to a positive EMG phenomenon. The EMG silent periods underlying the brief jerky movements of asterixis are, to use the same terminology, negative phenomena. We prefer to call brief, lightning-like movements of the former type *positive myoclonus* and identically appearing movements of the latter type *negative myoclonus*. In either case, the movements produced appear to be myoclonic jerks; appearances, after all, were the only phenomena available to be used for categorization by those who, like Friedreich, originally defined myoclonus long before the advent of EMG. Although EMG does now permit us to differentiate negative from positive myoclonus, is that sufficient reason to categorize the former as something other than myoclonus?

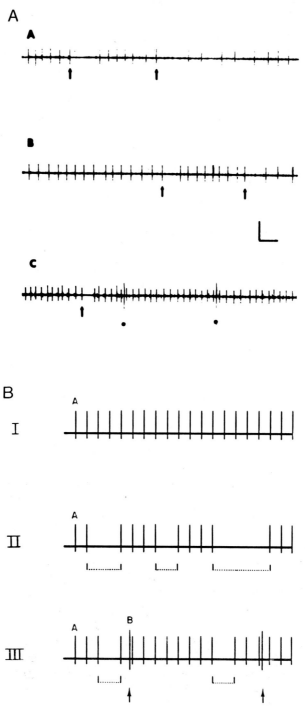

The term asterixis is an excellent one to describe the gross jerky, flapping movements; as noted above, however, lesser varieties of this same disorder result in a tremulous movement that looks more like tremor than asterixis. In fact, it is possible that essential-familial tremor may be attributable to a phenomenon such as asterixis (i.e., EMG silent periods) which occurs at regular intervals. With EMG recordings, however, these smaller tremulous movements, which are difficult to recognize clinically as asterixis, are easily identifiable as negative myoclonus. Why should we describe yet a third phenomenon when all three (ordinary myoclonus, asterixis, and its associated tremor) have much in common? Asterixis means EMG silent periods, but these latter are also quite prominent in patients with asterixis tremor, posthypoxic intention myoclonus, myoclonic epilepsy, or rhythmic positive myoclonus in myoclonic dystonia (see ref. 21, Fig. 4). Asterixis and myoclonus are often confused; that is, what turns out to be asterixis in the EMG laboratory is called myoclonus at the bedside. Plum and Posner (23) agree "it sometimes becomes difficult to distinguish between intense asterixis and myoclonus." Those earlier clinicians who described myoclonus according to the appearance of the movement could not determine whether the movement was due to excessive or insufficient EMG activity.

Negative and positive myoclonus also have other similarities. Both occur with unusual synchrony in all muscle groups in one limb (in both agonists and antagonists) but do not occur simultaneously in both arms, for example. Both are seen in a number of similar situations. Both are seen with various metabolic encephalopathies. Both are produced by agents, such as intrathecal metrizamide (3,7,31), that can also cause seizures. Both are present together in patients who are affected by several of the epilepsies noted above. Both occur normally during drowsiness and light sleep when one experiences "sleep starts" or "hypnic jerks" (which are bursts of excessive EMG activity) and negative myoclonic jerks as mentioned above. Although Marsden and colleagues (16) lump both together as "physiological myoclonus" (hypnic jerks are said to be generalized myoclonus if the individual is lying down, and those involving the neck when a person is sitting upright are called segmental myoclonus), we prefer to treat them independently. In any case, it is reasonable to keep the core phenomenon referred to as asterixis within the general framework of myoclonus, and it is equally reasonable to define asterixis and related brief myoclonic-like pauses in EMG activity as negative myoclonus. As our knowledge of the pathophysiology of these phenomena advances, such categorizations will be reassessed. All EMG silent periods are certainly not asterixis (or even

FIG. 7. A: Single motor unit potentials recorded from M. extensor indicis proprius in a patient who is maintaining a tonic contraction at three increasing levels of force (A, B, and C, respectively). Note the apparently random occurrence of pauses in firing following each arrow. A second larger unit is recruited in C above the dots. Time calibration, 200 msec. (Reprinted with permission from Young and Shahani, ref. 40.) **B:** Cartoons of a single motor unit firing tonically (I), irregular pauses in this firing (II) similar to those seen in (A) and irregular pauses plus a newly recruited unit (B) at the arrows (III). Unit B may represent positive myoclonus. Each of the lines (I, II, and III) represents 2 sec.

negative myoclonus), but in our present primitive state of knowledge, why not consider those involuntary ones which are associated with irregular jerky movements as myoclonus?

The best hypotheses accounting for positive myoclonus (including that seen with seizures or transcutaneous electrical shocks administered to the head) involve brief excessive bursts of excitation manifest as excitatory postsynaptic potentials (EPSPs) (or depolarizing shifts in potential) produced in spinal motor neurons by activity in descending fiber systems. Within the CNS, inhibitory activity is as "active" and prominent as excitatory activity; in fact, there may be more types of inhibition [inhibitory postsynaptic potentials (IPSPs), remote or presynaptic inhibition, increased chloride and/or potassium conductances] than of excitation. If neural activity in descending tracts produces brief involuntary bursts of inhibition (such as IPSPs) on appropriately placed interneurons or motor neurons, the latter would suddenly fall silent, and asterixis or negative myoclonus would be produced. If one acknowledges the inevitability of excessive excitatory activity underlying positive myoclonus, at least at the spinal motor neuron level, it seems equally probable that bursts of excessive inhibitory activity (either at spinal or some higher level) with a similar short time span should produce asterixis or negative myoclonus.

In conclusion, we believe it important to dissociate the phenomenon of asterixis from other signs and symptoms of a generalized, nonspecific metabolic encephalopathy. As an example of the conceptual difficulties that arise if one fails to do that, Bertoni and colleagues (3) treat asterixis as just another sign of the "depressive metabolic encephalopathy" produced by metrizamide. They emphasize the "unusual degree of depressive rather than irritative effects," whereas we suggest the EMG silent periods are a result of excessive bursts of specific inhibitory activity rather than a generalized depression of CNS activity.

SUMMARY

Asterixis is a disorder of motor control characterized by irregular myoclonic lapses of posture affecting various parts of the body independently. These lapses are caused by involuntary 50- to 200-msec silent periods appearing in muscles (even antagonistic groups of muscles) which are tonically active. That is, the silent periods and postural lapses occur in muscles that have been contracting for a time whether or not there has been slow shortening or lengthening but probably do not occur during or immediately after a sudden movement at a joint. What constitutes a sudden as opposed to a slow movement remains to be defined.

When bilateral asterixis is present, one cannot rule out the possibility of a focal lesion (see Table 2), but it is almost always due to a metabolic encephalopathy (with a wide variety of possible causes). Unilateral asterixis is due to a localized lesion, perhaps otherwise not clinically evident, in the contralateral cerebral hemisphere. This episodic dysfunction within neural circuits which are normally concerned with maintenance of sustained or tonic muscle contraction may be released by focal lesions only in specific CNS areas (such as ventrolateral thalamus) or by a more generalized neurochemical imbalance (metabolic encephalopathies of various kinds). The system, a lesion or metabolic dysfunction which produces asterixis, is presumably an anatomically and/or pharmacologically distinct one; asterixis is not the result of a nonspecific disorder any more than are seizures. Presumably, those aspects of each of the different factors (e.g., subdural hematomas, drugs, electrolyte imbalance, cerebrovascular accidents, intracerebral tumors) that may produce asterixis or a seizure are mediated through some fundamental neuronal or neural systems process. To label asterixis or seizures nonspecific results of CNS disorders or results of nonspecific CNS disorders may be simply to avoid confronting our ignorance of the specific pathophysiologic mechanisms involved.

Although the anatomy, neurochemistry, and physiologic function of this asterixogenic system remain to be elucidated, observations that asterixis may be caused by discrete anatomic or pharmacologic (e.g., phenytoin) lesions should tell us something important about mechanisms underlying sustained muscle contraction in humans. Unfortunately clinicoanatomic correlations alone cannot provide precise answers because even those reasonably focal vascular lesions that cause asterixis are too gross to permit localization or identification of the neural systems involved. The most discrete, best localized asterogenic lesions are ventrolateral thalamotomies, but thalamic, parietal, or medial hemisphere (anterior cerebral artery territory) infarcts, hemorrhages, or tumors, and rare midbrain lesions have also produced asterixis. What these different areas have in common remains to be demonstrated. Although some patients with unilateral asterixis also have a hemiparesis, hemisensory loss, or hemiataxia, these other deficits are not necessary for asterixis to be present. Sensory loss (particularly affecting joint position sense) or very mild hemiparesis (partial pyramidal lesions) have been postulated as crucial to the pathophysiology of asterixis. If sensory loss is necessary for asterixis, it is sensation of such a complex type or at such a high level of integration that we cannot test for it clinically or in any other way. Similarly, there need be no other evidence of a pyramidal syndrome for asterixis to be present. These hypotheses concerning its pathophysiology remain speculative.

Our hypotheses regarding asterixis are as follows: (a) Circuitry constituting that neural subsystem concerned with sustained muscle contraction (posture) exists within medial frontal cortex (? supplementary motor area), parietal lobe, ventrolateral thalamus, and perhaps adjacent internal capsule and midbrain. (b) Asterixis and not paralysis results from (i) a lesion of (a), or (ii) abnormal activity within a separate arousal system caused by a large number of factors, each of which makes the person less alert. (c) Lesions of (a) may be (i) of a variety of anatomic types, or (ii) due to specific biochemical agents, such as DPH, which can produce asterixis without depressing alertness. (d) Continuous input from an arousal system into the tonic motor subsystem outlined in (a) is necessary for the maintenance of posture. Osawa has recently reported that 1 mg i.v. TRH reduces the frequency of unilateral asterixis for as long as 2 hr (21c). He postulates that TRH enhances the function of pyramidal tracts and brainstem reticular formation. He therefore suggests (21b,c) that these two structures are the ones we refer to above (item d).

The term asterixis refers to a now well-recognized neurologic sign. Negative myoclonus is a more inclusive term encompassing asterixis and tremor in patients with metabolic encephalopathy and other circumstances in which brief periods of EMG silence produce an abnormal movement. Asterixis is one type of negative myoclonus. Lesser variants (miniasterixis, for example) include those tremors seen in patients who also have asterixis. The term metabolic tremor is not synonymous with negative myoclonus because other metabolic tremors, due, for example, to thyrotoxicosis, adrenergic overactivity, or lithium, are not related to asterixis or myoclonus (42).

Although little is known of the fundamentals of this interesting phenomenon, asterixis-negative myoclonus has become well recognized clinically and is separable from the mental changes and other complexities of metabolic encephalopathies. More intelligent use of the opportunities for investigation provided by these observations should advance our understanding of the motor system and help provide more effective techniques in restorative neurology.

This has been a review of asterixis based on reports in the literature and our own experience. In addition to describing asterixis, we have listed those toxic–metabolic encephalopathies that have been associated with it. Although it is bilateral and accompanied by decreased alertness when it is encephalopathic in origin, asterixis can also be produced by discrete CNS lesions of which it may be the only symptom, unassociated with changes in alertness, sensation, or corticospinal function. Hemorrhages, infarcts, tumors, and other anatomically demonstrable lesions (including ventrolateral thalamotomies) that affect thalamus, adjacent internal capsule, parietal or medial frontal cerebral cortex or midbrain can produce asterixis. Typically, this is unilateral (contralateral to the lesion), but bilateral asterixis has been caused by bilateral or diffuse lesions (such as subdural hematomas), or even a single midbrain lesion. Small amounts of phenytoin can markedly exacerbate unilateral asterixis, whereas toxic levels of many anticonvulsants often produce bilateral asterixis. Asterixis, as described by patients, is often mistaken for focal seizures. The clinical relevance of this situation has been emphasized, as well as the conclusion that unilateral asterixis is always due to a focal cerebral lesion, which may otherwise not be evident clinically.

By careful analysis of lesions producing focal asterixis, it should be possible to delineate the anatomy of those CNS structures, if not their biochemistry, which are responsible for asterixis. We assume that one motor subsystem is responsible for the maintenance of tonic muscle contraction so that lesions affecting it produce the lapses of EMG activity and posture known as asterixis. Various metabolic disturbances may also affect this system directly (e.g., phenytoin), or indirectly perhaps by affecting those CNS systems responsible for alerting or arousal, whose activity is necessary for action of the tonic motor subsystem and maintenance of posture. Drowsiness in normal people (the varied toxic–metabolic encephalopathies have been listed above) and diffuse CNS lesions all can produce asterixis, perhaps by their effects upon alerting or arousal mechanisms rather than by "nonspecific" CNS actions.

We have also characterized asterixis as one type of negative myoclonus, thereby attempting to establish its place in a general schema of motor disorders.

ACKNOWLEDGMENTS

This work was supported by the Louise Ingalls and Dewey D. Stone Funds of the Parkinson's Disease Project at Massachusetts General Hospital. We also thank Susan Wyoral and Barbara Marino for their invaluable help during the preparation of this manuscript. Dr. Raymond Adams generously read an early draft of this work and made many helpful suggestions.

REFERENCES

1. Adams RD, Foley JM. The neurological changes in the more common types of severe liver disease. *Trans Am Neurol Assoc* 1949; 74:217–9.
2. Adams RD, Foley JM. The neurological disorders associated with liver disease. In: Merritt HH, Hare CC, eds. Metabolic and toxic diseases of the nervous system. Baltimore: Williams & Wilkins, 1953:198–237.
3. Bertoni JM, Schwartzman RJ, Van Horn G, Partin J. Asterixis and encephalopathy following metrizamide myelography: investigations into possible mechanisms and review of the literature. *Ann Neurol* 1981; 9:366–70.
4. Bodensteiner JB, Morris HH, Golden GS. Asterixis associated with sodium valproate. *Neurology* 1981; 31:186–90.
5. Bril V, Sharpe JA, Ashby P. Midbrain asterixis. *Ann Neurol* 1979; 6:362–4.
6. Calzetti S, Gemignani F, Salati MR, Terzano MG. Unilateral asterixis due to thalamic tumor. Case report. *Ital J Neurol Sci* 1983; 1:87–90.
7. Chehrazi B, Virapongse C. Transient encephalopathy and asterixis following metrizamide myelography. *J Neurosurg* 1981; 55:826–9.
8. Conn HO. Asterixis in non-hepatic disorders. *Am J Med* 1960; 29:647–61.
9. Degos J-D, Verroust J, Bouchareine A, Serdaru M, Barbizet J. Asterixis in focal brain lesions. *Arch Neurol* 1979; 36:705–7.
10. Donat JR. Unilateral asterixis due to thalamic hemorrhage. *Neurology* 1980; 30:83–4.
11. Ericson G, Warren SE, Gribik M, Channick M, Steinberg SM. Unilateral asterixis in a dialysis patient. *JAMA* 1978; 240:671.
12. Glantz R, Weiner WJ, Goetz CG, Nausieda PA, Klawans HL. Drug-induced asterixis in Parkinson disease. *Neurology* 1982; 32:553–5.
13. Goldblatt D, Griggs RC. Unilateral asterixis in a paretic limb: an involuntary movement accentuated by upper motor neuron lesion. *Neurology* 1979; 29:541–2.
14. Lance JW, Adams RD. The syndrome of intention or action myoclonus as a sequel to hypoxic encephalopathy. *Brain* 1963; 86:111–36.
15. Leavitt S, Tyler HR. Studies in asterixis. *Arch Neurol* 1964; 10:360–8.
16. Marsden CD, Hallett M, Fahn S. The nosology and pathophysiology of myoclonus. In: Marsden CD, Fahn S, eds. Movement disorders. London: Butterworths, 1982:196–248.
17. Massey EW, Goodman JC, Stewart C, Brannon WL. Unilateral asterixis: motor integrative dysfunction in focal vascular disease. *Neurology* 1979; 29:1188–90.
18. Merton PA, Morton HB. Stimulation of the cerebral cortex in the intact human subject. *Nature* 1980; 285:227.
19. Morrey EW, Goodman JC, Stewart T, Brannon WL. Unilateral asterixis: motor integrative dysfunction in focal vascular disease. *Neurology* 1979; 29:1180–2.
20. Murphy MJ, Goldstein MN. Diphenylhydantoin-induced asterixis. *JAMA* 1974; 299:538–40.
20a. Narayabashi H, Ohye C. Importance of microstereoencephalotomy for tremor alleviation. *Appl Neurophysiol* 1980; 43:222–7.
21. Obeso JA, Rothwell JC, Lang AE, Marsden CD. Myoclonic dystonia. *Neurology* 1983; 33:825–30.
21a. Osawa M. Clinical studies in asterixis. I. Clinical investigation on asterixis by surface electromyographic and accelerometric recordings. *J Tokyo Women's Med Coll* 1983;53:1137–48.

21b. Osawa M. Clinical studies in asterixis. II. Clinical evaluations of unilateral asterixis. *J Tokyo Women's Med Coll* 1983;53:1149–61.

21c. Osawa M. Clinical studies in asterixis. III. Effects of thyrotropin-releasing hormone (TRH) on asterixis. *J Tokyo Women's Med Coll* 1983;53:1162–6.

21d. Osawa M, Hashino M, Aikawa K, Maruyama S. A case of carbamazepine-induced asterixis. *Neurol Med* 1981;15:484–6.

22. Pagni CA, Ettorre G, Infuso L, Marossero F. EMG responses to capsular stimulation in the human. *Experientia* 1964; 20:691–2.

23. Plum F, Posner JB. *The diagnosis of stupor and coma*, 2nd ed. Philadelphia: FA Davis, 1972:108, 162.

24. Reinfeld H, Louis S. Unilateral asterixis—clinical significance of the sign. *NY State J Med* 1983; 83:206–8.

25. Santamaria J, Graus E, Genis D. Bilateral asterixis in unilateral subdural hematoma. *J Neurol* 1983; 229:87–9.

26. Santamaria-Cano J, Graus-Ribas F, Martinez-Matos J, Rubio-Borrero F, Arbizu-Urdiain T, Peres-Serra J. Asterixis en lesiones focales del sistema nervioso central. *Rev Clin Espan* 1983; 168:37–9.

27. Shahani BT, Young RR. Studies of normal human silent period. In: Desmedt JE ed. New developments in electromyography and clinical neurophysiology, vol. 3. Basel: Karger, 1973:589–602.

28. Shahani BT, Young RR. Asterixis—a disorder of the neural mechanisms underlying sustained muscle contraction. In: Shahani M, ed. The motor system—neurophysiology and muscle mechanisms. Amsterdam: Elsevier, 1976:301–16.

29. Shahani BT, Young RR. Physiological and pharmacological aids in the differential diagnosis of tremor. *J Neurol Neurosurg Psychiatry* 1976; 39:772–83.

30. Shibasaki H, Motomura S, Yamashita Y, Shii H, Kuroiwa Y. Periodic synchronous discharge and myoclonus in Creutzfeldt-Jacob disease: diagnostic application of jerk-locked averaging method. *Ann Neurol* 1981; 9:150–6.

31. Smith MS, Laguna JF. Confusion, dysphasia and asterixis following metrizamide myelography. *Can J Neurol Sci* 1980; 7:309–11.

32. Tarsy D. Unilateral asterixis. *Arch Neurol* 1977; 34:723.

33. Tarsy D, Lieberman B, Chirico-Post J, Benson F. Unilateral asterixis associated with a mesencephalic syndrome. *Arch Neurol* 1977; 34:446–7.

34. Tyler HR, Leavitt S. Asterixis. *J Chronic Dis* 1965; 18:409–11.

35. Vallat JM, Rkina M, Bokor J. Unilateral asterixis due to subdural hematoma. *Arch Neurol* 1981; 38:535.

36. Watts RL, Williams RS, Young RR. The anatomy of cerebral lesions responsible for unilateral asterixis. (In press.)

37. Weinreb WH, Perry RJ, Jenkyn LR. Rhythmic alternating asterixis. *J Neurol Neurosurg Psychiatry* 1982; 45:857–8.

38. Yagnik P, Dhopesh V. Unilateral asterixis. *Arch Neurol* 1981; 38:601–2.

39. Young RR, Shahani BT. Anticonvulsant asterixis. *Electroencephalogr clin Neurophysiol* 1973; 34:760a.

40. Young RR, Shahani BT. Clinical neurophysiological aspects of post-hypoxic intention myoclonus. In: Fahn S, Davis JN, Rowland LP, eds. Cerebral hypoxia and its consequences. New York: Raven Press, 1979:85–105.

41. Young RR, Shahani BT, Kjellberg RN. Unilateral asterixis produced by a discrete CNS lesion. *Trans Am Neurol Assoc* 1976; 101:306–7.

42. Young RR, Wiegner AW. Tremor. In: Swash M, Kennard C, eds. Scientific basis of clinical neurology. Edinburgh: Churchill-Livingstone, 1985.

Advances in Neurology, Vol. 43: Myoclonus,
edited by S. Fahn et al. Raven Press,
New York © 1986.

Posthypoxic Action Myoclonus: Literature Review Update

Stanley Fahn

Department of Neurology, Columbia University College of Physicians and Surgeons, and The Neurological Institute of New York, New York, New York 10032

The syndrome of posthypoxic action myoclonus was first reported in 1963 by Lance and Adams (13). They described four patients who recovered from hypoxic coma with a permanent neurologic sequela of action or intention myoclonus. The characteristic feature of this syndrome is the induction of myoclonic jerks (both positive and negative myoclonus) by voluntary motor activity. Myoclonus is predominantly activated by walking and by motor tasks requiring precision. In 1979 a review of the literature on this subject revealed a total of 59 cases at that time (9). The purpose of this chapter is to update that review. A total of 23 additional cases have been reported. In addition, six other cases seen at our institution since the 1979 review are also presented.

CASE REPORTS

Case 1

On October 21, 1980, the patient, a 50-year-old businessman, had a myocardial infarction followed by a cardiopulmonary arrest. He was brought to an emergency room and was resuscitated; he was in coma for the following 2 days. He gradually became more alert and was eventually able to walk with assistance. A pronounced intellectual deficit was noticed. At the time of his transfer to a rehabilitation hospital, it was noticed that he had generalized myoclonus. Treatment with diazepam and phenobarbital produced lethargy. Clonazepam 3 mg/day suppressed the myoclonus. On March 13, 1981, he was admitted to the Neurological Institute of New York. He was alert, but not oriented to time or place. Speech was fluent. He could not do simple calculations, recite the names of the presidents, nor recall any of three names after 5 min. Neurological examination revealed increased muscle tone in the legs, mild ataxia with spontaneous falling, inability to tandem-walk, dysmetria of the legs, increased tendon reflexes, and extensor plantar reflexes. On admission, myoclonus was infrequent. An electromyogram (EMG) showed rare myoclonic jerking movements. Sensory, visual, and brainstem auditory-evoked potentials were all normal.

Clonazepam was discontinued, and myoclonus of face, trunk, and all limbs became more pronounced. This increased with action, especially with walking. There were both synchronous generalized myoclonic jerks and asynchronous focal jerks. A repeat EMG showed irregular (0.5–3 sec) contractions of arm and leg muscles. There was synchronous firing of arm flexors and extensors and of leg flexors and extensors, as well as asynchronous firing of these muscles. Removal of clonazepam did not enhance any intellectual function. Clonazepam was reinstated, and the severity of the myoclonus was reduced in a dose-responsive manner. At a dosage of 7 mg/day, the myoclonus was almost eliminated.

Follow-up examination on April 19, 1982, revealed the virtual absence of myoclonus on a dosage of 8 mg/day of clonazepam. There were occasions during walking when some myoclonus appeared, resulting in a tendency to fall. There were mild myoclonic jerks of the right arm when he wrote. He was able to take care of his daily activities of living except for shaving. Mentation remained markedly impaired.

Case 2

On February 9, 1977, the patient, a 56-year-old woman with a history of aspirin sensitivity, took some nonsteroidal anti-inflammatory drug and developed an acute asthmatic attack with a loss of consciousness. When seen in an emergency room, her pulse was palpable, but she was not breathing and her pupils were fixed and dilated. Ventricular fibrillation developed. She was defibrillated and resuscitated. She had several generalized seizures over the next few days, and subsequently myoclonic jerking was seen when she attempted to use her hands. Treatment with clonazepam reduced the severity of the myoclonus, but she was unable to feed herself or to walk unassisted. In March 1979, valproate was added. A dosage of 1 g/day further reduced the myoclonic jerking in the presence of clonazepam 14 mg/day. The patient was maintained on these medications.

Case 3

In August 1979, the patient, a 56-year-old woman, had a myocardial infarction followed by a cardiopulmonary arrest. She was in coma for 12 days. On recovery she had difficulty learning but could read and comprehend. She also had spontaneous myoclonic jerks of the left arm. She was admitted to the Neurological Institute of New York in January 1980 (Dr. Richard Mayeux). Examination revealed that the patient had immediate recall in the digit span test, but there was a loss of recall of all items to remember after a few minutes. Calculations were severely impaired. There were spontaneous and action myoclonic jerks of the limbs. Gait was ataxic, and the patient was unable to stand without assistance. She had almost continuous eyelid closure. Trials of vasopressin, lecithin, amantadine, and 5-hydroxytryptophan (5-HTP) were without effect. Sinemet reduced myoclonus slightly. Piracetam made it worse. Valproate and clonazepam helped moderately so that she was able to walk approximately 15 ft without assistance.

Case 4

In November 1977, the patient, a 47-year-old woman, suffered burns affecting almost 50% of her body. Approximately 36 hr later, she developed respiratory distress, culminating in respiratory arrest. She was in coma for 4 days, during which seizures occurred. On recovery, she had action myoclonus, particularly in the legs. She was unable to walk. L-Tryptophan was questionably effective. She was admitted to the Neurological Institute of New York (Dr. Robert Barrett) in February 1979. Examination revealed dysmetria of the legs: wide-based gait interrupted by myoclonus leading to falls. Myoclonus of all extremities was present at rest, with startle and with action. L-Tryptophan was discontinued without worsening of the myoclonus. Valproate up to 750 mg/day produced marked benefit. Protriptylline interfered with the effectiveness of valproate. She continues on valproate and is able to walk with occasional falling.

Case 5

In February 1982, the patient, a 39-year-old man, was shot in the neck. He was able to drive himself to an emergency room before losing consciousness. He was later informed that he had a respiratory arrest and was in a coma for 9 days. During that time he had seizures. Two weeks after the gunshot injury, he developed myoclonic jerking of the arms and legs. He had difficulty walking. In March 1982 he was transferred to a rehabilitation hospital. Treatment with phenytoin 400 mg/day and clonazepam 8 mg/day suppressed the seizures and reduced the myoclonus. Within 6 months he was able to walk approximately 30 ft unassisted and was able to feed himself by using weights on his wrists. He subsequently worsened and was admitted to the Neurological Institute of New York on January 16, 1983. Examination revealed dysarthric, halting speech and action myoclonus of the arms and legs with inability to walk, write, or feed himself because of the myoclonus. Electroencephalogram (EEG) showed background slowing and frequent low-voltage spikes and polyspikes that occurred symmetrically in the frontal and frontoparasagital areas. Median nerve sensory-evoked potentials were normal. Jerk-locked averaging of cortical potentials (Dr. Wayne Hening) failed to reveal any clearcut cortical spikes.

Increasing the dosage of clonazepam to 20 mg/day did not bring additional improvement. Valproate was then added, and the myoclonus was reduced. At a dosage of valproate 3,000 mg/day and clonazepam 18 mg/day, the patient was able to walk by using a walker and climb stairs by holding onto a railing. He was able to write his name and could hold a partially filled cup with his left hand but not his right.

Follow-up examination on April 12, 1983, revealed further improvement. Myoclonus was less severe. He could brush his hair, brush his teeth, feed himself with a cup and spoon, and bathe and dress himself. He walked short distances unassisted, but with a tendency to fall.

Case 6

In 1977 the patient, a 28-year-old woman, suffered hypoxic brain injury during a surgical procedure. She was comatose for 4 months. On recovery, she had some intellectual impairment and action myoclonus of the face, neck, arms, legs, and trunk. There was dysmetria of the arms. The myoclonus prevented her from walking. Phenytoin, valproate, and clonazepam were given in combination with little benefit. She was admitted to the Neurological Institute of New York (Dr. Susan Bressman) in September 1983. Examination revealed obesity, kyphosis, slowness in response to commands, and a paucity of spontaneous movement. There was dysarthria, a nasal quality, and unusual pauses and hesitation of her speech. Ocular movements showed jerky pursuit and horizontal nystagmus. The eyelids tended to close. There was mild quadriparesis. She could not sit or stand without support. Even with support, she tended to fall when standing due to myoclonic jerks, which were greater in the legs than in the arms. There was mild ataxia of all limbs. Tendon reflexes were brisk, and the plantar reflexes were extensor. Brainstem auditory- and somatosensory-evoked potentials were normal.

A trial of decreasing the dosage of clonazepam resulted in a worsening of myoclonus without altering the mental state. Phenytoin was discontinued without any clinical effect. 5-HTP (increased to 500 mg/day) was added to the clonazepam (10 mg/day) and valproate (3,500 mg/day) and resulted in a lessening of the myoclonic jerks but without any improvement of her functional activities.

LITERATURE REVIEW

The earlier review of cases of posthypoxic action myoclonus summarized the findings of 59 cases that had been reported (9). A further 29 cases have been described, including the six new cases in this report. These are summarized in Tables 1 and 2. Additional historical information is available about case 30 (11), which was covered in the previous review (9), and this is included in Tables 1 and

TABLE 1. Reported cases of posthypoxic action myoclonus: acute stage[a]

Year reported	Case No.	Age at onset (years)	Sex	Duration of syndrome[b] (years)	Etiology	Duration of coma (days)	Seizures during coma	Myoclonus during coma	Ref.
1978	60	43	M	10	Compressed chest	3	+	0	14
	61	30	F	?	Asthma (RA)	18	+	+	3
	62	26	F	1	Asthma (CA)	3 months	?	?	17
	63	43	F	1	Hemorrhagic shock	?	?	?	17
	64	42	M		Insulin coma	?	?	?	17
	65	44	F		Cardiac arrest	3	?	?	21
1979	66	48	F	2	Postoperative (RA)	?	+	?	7
	67	54	M	?	Aspirated (RA)	Hours	+	+	8
	68	26	F	?	Drowning (RA)	3	?	?	19
	30	37	F	2	Drug overdose (RA)	1	?	?	11c
	69	56	M	1	Arrhythmia → CA	4	?	+	2
1980	70	43	F	5	Anesthesia	14	?	?	6
1981	71	60	M	3	Anesthesia (CA,-RA)	5	0	?	1
	72	58	M	1	?	?	0	?	12

1982	73	52	M		Cardiac tamponade	2 Weeks	?	?	20
	74	35	M	1	Dextropropoxiphene overdose (CA,-RA)	?	?	?	15
1983	75	24	M	4 Months	Diving (CA,-RA)	5 Weeks	?	?	15
	76	42	F	3.5	Anesthesia	1	?	?	22
	77	65	M	?	Surgery	?	?	?	22
	78	4	F	11	Birth anoxia	<1	0	0	16
	79	2	M	7	Postnatal CA	<1	0	0	16
	80	45	M	4	Asthma (RA)	3	+	?	5
	81	24	F	5 Months	Pneumothorax	3	?	?	5
	82	54	F	1	Asthma (RA)	3	?	?	5
	83	50	M	1	MI (CA,-RA)	2	?	?	TC[d]
	84	56	F	5	Asthma (RA)	5	?	?	TC
	85	56	F	3	MI (RA)	12	?	?	TC
	86	49	F	5	Burns (RA)	4	?	?	TC
	87	39	M	1	Gunshot wound (RA)	9	+	?	TC
	88	27	F	8	Surgery	4 Months	?	?	TC

[a](+) Present; (?) not mentioned; (RA) respiratory arrest; (CA) cardiac arrest; (MI) myocardial infarction.
[b]Duration of syndrome refers to time between onset and year of publication of the report.
[c]Update of case 30.
[d](TC) This chapter.

TABLE 2. *Reported cases of posthypoxic action myoclonus: chronic stage[a]*

Case No.	Seizures	Dysarthria	CSF HIAA (ng/ml)	Ataxia	Predominant side affected	Gait affected[b]	Results of treatment	
							Drug	Improvement[c]
60	?	+		−	L	RA	Thalamotomy	0
							Primidone	0
							Baclofen	0
							Nortriptylline	0
							Diazepam, nitrazepam	0
							Clonazepam	0
							Anticonvulsants	0
							Tetrabenazine	0
							5-HTP	ΔΔΔ → 0
							Paroxetine + 5-HTP	0
61	?	?	49	+		RA	Diazepam, nitrazepam	0
							Clonazepam	ΔΔ
							Anticonvulsants	0
							Valproate	ΔΔ
							5-HTP	ΔΔΔ
62	?	+		?	L	RA	5-HTP	ΔΔΔ
63	?	?		?		?	5-HTP	ΔΔΔ
64	?	?		?		?	5-HTP	ΔΔΔ
65	?	?		−	R	RA	Piracetam	ΔΔΔ
66	?	+		?		RA	5-HTP	0
							Diazepam	Δ
							Clonazepam	Δ
							Tiapride	0
							Piracetam	ΔΔΔ
67	+	?		?		RA	Clonazepam	ΔΔ
68	?	?	<10	?		RA	Diazepam, nitrazepam	0
							Carbamazepine	0
							Methysergide	0
							Valproate	ΔΔΔ
							L-DOPA	Δ
30	+	?	15.2	?		WD	Same as previously reported	
69	?	+		+		RA	Anticonvulsants	0
							Valproate	ΔΔ
70	?	?		?		RA	Diazepam	ΔΔ
							Nitrazepam	0
							Clonazepam	0
							Carbamazepine	0
							Phenobarbial	0
							Baclofen	ΔΔΔ
							L-DOPA	ΔΔΔ
71	?	?	25	+	R	RA	5-HTP	ΔΔ
72	?	+		+			Clonazepam	Δ
							Valproate	Δ
73	?	?		?		RA	Barbiturates	0
							Diazepam	0
							Valproate	ΔΔΔ
74	?	−		?	L		Paroxetine	ΔΔΔ
							Clonazepam	Δ

TABLE 2. *(continued)*

Case No.	Seizures	Dysarthria	CSF HIAA (ng/ml)	Ataxia	Predominant side affected	Gait affected[b]	Results of treatment Drug	Improvement[c]
75	?	+		?			Biperidine	0
							Phenytoin	0
							Clonazepam	Δ
							Antipsychotics	0
							Tetrabenazine	0
							Baclofen	0
							Paroxetine	Δ
76	?	+		?	R	RA	Clonazepam	ΔΔ
							Valproate	0
							5-HTP	ΔΔ → Δ
							Fluoxetine + 5-HTP	ΔΔΔ
77	+	+		?		RA	5-HTP	ΔΔ → Δ
							Fluoxetine + 5-HTP	ΔΔΔ
78	−	+		−	L	WD	Lisuride	0
							Clonazepam	0
79	+	+		?		WD	None reported	
80	−	?		?		RA	Clonazepam	ΔΔΔ
81	?	?		?		RA	Clonazepam	ΔΔΔ → normal in 3 months
82	?	?		?		RA	Clonazepam	ΔΔΔ
83	+	−		+		RA	Diazepam, phenobarbital	0
							Clonazepam	ΔΔΔ
84	+	−		+		WD	5-HTP	0
							Valproate	ΔΔ
							Clonazepam	ΔΔ
85	−	+		+		RA	Vasopressin	0
							Piracetam	Worse
							Valproate	ΔΔ
							Clonazepam	ΔΔ
							Lecithin	0
							L-DOPA	Δ
							Amantadine	0
86	+	−		+	L	WD	Diazepam	0
							Anticholinergic	0
							Antihistaminic	0
							L-Tryptophan	0
							Phenytoin	0
							Valproate	ΔΔΔ
87	+	+		+		RA	Clonazepam	ΔΔ
							Valproate	ΔΔ
88	−	+		+		RA	Phenytoin	0
							Clonazepam	Δ
							Valproate	0
							5-HTP	Δ

[a](+) Present; (−) absent; (?) not mentioned.
[b](WD) walks with difficulty; (RA) requires assistance or walker.
[c](0) Normal gait or no effect of treatment; (Δ) mild to moderate improvement; (ΔΔ) marked improvement; (ΔΔΔ) improvement to an almost normal level.

2. The new cases summarized in this chapter, plus the 59 reviewed previously, brings the total to 88.

The causes of anoxia in the 88 cases are listed in Table 3. Anesthesia accidents constitute the most common cause in these 88 cases: 31 of the patients (35%) fall in this category. This is a reduction from the 44% in this category reported in 1979 (9). Myocardial damage, obstructed airway, and drug overdosages occur almost equally in the list of causes, and each accounts for 10% to 14% of the cases. The miscellaneous causes make up the remainder, with asthma leading the list in this group (Table 3). Birth anoxia and perinatal cardiac arrest are new to the list (cases 78 and 79) (16).

The duration of anoxic coma was reported for 49 patients and ranged from less than 1 day to 120 days (Table 4). The long durations of more than 1 month were possibly not rigidly defined and represent what the patients were later told by their physicians. The median duration of coma was 4 days. As mentioned previously (9), it is not possible to correlate severity of myoclonus with duration of coma because the lack of quantitative ratings of severity in the case reports precludes comparison of patients.

At least 23 patients had seizures during the comatose state, and seven did not have seizures (Table 5). There was no mention of seizures in the remaining 58 patients. The presence or absence of myoclonus during the period of coma was specifically reported for 23 cases; of these, 16 (70%) had myoclonus during coma (Table 5). The two cases of perinatal anoxia had neither seizures nor myoclonus at the time of the coma.

There were 47 women and 41 men affected, and all but 12 were older than 20 years at the onset of hypoxia (the age was not stated in three cases) (Table 6). In addition to the two with perinatal anoxia, only one child has been reported with this syndrome, a boy of 6 years (case 12 in ref 9). The two with the perinatal anoxia did not develop myoclonus until the ages of 2 and 4 years. In general, the syndrome of posthypoxic action myoclonus appears to be permanent. Only one patient had a spontaneous remission after 5 months (case 81), although lessening of ataxia and dysarthria has been seen.

One uniform characteristic clinical feature of all 88 patients reported is the presence of action myoclonus. The two children with perinatal anoxia had in addition oscillatory myoclonus (16), in which myoclonus-at-rest occurred as oscillatory jerks in transient bursts that then faded (10). The severity of action myoclonus in the 88 patients varied, but that induced by walking appeared to be the most affected and the most resistant to treatment.

The neuropharmacology, cerebrospinal fluid (CSF) biochemistry, and physiology of posthypoxic action myoclonus have been discussed in the previous review (9), and there is little new information to add. Patients can be divided into two groups having either cortical reflex myoclonus or reticular reflex myoclonus. Perhaps as future physiologic analyses are carried out, further subdivisions will become known. The pathology of posthypoxic action myoclonus has also been discussed in the previous review, and only two cases have been reported. One of these (case 42)

TABLE 3. *Causes of anoxia (88 cases)*

Causes of anoxia	No. of patients
Associated with anesthesia and surgery	
Cardiac arrest	15
Obstructed airway	5
Postoperative respiratory arrest	3
Pneumothorax	1
Faulty valve (no O_2)	1
Not specified	7
	32
Myocardial	
Infarction (cardiac arrest)	9
Arrhythmia (cardiac arrest)	1
Cardiac tamponade	1
Postnatal cardiac arrest	1
	12
Obstructed airway	
Tracheal edema	3
Hanging	2
Peritracheal hemorrhage	1
Trauma	1
Aspiration	3
Chest compression	1
	11
Drug intoxication	
Heroin	2
Barbiturate	1
Insecticide	1
Multiple drugs	1
Insulin coma	1
Dextropropoxiphene	1
Not specified	2
	9
Miscellaneous	
Asthma	8
Anaphylaxis	2
Chest trauma	1
Face trauma	1
Syncope	1
Hemorrhagic shock	1
Drowning	1
Deep-sea diving	1
Gunshot wound of neck	1
Burning	1
Respiratory arrest	1
Birth anoxia	1
Pneumothorax	1
	21
Not stated	3
Total	88

TABLE 4. *Duration of anoxic coma*

Days in coma	No. of patients
<1	6
1	4
2	6
3	13
4	4
5	2
7	2
>7	1
8	2
9	1
12	2
14	3
16	1
18	1
35	1
90	1
120	1
Total stated:	51
Not stated:	37
	88

TABLE 5. *Seizures and myoclonus during anoxic coma*

	Present	Absent	Not stated
Seizures	23	7	58
Myoclonus	16	7	65

TABLE 6A. *Age at time of coma*

Sex	?	At birth	6	15–20	21–30	31–40	41–50	51–60	61–70	71+	Total
F		1		2	13	7	11	9	2	2	47
M	3	1	1	4	5	6	6	9	4	2	41
Total:	3	2	1	6	18	13	17	18	6	4	88

has been further elaborated in a publication by Richardson and his colleagues (18). There was a paucity of structural alterations in this case. Prominent astrocytosis was seen in the supratrochlear nucleus, the lateral subnucleus of the mesencephalic gray matter, and the adjacent cuneiform and subcuneiform nuclei. These regions may have had neuronal loss as well; however, these authors found no alterations in

TABLE 6B. *Incidence by age group*

Sex	Children	15–40	41–60	61+	?
F	1	22	20	4	
M	2	15	15	6	3
Total:	3	37	35	10	3

TABLE 7. *Drugs evaluated in posthypoxic action myoclonus in the literature cited in this chapter*

Drug	Reference number		
	Improvement	No effect	Worse
Anticonvulsants			
Phenobarbital		6, 20, TC	
Carbamazepine		6, 19	
Primidone		14	
Phenytoin		15, TC	
Valproate	2, 3, 12, 19, 20, 22, TC[a]	TC	
Miscellaneous		2, 3, 14	
Benzodiazepines			
Nitrazepam		3, 6, 14, 19	
Diazepam	6, 7	3, 14, 19, 20, TC	
Clonazepam	3, 5, 7, 8, 12, 15, 16, 22, TC	6, 14	
Dopamine agonists			
Levodopa	6, 19, TC		
Amantadine		TC	
Lisuride		16	
Dopamine antagonists			
Tetrabenazine		7, 14, 15	
Antipsychotics		15	
Anticholinergics		15, TC	
Serotonin precursors			
5-HTP	1, 3, 14, 17, 22, TC	7, TC	
L-Tryptophan		TC	
Serotonin-uptake blockers			
Paroxetine	15	14, 15	
Fluoxetine	22		
Serotonin antagonists			
Methysergide		19	
Antidepressants			
Nortriptylline		14	
Miscellaneous			
Piracetam	7, 21		TC
Baclofen	6	14, 15	
Vasopressin		TC	
Antihistaminic		TC	
Lecithin		TC	

[a](TC) this chapter.

the basal ganglia, subthalamic nuclei, thalamus, tectum, pons, or medulla. The cerebral cortex, hippocampus, cerebellar cortex, and deep cerebellar nuclei were normal. When compared to the pathology of the case reported by Castaigne et al. (4), which had more extensive damage, the affected regions in common were the midbrain periaqueductal gray matter and dorsolateral gray matter of the tegmentum.

Drugs used in the treatment of posthypoxic action myoclonus in the latest 29 case reports (Table 2) were fairly similar to those evaluated previously (9). The most consistently effective agents were clonazepam, valproate, and 5-HTP (Table 7). Newer drugs with some efficacy, however, have also been proposed, particularly piracetam and fluoxetine (Table 7). It is interesting to note that benzodiazepines other than clonazepam are rather ineffective. It is not clear what action of clonazepam renders it useful for myoclonus. In Table 7, lisuride is listed as a dopamine agonist; it is also a serotonin agonist, which may be relevant to its potential role in the treatment of myoclonus. Yet, there are reports of some efficacy from levodopa. It would be helpful to learn more about the mechanisms of action of both clonazepam and valproate since this might shed light on the pathophysiology of myoclonus.

ACKNOWLEDGMENTS

I am grateful to Drs. Robert Barrett, Richard Mayeux, and Susan Bressman for allowing me to evaluate and report their patients.

REFERENCES

1. Beretta E, Regli F, de Crousaz G, Steck AJ. Postanoxic myoclonus: treatment of a case with 5-hydroxytryptophane and a decarboxylase inhibitor. *J Neurol* 1981;225:57–62.
2. Bruni J, Willmore LJ, Wilder BJ. Treatment of postanoxic intention myoclonus with valproic acid. *Can J Neurol Sci* 1979;6:39–43.
3. Carroll WM, Walsh PJ. Functional independence in postanoxic myoclonus: contribution of L-5-HTP, sodium valproate and clonazepam. *Br Med J* 1978;2:1612.
4. Castaigne P, Cambier J, Escourolle R, Cathola HP, Lecasble R. Observation anatomo-clinique d'un syndrome myoclonique post-anoxique. *Rev Neurol (Paris)* 1964;111:60–73.
5. Chee YC, Poh SC. Myoclonus following severe asthma: clonazepam relieves. *Aust NZ J Med* 1983;13:285–6.
6. Coletti A, Mandelli A, Minoli G, Tredici G. Postanoxic action myoclonus (Lance–Adams syndrome) treated with levodopa and GABAergic drugs. *J Neurol* 1980;223:67–70.
7. Cremieux C, Serratrice G. Myoclonie d'intention et d'action post-anoxique: amelioration par le piracetam. *Nouvelle Presse Medicale* 1979;41:3357–8.
8. DeLisa JA, Stolov WC, Troupin AS. Action myoclonus following acute cerebral anoxia. *Arch Phys Med Rehabil* 1979;60:32–6.
9. Fahn S. Posthypoxic action myoclonus: review of the literature and report of two new cases with response to valproate and estrogen. *Adv Neurol* 26:49–84, 1979.
10. Fahn S, Singh N. An oscillating form of essential myoclonus. 2. *Neurology* 1981;31(4):80.
11. Hallett M, Chadwick D, Marsden CD. Cortical reflex myoclonus. *Neurology* 1979;29:1107–25.
12. Kelly JJ Jr, Sharbrough FW, Daube JR. A clinical and electrophysiological evaluation of myoclonus. *Neurology* 1981;31:581–9.
13. Lance JW, Adams RD. The syndrome of intention or action myoclonus as a sequel to hypoxic encephalopathy. *Brain* 1963;86:111–36.
14. Magnussen I, Dupont E, Engbaek F, de Fine Olivarius B. Posthypoxic intention myoclonus treated with 5-hydroxytryptophan and an extracerebral decarboxylase inhibitor. *Acta Neurol Scand* 1978;57:289–94.

15. Magnussen I, Mondrup K, Engbaek F, Lademann A, de Fine Olivarius B. Treatment of myoclonic syndromes with paroxetine alone or combined with 5-HTP. *Acta Neurol Scand* 1982;66:276–82.
16. Obeso JA, Lang AE, Rothwell JC, Marsden CD. Postanoxic symptomatic oscillatory myoclonus. *Neurology* 1983;33:240–3.
17. Rascol A, Guiraud-Chaumeil B, Laboucarie J, Montastruc JL, El-Hage W: Utilisation du 5-hydroxytryptophane levogyre dans les myoclonies post-anoxiques. *Therapie* 1978;33:623–8.
18. Richardson JC, Rewcastle NB, De Lean J: Hypoxic myoclonus: clinical and pathological observations. In: Rose FC, ed. Physiological aspects of clinical neurology. Oxford: Blackwell Scientific, 1977:231–45.
19. Rollinson RD, Gilligan BS. Postanoxic action myoclonus (Lance–Adams syndrome) responding to valproate. *Arch Neurol* 1979;36:44–5.
20. Sotaniemi K. Valproic acid in the treatment of nonepileptic myoclonus: report of three cases. *Arch Neurol* 1982;39:443–91.
21. Terwinghe G, Daumerie J, Nicaise C, Rosillon O. Effet therapeutique du piracetam dans un cas de myoclonie d'action postanoxique. *Acta Neurol Belg* 1978;78:30–6.
22. Van Woert MH, Magnussen I, Rosenbaum D, Chung E. Fluoxetine in the treatment of intention myoclonus. *Clin Neuropharmacol* 1983;6:49–54.

Advances in Neurology, Vol. 43: Myoclonus,
edited by S. Fahn et al. Raven Press,
New York © 1986.

Biochemistry and Therapeutics of Posthypoxic Myoclonus

Melvin H. Van Woert, David Rosenbaum, and Eunyong Chung

Departments of Neurology and Pharmacology, Mount Sinai School of Medicine, New York, New York 10029

Myoclonus has been considered to be an epileptic phenomenon because of its frequent concomitant occurrence in idiopathic epilepsy and other seizure disorders. A progressive increase in myoclonus will frequently precede tonic–clonic major motor seizures. Furthermore, numerous convulsant chemicals [e.g., metrazol, dichlorodiphenyltrichloroethane (DDT)] will produce only myoclonus at low doses and both myoclonus and generalized seizures at higher doses. Like epilepsy, myoclonus also may be due to hyperexcitable neurons produced by either a primary metabolic abnormality or a decreased inhibitory input, such as from γ-aminobutyric acid (GABA)-ergic or glycinergic neurons.

Myoclonus can occur alone without major or minor seizures or electroencephalogram (EEG) abnormalities (e.g., hereditary essential myoclonus). Furthermore, the serotonin (5-HT) precursor L-5-hydroxytryptophan (L-5-HTP), which is not an anticonvulsant, has potent antimyoclonic action. Of the standard anticonvulsants, barbiturates produce only minimal reduction in myoclonus (45,57), and trials of phenytoin and succinimides, in general, also have been disappointing. Among the anticonvulsants, only benzodiazepine compounds, particularly clonazepam (Clonopin) and valproic acid (Depakene) have impressive antimyoclonic action.

(L-5-HTP) WITH CARBIDOPA

Clinical and laboratory investigations have suggested that there may be an impairment in brain 5-HT metabolism in certain types of myoclonus. It is not yet known whether this biochemical abnormality is due to the loss of a specific serotonergic pathway or to a functional deficiency in 5-HT synthesis and/or release.

Serotonin is a neurotransmitter in the central nervous system (CNS) that is synthesized from the essential amino acid L-tryptophan (Fig. 1). Tryptophan is hydroxylated, by the enzyme tryptophan hydroxylase (TH) to form L-5-HTP, which is decarboxylated by L-aromatic amino acid decarboxylase (L-AAAD) to form 5-HT. This decarboxylase may be the same enzyme that converts levodopa to dopamine and is inhibited in extracerebral tissues by carbidopa. Serotonin is degraded primarily by monoamine oxidase (MAO) to form 5-hydroxyindoleacetic acid (5-HIAA), an inactive metabolite.

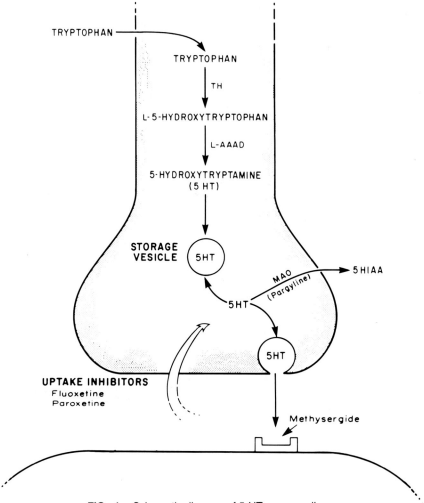

FIG. 1. Schematic diagram of 5-HT nerve ending.

The following evidence suggests that brain 5-HT deficiency may produce certain types of myoclonus:

1. Cerebrospinal fluid (CSF) 5-HIAA, the major metabolite of 5-HT, is decreased in myoclonic disorders, such as postanoxic and post-traumatic intention myoclonus, progressive myoclonus epilepsy, and essential myoclonus. In one study, basal CSF 5-HIAA was 67% of control (6), and in two studies using probenecid to block 5-HIAA excretion from the CNS, CSF 5-HIAA was reduced to 60% (65); and 51% (61) of normal values.

2. Drugs that enhance brain serotonergic action reduce myoclonic activity:

(a) High doses of L-5-HTP (1,000–2,000 mg/day) in combination with the peripheral decarboxylase inhibitor carbidopa is effective therapy for the above myoclonic syndromes with low CSF 5-HIAA (6,18,25,37,42,61,65).

(b) Low doses of L-5-HTP (400–500 mg/day) and carbidopa with fluoxetine (30–40 mg/day), a specific 5-HT uptake blocker, is also effective antimyoclonic therapy. In two patients with intention myoclonus responsive to L-5-HTP and carbidopa, fluoxetine reduced the required dose of L-5-HTP to approximately one-third, with greater antimyoclonic activity, decreased side effects, and reduction in platelet 5-HT and plasma 5-HIAA and L-5-HTP concentrations (64) (Fig. 2). Since fluoxetine only potentiates 5-HT released from serotonergic neurons, this clinical study further supports the hypothesis that the antimyoclonic action of L-5-HTP is due to replenishment of a specific 5-HT deficiency. Magnussen et al. (44) reported that paroxetine, another specific 5-HT reuptake inhibitor, when given alone or in combination with L-5-HTP with carbidopa, ameliorated posthypoxic intention myoclonus in two of three patients.

(c) L-Tryptophan, in combination with a MAO inhibitor, which prevents degradation of 5-HT, has been found to have a moderate therapeutic response in patients with postanoxic intention myoclonus (6,18). Since the synthesis of 5-HT from L-tryptophan occurs only in serotonergic neurons, this evidence also supports the 5-HT deficiency hypothesis of certain myoclonic disorders.

3. Methysergide, 5-HT receptor antagonist, has had mixed clinical effects in patients with postanoxic myoclonus when administered alone, but it blocked the therapeutic action of L-5-HTP and carbidopa (42).

4. Several animal models of myoclonus are responsive to therapy with 5-HT agonists:

(a) Stimulus-sensitive myoclonus produced by injection of the insecticide p,p'-DDT, intragastrically or into the medullary reticular formation (MRF) in rats, is

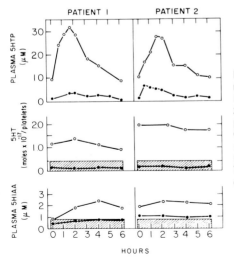

FIG. 2. Pharmacokinetics of L-5-HTP and its metabolites after morning dose. ○, after a L-5-HTP dose (350 mg in patient 1, 400 mg in patient 2); ●, after L-5-HTP (50 mg in patient 1, 75 mg in patient 2) in combination with fluoxetine (10 mg). Carbidopa (50 mg) was given in all four studies. *Hatched bars*, normal range. Plasma L-5-HTP is not detectable in untreated patients. (From Van Woert et al., ref. 64. Reproduced with permission of publisher.)

improved by 5-HT agonists and aggravated by 5-HT antagonists (9). Myoclonus induced by injection of DDT into the MRF is an example of reticular reflex myoclonus produced by enhancement of the physiological spinoreticular-spinal reflex. In this DDT animal model of myoclonus, the antimyoclonic action of L-5-HTP appears to be due to enhanced action at the inferior olive, which stimulates climbing fiber projections to cerebellar Purkinje cells (12). We postulate that, by this mechanism, 5-HT modifies cerebellar control over the MRF through the Purkinje-fastigial-MRF pathway.

(b) In the photosensitive baboon Papio papio, intermittent light stimulation produces bilateral myoclonus (31). Various 5-HT agonists and L-5-HTP suppress myoclonic responses to photic stimulation, whereas D,L-*p*-chlorophenylalanine, which decreases brain 5-HT levels, lowers seizure threshold and increases myoclonus (66).

(c) Subconvulsant doses of metrazol (60 mg/kg i.p.) produce stimulus-sensitive myoclonic jerks and a startle response in rats which can be prevented by pretreatment with L-5-HTP in combination with carbidopa and aggravated by pharmacological agents that decrease brain 5-HT (17,63). The cerebral cortex contributes to but is not essential for metrazol-induced myoclonus, since complete decortication raises the threshold but does not abolish the bilateral myoclonic response to subconvulsant doses of metrazol (38). It is of interest that intravenously injected metrazol combined with intermittent photic stimulation produced precentral and frontal polyspikes and myoclonic jerks, particularly in the upper extremities in normal human subjects (23).

(d) There have also been numerous reports indicating that decreased brain 5-HT is associated with enhanced seizure susceptibility, whereas increased brain 5-HT levels attenuate convulsions in various animal models of epilepsy. Treatment with *p*-chlorophenylalanine, an inhibitor of brain 5-HT synthesis, facilitates the rate of development of amygdaloid-kindled seizures in the rat (48), increases susceptibility to audiogenic seizures in mice (2), and decreases seizure threshold in electroconvulsive shock in mice and rats (30). On the other hand, L-5-HTP was found to retard the evolution of the kindling process (48), decrease seizure susceptibility in audiogenic mice (2), and raise the threshold for electroconvulsive shock-induced seizures (30). Amygdaloid kindling produces selectively significant decreases in the concentrations of 5-HT and 5-HIAA in the midbrain region where 5-HT-containing raphe nuclei are located (48).

In clinical studies, patients with postanoxic intention myoclonus have derived the greatest degree of symptomatic improvement during L-5-HTP and carbidopa therapy. Intention myoclonus associated with head trauma, methyl bromide toxicity, postencephalitic brain damage, progressive familial myoclonus epilepsy, and essential myoclonus also have improved with this therapy. In our 18 patients with intention myoclonus, 61% derived greater than 50% overall improvement during treatment with L-5-HTP in combination with carbidopa (65). Palatal myoclonus has also been reported to respond to therapy with L-5-HTP and carbidopa (43,67).

The optimum dosage of L-5-HTP should be determined by gradual titration according to adverse and therapeutic effects in each patient. The patient should be started on 25 mg L-5-HTP four times a day and the dosage increased by 100 mg/day in divided doses every 3 to 5 days if there are no significant side effects. If significant gastrointestinal side effects (nausea, diarrhea, anorexia, and, rarely, vomiting) develop, the rate of L-5-HTP daily dose increase (100 mg in four divided doses) may be delayed to every 1 to 2 weeks. A reduction in myoclonus is usually first observed at a L-5-HTP dose of 600 to 1,000 mg/day (with carbidopa), and the usual optimal therapeutic dose of L-5-HTP is between 1,000 and 2,000 mg/day in four divided doses. Carbidopa should be started with L-5-HTP and discontinued only when the L-5-HTP has been stopped. The total daily dose of carbidopa usually ranges from 100 to 200 mg in four divided doses.

5-HT-Induced Myoclonus

In guinea pigs, large doses of L-5-HTP, a 5-HT precursor, or 5-HT agonists produce myoclonus that is not stimulus sensitive (34). Clinically, a myoclonic syndrome resembling infantile spasms was also observed in 15% of human infants with Down's syndrome treated with L-5-HTP (13). Myoclonus occasionally observed during therapy with tricyclic antidepressants or MAO inhibitors (Liberman, *this volume*) also may be related to increased serotonergic neurotransmission. Methysergide, a 5-HT receptor blocker, may reduce these putative 5-HT-induced myoclonic syndromes (33). Thus it has been postulated that increased serotonergic neurotransmission may produce myoclonus that is pharmacologically and biochemically opposite from the stimulus-sensitive myoclonus which responds to therapy with 5-HT precursors.

BENZODIAZEPINES

The most effective benzodiazepine drug for the treatment of myoclonus is clonazepam (Clonopin). It has a broad spectrum of activity against various types of epilepsy, and its major use is in petit mal absences, infantile spasms, and myoclonic epilepsies (53). The following myoclonic disorders have been reported to respond to clonazepam therapy: infantile spasms, progressive myoclonus epilepsy, Ramsay Hunt syndrome, postencephalitic myoclonus, epilepsia partialis continua, postanoxic intention myoclonus, Lennox–Gastaut syndrome, status myoclonus, juvenile myoclonic epilepsy, and photosensitive myoclonic seizures.

Effect on GABA

Pharmacologic and neurophysiological evidence has accumulated which suggests that benzodiazepine compounds enhance GABAergic neurotransmission and that the anticonvulsant action of benzodiazepines may be mediated through GABA (15,26,55). Drugs that interfere with GABAergic neurotransmission produce epileptic seizures in animals and humans. Benzodiazepine drugs block the seizures elicited by GABA receptor antagonists (e.g., picrotoxin, bicuculline) and drugs that reduce GABA synthesis (e.g., isoniazid, thiosemicarbazide, 3-mercaptopropionic acid) (16,26). Furthermore, CSF GABA has been found to be decreased in patients with epilepsy (20,68), and the concentration of GABA and glutamic acid decarboxylase (GAD) is reduced in human focal epileptogenic brain tissue (39,62).

The evidence that the mechanism of anticonvulsant activity of benzodiazepines is by enhancement of GABAergic neurotransmission is impressive. However, the mechanism of antimyoclonic action of benzodiazepines is not clear, and the evidence for a role of GABA in modifying myoclonic phenomena is conflicting.

The level of CSF GABA was determined in seven patients with postanoxic intention myoclonus and in three patients with progressive myoclonus epilepsy (without Lafora bodies) (19). The CSF GABA in both groups of patients with myoclonus was reduced approximately 50% compared to controls consisting of patients with various other neurological disorders. Whole blood GABA in the two myoclonic groups, however, did not differ significantly from controls. Recently, CSF GABA was found to be decreased by 24% in a group of 15 patients with progressive myoclonus epilepsy (without Lafora bodies); the more severely afflicted patients had lower CSF GABA than the ones with lesser involvement (1).

Agonists of GABA inhibit the focal rhythmic myoclonus produced by unilateral injections of the GABA antagonists picrotoxin and bicuculline into the caudate nucleus of the rat (60) but have no effect on the stimulus-sensitive, 5-HT-responsive DDT animal model of myoclonus (9). Progabide is a potent and specific GABA agonist which directly interacts with GABA receptor site as well as being a GABA precursor (40). It has been found to be an effective anticonvulsant particularly useful in partial complex seizures (46). We have initiated a clinical trial of progabide in patients with intention myoclonus. Progabide (1,800 mg/day) has had no effect in a 51-year-old man with generalized intention myoclonus due to postoperative respiratory arrest and supraventricular tachycardia and in a 22-year-old man with progressive myoclonus epilepsy.

Effect on 5-HT

Since clonazepam is a potent antimyoclonic agent in 5-HT-responsive postanoxic intention myoclonus, its effect on brain 5-HT metabolism has been investigated. Although there may be some species differences, clonazepam has had minimal to no effect on brain concentrations of 5-HT and 5-HIAA in mice and rats (10,56). In fact, clonazepam has been shown to decrease 5-HT utilization in brain (Jenner et al., *this volume*), which provides further evidence that the antimyoclonic action of clonazepam is not attributable to enhancement of brain 5-HT metabolism.

Behavioral studies in mice have indicated that benzodiazepines can have an action on the motor system similar to that of 5-HT agonists. Drugs that stimulate the central serotonergic system produce head twitching and a pinna response in mice (14). Nakamura and Fukushima (49) and Chadwick et al. (5) have reported that clonazepam produces head twitching and a pinna response in mice, which they attribute to stimulation of 5-HT neuronal pathways. Fludiazepam and diazepam have been reported to potentiate head twitches in mice induced by intracerebrally injected 5-HT and intraperitoneally injected 5-methoxytryptamine, a potent 5-HT receptor agonist; cyproheptadine, a 5-HT receptor blocker, counteracted this potentiating action of benzodiazepines (50,51). Similarly, in the DDT model of myoclonus in mice, clonazepam reduces the myoclonus; this antimyoclonic action is blocked by the 5-HT receptor antagonists methysergide, metergoline, and cinnanserin (10). Although clonazepam does not enhance 5-HT metabolism or interact with the 5-HT receptor site, it might activate 5-HT receptor-coupled reactions (e.g., second messenger) in some regions of the brain. This hypothesis warrants further investigation since it could explain the behavioral similarities of the benzodiazepines and 5-HT.

VALPROIC ACID

Valproic acid (Depakene) is an anticonvulsant that is particularly effective in the therapy of progressive myoclonus epilepsy and somewhat less useful in the treatment of postanoxic intention myoclonus (21,54). It has multiple pharmacological actions in the CNS, and it is not clear which of the known actions, if any, are responsible for the antimyoclonic effect.

Effect on GABA

Valproic acid is a weak inhibitor of GABA-transaminase (GABA-T) and a more potent inhibitor of succinic semialdehyde dehydrogenase (SSADH) (3,24,27):

$$
\begin{array}{l}
\qquad\quad \text{GAD} \\
\text{glutamate} \longrightarrow \text{GABA} \\
\qquad\qquad\quad \uparrow\downarrow \;\; \text{GABA-T} \\
\qquad\qquad\quad \text{succinic semialdehyde} \\
\qquad\qquad\quad \downarrow \text{SSADH} \\
\qquad\qquad\quad \text{succinic acid}
\end{array}
$$

Inhibition of these enzymes, which catabolize GABA, increases the concentration of this inhibitory neurotransmitter in the CNS. Electrophysiological studies show that valproic acid can also potentiate the inhibition of neuronal firing by GABA in certain regions of the brain (4,41). The evidence that the therapeutic effect of valproic acid is due to an increase in GABAergic neurotransmission is not totally convincing, however, since the doses of valproic acid necessary to increase GABA levels in rat brain are much greater than those used in clinical treatment (3,58). Furthermore, as described above, it is questionable whether increasing brain GABA would have any effect on myoclonus.

Effect on 5-HT

Valproic acid elevates freely diffusible serum tryptophan by displacing it from binding sites on serum albumin (11,36). This in turn raises brain tryptophan levels.

Since TH is normally not saturated with its substrate, elevated brain tryptophan concentration may produce an increase in 5-HT synthesis. However, the valproic acid-induced increase in 5-HT synthesis is marginal and does not appear to be an adequate mechanism to explain the antimyoclonic action of valproic acid.

Effect on Aspartic Acid

Valproic acid decreases the concentration of the excitatory amino acid aspartic acid in the CNS (7,59). The reduction in brain aspartate concentration by valproic acid has temporal correlation with its anticonvulsant activity. A reduction in the excitatory neurotransmitter pool of aspartate could be associated with a decreased excitatory state in the CNS. The possible role of aspartate in myoclonic disorders warrants further investigation.

Effect on Glycine

Glycine is an inhibitory neurotransmitter which, like GABA, may modulate neuronal excitability and seizure threshold. Iontophoretically applied valproic acid augments the inhibitory effects of glycine on retinal ganglion cells *in vitro* (28) and increases plasma and urinary glycine by inhibiting hepatic glycine cleavage enzymes (47). However, valproic acid has no effect on cortical, medullary, and spinal cord glycine levels (7,36; Van Woert et al., *this volume*). Thus although myoclonus can be produced by inhibition of glycine receptors, such as by strychnine and urea (Chung et al., *this volume*), there is currently no evidence that valproic acid acts by increasing glycinergic neurotransmission.

In conclusion, valproic acid has multiple biochemical and physiological effects in the brain that could decrease neuronal excitability; however, the mechanism of its antimyoclonic and anticonvulsant action remains to be determined.

MISCELLANEOUS DRUGS

Adrenocorticotropic hormone and prednisone have been used to treat infantile myoclonic spasms and polymyoclonia and opsoclonus associated with neuroblastoma and myoclonic encephalopathy of infants (8,29,32). The mechanisms responsible for the therapeutic effects of adrenocorticosteroids in these conditions are not known, but it has been suggested that they may counteract the adverse effects of autoimmune phenomena or viral infections in some cases.

Both 4B-phenyl-GABA (Lioresal, Baclofen) and alcohol have been reported to reduce myoclonus in patients with hereditary essential myoclonus (35).

Respiratory myoclonus has been treated by phrenicectomy when the diaphragmatic contractions become very uncomfortable. A single report indicates that phenytoin may be an effective pharmacological mode of therapy for some patients with this disorder (52).

Intention myoclonus may be worse premenstrually and improve during the first two trimesters of pregnancy. Fahn (22) reported an inverse correlation between the intensity of myoclonus and the level of plasma estrogen during the menstrual cycle in one patient with postanoxic intention myoclonus. This patient's myoclonus improved during therapy with the conjugated estrogen premarin, suggesting that the estrogen/progesterone ratio may be important in regulating neuronal excitability.

CONCLUSIONS

Myoclonus may be attributable to hyperexcitable neurons in the spinal cord, MRF, or cerebral cortex. These neurons may be hyperexcitable due to a primary metabolic abnormality which might alter ionic channels, or to a decrease of inhibitory input from GABAergic, glycinergic, or serotonergic neurons. The mechanism of antimyoclonic action of L-5-HTP with carbidopa appears to be due to the correction of a biochemical or functional deficiency of brain 5-HT. Although considerable information about the pharmacological actions of clonazepam and valproic acid is available, the mechanisms of their antimyoclonic actions require further elucidation.

ACKNOWLEDGMENTS

This work was supported by USPHS grant NS-12341 and in part by NIH grant RR-71, Division of Research Resources, General Research Centers Branch.

REFERENCES

1. Airakainen EM, Leino E. Decrease of GABA in the cerebrospinal fluid of patients with progressive myoclonus epilepsy and its correlation with the decrease of 5HIAA and HVA. *Acta Neurol Scand* 1982; 66:666–72.
2. Alexander GJ, Kopeloff LM. Audiogenic seizures in mice: influence of agents affecting brain serotonin. *Res Commun Chem Pathol Pharmacol* 1976; 14:437–48.
3. Anlezark GM, Horton RW, Meldrum BS, Sawaya MCB. Anticonvulsant action of ethanolamine-o-sulphate and di-n-propylacetate and the metabolism of γ-aminobutyric acid (GABA) in mice with audiogenic seizures. *Biochem Pharmacol* 1976; 25:413–6.
4. Baldino F, Geller HM. Sodium valproate enhancement of γ-aminobutyric acid (GABA) inhibition: electrophysiological evidence for anticonvulsant activity. *J Pharmacol Exp Ther* 1981; 217:445–50.
5. Chadwick D, Gorrod JW, Jenner P, Marsden CD, Reynolds EH. Functional changes in cerebral 5-hydroxytryptamine metabolism in the mouse induced by anticonvulsant drugs. *Br J Pharmacol* 1978; 62:115–24.
6. Chadwick D, Hallett M, Harris R, Jenner P, Reynolds EH, Marsden CD. Clinical, biochemical and physiological features distinguishing myoclonus responsive to 5-hydroxytryptophan, tryptophan with a monoamine oxidase inhibitor, and clonazepam. *Brain* 1977; 100:455–87.
7. Chapman AG, Riley K, Evans MC, Meldrum BS. Acute effects of sodium valproate and γ-vinyl GABA on regional amino acid metabolism in the rat brain. *Neurochem Res* 1982; 7:1089–105.
8. Christoff N. Myoclonic encephalopathy of infants. A report of two cases and observations on related disorders. *Arch Neurol* 1969; 21:229–34.
9. Chung Hwang E, Van Woert MH. p,p'-DDT-induced neurotoxic syndrome: experimental myoclonus. *Neurology* 1978; 28:1020–5.
10. Chung Hwang E, Van Woert MH. Antimyoclonic action of clonazepam: the role of serotonin. *Eur J Pharmacol* 1979; 60:31–40.
11. Chung Hwang E, Van Woert MH. Effect of valproic acid on serotonin metabolism. *Neuropharmacology* 1979; 18:391–7.
12. Chung Hwang E, Plaitakis A, Magnussen I, Van Woert MH. Relationship of inferior olive-climbing fibers to p,p'-DDT-induced myoclonus in rats. *Neurosci Lett* 1981; 24:103–8.
13. Coleman M. *Serotonin in Down's Syndrome*. Amsterdam: Elsevier-North Holland, 1973.

14. Corne JJ, Pickering RW, Warner BT. A method for assessing the effects of drugs on the central action of 5-hydroxytryptamine. *Br J Pharmacol Chemother* 1963; 20:106–20.

15. Costa E, Guidotti A, Mao CC. Evidence for involvement of GABA in the action of benzodiazepines: studies on rat cerebellum. *Adv Biochem Pharmacol* 1975; 14:113–30.

16. Costa E, Guidotti A, Mao CC, Suria A. New concepts on the mechanism of action of benzodiazepines. *Life Sci* 1975; 17:167–186.

17. De La Torre JC, Kawanaga HM, Mullan S. Seizure susceptibility after manipulation of brain serotonin. *Arch Int Pharmacodyn Ther* 1970; 188:298–304.

18. De Lean J, Richardson JC, Hornykiewicz O. Beneficial effects of serotonin precursors in post-anoxic action myoclonus. *Neurology* 1976; 26:863–8.

19. Enna SJ, Ferkany JW, Van Woert M, Butler IJ. Measurement of GABA in biological fluids: effect of GABA transaminase inhibitors. *Adv Neurol* 1979; 23:741–50.

20. Enna SJ, Stern LZ, Wastek GJ, Yamamura HI. Cerebrospinal fluid γ-aminobutyric acid variations in neurological disorders. *Arch Neurol* 1977; 34:683–5.

21. Fahn S. Post-anoxic action myoclonus: improvement with valproic acid. *N Engl J Med* 1978; 299:313–4.

22. Fahn S. Posthypoxic action myoclonus: review of the literature and report of two new cases with response to valproate and estrogen. *Adv Neurol* 1979; 26:49–84.

23. Gastaut H. Combined photic and metrazol activation of the brain. *Electroencephalogr Clin Neurophysiol* 1950; 2:249–61.

24. Godin Y, Heinler HL, Mark J, Mandel P. Effect of dipropylacetate, an anticonvulsant compound, on GABA metabolism. *J Neurochem* 1969; 16:869–73.

25. Growdon JH, Young RR, Shahani BT. L-5-hydroxytryptophan in the treatment of syndromes in which myoclonus is prominent. *Neurology* 1976; 26:1135–40.

26. Haefely W, Kulcsar WA, Mohler H, Pieri L, Polc P, Schaffner R. Possible involvement of GABA in the central action of benzodiazepines. *Biochem Pharmacol* 1975; 14:131–51.

27. Harvey PKP, Bradford HF, Davison AN. The inhibitory effect of sodium-n-dipropyl acetate on the degradative enzymes of the GABA shunt. *FEBS Lett* 1975; 52:251–4.

28. Hayashi T, Negishi K. Suppression of retinal spike discharge by dipropylacetate (depakene); a possible involvement of GABA. *Brain Res* 1979; 175:271–8.

29. Jeavons PM, Bower BD. Infantile spasms. A review of the literature and a study of 112 cases. In: *Clinics in developmental medicine*, no. 15. London: W. Heinemann Medical Books, 1964:1.79.

30. Kilian M, Frey H-H. Central monoamine and convulsive threshold in mice and rats. *Neuropharmacology* 1973; 12:681–92.

31. Killam KF, Killam EK, Naquet R. Mise en evidence chez certains d'un syndrome photomyoclonique. *CR Acad Sci* 1966; 262:1010–2.

32. Kinsbourne M. Myoclonic encephalopathy of infants. *J Neurol Neurosurg Psychiatry* 1962; 25:271–6.

33. Klawans HL, Goetz C, Bergen D. Levodopa-induced myoclonus. *Arch Neurol* 1975; 32:331–4.

34. Klawans HL, Goetz C, Westheimer R, Weiner WJ. 5-Hydroxytryptophan induced behavior in intact guinea pigs. *Res Commun Chem Pathol Pharmacol* 1973; 5:555–9.

35. Korten JJ, Notermans SLH, Frenken CWGM, Babreels FJM, Joosten EMG. Familial essential myoclonus. *Brain* 1974; 97:131–8.

36. Kukino K, Deguchi T. Effects of sodium dipropylacetate on γ-aminobutyric acid and biogenic amines in rat brain. *Chem Pharm Bull* 1977; 25:2257–62.

37. Lhermitte F, Marteau R, Degos CF. Analyse pharmacologique d'un noveau cas de myoclonies d'intenion et d'action postanoxique. *Rev Neurol (Paris)* 1972; 126:107–14.

38. Lorentz de Haas AM, Lombroso C, Merlis JK. Participation of the cortex in experimental reflex myoclonus. *Electroencephalogr Clin Neurophysiol* 1953; 5:177–86.

39. Lloyd KG, Munari C, Worms P, Bossi L, Bancaud J, Talairach T, Morselli PL. The role of GABA mediated transmission in convulsive states. In: Costa E, Diehiara GL, Gessa GL, eds. *GABA and benzodiazepine receptors*. New York: Raven Press, 1980:199–206.

40. Lloyd KG, Worms P, Depoortere H, Bartholini G. Pharmacological profile of SL 76 002, a new GABA-mimetic drug. In: Krogsgaard-Larsen P, Scheel-Kruger J, Kofod H, eds. *GABA-neurotransmitters*, Copenhagen: Munksgaard, 1979:308–25.

41. Macdonald RL, Bergey GK. Valproic acid augments GABA-mediated postsynaptic inhibition in cultured mammalian neurons. *Brain Res* 1979; 170:558–62.

42. Magnussen I, Dupont E, Engbaek F, de Fine Olivarius B. Post-hypoxic intention myoclonus

treated with 5-hydroxytryptophan and an extracerebral decarboxylase inhibitor. *Acta Neurol Scand* 1978; 57:289–94.

43. Magnussen I, Dupont E, Prange-Hansen AA, de Fine Olivarius B. Palatal myoclonus treated with 5-hydroxytryptophan and a decarboxylase inhibitor. *Acta Neurol Scand* 1977; 55:251–3.

44. Magnussen I, Mondrup K, Engbaek F, Lademann A, de Fine Olivarius B. Treatment of myoclonic syndrome with paroxetine alone or combined with 5HTP. *Acta Neurol Scand* 1982; 66:276–82.

45. Martin A, Hirt HR. Clinical experience with clonazepam (Rivotril) in the treatment of epilepsia in infancy and childhood. *Neuropaediatrie* 1973; 4:245–66.

46. Morselli PL, Bossi L. Antiepileptic efficacy of GABA agonists in man. In: Fariello RG, Engel Jr J, Morselli PL, Quesney LF, eds. *Neurotransmitters, seizures and epilepsy II*. New York: Raven Press, 1984, pp. 253–61.

47. Mortensen PB, Kolvraa S, Christensen E. Inhibition of the glycine cleavage system: hyperglycinemia and hyperglycinuria caused by valproic acid. *Epilepsia* 1980; 21:563–9.

48. Munkenbeck KE, Schwark WS. Serotonergic mechanisms in amygdaloid-kindled seizures in the rat. *Exp Neurol* 1982; 76:246–53.

49. Nakamura M, Fukushima H. Head twitches induced by benzodiazepines and the role of biogenic amines. *Psychopharmacology* 1976; 49:259–61.

50. Nakamura M, Fukushima H. Effect of benzodiazepines on central neuron systems. *Psychopharmacology* 1977; 53:121–6.

51. Nakamura M, Fukushima H. Effects of reserpine, parachlorophenylalanine, 5,6-dihydroxytryptamine and fludiazepam on the head twitches induced by 5-hydroxytryptamine or 5-methoxytryptamine in mice. *J Pharm Pharmacol* 1978; 30:254–6.

52. Phillips JR, Eldridge FL. Respiratory myoclonus. (Leewenhoek's disease.) *N Engl J Med* 1973; 289:1390–5.

53. Pinder RM, Brogden RN, Spright TM, Avery GS. Clonazepam: a review of its pharmacological properties and therapeutic efficacy in epilepsy. *Drugs* 1976; 12:321–61.

54. Pinder RM, Brogden RN, Speight TM, Avery GS. Sodium valproate: a review of its pharmacological properties and therapeutic efficacy in epilepsy. *Drugs* 1977; 13:81–123.

55. Polc P, Mohler H, Haefely W. The effect of diazepam on spinal cord activities: possible sites and mechanisms of action. *Naunyn Schmiedebergs Arch Pharmacol* 1974; 284:319–37.

56. Pratt J, Jenner P, Reynolds EH, Marsden CD. Clonazepam induces decreased serotonergic activity in the mouse brain. *Neuropharmacology* 1979; 18:791–9.

57. Rosen AD, Berenyi K, Laurenceau V. Intention myoclonus. Diazepam and phenobarbital treatment. *JAMA* 1969; 209:772–3.

58. Sawaya MCB, Horton RW, Meldrum BS. Effects of anticonvulsant drugs on the central enzymes metabolizing GABA. *Epilepsia* 1975; 16:649–52.

59. Schecter PJ, Trainer Y, Grove J. Effect of n-dipropylacetate on amino acid concentrations in mouse brain: correlation with anticonvulsant activity. *J Neurochem* 1978; 31:1325–7.

60. Tarsy D, Pycock CJ, Meldrum BS, Marsden CD. Focal contralateral myoclonus produced by inhibition of GABA action in the caudate nucleus of rats. *Brain* 1978; 101:143–62.

61. Thal LJ, Sparpless NS, Wolfson L, Katzman R. Treatment of myoclonus with L-5-hydroxytryptophan and carbidopa: clinical, electrophysiological and biochemical observations. *Ann Neurol* 1980; 7:570–6.

62. Van Gelder NM, Sherwin AL, Rasmussen T. Amino acid content of epileptogenic human brain focal versus surrounding regions. *Brain* 1972; 40:385–93.

63. Van Woert MH, Chung Hwang E. Animal models of myoclonus. *Adv Neurol* 1979; 26:173–80.

64. Van Woert MH, Magnussen I, Rosenbaum D, Chung E. Fluoxetine in the treatment of intention myoclonus. *Clin Neuropharmacol* 1983; 6:49–54.

65. Van Woert MH, Rosenbaum D, Howieson J, Bowers MB. Long term therapy of myoclonus and other neurological disorders with L-5-hydroxytryptophan and carbidopa. *N Engl J Med* 1977; 296:70–5.

66. Wada JA, Balzano E, Meldrum BS, Naquet R. Behavioral and electrographic effects of L-5-hydroxytryptophan and D,L-parachlorophenylalanine on epileptic Senegalese baboon (Papio papio). *Electroencephalogr Clin Neurophysiol* 1972; 33:520–6.

67. Williams A, Goodenberg D, Calne D. Palatal myoclonus following herpes zoster ameliorated by 5-hydroxytryptophan and carbidopa. *Neurology* 1978; 28:358–9.

68. Wood JH, Hare TA, Glaeser BS, Ballenger JC, Post RM. Low cerebrospinal fluid γ-aminobutyric acid content in seizure patients. *Neurology* 1979; 29:1203–8.

Advances in Neurology, Vol. 43: Myoclonus,
edited by S. Fahn et al. Raven Press,
New York © 1986.

Treatment of Posthypoxic Action Myoclonus: Implications for the Pathophysiology of the Disorder

D. Chadwick, *M. Hallett, †P. Jenner, and †C. D. Marsden

*Mersey Regional Department of Medical and Surgical Neurology, Walton Hospital, Liverpool L9 1AE, England; *Department of Neurology, Brigham and Women's Hospital, Boston, Massachusetts 02215; and †Department of Neurology, Institute of Psychiatry, De Crespigny Park, London SE5 8AF, England*

There is general agreement that patients with posthypoxic and post-traumatic action myoclonus (21) have universally low lumbar cerebrospinal fluid (CSF) concentrations of 5-hydroxyindoleacetic acid (5-HIAA) (Table 1), the metabolite of serotonin (5-HT) (4,9,15,22,31) and respond, sometimes dramatically, to treatment with 5-hydroxytryptophan (5-HTP), the immediate precursor of 5-HT (Fig. 1) (4,9,14, 15,22,23,29,31). Levels of CSF 5-HIAA rise both with treatment and if the disability should resolve spontaneously (4). It is tempting to assume, therefore, that the syndrome is specifically related to a loss of 5-HT neurons, resulting in a deficiency of 5-HT (31). However, any hypothesis seeking to explain the patho-

TABLE 1. *CSF5-HIAA concentrations in posthypoxic action myoclonus*

Myoclonic patients ng/ml (± SEM)	Controls ng/ml (± SEM)	Ref.
10	?	23
10	39 ± 7.9 [34]	15
9	18 ± 2 [7]	9
12		
54 ± 9.5 [9][a]	90 ± 11 [10]	30[b]
12.9, 23.7, 23.8, 27.4, 15.2, 21.9, 24.6	32 ± 1.7 [32]	4
Undetectable	?	11
26	?	3
59 ± 8 [6]	115 ± 13 [12]	29[c]

[a]Numbers in brackets are the number of observations.
[b]Values are following probenecid. Some of the myoclonic patients did not have a history of hypoxia.
[c]Values are following probenecid. In only two of the six myoclonic patients was there a history of hypoxia.

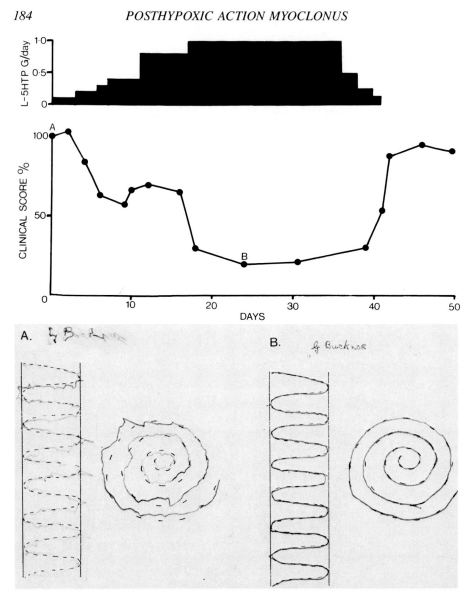

FIG. 1. Upper: Alteration in disability score (ref. 4) following oral administration of incremental doses of 5-HTP and its subsequent withdrawal in a patient with posthypoxic action myoclonus receiving carbidopa (75–150 mg/day). **Lower:** Specimens of handwriting and drawing are shown for points A and B.

physiology of posthypoxic action myoclonus must also take into account the responsiveness of this disorder to other neurotransmitter precursors and to other drugs. It is the purpose of this chapter to reexamine this hypothesis in the light of observations made in patients studied at Kings College and the Maudsley hospitals (4,5) and other published data.

EFFECTS OF OTHER SEROTONERGIC MANIPULATIONS

If the therapeutic effect of 5-HTP is dependent on its ability to cause an elevation of brain 5-HT (25), then other agents having a similar pharmacological effect should also have a therapeutic action against posthypoxic action myoclonus (Table 2).

There is agreement that both monoamine oxidase inhibitors (MAOIs) and L-tryptophan (the physiological precursor of 5-HT) given in combination with a MAOI have a therapeutic effect (Fig. 2), although this is less striking than with 5-HTP (4,9,22,23). There is disagreement as to whether L-tryptophan alone is effective, however. Chadwick et al. (4) found no response to oral L-tryptophan in doses up to 16 g/day in four posthypoxic patients, all of whom did show a moderate therapeutic response when L-tryptophan was combined with a MAOI. Similarly, Van Woert and Sethy (31) found L-tryptophan to be ineffective in a single patient at doses up to 6 g/day. De Lean et al. (9), however, reported a moderate therapeutic response to 10 g/day in two patients.

Methysergide, a 5-HT antagonist, has been reported to exacerbate posthypoxic myoclonus (9,22,23,27). Others have found it to have little functional effect (4,31) or even, in some instances, to improve posthypoxic myoclonus (1,9). The latter group found a therapeutic action in one patient receiving a dose of 6 mg/day but an exacerbating effect when the same patient received 12 mg/day. Difficulties arise in interpreting these results because methysergide crosses the blood-brain barrier poorly (10) and may possess both 5-HT agonist (24) and antagonist (18) properties.

Parachlorophenylalanine (PCPA), an inhibitor of tryptophan hydroxylase, did not exacerbate myoclonus in two patients (9), despite the fact that lumbar CSF concentrations of 5-HIAA were reduced in one of the patients. It is uncertain whether this drug produces functionally significant depletion of brain 5-HT in the doses given.

Thus although there are some inconsistencies, the overall evidence supports a hypothesis that posthypoxic myoclonus may be causally related to a deficiency of cerebral 5-HT. Other drugs may also be effective in controlling posthypoxic myoclonus.

TABLE 2. *Effects of other drugs influencing 5-HT on posthypoxic myoclonus*[a]

| Increase of 5-HT | | | Depletion of 5-HT (PCPA) | 5-HT receptor antagonists (methysergide) | Ref. |
MAOIs	L-tryptophan	L-tryptophan + MAOI			
+[1][b]				−[1]	22,23
				−[1]	27
				+[1]	1
	0[1]			0[1]	31
+[1]	+[2]	+[2]	0[2]	+/−[1]	9
				0/−[1]	9
+[4]	0[4]	++[4]		0[1]	4

[a] + +, Excellent response; +, moderate response; 0, no change; −, worse.
[b] Numbers in brackets are number of cases studied.

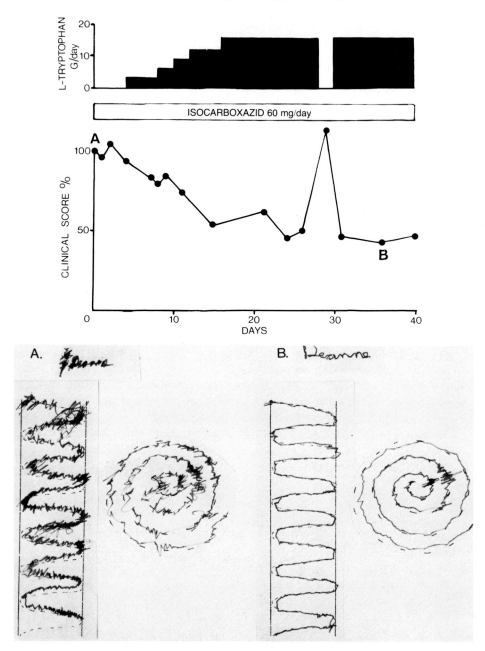

FIG. 2.   Upper: Alteration in disability score (ref. 4) following oral administration of incremental doses of L-tryptophan (plus isocarboxazid, 60 mg/day) and its subsequent placebo substitution in a patient with posthypoxic action myoclonus.   **Lower:** Specimens of handwriting and drawing are shown for points A and B.

EFFECTS OF BENZODIAZEPINES AND OTHER ANTICONVULSANT AGENTS

Prior to the growth of interest in the biochemical basis of posthypoxic myoclonus, this disorder was most frequently treated with conventional anticonvulsant drugs, which had a mild to moderate effect. In 1971, Boudouresques et al. (2) reported the dramatic effect of clonazepam, a benzodiazepine derivative, in a patient with posthypoxic myoclonus. Chadwick et al. (5) and Goldberg and Dorman (12) confirmed this observation (Fig. 3). It seems that those patients responsive to 5-HTP also respond in an equally dramatic way to clonazepam (4,29). Newer anticonvulsant drugs, such as valproate (3,11,28) and carbamazepine (16), may also be effective in suppressing action myoclonus in patients who respond only partially or not at all to 5-HTP and clonazepam.

Can the antimyoclonic effects of these other drugs be related to actions on cerebral 5-HT? Benzodiazepines are capable of elevating CSF 5-HIAA in humans (4) and brain concentrations of 5-HT in animals (7). Furthermore, anticonvulsant drugs may have effects on cerebral 5-HT in the clinical situation (6), and valproate may elevate cerebral 5-HT in animals (17) and CSF 5-HIAA in humans (11). However, the overall effects of anticonvulsants and benzodiazepines are to diminish the rate of turnover of 5-HT rather than to increase its functional activity (see Jenner, *this volume*).

The therapeutic action of benzodiazepines and other anticonvulsant drugs in posthypoxic myoclonus may be mediated via other neurotransmitter systems rather than by a direct effect on 5-HT neurons. It seems most likely that γ-aminobutyric acid (GABA)-ergic mechanisms may be involved in view of the increasing evidence of interactions between both benzodiazepines and conventional anticonvulsant agents at or around the GABA receptor–chloride ionophor membrane complex (26).

NEUROCHEMICAL BASIS OF POSTHYPOXIC ACTION MYOCLONUS AND ITS RESPONSIVENESS

The universal finding of low CSF concentrations of 5-HIAA in patients suffering posthypoxic myoclonus and the suppression of myoclonus associated with agents elevating brain 5-HT suggests that the syndrome may be due to a relative or absolute deficiency of 5-HT. A 5-HT deficiency might be produced by a number of mechanisms.

A deficiency of the physiological precursor L-tryptophan is an unlikely cause as CSF concentrations of tryptophan are normal in patients with myoclonus, and L-tryptophan itself has dubious therapeutic effects (4).

A 5-HT deficiency might be caused by loss of tryptophan hydroxylase, the rate-limiting enzyme in the synthesis of 5-HT (31). Animal evidence does show a decreased rate of tryptophan hydroxylase activity following cerebral hypoxia (8), and such a hypothesis would be in keeping with the observation that 5-HTP but not L-tryptophan alone is effective in controlling posthypoxic myoclonus. The conversion of L-tryptophan to 5-HT (via 5-HTP) requires an intact 5-HT system, as tryptophan hydroxylase is found only within 5-HT neurons (20). In contrast,

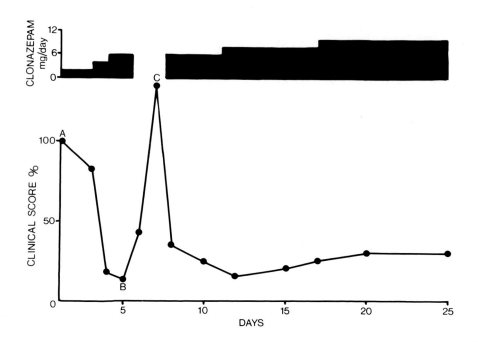

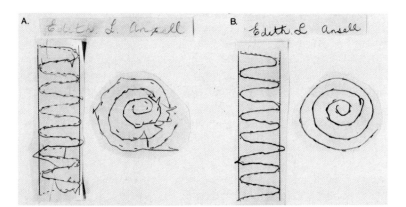

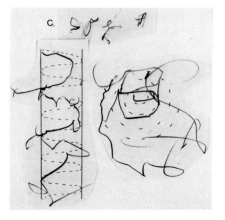

FIG. 3. **Upper:** Alteration in disability score (ref. 4) following oral administration of incremental doses of clonazepam and its subsequent placebo substitution in a patient with posthypoxic action myoclonus. **Lower:** Specimens of handwriting and drawing are shown for points A, B, and C.

aromatic acid decarboxylase, which is necessary to convert 5-HTP to 5-HT, is found in other monoamine neurons. Thus if hypoxia were to cause a selective loss of 5-HT neurons, this would offer an explanation of this syndrome and its responsiveness.

Not all observations are consistent with this. Korf et al. (19) administered 5-HTP to rats in doses of 12.5 mg/kg (a dose greater than that administered in human studies) in combination with a peripheral decarboxylase inhibitor. The formation of 5-HT remained dependent on a specific 5-HTP decarboxylase related to 5-HT neurons. The administration of L-tryptophan alone is capable of elevating 5-HIAA (although producing little therapeutic effect) in patients with 5-HTP-responsive myoclonus (4,9). Furthermore, there is general agreement that L-tryptophan may have a therapeutic effect when combined with a MAOI, again suggesting that 5-HT neurons are indeed capable of synthesizing 5-HT from L-tryptophan. These facts suggest that an intact 5-HT system, with its associated tryptophan hydroxylase and 5-HTP decarboxylase, may be present in patients with posthypoxic action myoclonus and may indeed be necessary for the therapeutic action of 5-HTP and L-tryptophan given in combination with MAOIs.

The finding that 5-HTP, but not L-tryptophan, is effective in treating myoclonus probably reflects the fact that 5-HT formed following L-tryptophan loading does not become functionally active (13). It may be that the low CSF 5-HIAA found in patients with posthypoxic myoclonus results from a hypoactive but intact 5-HT neuronal system, caused by a loss of drive from other, unidentified neuronal systems (4). This latter hypothesis gains some support from the observations that other drugs (e.g., benzodiazepines) have therapeutic effects against myoclonus which are probably independent of a direct action on 5-HT systems. We should consider the possibility that other neurotransmitter systems, perhaps GABAergic, may be capable of interacting with the 5-HT system to suppress posthypoxic myoclonus.

REFERENCES

1. Bedard P, Bouchard R. Dramatic effect of methysergide on myoclonus. *Lancet* 1974; 1:738.
2. Boudouresques J, Roger J, Khalu R, Vigouroux RA, Gossett A, Pellisier JF, Tassinari CA. A propos de 2 observations de syndrome de Lance et Adams. Effet therapeutique du RO-05-4023. *Rev Neurol (Paris)* 1971; 125:306–9.
3. Carroll WM, Walsh PJ. Functional independence in post-anoxic myoclonus: contribution of L-5-HTP, sodium valproate and clonazepam. *Br Med J* 1978; 2:1616.
4. Chadwick D, Hallett M, Harris R, Jenner P, Reynolds EH, Marsden CD. Clinical, biochemical and physiological features distinguishing myoclonus responsive to 5-hydroxytryptophan, tryptophan with a monoamine oxidase inhibitor, and clonazepam. *Brain* 1977; 100:455–87.
5. Chadwick D, Harris R, Jenner P, Reynolds EH, Marsden CD. Manipulation of brain serotonin in the treatment of myoclonus. *Lancet* 1975; ii:434–5.
6. Chadwick D, Jenner P, Reynolds EH. Serotonin metabolism in human epilepsy: the influence of anticonvulsant drugs. *Ann Neurol* 1977; 1:218–24.
7. Chase TM, Katz RI, Kopin IJ. Effect of anticonvulsants on brain serotonin. *Trans Am Neurol Assoc* 1969; 94:236–8.
8. Davis JN, Carlsson A. Effect of hypoxia on tyrosine and tryptophan hydroxylation in unanaesthetised rat brain. *J Neurochem* 1972; 20:913–5.

9. De Lean J, Richardson JC, Hornykiewicz O. Beneficial effects of serotonin precursors in post-anoxic action myoclonus. *Neurology* 1976; 26:863–8.
10. Doepfner W. Biochemical observations on LSD 25 and deseril. *Experientia* 1962; 18:256–7.
11. Fahn S. Post-anoxic action myoclonus: improvement with valproic acid. *N Engl J Med* 1978; 299:313–4.
12. Goldberg MA, Dorman JD. Intention myoclonus: successful treatment with clonazepam. *Neurology (Minneap)* 1976; 26:24–6.
13. Grahame-Smith DG. Studies in vivo on the relationship between brain tryptophan, brain 5HT synthesis and hyperactivity in rats treated with a monoamine oxidase inhibitor and L-tryptophan. *J Neurochem* 1971; 18:1053–66.
14. Growdon JH, Young RR, Shahani BT. L-5-hydroxytryptophan in the treatment of syndromes in which myoclonus is prominent. *Neurology (Minneap)* 1976; 26:1135–40.
15. Guilleminault C, Tharp BR, Cousin D. HVA and 5HIAA CSF measurements and 5HTP trials in some patients with involuntary movements. *J Neurol Sci* 1973; 18:435–41.
16. Hirose G, Singer P, Bass NH. Successful treatment of posthypoxic action myoclonus with carbamazepine. *JAMA* 1971; 218:1432–3.
17. Horton RW, Anlezark GM, Sawaya CD, Meldrum BS. Monoamine and GABA metabolism and the anticonvulsant actions di-N-propylacetate and etholamine-O-sulphate. *Eur J Pharmacol* 1977; 41:387–97.
18. Klawans HL, Goetz C, Weiner WJ. 5-Hydroxytryptophan-induced myoclonus in guinea pigs and the possible role of serotonin in infantile myoclonus. *Neurology (Minneap)* 1973; 23:1234–40.
19. Korf J, Venema K, Postema F. Decarboxylation of exogenous L-5-hydroxytryptophan after destruction of the cerebral raphe system. *J Neurochem* 1974; 23:249–52.
20. Kuhar MJ, Roth RH, Aghajanian GK. Selective reduction of tryptophan hydroxylase activity in rat forebrain after midbrain raphe lesions. *Brain Res* 1971; 35:167–76.
21. Lance JW, Adams RD. The syndrome of intention or action myoclonus as a sequel to hypoxic encephalopathy. *Brain* 1963; 86:111–36.
22. Lhermitte F, Marteau R, Degos CF. Analyse pharmacologique d'un nouveau cas de myoclonies d'intention et d'action postanoxique. *Rev Neurol (Paris)* 1972; 126:107–14.
23. Lhermitte F, Peterfalvi M, Marteau R, Gazengel J, Serdaru M. Analyse pharmacologique d'un cas de myoclonies d'intention et d'action postanoxique. *Rev Neurol (Paris)* 1971; 124:21–31.
24. Martin WR, Eades CG. Action of tryptamine on the dog spinal cord and its relationship to the agonist actions of LSD like agents. *Psychopharmacologia* 1970; 17:242–57.
25. Modigh K. Functional aspects of 5-hydroxytryptamine turnover in the central nervous system. *Acta Physiol Scand [Suppl]* 1974;403:1–56.
26. Olsen RW, Leeb-Lundberg F. Convulsant and anticonvulsant drug binding sites related to the GABA receptor/Ionophore system. In: Morselli PL, Lloyd KG, Loscher W, Meldrum B, Reynolds EH, eds. Neurotransmitters, seizures and epilepsy. New York: Raven Press, 1981:151–60.
27. Romero F, Gonzalez F, Codina A, De Castro JL. Methysergide and myoclonus. *Lancet* 1975; 1:395–6.
28. Sotaniemi K. Valproic acid in the treatment of nonepileptic myoclonus. *Arch Neurol* 1982; 39:448–9.
29. Thal LJ, Sharpless NS, Wolfson L, Katzman R. Treatment of myoclonus with L-5-hydroxytryptophan and carbidopa: clinical, electrophysiological and biochemical observations. *Ann Neurol* 1980; 7:570–6.
30. Van Woert MH, Rosenbaum D, Howieson J, and Bowers MB. Long-term therapy of myoclonus and other neurological disorders with L-5-hydroxytryptophan and carbidopa. *N Engl J Med* 1977; 296:70–5.
31. Van Woert MH, Sethy VH. Therapy of intention myoclonus with L-5-hydroxytryptophan and a peripheral decarboxylase inhibitor, MK486. *Neurology (Minneap)* 1975; 25:135–40.

Advances in Neurology, Vol. 43: Myoclonus,
edited by S. Fahn et al. Raven Press,
New York © 1986.

Lisuride in the Treatment of Myoclonus

*J. A. Obeso, †J. C. Rothwell, †N. P. Quinn, ‡A. E. Lang,
*J. Artieda, and †C. D. Marsden

*Department of Neurology, Clinica Universitaria, University of Navarra Medical School,
Pamplona, Spain; †University Department of Neurology, Institute of Psychiatry and
King's College Hospital Medical School, London, England; and ‡Department of
Neurology, Toronto Western Hospital, Toronto, Ontario, Canada

Despite important advances in the clinical, pathophysiological, and pharmacological understanding of myoclonus, treatment of this condition remains difficult. In recent years, particular attention has been placed on the therapeutic action of serotonin and dopamine agonists. Intravenous or oral treatment with 5-hydroxytryptophan (5-HTP) plus carbidopa to increase brain serotonin can produce improvement in patients with action and reflex myoclonus of different etiologies (2,6,10). In patients with photosensitive epilepsy, the dopamine agonist apomorphine can abolish spike–wave electroencephalogram (EEG) activity induced by photic stimulation (8). Anlezark et al. (1) have demonstrated a protective effect of apomorphine against auditory and visually induced seizures in animals. Apomorphine, lisuride, bromocriptine, and dopamine decreased spontaneous focal spikes in rats with chronic cobalt implanted in the motor cortex (3). Thus, both serotonin and dopamine agonists appear capable of reducing different types of myoclonus.

Lisuride hydrogen maleate is a semisynthetic ergot alkaloid which acts as a potent postsynaptic dopaminergic and serotonergic central agonist (4,5). In previous reports (7,9), we showed a beneficial effect of intravenous lisuride in six patients with cortical reflex myoclonus. Such observations have been extended to a total of 14 patients with different varieties of myoclonus.

PATIENTS

The clinical and electrophysiological characteristics of the 14 patients studied are summarized in Tables 1, 2, and 3. In most patients, the etiology of the myoclonus was not known despite extensive investigation. Muscle jerking was focal in four patients and multifocal and/or generalized in 10. Somesthetic stimulation (muscle stretching, touching, pinpricking, or electrical stimulation of nerve) evoked reflex muscle jerking in ten patients. Visual stimulation (flash) induced generalized rhythmic myoclonic jerking in two patients (J.D. and P.R.L.).

Multichannel electromyographic recording of spontaneous, action, and reflex myoclonus was undertaken in all patients. Somatosensory cortical evoked potentials also were recorded (normal amplitude of the P1-N1 complex usually ranges between

TABLE 1. *Clinical features of patients treated with intravenous lisuride*

Patient	Sex	Age (years)	Etiology/Diagnosis	Clinical features of myoclonus[b]			Focal/generalized
				Spontaneous	Action	Reflex	
E.A.	F	56	Head trauma	+ +	+ + +	+ + +	Multifocal and generalized
C.G.	F	52	Ramsay–Hunt	−	+ + +	+ +	Multifocal
J.A.	F	22	Ramsay–Hunt	−	+ + +	−	Multifocal and generalized
J.D.[a]	F	15	Ramsay–Hunt	+	+ + +	+	Multifocal and generalized
P.R.L.[a]	F	62	OPCA	−	−	+ + +	Multifocal and generalized
C.M.	F	62	Unknown	+	+ + +	+ + +	Multifocal
J.B.	F	34	Unknown	+ + +	+ +	+ + +	Focal (hand)
P.M.	M	19	Unknown	+ +	+ + +	+ + +	Focal (hand)
J.M.	M	70	Unknown	−	+ + +	+ + +	Focal (hand)
E.R.	F	58	Unknown	+ + +	−	−	Focal (hand)
G.A.	F	15	Anoxia/oscillatory myoclonus	+	+ + +	−	Multifocal
D.D.	F	62	Induced by L-DOPA Parkinson's disease	+ + +	−	−	Generalized
M.V.	M	51	Unknown	−	−	+ + +	Segmental (neck and facial muscles)
R.L.	M	72	Creutzfeldt–Jakob	+ + +	+ +	+ + +	Generalized/multifocal

[a]These two patients also had visually sensitive myoclonus.
[b]Clinical features: (−), none; (+), mild; (++), moderate; (+++), severe.

TABLE 2. *Electrophysiological characteristics of myoclonus[a] in patients responding to lisuride*

Patient	Duration of EMG burst (msec)	Latency from EEG positive peak time locked to muscle jerks	Amplitude of SEP (P1–N2) (μV)
E.A.	25–50	17-msec finger flexors	10
C.G.	50–60	Not done	25
J.A.	20–30	20-msec finger flexors	40
J.D.	10–30	Not done	45
P.R.L.	30–50	Not done	25
C.M.	25–50	Not done	8
J.B.	25–50	22-msec finger flexors	30
P.M.	25–75	25-msec first dorsal interosseous	45
J.M.	25–50	No EEG peak	8

[a]Origin of myoclonus presumed to be cortical.

TABLE 3. *Electrophysiological characteristics of myoclonus[a] in patients not responding to lisuride*

Patient	Duration of EMG burst (msec)	Latency from EEG positive peak time locked to muscle jerks	Amplitude of SEP (P1–N2) (μV)
E.R.	200–400	No EEG peak	2.5
G.A.	60–120	No EEG peak	2.0
D.D.	200–400	No EEG peak	1.8
M.V.	50–100	No spontaneous or action myoclonus	1.5
R.L.	200–300	No EEG peak	3.2

[a]Origin of myoclonus presumed to be subcortical.

1 and 5 μV). Back averaging of the cortical activity preceding muscle jerking was performed in most cases but could not be undertaken in patients C.G., J.D., P.R.L., C.M., and R.L. (For detailed techniques, see Obeso et al. and Rothwell et al., *this volume*.)

Lisuride (0.1–0.15 mg) was given intravenously to all patients after prior oral administration of 20 mg domperidone to prevent nausea and vomiting. The severity of the myoclonus was assessed prior to and at 15 min- to 1-hr intervals after injection using a modification of the scale previously described (4). This scale, on a grading of 0 to 3, rated frequency and intensity of myoclonus in the affected area of the body and the extent to which it interfered with a series of simple motor tasks. The effect of lisuride on spontaneous and action myoclonus was assessed, as was its effect on jerks reflexively triggered by electrical stimulation of peripheral nerves in the arm. Clinical response was graded as follows: mild, <20% improvement; moderate, obvious benefit with demonstrable (>50%) reduction of disability; dramatic, striking reduction of myoclonus (>90%) resulting in considerable improvement of disability.

RESULTS AND DISCUSSION

Nine of the fourteen patients improved when given intravenous lisuride (Table 4; Fig. 1). All nine patients had reflex muscle jerks (eight cases) and/or action myoclonus (nine cases), as well as electrophysiological features distinctive of cortical myoclonus (Table 2).

In contrast, of those five cases who showed no response to lisuride, three patients had no reflex myoclonus. Two had only spontaneous muscle jerks, and one patient had myoclonus mainly on action with occasional spontaneous jerks. The two patients who did have reflex myoclonus, with somesthetic stimulation provoking focal or generalized myoclonus, appeared to have a subcortical source for their muscle jerks. In one of these last two cases (M.V.), electrophysiological studies indicated a subcortical reticular reflex type of myoclonus. In the other (R.L.), clinical and EEG findings were suggestive of Creutzfeldt–Jakob disease. Somatosensory evoked potentials (SEPs) were not enlarged in this case, nor was there a constant relationship between EEG activity and myoclonic jerking. These findings suggest that the myoclonus did not arise at the cortical level. The conclusion from study of these 14 patients was that lisuride was particularly active against cortical reflex myoclonus.

The mechanism of action of lisuride has been investigated in detail in two patients (Table 5). The pharmacological results suggest that lisuride exerted its antimyoclonic effect as a result of a central serotonergic action. Thus, L-DOPA (plus carbidopa) and apomorphine had no effect on their myoclonus, but 5-HTP replicated the actions of lisuride. The beneficial actions of lisuride were abolished by prior treatment with methysergide but not haloperidol or sulpiride.

It is of interest that in the two patients who also had visually sensitive muscle jerking, this too improved with lisuride. Dopamine agonists are known to reduce

TABLE 4. *Response of myoclonus to intravenous lisuride*

Patient	Lisuride (mg/kg)	Overall clinical assessment[a]	Myoclonus[b]		
			Action	Reflex	Spontaneous
E.A.	0.15	Dramatic	+ + +	+	+
C.G.	0.10	Moderate	+ +	+ + +	Nil
J.A.	0.10	Dramatic	+ + +	Nil	Nil
J.D.	0.10	Dramatic	+ + +	+ + +	—
P.R.L.	0.15	Moderate	Nil	+ +	Nil
C.M.	0.10	Dramatic	+	+ + +	+
J.B.	0.10	Dramatic	+ +	+ + +	+ +
P.M.	0.10	Moderate	+ +	+ + +	+ +
J.M.	0.10	Moderate	+ +	+ + +	Nil

[a]Clinical response: moderate, obvious benefit with demonstrable (>50%) reduction in disability; dramatic, striking reduction in myoclonus with almost complete improvement (>90% in disability).
[b]Response: + + +, dramatic; + +, moderate; +, mild; —, no response; nil, no myoclonus of this type.

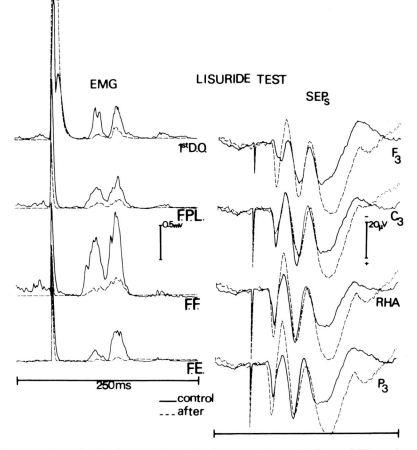

FIG. 1. Effect of lisuride (0.1 mg i.v.) on the reflex muscle jerks (EMG) and SEPs produced by electrical stimulation of the cutaneous nerves of the index finger at twice sensory threshold in patient J.B. Traces are the superimposed average of 128 trials before *(solid lines)* and after *(dotted lines)* lisuride. EMGs are surface rectified records from the right first dorsal interosseous (1st D.O.), flexor pollicis longus (F.P.L.), forearm flexor muscles (F.F.), and forearm extensor muscles (F.E.). SEPs recorded monopolarly to a linked mastoid reference: RHA is the somatosensory area of the right hand located 7 cm lateral on a line joining the external auditory meatus to a point 2 cm behind the vertex. Stimuli were introduced 50 msec after the start of the sweep (see stimulus artifact). After lisuride, the reflex muscle jerks almost disappear, while the SEPs are slightly increased in size.

visually triggered myoclonus (8a), so it may be that a combined serotonergic and dopaminergic action was effective in these two patients in reducing both the somatosensory and visual myoclonus.

To date, we have treated only one patient with lisuride orally. Patient J.A. received up to 5 mg lisuride added to her therapeutic regimen, which included clonazepam (2 mg t.i.d.) and sodium valproate (200 mg t.i.d.). There was a marked improvement of her action myoclonus after lisuride was introduced, but

TABLE 5. *Clinical and electrophysiological response of cortical reflex myoclonus to dopamine and serotonin agonists and antagonists*

Drug	Dosage	Patient[a]	
		C.M.	J.D.
Lisuride	0.1–0.15 mg i.v.	Dramatic	Dramatic
L-DOPA + carbidopa	250 mg q.i.d. for 3 days p.o.	Nil	Nil
Apomorphine	1 mg s.c.	Nil	Nil
5-HTP + carbidopa	180 mg iv + 50 mg p.o.	Dramatic	Dramatic
Effect of Lisuride following pretreatment with	0.1–0.15 mg i.v.		
Haloperidol	3 mg/day for 3 days p.o.	Dramatic	—
Sulpiride	200 mg i.v. stat	—	Moderate
Methysergide	3 mg/day for 3 days p.o.	Nil	Nil

[a]Moderate, improvement in action and reflex myoclonus was >50% compared with control; dramatic, improvement >90% compared with control.

nausea and vomiting prevented continued treatment. The role of oral lisuride in the treatment of myoclonus, either as a sole agent or in combination with other antimyoclonic drugs, remains to be established by long-term studies.

REFERENCES

1. Anlezark M, Marrosu F, Meldrum B. Dopamine agonists in reflex epilepsy. In: Morselli PL, Lloyd KG, Loscher W, Meldrum B, Reynolds E, eds. Neurotransmitters, seizures and epilepsy. New York: Raven Press, 1981:251–62.
2. Chadwick D, Hallett M, Harris R, Jenner P, Reynolds EH, Marsden CD. Clinical, biochemical, and physiological features distinguishing myoclonus responsive to 5-hydroxytryptophan, tryptophan with a monoamine oxidase inhibitor, and clonazepam. *Brain* 1977; 100:455–87.
3. Farjo IB, McQueen JK. Dopamine agonists and cobalt-induced epilepsy in the rat. *Br J Pharmacol* 1979; 67:353–60.
4. Horowski R, Wachtel H. Direct dopaminergic action of lisuride hydrogen maleate, an ergot derivative in mice. *Eur J Pharmacol* 1976; 36:373–83.
5. Kehr W. Effect of lisuride and ergot derivatives on monoaminergic mechanisms in rat brain. *Eur J Pharmacol* 1977; 41:261–73.
6. L'Hermitte F, Petrafaldi M, Marteau R, Gazengel J, Serdaru M. Analyse pharmacologique d'un cas de myoclonies d'intention et d'action post-anoxiques. *Rev Neurol* 1971; 124:21–31.
7. Obeso JA, Rothwell JC, Quinn NP, Lang AE, Thompson C, Marsden CD. Cortical reflex myoclonus responds to intravenous lisuride. *Clin Neuropharmacol* 1983; 6:231–40.
8. Quesney LF, Anderman F, Lal F, Prelevic S. Transient abolition of generalised photosensitive epileptic discharge in humans by apomorphine, a dopamine receptor agonist. *Neurology* 1980; 30:1169–74.
8a. Obeso JA, Artieda J. Dopamine agonists suppress visual cortical reflex myoclonus. *J Neurol Neurosurg Psychiatry (in press)*.
9. Rothwell JC, Obeso JA, Marsden CD. On the significance of giant somatosensory evoked potentials in cortical myoclonus. *J Neurol Neurosurg Psychiatry* 1984;47:33–42.
10. Van Woert MH, Sethy VH. Therapy of intention myoclonus with L-5-hydroxytryptophan and a peripheral decarboxylase inhibitor, MK 486. *Neurology [Suppl]* 1972; 12:72–81.

Advances in Neurology, Vol. 43: Myoclonus,
edited by S. Fahn et al. Raven Press,
New York © 1986.

Newer Drugs for Posthypoxic Action Myoclonus: Observations from a Well-Studied Case

Stanley Fahn

Department of Neurology, Columbia University College of Physicians and Surgeons, and The Neurological Institute of New York, New York, New York 10032

The introduction of new drugs for the treatment of medical conditions is often brought about by serendipity—the chance discovery by the observant, prepared individual. Another approach, especially in the treatment of patients with movement disorders, is by the logically planned open-label trials of pharmacotherapy. Careful observations of the effects of many drugs have led to the introduction of useful therapies for a number of conditions. Not uncommonly the alert, observant patient or relative of the patient makes an association that leads to the development of new, beneficial drugs. Such was the situation that led Schwab et al. (2) to study and introduce amantadine for parkinsonism.

As documented in a review of posthypoxic action myoclonus (1), the husband of a patient made the observation that the severity of his wife's myoclonus fluctuated with her menstrual periods. This led to the introduction of estrogen to partially suppress the myoclonic jerks. His observation was based on his own creation and daily utilization of a detailed scoring system of his wife's functioning and her severity of myoclonus (Table 4 in ref. 1). He has continued this activity. Such detailed observations can be most useful when testing new drugs, and this chapter shows how this has led to the reduction of this patient's myoclonus.

CASE HISTORY

Details of the medical history have already been presented (1), so only a summary is necessary.

In January 1976, at the age of 52, the patient had an anesthesia accident and went into hypoxic coma that lasted 16 days. On recovery, she had severe generalized myoclonus that interfered with talking, eating, walking and carrying out any daily activities, especially in the morning hours. The introduction of valproate in the presence of clonazepam dramatically controlled her myoclonus, except when she was attempting to walk. Cerebrospinal fluid (CSF) concentration of 5-hydroxyindoleacetic acid (5-HIAA) was undetectable before the introduction of valproate and became normal afterward. This suggested that the serotonergic fibers were inhibited and that they became disinhibited after treatment with valproate. Subsequent evaluation of clonazepam and valproate separately revealed that the combination

197

of the two drugs was essential, otherwise the myoclonic jerks could not be controlled. Later, the discovery was made by her husband that the severity of myoclonus followed the menstrual cycle, as mentioned above (see Fig. 3 in ref. 1). This led to the addition of Premarin to her treatment regimen. Since then, a number of other drugs were tried, with the results quantitatively measured using the scoring system derived by her husband.

RESULTS

By following the daily quantitative scores of the severity of myoclonus, it was found that the plasma levels of clonazepam and valproate never correlated with the clinical state. Without changing the dosage of clonazepam, valproate, or Premarin, the myoclonus and functional state steadily worsened. Sometimes this was due to increased toxicity to the first two drugs, necessitating a decrease in dosage. At other times, an increase of dosage was necessary to obtain improvement over a declining state. It appeared that altering dosage, first down and then up, could overcome a declining clinical state. This was one factor that spurred attempts to find additional effective medications. Another factor was that the patient was still not able to walk independently because of myoclonus in the thigh muscles. A series of medications was evaluated between 1979 and 1983 (Table 1).

Transient benefit was seen consistently with pemoline (increased alertness) and with dieting or fasting (decreased myoclonus); however, the benefit did not last. Of all medications tested since 1979, only piracetam showed persistent benefit. Piracetam was first shown to ameliorate myoclonus by Terwinghe et al. (3). Table 2 shows improvement over time in the presence of piracetam, despite lower dosages of clonazepam and valproate. The higher the score, the better the function (see Table 4 in ref. 1).

It seems worthwhile for piracetam to be tested on a series of patients with myoclonus to determine its role in the treatment of this condition. If drugs are moderately effective, they may be detected only by careful clinical monitoring in as quantitative a manner as possible. The scoring system devised (1) is a means of achieving this.

TABLE 1. *New medication tested*

Year	Drug tested	Result
1979	Phenytoin	No effect
	Baclofen ×2	No effect
1981–82	Propranolol ×2	No effect
1980	L-Tryptophan	Worse
	Acetazolamide	Worse
	Clonidine	Worse
1981	Amantadine	Worse
1982	Isoniazid	Worse
	Pemoline ×2	Transient benefit
1978–81	Dieting + ketogenic diet ×5	Transient benefit
1980–83	Piracetam	Better

TABLE 2. *Medication trend over a five-year period[a]*

Year	Month	CLON (mg/day)	VAL (g/day)	PREM (mg/day)	PIR (g/day)	Score
1978	July	8.0	2.5	6.25	—	16.5
	Oct	8.0	2.0	5.0	—	15.3
1979	Jan	8.0	2.0	5.0	—	17.0
	April	8.0	1.75	5.0	—	16.9
	July	7.0	1.75	5.0	—	14.0
	Oct	7.0	1.75	3.75	—	16.3
1980	Jan	6.5	3.0	3.75	—	21.1
	April	6.5	1.5	3.75	—	18.9
	July	4.5	1.25	3.75	—	21.9
	Oct	5.5	1.25	3.75	—	24.6
1981	Jan	5.5	1.0	3.75	7.2	22.6
	April	4.5	1.5	3.75	4.0	23.7
	July	4.5	1.75	3.75	4.8	23.9
	Oct	4.5	1.75	2.5	4.0	24.5
1982	Jan	3.5	1.75	1.25	4.0	23.6
	April	4.5	1.75	3.75	0	23.9
	July	5.0	1.25	3.75	8.0	24.1
	Oct	4.5	1.5	2.5	2.4	23.9
1983	Jan	5.0	1.5	2.5	5.0	24.4
	April	5.0	1.5	2.5	4.0	22.6

[a](CLON) clonezepam; (VAL) valproate; (PREM) Premarin; (PIR) piracetam.

ACKNOWLEDGMENTS

Mr. Norman Seiden developed the scoring system to quantitate the severity of myoclonus present in his wife. A running graph of the medication dosages and the clinical state provided daily information on the effectiveness of any medication change.

REFERENCES

1. Fahn S. Posthypoxic action myoclonus: review of the literature and report of two new cases with response to valproate and estrogen. *Adv Neurol* 1979;26:49–84.
2. Schwab RS, England AC Jr, Poskanzer DC. Amantadine in the treatment of Parkinson's disease. *JAMA* 1969;208:1168–1170.
3. Terwinghe G, Daumerie J, Nicaise C, Rosillon O. Effet therapeutique du piracetam dans un cas de myoclonie d'action postanoxique. *Acta Neurol Belg* 1978;78:30–36.

Advances in Neurology, Vol. 43: Myoclonus,
edited by S. Fahn et al. Raven Press,
New York © 1986.

Postmortem Studies on Posthypoxic and Post-Methyl Bromide Intoxication: Case Reports

*J. J. Hauw, *R. Escourolle, *,**M. Baulac, †A. Morel-Maroger, ‡M. Goulon, and **P. Castaigne

*Charles Foix Neuropathology Laboratory, and **Clinique des Maladies du Système Nerveux, Hôpital de la Salpêtrière, F-75651 Paris Cedex 13; †Neurology Department, Corbeil Essonnes Hospital, F-91110 Corbeil-Essonnes; and ‡Intensive Care Department, Raymond Poincaré Hospital, F-92380 Garches, France*

Few reports of pathological examinations of the brain in posthypoxic myoclonus and in related conditions have been published (4,5,6,14,20,26,30) since the detailed description of the syndrome by Lance and Adams (15). Five case reports, two of which were previously reported (4,5,14), are summarized here. Three cases can be classified as "chronic intention or action myoclonus as a sequel to hypoxic encephalopathy" in conscious patients. Another case report is concerned with oscillatory myoclonus in a patient recovering from coma related to cardiocirculatory failure, with a "chronic stupor" type level of consciousness. In the last case report, this syndrome is a result of acute methyl bromide intoxication.

PATIENTS AND METHODS

Pathological Methods

In every case, the brain was studied after formalin fixation. Coronal section of the hemispheres and sections perpendicular to the axis of the brainstem including the cerebellum were macroscopically examined. Numerous blocks representative of main structures of hemispheres, brainstem, and cerebellum were embedded in celloidin (and often in paraffin as well). Sections of each celloidin-embedded block, cut when necessary in semiserial series, were stained with hematoxylin and eosin, with the Loyez technique for myelin (and occasionally with Nissl's thionin technique). Sections from paraffin-embedded blocks were stained with hematoxylin and eosin and with Bodian's protargol impregnation associated with luxol fast blue stain. No quantitative studies were performed. The nomenclature and abbreviations used were those of Nieuwenhuys et al. (21). For brainstem nuclei, the nomenclature of Olszewski and Baxter (23) was applied when necessary.

Case Reports

Case 1

This 80-year-old woman (CF 3078), afflicted with gastric carcinoma, has already been reported in detail (4,5). She underwent general anesthesia for gastrostomy on June 20, 1963. Cardiopulmonary arrest and tracheal aspiration induced severe hypoxia for 10 to 20 min. She remained unconscious for 5 to 6 hr but quickly recovered a normal level of consciousness upon awakening. Movement disorders were observed immediately and persisted until death without any significant degree of improvement. These consisted of characteristic myoclonus of the action type. All four limbs were affected, especially the left side and the upper limbs, as well as the trunk, without any facial, velopalatal, or diaphragm muscle involvement. There was no other relevant neurological sign or symptom except for dysarthria ascribed to myoclonic jerks. The patient was unable to walk. No patent cerebellar tremor could be distinguished from the myoclonus. An electroencephalogram (EEG) showed apparently spontaneous, paroxysmal crises with spike activity (15 Hz) sometimes associated with myoclonus of the left limbs. Attempts at voluntary movements induced rhythmic cortical discharges preceding the myoclonus. The patient died on July 9, 1963 of bronchopneumonia and purulent meningitis.

Pathological examination

Macroscopic examination of the brain (1,220 g) was normal. The microscopic findings are given in Fig. 1 and Table 1. Changes were roughly symmetric. The most marked ones were found in certain amygdala nuclei (nucleus lateralis and pars medialis of nucleus basalis); nucleus subthalamicus, nuclei ventrolateralis, medialis (dorsomedialis), and parafascicularis of thalamus; striatum; nuclei pontis and nuclei of tegmentum pontis; inferior colliculi, griseum centrale mesencephali (subnucleus dorsalis of griseum centrale mesencephali and nucleus supratrochlearis were affected), and the nucleus centralis superior; and subnucleus medialis at the rostal pons level. They consisted of neuronal loss, with infrequent vacuolation, and mild astrogliosis. The only other significant change was a small necrotic area of the right pes pontis (lacuna). It should be emphasized that the cerebral and cerebellar cortex were nearly normal, with the exception of several recent ischemic changes which could not account for myoclonus. In the same way, globus pallidus, hypothalamus, substantia nigra, nucleus interpeduncularis, nucleus ruber, cerebellar deep nuclei and tracts, and medulla oblongata were normal.

In brief, after a postanesthesic hypoxic action myoclonus, the neuropathological study, performed on the 20th day, showed widespread symmetric changes involving, in particular, thalamus, nucleus subthalamus, striatum, griseum centrale mesencephali, and some brainstem raphe nuclei.

Case 2

This 68-year-old man (CF E 196) suffered osteitis of the left inferior maxillary which was treated by surgery and antibiotics in December, 1966. On January 2,

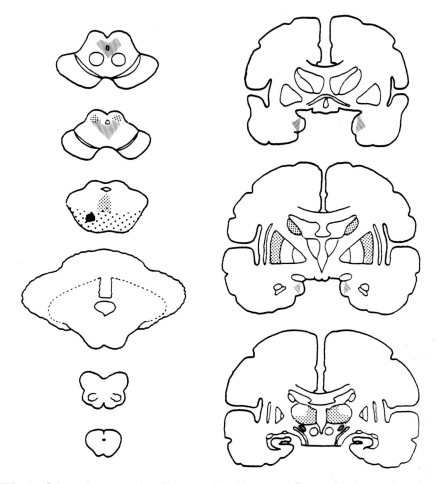

FIG. 1. Schematic topography of changes found in case 1. Severe *(black areas)*, moderate *(gray areas)* and mild *(dotted areas)* changes are shown.

1967, he experienced shivering, fever (40° C), and shock attributed to gram-negative sepsis. On January 3, movement disorders and anuria were noted. On January 7, he was hospitalized. General examination showed heart failure with electrocardiographic changes indicative of ischemia. The patient was conscious, with a varying level of awareness (phases of hypervigilancy and alertness alternating with periods of bradypsychia). Intense myoclonus involved the four limbs and facial muscles, especially on the right side, without palatal or diaphragm contraction. They were either spontaneous or, frequently, evoked by action and sensory stimuli. These signs, present since the onset of the disease, did not vary after normalization of blood chemistries under periodic hemodialysis. They were interpreted as a consequence of the initial systemic shock. Other neurological signs and symptoms included station and gait disorders which were thought to be cerebellar, adiado-

TABLE 1. *Main pathological changes in five cases of postanoxic and post-methyl bromide intoxication myoclonus*

	Case[a]				
	1 (Anesth)	2 (Shock)	3 (Anesth)	4 (Shock)	5 (Methyl bromide)
Time from onset to death	20 days	10 days	40 days	70 days	4 years 8 months
Cerebral cortex	−	−	−	−	+
Cornu amm	−	+ +	−	−	+
Amygd	+ +	+	−	+	−
N caudatus	+	−	−	−	−
Put	+	−	−	−	−
Pal	−	+	−	−	−
Thalamus					
V lat	+	+	−	−	−
Medial	+	−	+	+	+
Parafasc	+	−	−	−	−
Hypoth	−	−	−	−	−
C mam	−	+	+ + +	−	−
N subthal	+ +	−	−	−	−
N sept		−			
N basalis	−	−	−	−	−
N ruber	−	−	−	−	−
Subs nigra	−	−	−	−	−
N interped	−	−	−	−	−
Gris centr mesenc	+ +	+ +	−	+	+ +
Sup collicul	−	−	−	−	−
Inf collicul	+	−	−	−	+ + +
N centr sup	+	+	−	−	+ +
N pontis	+ +	+	−	−	+
Lc cer	−	−	−	−	−
Cerebellar cortex	−	+	−	+ + +	−
N dent	−	−	−	+ + +	+
N ol inf	−	−	−	+	−
N rp magnus	−	−	−	−	−
Sp cord					−

[a] + + +, Severe; + +, moderate; +, mild. Anesth, postanesthesia; Cornu amm, cornu ammonis; Amygd, amygdala; put, putamen; Pal, pallidum; V lat, nucleus ventrolateralis; medial, nucleus medialis; Parafasc, nucleus parafascicularis; Hypoth, hypothalamus; C mam, corpus mamillare; N Subthal, nucleus subthalamus; N sept, nuclei septi; Subs nigra, substantia nigra; N interped, nucleus interpeduncularis; Gris centr mesenc, griseum centrale mesencephali; Sup collicul, superior colliculus; Inf collicul, inferior colliculus; N pontis, nuclei pontis; Lc cer, Locus ceruleus; N dent, nucleus dentatus; N ol inf, nucleus olivaris inferior; N rp magnus, nucleus raphe magnus; Sp cord, spinal cord.

chokinesia, with some propensity to a right grasping reflex, and a few difficulties in denominating. These signs did not significantly vary until death. The EEG showed bilateral delta waves (sensitive to hemineurin which had no effect on myoclonus) and no spike activity. The patient died suddenly on January 13, 1967.

Pathological examination

No macroscopic abnormalities of the brain were noted. Microscopic examination showed few marked changes (Fig. 2, Table 1). These included patent focal neuronal

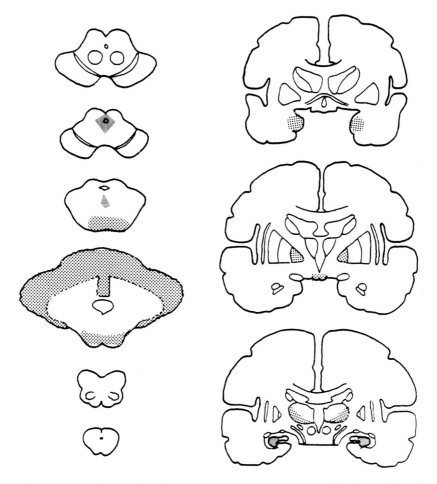

FIG. 2. Schematic topography of changes found in case 2. Severe *(black areas)*, moderate *(gray areas)* and mild *(dotted areas)* changes are shown.

loss and astrogliosis in some anterior fields of the pyramidal layer of hippocampus (HE2-HE3) and moderate gliosis in the griseum centrale mesencephali (subnuclei dorsalis, medialis, and lateralis); nuclei intercollicularis; supratrochlearis; nucleus centralis superior; and subnucleus medialis. Ischemic neurons and scattered microglial cells were found in hippocampus, globus pallidus, nucleus ventrolateralis of thalamus, corpus mamillare, and nuclei pontis. The most numerous ischemic cells were found in the cerebellar Purkinje cell layer, both in the vermis and in the hemispheres. The other layers of the cerebellar cortex and the deep cerebellar nuclei, as well as the medulla oblongata, appeared normal. The only other significant changes were numerous calcifications of the pallidal blood vessels.

In summary, after a shock-induced action myoclonus, the neuropathological study, performed on the 10th day, revealed mild scattered symmetric changes involving the hippocampus, thalamus, griseum centrale mesencephali, and some raphe nuclei, as well as nuclei pontis and cerebellar cortex.

Patient 3

This 50-year-old man (CF 5141) had a history of pleuropulmonary tuberculosis and chronic alcoholism. He was treated by surgery and radium implants for a tongue epithelioma. On September 20, 1973, he was given general anesthesia for surgical treatment of an inferior maxillary radionecrosis. He suffered cardiopulmonary arrest at intubation. He recovered after cardiac massage, but the exact duration of hypoxia was unknown. He was unconscious (stage II coma) for 3 days and had repeated general seizures. The level of consciousness progressively came back to normal within a few days. Severe myoclonus of the intention or action type of all four limbs, trunk, and facial muscles was induced by any movement or sensory stimuli. Speech was rendered nearly impossible by the tumor recurrence, tracheotomy, and myoclonus. He was unable to walk. Neurological examination, when made possible by drug administration, showed mild cerebellar limb ataxia and normal eye movements. The EEG did not show spikes associated with myoclonus. The patient suffered from tracheal aspiration and bronchopneumonia and died on November 2, 1973 from a poorly explained pneumothorax with subcutaneous emphysema.

Pathological examination

Macroscopic study of the brain (1,250 g) showed bilateral atrophy and necrosis of corpus mamillare. Microscopic examination (Fig. 3; Table 1) showed focal changes in corpus mamillare. Neuronal loss and glial and vascular proliferation were evident. Mild neuronal loss and glial proliferation were present in nuclei medialis of thalamus. Subtle changes (mild gliosis) were found in griseum centrale mesencephalis (subnucleus medialis), but their significance could not be ascertained. Cerebellum, other basal ganglia, and brainstem structures appeared normal.

In brief, after a postanesthesic hypoxic intention or action myoclonus in an alcoholic patient, the neuropathological study, performed on the 40th day, showed focal symmetric changes of corpus mamillare which where identical to those of Wernicke-Korsakoff encephalopathy. The mild related thalamus changes are frequently described in this disease.

Case 4

This 56-year-old woman (CF 4206) suffered from angina pectoris. In October of 1968, numerous attacks led to her admission to the hospital where heparin and corticoid treatment were instituted. On October 20, abdominal pain preceded shock with a loss of consciousness that lasted for 40 min. Arterial pressure returned to normal after 24 hr of norepinephrine treatment. On October 23, a second shock

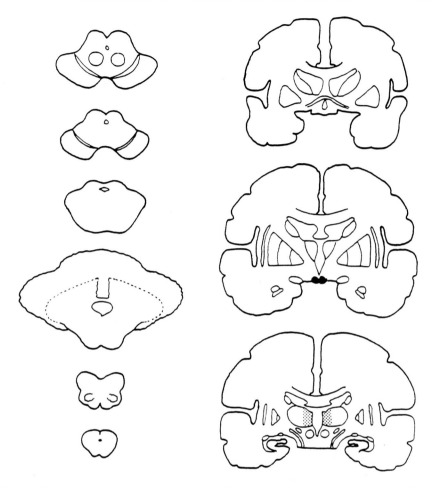

FIG. 3. Schematic topography of changes found in case 3. Severe *(black areas)* and mild *(dotted areas)* changes are shown.

with hyperthermia (>41° C) was associated with left-sided seizures and coma. The patient remained unconscious for 24 hr. During the next few days, she was able to answer simple questions but could not speak fluently. On October 27 and November 1, new shocks occurred with hyperthermia. On October 30, on admission to La Salpêtrière Hospital, the patient was in a mental state of chronic stupor. She had difficulty answering simple questions and orders. The voluntary motility of all four limbs was markedly reduced. She evidenced obvious movement disorders of the hands and the chin primarily caused by myoclonus of the shoulder and arm musculature. Although absent at rest, this was induced by muscular stretch and appeared to be rhythmic (3 Hz). The EEG showed slow waves of 4 to 5 Hz with intermittent paroxysmal potentials. The patient died suddenly on January 13, 1969.

Pathological examination

Macroscopic study of the brain (1,190 g) was normal. The main microscopic changes (Fig. 4; Table 1) were located in the cerebellum. They involved the cortex, with massive Purkinje cell loss, proliferation of Bergmann's glial cells, and an abundance of microglial cells in the molecular layer. The deep cerebellar nuclei, in particular dentatus nuclei, exhibited marked changes (neuronal loss and gliosis). Mild gliosis was found in nuclei medialis of thalamus and in the griseum centrale mesencephali. In addition, a few ischemic changes were seen in the cerebral cortex (especially in parietooccipital lobes) and in inferior olive nuclei.

In summary, after shock-induced rhythmic myoclonus triggered or revealed by muscle stretch, the neuropathological study, performed 73 days after the onset of

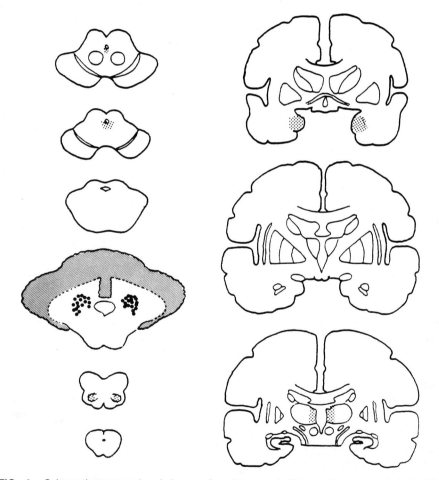

FIG. 4. Schematic topography of changes found in case 4. Severe changes are indicated by black (nucleus dentatus) and dark gray (cerebellar cortex). *Dotted areas,* mild changes.

the movement disorder, showed marked cerebellar changes, involving the Purkinje cell layer and, above all, the cerebellar deep nuclei, and mild gliosis of nuclei medialis of thalamus and of inferior olive nuclei.

Case 5

Patient 5 (CF E 775) has already been reported in detail (14). This 45-year-old woman suffered acute methyl bromide intoxication on February 16, 1966, due to a fire extinguisher leak. She was found unconscious in deep coma with initial depressed blood pressure, hypothermia, and generalized clonus. After 3 weeks of respiratory assistance, consciousness improved to chronic stupor with generalized myoclonus of the intention or action type. It involved the four limbs and the face without palatal or diaphragmatic myoclonus. The EEG showed spikes, multiple spikes, and slow waves, sometimes in relation to myoclonic jerks. The patient died on October 30, 1971, from purulent pleurisy.

Pathological examination

No macroscopic abnormality of the brain and spinal cord was seen. Microscopic study (Fig. 5; Table 1) showed marked, symmetric changes in the inferior colliculi. These consisted of old cavitated necrotic foci containing a few compound granular cells and some hemosiderin. They were surrounded by astrocytic gliosis with Rosenthal fibers and neuronal loss extending toward the lemniscus lateralis but sparing the superior cerebellar peduncle. On the other hand, the griseum centrale mesencephali (subnuclei dorsalis, medialis, and lateralis), the nuclei cuneiformis and subcuneiformis, the nucleus supratrochlearis, the nucleus centralis superior, and the subnucleus medialis were affected. The superior colliculi were normal. In contrast, the changes found in the griseum centrale mesencephali (nuclei medialis and lateralis) were marked at this level. They involved the medial part of the nucleus of the third nerve. However, the nucleus interpeduncularis was spared. At more caudal levels, the nucleus centralis superior and the nucleus reticularis tegmenti ponti were more affected than the nucleus reticularis pontis oralis. There was degeneration of the tectospinal tract. Moderate to mild changes were seen in nuclei pontis, nuclei dentatus, and nuclei medialis of thalamus. These consisted of scattered neuronal loss and astrogliosis. The cerebral cortex exhibited some laminar changes of the third and fifth layers and mild neuronal loss in the hippocampus.

In brief, acute methyl bromide intoxication with shock was followed by a chronic stupor and persistent action myoclonus. Neuropathological examination, performed 5 years and 8 months later, showed marked changes in inferior colliculi and moderate changes in griseum centrale mesencephali, nuclei cuneiformis and subcuneiformis, nuclei supratrochlearis, nucleus centralis superior and nucleus reticularis tegmenti ponti, and in nuclei medialis of thalamus, nuclei pontis, and nuclei dentatus.

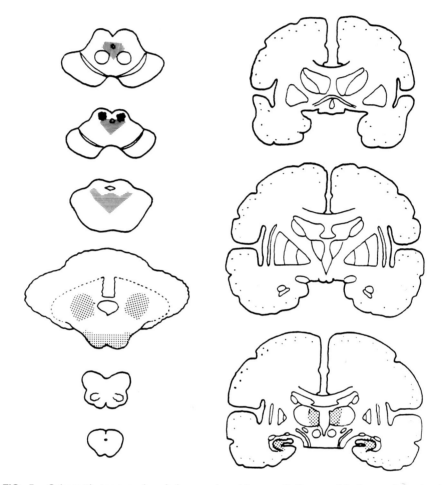

FIG. 5. Schematic topography of changes found in case 5. Severe *(black areas)*, moderate *(gray areas)* and mild *(dotted areas)* changes are shown.

DISCUSSION

On clinical grounds, these five patients differed somewhat. Three of them could be classified as postanoxic action myoclonus (due in cases 1 and 3 to anesthetic anoxia and in case 2 to septic shock), one (case 4) as rhythmic stimulus-sensitive (oscillatory) posthypoxic myoclonus, and the remaining one (case 5) as action myoclonus due to methyl bromide intoxication (2,6,10,12,19).

Pathological changes varied significantly from case to case. This could be due to differences between the onset of myoclonus and death; different types of myoclonus; or different mechanisms.

The amount of time from the onset of myoclonus to the pathological examination was important in assessing the significance of the changes. Short-lasting ischemic changes, particularly when scattered and mild, were often difficult to distinguish from agonal or nonspecific changes in patients subjected to resuscitation and/or intensive care. From this point of view, the findings in long-lasting myoclonus (cases 5, 4, and 3) were more significant than those in short-lasting myoclonus (cases 1 and 2).

Different types of myoclonus could be distinguished. It might be of significance, although data from a few cases must be considered with reservation, that the only marked cerebellar changes to be found were in the single case of rhythmic stimulus-sensitive posthypoxic myoclonus.

In addition, although similar to posthypoxic action myoclonus on clinical grounds, the sequelae of acute methyl bromide intoxication seem to have characteristic features. In two long-lasting cases (11; case 5), changes were seen in both colliculi inferiores and griseum centrale mesencephalis, although in the case of Franken (11), they were more diffuse.

The significance of pathological changes to the understanding of the pathogenesis of the action myoclonus is dubious. It must be emphasized that some cases are practically devoid of recognizable changes that are likely to explain the syndrome. In our case 3, the pathology was limited to lesions of corpus mamillare, mild changes of medialis nucleus of thalamus, and dubious abnormalities of griseum centrale mesencephalis. The presence of some degree of gliosis in this area is frequent in the absence of any significant clinical or pathological abnormality. It might be mentioned, however, that negative findings concern principally nerve cell bodies and main myelinated tracts. Slight neuronal loss or fiber degeneration which could induce only mild gliosis is undetectable unless morphometric methods are used. This was not the case in this observation (or in any one either of this series or thus far reported). It should be pointed out, however, that these cases are characterized by relatively limited changes and therefore enable better correlations than do those with more widespread damage (6,30).

The changes, although sometimes subtle, appear multifocal and symmetric. This symmetry could be a condition for the onset of the myoclonus. Although the other published pathological reports do not rule out this hypothesis, the case of Avanzini et al. (1) does not favor it. They report the unilateral myoclonus to be related to a contralateral thalamic arteriovenous malformation. It may be argued that the hemodynamic consequences of such a lesion can be bilateral.

The analysis of our cases and other published case reports (6,20,26,30) (Table 2) focuses the discussion on the localization of changes that can induce action myoclonus on three main putative areas. First, the thalamus was slightly affected in all five cases in our study. The changes were found either in nucleus medialis or in nucleus ventrolateralis. The latter was considered previously by Lance and Adams (15) to have etiological significance, but their hypothesis later proved insufficient (10,17). No significant abnormality of the thalamus was described in the two other reported cases with limited changes (20,26).

Second, the brainstem raphe was found to be affected in cases 1, 2, 4, and 5 of our study and in the case reported by Richardson et al. (26). Such findings are of

TABLE 2. *Other pathological reports*

Case no.	Findings	Ref.
1	Astrogliosis of the midbrain periaqueductal gray and dorsolateral gray of tegmentum	26
3	Very severe diffuse anoxic brain damage	30
2	Widespread anoxic damage in cerebral cortex boundary zones and the hippocampus	6
1	Parietooccipital laminar damage; necrosis of putamen and head of nucleus caudatus	20

interest, as these areas are thought to contain the serotonergic nuclei of brainstem, and serotonin precursors can improve the myoclonus (16). Furthermore, the serotonin turnover was found to decrease in some cases (13). Precise topographic data concerning the location and the projections of serotonergic neurons in humans are not currently available. However, animal studies, especially in monkeys (27–29), have shown the presence of serotonergic neurons in mesencephalic raphe (nucleus raphe dorsalis, subnucleus lateralis of griseum centralis mesencephalis, raphe pontis, nucleus centralis superior, nucleus raphe magnus). Some scattered serotonergic neurons have also been found in various parts of the brainstem (29). Parent et al. (24) have shown that, in rats, two ascending tracts originated from the nucleus raphe dorsalis [B7 area of Dahlström and Fuxe (8)]: a ventral transtegmental tract toward median forebrain bundle and a more dorsal periventricular tract which runs along the colliculus toward habenula and thalamus. In our cases 1, 2, 4, and 5, as well as in the case of Richardson et al. (26), the lesion of serotonergic cells or tracts could explain myoclonus. Such was not true in our case 3, in the case of Masson et al. (20), and in the cases of Wolf (30) and Chadwick et al. (6), as emphasized by Marsden (18).

Third, the last site of these changes could be the cerebellum, as suggested by our case 2 and, in particular, by case 4, as well as by the observation (proven by biopsy) of Cooper et al. (7) and that of Oka et al. (22) (of intention myoclonus in acute leukemia). However, the myoclonus of patient 4 differed from that of characteristic Lance and Adams action myoclonus. The latter resembles more that of the Ramsay Hunt (23) syndrome. It must be emphasized, however, that in this syndrome, the changes did not always involve the cerebellum and were frequently widespread (9).

The changes found in other brain structures, in some of our cases and in some of those reported, do not seem relevant to myoclonus. It can be emphasized that involvement of these structures did not prevent the occurrence of action myoclonus. Multiple widespread lesions induced by deep hypoxia have frequently been found in patients with no myoclonus. However, the pathological human brain is a very complicated model, which is obviously necessary yet poorly suitable to the study of the physiopathology of myoclonus. Additional experimental evidence and pathological case reports are required.

SUMMARY

In two cases of action myoclonus following hypoxic or shock encephalopathy, neuropathological examination disclosed mild or moderate scattered changes involving thalamus, griseum centrale mesencephali, and nucleus centralis superior. Other areas were affected only in one of these cases (striatum, nucleus subthalamicus or hippocampus, nuclei pontis, and cerebellar cortex). In another case (an alcoholic patient), the changes, which involved only corpus mamillare and thalamus, were those of Wernicke–Korsakoff encephalopathy. In one case of oscillatory myoclonus following septic shock, there were marked cerebellar changes involving deep nuclei and mild abnormalities in the thalamus and inferior olive. The last case of action myoclonus following acute methyl bromide intoxication was characterized by marked changes in the inferior colliculi and moderate or mild abnormalities of thalamus, griseum centrale mesencephali, nucleus centralis superior, nucleus reticularis tegmenti pontis, nuclei pontis, and dentatus. The findings are compared with the data of seven previously reported neuropathological examinations in action myoclonus following hypoxic encephalopathy.

ACKNOWLEDGMENTS

We thank Mrs. Bethermin, Mrs. Coestesquis, Mrs. Raiton, and Mr. Miele for technical assistance. Mrs. M. A. Warrick kindly reviewed the English manuscript.

REFERENCES

1. Avanzini G, Broggi G, Caraceni T. Intention and action myoclonus from thalamic angioma. *Eur Neurol* 1977;15:194–202.
2. Bonduelle M. The myoclonias. In: Vinken PJ, Bruyn GW, eds. Handbook of clinical neurology, vol. 6. Amsterdam: North Holland, 1968:761–81.
3. Brierley JB, Graham DI. Hypoxia and vascular disorders of the central nervous system. In: Hume Adams J, Corsellis JAN, Duchen LW, eds. Greenfield's neuropathology. London: Edward Arnold, 1984;125–207.
4. Castaigne P, Cambier J, Escourolle R. Les myoclonies d'intention et d'action. In: Bonduelle M, Gastaut H, eds. Les myoclonies. Paris: Masson, 1968:107–20.
5. Castaigne P, Cambier J, Escourolle R, Cathala HP, Lecasble R. Observation anatomo-clinique d'un syndrome myoclonique post-anoxique. *Rev Neurol (Paris)* 1964;111:60–73.
6. Chadwick D, Hallett M, Jenner P, Marsden CD. Serotonin and action myoclonus—a review. In: Legg NJ, ed. Neurotransmitter systems and their clinical disorders. London: Academic Press, 1978:151–65.
7. Cooper TS, Amin I, Riklan M, Waltz JM, Poon TP. Chronic cerebellar stimulation in epilepsy. Clinical and anatomical studies. *Arch Neurol* 1970;33:559–70.
8. Dahlström A, Fuxe K. Evidence for the existence of monoamine containing neurons in the central nervous system. I. Demonstration of monoamines in the cell bodies of brain stem neurons. *Acta Physiol Scand* 1964;62:1–55.
9. Escourolle R, Gray F, Hauw J-J. Les atrophies cérébelleuses. *Rev Neurol (Paris)* 1982;138:953–65.
10. Fahn S. Posthypoxic action myoclonus: review of the literature and report of two new cases with response to valproate and estrogen. In: Fahn S, Davis JN, Rowland LP, eds. Advances in neurology vol. 26. New York: Raven Press, 1979:49–84.
11. Franken L. Etude anatomique d'un cas d'intoxication par le bromure de méthyle. *Acta Neuropsychiatr (Belg)* 1959;59:375–83.
12. Gastaut H. Séméiologie des myoclonies et nosologie analytique des syndromes myocloniques. In: Bonduelle M, Gastaut H, eds. Les myoclonies. Paris: Masson, 1968:1–30.

13. Guilleminault C, Tharp BR, Cousin D. HVA and 5-HIAA CSF measurements and 5-HTP trials in some patients with involuntary movements. *J Neurol Sci* 1973;18:435–41.
14. Goulon M, Nouailhat F, Escourolle R, Zarranz-Imirizaldu JJ, Grosbuis S, Lévy-Alcover MA. Intoxication par le bromure de méthyle. Trois observations, dont une mortelle. Etude neuro-pathologique d'un cas de stupeur avec myoclonies, suivi pendant cinq ans. *Rev Neurol (Paris)* 1975;131:445–68.
15. Lance JW, Adams RD. The syndrome of intention or action myoclonus as a sequel to hypoxic encephalopathy. *Brain* 1963;86:111–36.
16. Lhermitte F, Peterfalvi M, Marteau R, Gazengel J, Serdaru M. Analyse pharmacologique d'un cas de myoclonies d'intention et d'action postanoxiques. *Rev Neurol (Paris)* 1971;124:21–31.
17. Lhermitte F, Talairach J, Buser P, Gautier J-C, Bancaud J, Gras R, Truelle J-L. Myoclonies d'intention et d'action post-anoxiques. Etude stéréotaxique et destruction du noyau ventral latéral du thalamus. *Rev Neurol (Paris)* 1971;124:5–20.
18. Marsden CD. Discussion. In: Fahn S, Davis JN, Rowland LP, eds. Advances in neurology vol. 26. New York: Raven Press, 1979:85.
19. Marsden CD, Hallett M, Fahn S. The nosology and pathophysiology of myoclonus. In: Marsden CD, Fahn SF, eds. Movement disorders. New York: Raven Press, 1982:196–248.
20. Masson M, Prier S, Hénin D. Etude neuropathologique d'un cas de myoclonies d'intention et d'action post-anoxiques. *Rev Neurol (Paris)* 1979;135:923–4.
21. Nieuwenhuys R, Voogd J, van Huijzen Chr. *The human central nervous system. A synopsis and atlas.* Berlin: Springer, 1979.
22. Oka H, Matsushima M, Ando K, Hoshizaki H. Intention myoclonus in acute leukaemia. *Brain* 1973;96:395–8.
23. Olszewski J, Baxter D. *Cytoarchitecture of the human brain stem.* Basel: Karger, 1982.
24. Parent A, Descarries L, Beaudet A. Organization of ascending serotonin systems in the adult rat brain. A radioautographic study after intraventricular administration of [3H]5-hydroxytriptamine. *Neuroscience* 1981;6:115–38.
25. Ramsay-Hunt J. Dyssynergia cerebellaris myoclonica. Primary atrophy of the dentate systems. A contribution to the pathology and symptomatology of the cerebellum. *Brain* 1921;44:490–538.
26. Richardson JC, Rewcastle NB, De Lean J. Hypoxic myoclonus: clinical and pathological observations. In: Rose FC, ed. Physiological aspects of clinical neurology. Oxford: Blackwell, 1977:231–45.
27. Schofield SPM, Everitt BJ. The organization of indoleamine neurons in the brain of the rhesus monkey. *J Comp Neurol* 1981;197:369–83.
28. Sladek JR Jr, Garver DL, Cummings JP. Monoamine distribution in the primate brain. IV. Indoleamine containing perikaria in the brain stem of Macaca arctoides. *Neuroscience* 1982; 7:477–93.
29. Takeuchi Y, Kimura H, Matsuura T, Sano Y. Immunohistochemical demonstration of the organization of serotonin neurons in the brain of the monkey (macaca fuscata). *Acta Anat* 1982; 114:106–24.
30. Wolf P. Periodic synchronous and stereotyped myoclonus with postanoxic coma. *J Neurol* 1977; 215:39–47.

Advances in Neurology, Vol. 43: Myoclonus,
edited by S. Fahn et al. Raven Press,
New York © 1986.

Pathological Findings in a Case of Hypoxic Myoclonus Treated with 5-Hydroxytryptophan and a Decarboxylase Inhibitor

J. De Léan, *J. C. Richardson, and **N. B. Rewcastle

*Laboratoire de Neurophysiologie clinique, Hôpital du St-Sacrement, Québec City, Québec, Canada, GIS 4L8; *Division of Neurology, Toronto General Hospital, Toronto, Ontario, Canada, M5G 1L7; and **Department of Pathology, Foothill General Hospital, Calgary, Alberta, Canada, T2N 2T9*

Action myoclonus is an unusual clinical manifestation of anoxic brain damage. Pharmacological studies have revealed a serotonergic disturbance in this unique syndrome (2,7,12) first reported by Lance and Adams (6). Two patients suffering this condition were studied clinically and investigated pharmacologically at the Toronto General Hospital (4). One did not survive, and the brain was subjected to a detailed neuropathological examination (11).

CASE HISTORY

On September 9, 1972, a 72-year-old woman took 25 capsules of Tuinal, 200 mg, in a suicide attempt. She arrived by ambulance at a hospital emergency room in a comatose, cyanosed, pulseless state; she was subsequently resuscitated. On regaining consciousness 36 hr later, she was found to have violent jerking movements of her trunk and limbs. These myoclonic jerks were triggered by voluntary activity and by auditory or tactile stimuli. Moderate improvement was obtained by oral diazepam, 100 mg/day. At this time her mental examination was normal except for memory loss for recent events surrounding the overdose. After several weeks she could walk with help and was discharged to a convalescent hospital. After 2 months, her myoclonic jerks worsened, and eventually she was transferred to a chronic care hospital where she remained bedridden for 2 years. Several years earlier, this patient had suffered repeated depressive states, requiring electroshock treatment on three occasions.

In December of 1974, she was transferred to the Toronto General Hospital for further investigation and drug trials. Her intellect and speech were normal. She was depressed and resigned to a state of helpless invalidism, which hampered our therapeutic efforts. She had no facial twitching or palatal myoclonus. On finger–nose testing, she had bilateral action myoclonus, as well as some intention tremor, more pronounced on the left. Heel–knee–shin test revealed similar myoclonus and intention tremor, more conspicuous in the right lower limb. She was confined to bed because attempts to sit, stand, and walk triggered uncontrollable myoclonic movements. Her deep tendon reflexes and plantar responses were normal. An electroencephalogram (EEG) revealed slow activity over the left hemisphere and failed to show any spike activity.

Pharmacological and Biochemical Findings

Drugs were given orally except for L-5-hydroxytryptophan (L-5-HTP), which also was administered intravenously over 15 min in a single dose. On daily neurological examination, speech, finger–nose test, and ability to sit up, stand, and walk were rated between 5 (no myoclonus) and 0 (severe jerking). Significant clinical changes were recorded by cinematography and controlled by substitution of placebo for sufficient periods of time. Initially and during the drug trials, 10 cc of cerebrospinal fluid (CSF) was collected by lumbar puncture and sent to the Department of Psychopharmacology, Clarke Institute of Psychiatry, Toronto (O. Hornykiewicz), for estimation of 5-hydroxyindoleacetic acid (5-HIAA).

Levodopa (2 g/day) and methysergide (12 mg/day) worsened the myoclonus (Fig. 1). L-Tryptophan (10 g/day) was of mild benefit. Parachlorophenylalanine (PCPA) (4 g/day) and methysergide (6 mg/day) failed to change the myoclonus. On a regimen of 1 g L-5-HTP and 100 mg carbidopa (l-α-methyldopa hydrazine), action myoclonus disappeared completely and intention tremor remained unchanged.

The patient became able to feed herself and to walk short distances unassisted. Because of her chronic underlying psychoneurotic personality disorder, she developed regressive hysterical reactions and returned to her usual deeply depressed, totally uncooperative state. Because little assistance was obtained from antidepressant medication, L-5-HTP was discontinued and the patient was discharged to a chronic hospital on her previous medication. Her physical condition continued as before, with severe myoclonus confining her to bed and wheelchair. In June of 1975, she was found unconscious and cyanosed. Resuscitation efforts failed. Autopsy showed death was caused by choking on food. The brain of the patient was fixed in formalin, and fresh tissue for chemical assay was not available.

Initially, the concentration of 5-HIAA in the CSF was found to be significantly low (Fig. 2). While on L-tryptophan, CSF 5-HIAA was twice the pretreatment value. A decrease in CSF 5-HIAA concentration to 30% of the pretreatment level was produced by PCPA. On L-5-HTP and MK 486, CSF 5-HIAA levels rose to four times the initial value.

Neuropathological Findings

Neuropathological examination was performed at the Banting Institute of Toronto, Division of Neuropathology, (Dr. Rewcastle). The fixed brain weighed 1,450 g, and no abnormalities were detected on the surface. Coronal slices of the cerebral

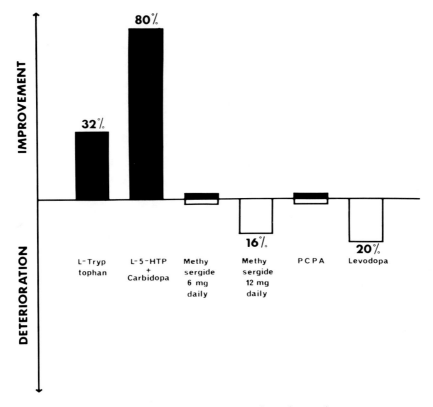

FIG. 1. Effects of various drugs on hypoxic myoclonus.

hemispheres revealed no lesion. The ventricles were of normal size. Transverse sections of the brainstem and cerebellum were unremarkable.

Microscopic examination was performed in detail using hematoxylin and eosin/ luxol fast blue, cresyl violet, phosphotungstic and hematoxylin, Holzer, and oil red O staining techniques. The basal ganglia and the diencephalic structures were studied in sections cut at 1-mm intervals at right angles to the anterior commissure– posterior commissure axes. Transverse sections from upper midbrain to lower medulla were cut at similar 1-mm intervals for comparison with the Olszewski– Baxter atlas (10). Representative areas of cerebral and cerebellar cortices as well as deep midline and lateral areas of the cerebellum were sampled to complete the study.

We were surprised by a paucity of structural changes which had proved difficult to differentiate from those usually seen in the aging nervous system. No evidence of hypoxic damage could be demonstrated in the cerebral cortex. Occasional clusters of fibrillary astrocytes were encountered within the cerebral cortex, slightly more frequently in the fifth and sixth layers. However, in the many areas studied, laminar type damage was not found, nor were lipid-containing macrophages present

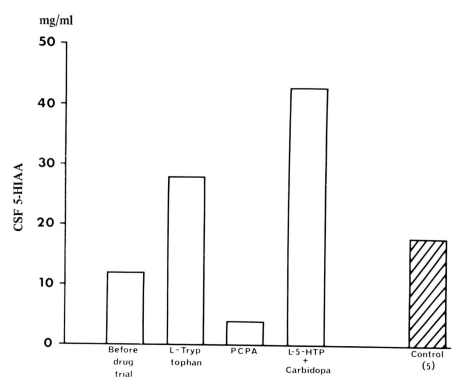

FIG. 2. Results of CSF 5-HIAA values (ng/ml).

in the cortical parenchyma on oil red O-stained frozen sections. The hippocampal formation was undamaged. The medial temporal lobes, including the hippocampal gyrus, showed occasional intraneuronal neurofibrillary tangles, granulovacuolar degeneration, and Hirano bodies, as well as very rare senile plaques which are encountered in brains of similar age.

No neuronal loss or glioses were evident in the caudate nucleus, putamen, pallidum, or subthalamic nucleus. No discernible abnormalities were found in the thalamus or other diencephalic areas.

In the lower brainstem, prominent astrocytic reaction involved the inferior olives, the parenchyma of the fourth ventricles corresponding to the vestibular nuclear areas. Such findings are not unusual in patients of advanced years. However, a marked astrocytic reaction of some duration, indicated by scattered hypertrophied cells and tight clusters of two or three such cells, was encountered in the midbrain tegmentum. This astrocytic prominence was present in the lateral parts of the supratrochlear nucleus, the lateral subnucleus of the mesencephalic gray, and the immediately adjacent cuneiform and subcuneiform nuclei of the caudal half of the midbrain. Actual neuronal loss was more difficult to assess, but in the dorsal and lateral parts of the supratrochlearis nucleus, sites of presumed nerve cell disintegration were indicated by tight clusters of macrophages distended by lipochrome pigment (Fig. 3). After comparison with age-matched controls, the astrocytic prominence in the midbrain periaqueductal gray matter and the sites of presumed neuronal loss represent changes in excess of age, although these changes were by no means marked. The neuronal populations of the supratrochlearis nucleus (Fig. 4) and the other raphe nuclei, centralis, linearis, magnus pallidus, and obscurus, were well maintained, although cell counting techniques were not performed. Neuronal populations throughout the midbrain tectum, pons, or medulla were well maintained for a brain of this age. The locus ceruleus was also well populated with neurons, allowing for the age of the patient. Incidental findings included an occasional midline brainstem neuron containing an intracytoplasmic neurofibrillary tangle and a small focus of mononuclear cell infiltration in the pontine tegmentum.

The cerebellar cortex, the deep cerebellar nuclei, and their outflow tracts were normal. Bielchowsky silver staining techniques demonstrated only a few collapsed basket cell arrangements revealing sites of rare Purkinje cell loss.

DISCUSSION

The anatomic basis of hypoxic myoclonus has not yet been established. Considering that hypoxic myoclonus is a permanent disability in most cases, it is con-

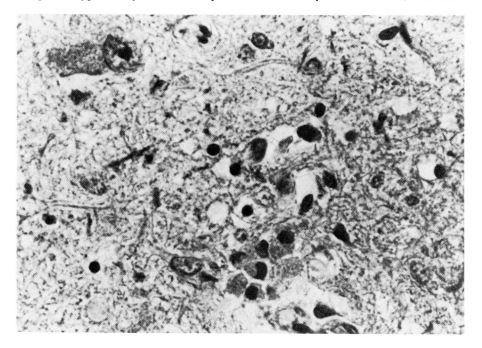

FIG. 3. Supratrochlear nucleus. Nerve cell damage indicated by astrocytic hypertrophy of some duration and tight clusters of macrophages in the lateral part of the nucleus. Hematoxylin and eosin/luxol fast blue. × 446. (Reproduced with permission from Blackwell Scientific Publications.)

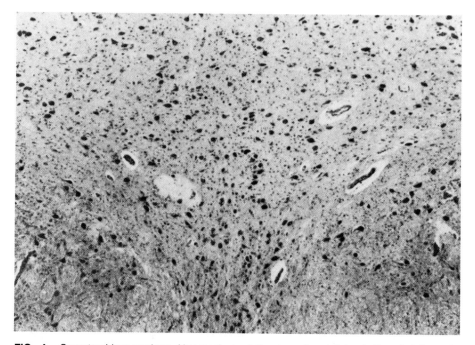

FIG. 4. Supratrochlear nucleus. Neuronal population is well maintained. Cresyl violet stain. ×25. (Reproduced with permission from Blackwell Scientific Publications.)

TABLE 1. *Pathological findings in hypoxic myoclonus*[a]

No. of cases	Telencephalon		Basal ganglia		Diencephalon		Midbrain	Cerebellum		Ref.
	Cerebral cortex	Hippocampus	Striatum	Pallidum	Thalamus	Subthalamus	(Raphe region)	Purkinje cells	Dentate nucleus	
1	+		+ +		+	+ + +	+	+		1
1							+			
2	+ +	+ +								3
1	+ +		+ + +							8
1										9
1	+ +		+	+	+ +	+ +		+	+	9

[a]Ischemic nerve cell damage: +, discrete; + +, moderate; + + +, severe.

ceivable that some neurons in the brain do suffer irreversible damage as a result of anoxia.

It is of interest to compare the neuropathological findings in our case with six other autopsy reports which are summarized in Table 1 (1,3,8,9). Of the five cases reported by Hauw et al. *(this volume)*, one has already been included in Table 1, whereas another case had involuntary movements suggesting a cerebellar lesion. The three remaining pathological reports of Hauw et al. *(this volume)* are discussed with the seven cases reviewed in Table 1.

These 10 pathological reports of hypoxic myoclonus fall into two distinct categories: (a) cases showing very few significant pathological changes, such as our case, the first case of Moreira Filho et al. (9), and one case of Hauw et al. *(this volume)* showing only evidence of a previous Wernicke encephalopathy; and (b) cases demonstrating multiple areas of anoxic damage, such as the case of Castaigne et al. (1), the second case of Moreira Filho et al. (9), and some cases reported by Hauw et al. *(this volume)*.

The widespread anoxic damage reported in the second group seems of dubious relevance to myoclonus, considering that similar findings are not unusual in non-myoclonic anoxic encephalopathy. Furthermore, myoclonus is reported in the first group in the absence of such destructive lesions.

Biochemical and pharmacological data support a possible disturbance of serotonergic mechanisms in hypoxic myoclonus. The brainstem is of special interest, considering that serotonergic neurons are probably located in this area. A destruction of serotonergic neurons in the brain has been proposed as a possible underlying mechanism for hypoxic myoclonus. This mechanism is not supported by our neuropathological findings. The neuronal population is well maintained in the supra-trochlearis nucleus, and the presumed neuronal loss encountered in some areas is by no means marked. Other studies (Table 1) also fail to demonstrate anoxic damage in the brainstem. Some pharmacological data suggest anatomically and functionally preserved serotonergic neurons in the brain of patients with hypoxic myoclonus. L-tryptophan plus a monoamine oxidase inhibitor were found to be beneficial in our other case (4) and in two other patients reported by Chadwick et al. (3).

It is difficult to correlate in any meaningful fashion the presumptive serotonergic disturbance in the patient, the presently known localization of serotonin in the human brainstem, and the minor structural changes evident in the caudal midbrain on our case. However, the limited evidence provided by our autopsy findings suggests that the anoxic damage suffered by the patient resulted, perhaps, in a functional derangement of serotonergic activity rather than a structural damage with significant reduction in the neuronal population.

CONCLUSION

Hypoxic myoclonus is a rare manifestation of brain anoxia. Our neuropathological findings fail to show the usual extent and distribution of nerve cell damage seen in anoxic encephalopathy and suggest that hypoxic myoclonus is not explained by demonstrable neuronal loss in motor structures, such as cerebellum, thalamus, or basal ganglia. The underlying disturbance of serotonergic mechanisms seems to be causally related to a functional derangement of anatomically intact serotonergic neurons rather than a destruction of the serotonin-containing neurons of the brain.

It is possible that nerve cell counts or other special histological techniques might reveal neuronal loss or changes which are undetectable by ordinary light microscopy.

Biochemical estimates of serotonin and 5-HIAA in the cortex and striatum of two cases with hypoxic myoclonus were found to be comparable to control values

(3). Similar measurements done in the diencephalon, brainstem, cerebellum, and spinal cord of patients with hypoxic myoclonus might help to elucidate the underlying disturbance of serotonergic mechanisms in postanoxic action myoclonus.

SUMMARY

A 72-year-old woman suffered a respiratory arrest following intoxication with barbiturates. Her examination 27 months after the anoxic incident revealed involuntary jerks of trunk and limb muscles triggered by willed movements. On a regimen of 1 g L-5-HTP and 100 mg *l*-α-methyldopa hydrazine (carbidopa), action myoclonus disappeared completely. This medication had to be discontinued because of a regressive hysterical reaction. Two months later, she was found unconscious; resuscitation efforts were unsuccessful. Autopsy showed death was caused by choking on food.

Coronal slices of the cerebral hemispheres and transverse section of the brainstem and cerebellum revealed no lesion. No evidence of hypoxic damage could be demonstrated in the cerebral cortex, hippocampus, striatum, pallidum, subthalamus, thalamus, or other diencephalic structures. In the caudal half of the midbrain tegmentum, a marked astrocytic reaction of some duration was encountered in the lateral parts of the supratrochlearis nucleus, the lateral subnucleus of the mesencephalic gray, and the immediately adjacent cuneiform and subcuneiform nuclei. In the former nucleus, sites of presumed nerve cell disintegration were found, but the neuronal populations of this nucleus and of the other raphe nuclei were well maintained. The other brainstem structures and the cerebellum were normal.

Our neuropathological findings suggest that hypoxic myoclonus (a) does not seem to be explained by demonstrable neuronal loss in motor structures, such as cerebellum, thalamus, or basal ganglia and (b) does not appear to be causally related to a detectable reduction in the serotonin-containing neurons of the brain but rather to a functional derangement of anatomically intact serotonergic pathways originating perhaps from other, as yet unidentified, damaged neuronal structures.

ACKNOWLEDGMENTS

We are indebted to Miss R. Levesque, Miss D. Baker, Mr. G. Langlois, and C. Marin for their valuable assistance.

REFERENCES

1. Castaigne P, Cambier J, Escourolle R, Cathala HP, Lecasble RO. Observation anatomo-clinique d'un syndrome myoclonique postanoxique. *Rev. Neurol. (paris)* 1964;111:60–73.
2. Chadwick D, Reynolds EH, Marsden CD. Relief of action myoclonus by 5-hydroxytryptophan. *Lancet* 1974;2:111–2.
3. Chadwick D, Hallet M, Jenner P, Marsden CD. Serotonin and action myoclonus—A review. In: Legg NJ, ed. Neuro-transmitter systems and their clinical disorders. London: Academic Press, 1978:151–65.
4. De Léan J, Richardson JC, Hornykiewicz O. Benefical effects of Serotonin precursors in postanoxic action myoclonus. *Neurology (Minneap)* 1976;26:863–8.

5. Guilleminault C, Tharp BR, Cousin D. HVA and 5-HIAA CSF measurements and 5HTP trials in some patients with involuntary movements. *J Neurol Sci* 1973;18:435–41.
6. Lance JW, Adams RD. The syndrome of intention or action myoclonus as a sequel to hypoxic encephalopathy. *Brain* 1963;86:111–36.
7. Lhermitte F, Peterfalvi M, Marteau R, Gazengel J, Serdaru M. Analyse pharmacologique d'un cas de myoclonies d'intention et d'action post-anoxiques. *Rev Neurol (Paris)* 1971;21–31.
8. Masson M, Prier S, Henin D. Etude neuropathologique d'un cas de myoclonies d'intention et d'action post-anoxiques. *Rev Neurol (Paris)* 1979;135:932–4.
9. Moreira Filho PG, Freitas MGR, Hahn MD, Cincinnatus D, Nascimento OJM. Encefalopatia mioclonica post-anoxica (sindrome de Lance-Adams). Estudo anatomopatologico de Dois Casos. *ARQ Neuropsiquatr* 1982; 40(2):146–55.
10. Olszewski J, Baxter D. *Cytoarchitecture of the human brainstem.* Philadelphia: Lippincott, 1954.
11. Richardson JC, Rewcastle NB, De Léan J. Hypoxic myoclonus: clinical and pathological observations. In: Rose FC, ed. Physiological aspects of clinical neurology. Oxford: Blackwell Scientific Publications, 1977:231–45.
12. Van Woert MH, Sethy VH. Therapy of intention myoclonus with L-5-hydroxytryptophan and a decarboxylase inhibitor, MK 486. *Neurology (Minneap)* 1975;25:135–40.

Advances in Neurology, Vol. 43: Myoclonus,
edited by S. Fahn et al. Raven Press,
New York © 1986.

Toxic Myoclonus

J. A. Obeso, C. Viteri, J. M. Martínez Lage, and *C. D. Marsden

*Movement Disorders Unit, Department of Neurology, Clínica Universitaria, University of
Navarra, Pamplona, Spain; and *Department of Neurology, Institute of Psychiatry,
London, England*

Transient muscle jerking may be present as part of a complex neurological picture following a variety of intoxications. Drug-induced myoclonus is discussed elsewhere in this volume. In this chapter, we consider only those exogenous toxins that may cause persistent and severe myoclonic jerking.

BISMUTH

General Considerations

In 1974, Burns et al. (5) described five patients from Australia with an encephalopathy characterized by confusion, ataxia, tremor, and intense myoclonic jerking. Each had had a colostomy for carcinoma of the colon and had received treatment with oral bismuth subgallate to improve stool consistency and odor for a period ranging between 6 months and 6 years. No cause was found for this encephalopathy, but all these patients improved when the intake of bismuth was stopped. Burns et al. (5) suggested that bismuth subgallate could produce a toxic encephalopathy. Immediately after this original report, Coffey and Graham (6) described another Australian patient with an encephalopathy similarly treated but without myoclonus and suggested that the subgallate radical could be the active toxic agent.

Bismuth encephalopathy was rapidly recognized at the same time in France, where it reached epidemic proportions (12). Buge et al. (3) studied six patients with an identical clinical presentation to the Australian cases and found highly elevated plasma levels of bismuth. These six patients were receiving bismuth subnitrate, and none had had a gastrointestinal operation. These data strongly suggested that bismuth itself was causing the encephalopathy, particularly because the degree of encephalopathy was correlated positively with the plasma level of the metal.

Between 1973 and 1977, approximately 50 cases were diagnosed in Australia (1), and more than 1,000 cases were detected in France, where 72 deaths were recorded (12,13). Six patients have been reported in Spain in the years from 1975 to 1980 (7,14,20).

The factors leading to absorption and toxic effects of bismuth have not been completely elucidated. The newer formulations of bismuth salts may have allowed easy intestinal absorption, thus achieving very high plasma levels. However, transient plasma levels of bismuth equal or even higher were probably obtained when administered via intramuscular injection for the treatment of syphilis, but side effects were not noticeable. A favored theory is that bismuth salts may be converted by some intestinal microorganism into an absorbable and toxic form, but definitive evidence for this hypothesis has not been obtained.

Clinical Characteristics

A general clinical picture emerges from the study of more than 1,000 patients. There is a prodromal phase lasting weeks or months, characterized mainly by depression, irritability, or apathy. This is followed by a rapid deterioration with confusion and hallucinations, intense myoclonic jerking, marked truncal ataxia, and dysarthria. Generalized convulsions may occur, and stupor and coma may ensue. Recovery is the rule when bismuth intake is stopped early in the evolution of the encephalopathy.

Buge et al. (4), from a study of 41 patients, have distinguished three clinical varieties of bismuth encephalopathy: (a) a benign form, (b) a severe form, and (c) a variety with long evolution.

Patients with the benign form showed subtle abnormalities during the prodromal phase. Excessive dreaming accompanied by nightmares, nocturnal myoclonus, and deterioration of handwriting were the main disturbances. In addition, these French authors paid special attention to the development of severe polydipsia and bulimia. During the acute phase, mental symptoms could dominate the clinical picture. For diagnostic purposes, it is important to recognize that myoclonus was not always obvious in these benign cases.

A severe form occurred in a smaller number of the cases reported by Buge et al. (4). The evolution of these cases was characterized by stupor and coma of rapid onset, severe and intense myoclonus, culminating in "myoclonic storms," seizures, and deterioration of cardiorespiratory function. Bismuth blood levels generally were very high (1,000–2,000 µg/liter). Death was not uncommon in this form.

Another type with a slower evolution starting with a prolonged phase of mild symptoms but culminating with a severe acute illness was recognized in approximately one-third of the patients with bismuth encephalopathy. In these cases, bismuth blood levels remained abnormally high for a long period of time. The subacute phase could last several months, while this acute phase continued for 10 to 16 weeks.

Although myoclonus is one of the most important features of bismuth encephalopathy, there has been no detailed analysis of its neurophysiological and pharmacological characteristics. According to most reports, myoclonus is mainly present on action, but it is also very sensitive to external stimuli. In a patient we studied, the jerks were multifocal, occurring spontaneously and on action. In addition, occasionally massive generalized myoclonus was observed, provoked particularly by visual stimuli. These clinical characteristics of myoclonus in bismuth encephalopathy are similar to those of postanoxic myoclonus.

The pathophysiology of myoclonus in bismuth intoxication is poorly understood. Degeneration of Purkinje cells of the cerebellar cortex was the only pathological finding in the original case reported by Burns et al. (5). However, autopsy of 12 patients studied by Escourolle et al. (8) revealed widespread perivascular lymphocytic infiltration and abundant intracytoplasmic lipofuscin, as well as high bismuth concentrations in cerebral tissue, mostly in the cortex, basal ganglia, and cerebellum. A similar distribution of bismuth deposits has been found by computerized tomography (CT) scan (14,15) (Fig. 1).

The electroencephalogram (EEG) usually showed a characteristic continuous generalized rhythm at a frequency of 3 to 5 Hz unaffected by eye opening. No specific EEG correlate associated with the myoclonus has been recorded in patients with bismuth encephalopathy (4,20); however, such correlation had not been sought by applying the back averaging technique. Somatosensory evoked potentials (SEPs) were enlarged bilaterally in one patient studied by Zarranz and Gadea in Spain (Fig. 2).

Treatment with clonazepam (up to 10 mg/day p.o.) and diazepam (20–60 mg/ day p.o.) has provided reasonable control of the jerks in our limited experience. Conventional antiepileptic drugs seem to be of no value, and 5-hydroxytryptophan (5-HTP) failed to improve the myoclonus in one patient (17).

METHYL BROMIDE

Methyl bromide poisoning has been observed mainly as a consequence of accidental leakage from fire extinguishers. It has almost disappeared since use of methyl bromide was prohibited in the construction of such equipment. In many patients, there has been a free interval of several days between the inhalation of methyl bromide and the onset of myoclonus or other neurological signs. Mental changes, cerebellar ataxia, and myoclonus were the main clinical characteristics of methyl bromide intoxication. The evolution could be extremely rapid in some patients, leading to coma and death within hours or a few days (9).

The myoclonus has been mainly of the action type, although spontaneous and stimulus-sensitive multifocal jerks also have been observed. The jerks were usually

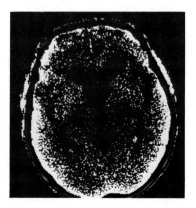

FIG. 1. CT brain scan from a patient with bismuth encephalopathy showing widespread dense bismuth deposits in cortex and basal ganglia.

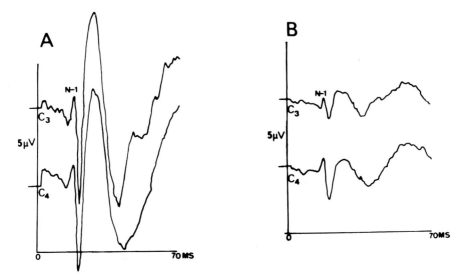

FIG. 2. Large SEPs (12.5 μV P_1-N_2) to digital nerve stimulation of the right hand recorded from an electrode at C_3 *(top trace)*, and from the left hand recorded from an electrode at C_4 *(bottom trace)* referred to as F_z, during the acute phase of bismuth intoxication **(A)**, and normal amplitude SEPs **(B)** recorded when the patient had recovered. The traces have been retouched for clarity. (J. J. Zarranz and A. G. Gadea, *unpublished observation.*)

of large amplitude, causing severe motor disability. Myoclonus could also become constant and generalized in certain cases who, in addition, developed generalized seizures. In some patients who showed a more benign course, however, the intense myoclonic jerking gave way to a postural tremor, clinically similar to that of benign essential tremor (18).

In three patients studied in detail by Goulon et al. (9), SEPs were enlarged bilaterally, and the EEG showed spikes and spike–wave activity preceding the myoclonus. These authors regarded the neurophysiological findings as identical to those described by Lance and Adams (11) in postanoxic myoclonus. The pathological findings in one of these patients, reported by Goulon et al. (9), who survived for 5 years in a state of stupor and intense myoclonic jerking, showed necrosis of both inferior colliculi, gliosis of the upper brainstem reticular formation, and moderate gliosis and degeneration of Purkinje cells in the cerebellum.

TOXIC COOKING OIL

In 1981, an outbreak of "atypical pneumonia" appeared in the center of Spain; 20,000 people were affected, and more than 350 deaths were recorded. Epidemiological studies led to the identification of rapeseed oil, which had been contaminated with anilines, as the responsible agent. The toxic oil was purchased from itinerant salesmen who sold the product unlabeled among lower class workers and peasants.

The respiratory and other systemic symptoms were soon followed by a plethora of neurological complaints in close to 80% of the affected patients. These include spontaneous muscle pain (76), muscular spasms (40%), muscle weakness (22%), and loss of visual acuity (30%). Generalized severe muscle wasting, absent tendon jerks, and inconstant patchy sensory loss were the most common neurological findings on examination.

Myoclonus has been a late complication in about 2 to 3% of the cases. The jerks have been multifocal and transient in most cases. In a small number of cases, however, continuous, repetitive, but irregular muscle jerking of multifocal distribution has been observed. Interestingly, treatment with lithium carbonate alone or associated with clonazepam or phenobarbital has been the most effective treatment for these severe cases.

MISCELLANEOUS

Gasoline Sniffing

Gasoline sniffing may cause an acute encephalopathy due to intake of tetraethyl lead. This has been characterized by visual hallucinations, ataxia, insomnia, irritability, and myoclonic jerking. The encephalopathy may become permanent after repeated exposures to the toxic agent, but recovery has been the rule in most cases. The myoclonus usually has been generalized, increased by action, and provoked by external stimuli (10). Pathological studies have shown nonspecific, widespread neuronal loss (2,19).

Choralose

Intense spontaneous and stimulus-sensitive myoclonus building up to generalized myoclonic status was described by Moene et al. (16) in six patients intoxicated with choralose. Most patients were agitated and in stupor or coma at the time of jerking.

CONCLUSIONS

A number of toxic agents may cause severe myoclonus. In most cases, the clinical presentation of muscle jerking is strikingly similar to postanoxic myoclonus, suggesting some common mechanism(s) of selective vulnerability in this type of myoclonus. In the future, cases of myoclonus due to external agents should be studied in detail, for they represent unfortunate but important clues to the pathophysiology and etiology of other spontaneous forms of myoclonus.

SUMMARY

Several toxins produce encephalopathies in which myoclonus can be a prominent feature. These include intoxications with bismuth, methyl bromide, cooking oil containing anilines, and tetraethyl lead. The clinical features in many cases resemble the action myoclonus syndrome of posthypoxic encephalopathy.

ACKNOWLEDGMENT

The authors are grateful to Mrs. M. L. Sola and Mrs. M. Obeso for their help in the preparation of this manuscript.

REFERENCES

1. Australian Drug Evaluation Committee. Adverse effects of bismuth subgallate. A further report from the Australian Evaluation Committee. *Med J Aust* 1974;2:664–6.
2. Bini L, Bollea G. Fatal poisoning by lead benzine (a clinico pathologic study). *J Neuropathol Exp Neurol* 1974;6:271–5.
3. Buge A, Rancurel G, Poisoon M, et al. Vingt observations d'encephalopathies aigües avec myoclonies au cours de traitements oraux par les sels de bismuth. *Ann Med Int* 1974;125:877–88.
4. Buge A, Rancurel G, Dechy H. Encephalopathies myocloniques bismuthiques formes évolutives, complications tardives durables ou definitives. *Rev Neurol (Paris)* 1977;133:401–15.
5. Burns R, Thomas DW, Barron VJ. Reversible encephalopathy possibly associated with bismuth subgallate ingestion. *Br Med J* 1974;1:220–3.
6. Coffey GL, Graham JW. Mental illness or metal illness bismuth subgallate. *Med J Aust* 1974;2:885–7.
7. Costa-Jussa F, Aguilar M, Martínez JA, et al. Encefalopatia por sales insolubles de bismuto. A propósito de tres observaciones clínicas. *Rev Neurol (Barcelona)* 1979;7:289–96.
8. Escourolle R, Bourdon R, Galli A, et al. Etude neuropathologique et toxicologique de douze cas d'encephalopathie bismuthique. *Rev Neurol (Paris)* 1977;133:153–163.
9. Goulon M, Nouailhat F, Escourolle R, et al. Intoxication par le bromure de methyle. *Rev Neurol (Paris)* 1975;131:445–468.
10. Hansen KS, Sharp FR. Gasoline sniffing, lead poisoning and myoclonus. *JAMA* 1978;240:1375–6.
11. Lance JW, Adams RD. The syndrome of intention or action myoclonus as a sequel to hypoxic encephalopathy. *Brain* 1963;86:111–36.
12. Le Quesne PM. Toxic substances and the nervous system: the role of clinical observation. *J Neurol Neurosurg Psychiatry* 1981;44:1–8.
13. Martin-Bouyer G. Intoxication par le sals de bismuth administré par voie orale. *Gastroenterol Clin Biol* 1975;2:349–56.
14. Martínez Lage JM, Viteri C, Artieda J, et al. Quinto caso español de encefalopatía mioclónica por bismuto. *Reunión Bianual Soc Esp Neurol Madrid, Mayo 1982.*
15. Metzger J, Buge A, Rancurel G, et al. Aspects tomodensitometrique de trois observations d'encephalopathie bismuthiques aigue. *Rev Neurol (Paris)* 1978;134:619–24.
16. Moene Y, Cuche M, Trillet M, et al Problemes diagnostiques posés par l'intoxication aigue a chloralose (a propos de 6 cas). *J Med Lyon* 1969;12:1483–93.
17. Passonant P, Bithard M, Besset A, et al. Encephalopathy associated with Bismuth salt ingestion and brain monoamine. *Int J Neurol* 1979;13:199–204.
18. Rondot P, Said G, Ferrey G. Les hyperkinesies volitionnelles. Etudes electrologiques. Classification. *Rev Neurol (Paris)* 1972;126:415–26.
19. Valpey R, Sumi M, Copass MK, et al. Acute and chronic progressive encephalopathy due to gasoline sniffing. *Neurology* 1978;28:507–10.
20. Zarranz JJ, Forcada I, Larracoechea J, et al. Encefalopatía mioclónica debido a intoxicación por sales insolubles de bismuto. *Med Clin (Barc)* 1977;68:78–80.

Advances in Neurology, Vol. 43: Myoclonus,
edited by S. Fahn et al. Raven Press,
New York © 1986.

Neuromuscular Effects of Monoamine Oxidase Inhibitors

Jeffrey A. Lieberman, John M. Kane, and Ross Reife

*Department of Psychiatry, The Long Island Jewish–Hillside Medical Center,
Glen Oaks, New York 11004*

The neuromuscular effects of the monoamine oxidase inhibitors (MAOIs) have received little attention perhaps because of the notoriety of the food interactions that cause hypertensive crises (5) and the hepatotoxic effects (16) associated with their use. In recent years, there has been a resurgence in the use of these drugs but following a period of disfavor. The renewed interest in MAOIs can be attributed to three factors: (a) demonstration of their therapeutic efficacy by acceptable scientific standards (61,62,64,66), (b) application and claims of selective efficacy in subtypes of affective and anxiety disorders (62,66,78), and (c) strict guidelines for their use to minimize the risk of potentially dangerous adverse effects (64,78).

MONOAMINE OXIDASE INHIBITORS

The MAOIs are most commonly used in the treatment of endogenous depression, atypical depression, panic disorder, and agoraphobia. They inhibit the enzyme MAO, thereby decreasing catabolism and increasing the concentrations of monoamines, including dopamine (DA), norepinephrine (NE), serotonin (5-HT), and phenylethylamine (PEA) (64). The pharmacologic effects of MAOIs are believed to be mediated by the increase in monoamine concentrations and the pharmacodynamic adaptations that consequently occur (6,64).

The MAIOs used in psychiatry can be divided into three main categories: hydrazines, nonhydrazines, and selective MAOIs (Table 1) (61). Evidence suggests that there are at least two forms of MAO (85). The first, MAO type A, preferentially deaminates 5-HT and NE; MAO type B preferentially deaminates PEA (85). Tyramine and DA are substrates for both forms of the enzyme (56,85). Both the A and B forms of MAO are present in the brains of various species, including humans (85). Human brain has been shown to have approximately 80% type B activity and 20% type A activity (85).

The onset of therapeutic effect has been reported to correlate with brain MAO inhibition (64). Ravaris et al. (62) have studied inhibition of platelet MAO as an index of brain MAO inhibition; however, the relationship of platelet (type B) to brain (types A and B) MAO is unknown. The authors suggest that approximately 85% inhibition of brain MAO is needed for increases in brain monoamine concentrations.

TABLE 1. *MOAI drugs*[a]

Generic name	Brand name	Status
Hydrazines		
Iproniazid	Marsalid	Not commercially available in U.S.
Isocarboxazid	Marplan	Available in U.S.
Mebanazine	Actomol	Not available
Nialamide	Niamid	Not commercially available in U.S.
Phenelzine	Nardil	Available in U.S.
Pheniprazine	Catron	Not available
Nonhydrazines:		
Tranylcypromine	Parnate	Available in U.S.
Selective MAOI		
Clorgyline	MAO-A inhibitor	Not commercially available in U.S.
L-Deprenyl	MAO-B inhibitor	Not commercially available in U.S.
Pargyline	Eutonyl-MAO-B inhibitor	Approved as an antihypertensive in U.S.

[a]Adapted from Quitkin et al. (61).

The commercially available MAOIs, phenelzine, isocarboxazid, and tranylcypromine, are nonspecific and inhibit both forms of MAO (61). Pargyline at low concentrations inhibits MAO type B (56). More recently, selective MAOI drugs have been developed. Clorgyline at low concentrations inhibits MAO-A, whereas L-deprenyl at low concentrations preferentially inhibits MAO-B (21,56). The relative efficacy and side effect profiles of these putative selective MAOIs are currently being investigated.

REPORTS IN THE LITERATURE

Neuromuscular effects have been observed clinically as a phenomenon of treatment with MAOIs since their earliest psychopharmacologic use (24). These have been described variously as muscle twitching, muscle tension, muscle or myoclonic jerks, tremor, and muscle and joint pain. There are few systematically collected data (Table 2) on the incidence of these effects, and reports of their frequency vary. Goldberg (24) reported that increased neuromuscular activity manifested by "muscular twitching, often accompanied by gross involuntary movement of the extremities" was a relatively common effect of large doses of any MAOI. Sheehan et al. (67) describe muscle twitching as occurring in most patients and suggest that it may indicate when a therapeutic dose has been reached. On the other hand, D. Robinson (*personal communication*, 1983), who has had extensive experience with phenelzine, suggests that myoclonic jerking in relation to sleep onset and sleep occurs in 10 to 15% of patients treated.

In a comparison trial of pargyline and clorgyline, Lipper et al. (44) reported side effects of muscle twitching and joint discomfort in subjects taking clorgyline, and joint discomfort, tremor, and stiffness in the pargyline group. They suggested that the complaint of joint discomfort was a marker for increased neuromuscular

TABLE 2. *Reports in the literature of MAOI-induced neuromuscular effects*

Drug	Neuromuscular effects	Ref.
Clorgyline	Muscle twitching, joint discomfort, tremor, stiffness	44
Pargyline		
Phenelzine	Muscle pain, tremor, muscle twitching	22
Phenelzine	Muscle twitching, (most common with phenelzine)	18
Isocarboxazid		
Pheniprazine		
Nialamide		
Clorgyline	Myoclonus	12
Pheniprazine +	Ataxia, hyperreflexia, clonus myoclonus, dysarthria	58
L-tryptophan		
Phenelzine +	Muscle twitching, hyperreflexia, clonus	23
L-tryptophan		
Tranylcypromine +	Myoclonus, ocular movements	3
L-tryptophan		
Clorgyline	Myoclonus, hyperreflexia, clonus, upper motor neuron symptoms (serotonin syndrome)	35
Phenelzine	Muscle tension, twitching, clonus	34
Tranylcypromine	Muscle twitching, hypertonia, hyperreflexia, myoclonus	10
Nialimide		

activity. Evans et al. (22) studied short-term (3–5 weeks of treatment) and long-term (6 months) effects of phenelzine (mean dose, 77 mg/day) in depressed patients. They reported incidences of side effects during short-term treatment of 2% for muscle pain and 15% for tremor, and a side effect incidence during long-term treatment of 28% for muscle pain and 14% for muscle twitching. Dally and Rhode (18), in an uncontrolled trial of several nonspecific MAOIs, reported that muscle twitching was a common side effect, particularly of phenelzine.

Cohen et al. (12) reported a case of myoclonus associated with hypomania. A 51-year-old man treated with clorgyline gradually developed sudden jerking movements in different body areas after 10 days of treatment. The contractions were so violent as to cause minor contusions; on one occasion, the patient was thrown to the floor from a sitting position by a sudden spasm of truncal muscles. These movements appeared worse in the late afternoon and evening, were exacerbated by anxiety, could be provoked by loud noises, and disrupted the patient's sleep. The movements and hypomania abated when the drug dose was decreased, but muscle pain persisted for the entire treatment period.

Other reported cases occurred as the result of the interaction of other drugs added to patients' MAOI regimens. Oates and Sjoerdsma (58) described neurologic alterations in seven patients treated with the MAOI pheniprazine when L-tryptophan (20–50 mg/kg) was added. The alterations included behavioral intoxication, ataxia, hyperreflexia (predominantly of the lower but also the upper extremities and masseteric muscles), ankle clonus, spontaneous jerking movements of the legs, diaphoresis, dysarthria, and paresthesias. These were dose related and subsided within 24 hr upon stopping the tryptophan. Glassman and Platman (23), in a controlled trial of phenelzine combined with tryptophan, reported that one patient, after ingesting 18 g tryptophan, abruptly developed muscle twitching, hyperreflexia, and clonus. The symptoms spontaneously abated within 24 hr upon stopping medication. Baloh et al. (3) described a 26-year-old woman treated with tranylcypromine (20 mg) for 4 days who developed muscle jerks of the mouth, trunk, and extremities 1 hr after taking 2 g L-tryptophan. The patient had no alteration of consciousness and on neurologic examination exhibited conjugate horizontal oscillations of the eyes in the primary position and all directions of gaze and intermittent asymmetric flexor jerks of upper and lower extremities that were not exacerbated by stimuli.

Insel et al. (35) described two cases of obsessive–compulsive disorder treated unsuccessfully with clorgyline. Following a 33-day washout period, a 35-year-old female received a single 100-mg dose of clomipramine (CMI) and became acutely excited, diaphoretic, and ataxic, and exhibited myoclonic leg movements. On examination she showed hyperreflexia, ankle clonus sustained for 10 sec bilaterally, and cardiovascular instability. The symptoms subsided over 3 hr. The second case, a 30-year-old male, reacted similarly after an identical sequence of drug administration, exhibiting upper motor neuron symptoms, myoclonus, and cardiac irritability that lasted 6 hr. The authors suggested that these drug-induced symptoms were comparable to the "serotonin syndrome" described in animals (36). Howarth (34) reported the occurrence of muscular tension, twitching, and clonus following a switch from phenelzine to imipramine.

Ciocatto et al. (10) reported two cases of overdose with MAOIs and other drugs (one trifluoperazine and one imipramine) that were characterized by extreme central nervous system (CNS) stimulation and neuromuscular activity. They also described two other cases of patients treated with MAOIs. A 47-year-old man treated with tranylcypromine took one dose of a benzodiazepine and developed excitement, headache, and diffuse muscular hypertonia. The patient was initially diagnosed as having a cerebrovascular accident; however, the symptoms rapidly and spontaneously disappeared. The second patient, a 40-year-old male, was treated with nialimide for depression without response. Medication was stopped; after a 4-day hiatus, he took one dose of amitriptyline, whereupon he developed confusion, headache, and muscle twitching.

The literature on adverse interactions between MAOI and TCA drugs has been reviewed by White and Simpson (83). They discuss a series of reports in which a single dose of a tricyclic antidepressant (TCA) given to patients receiving or previously treated with a MAOI produced a reaction characterized by muscular hyperactivity, rigidity, tremor, hyperthermia, convulsions, and coma.

CLINICAL ASPECTS

We have observed the occurrence of neuromuscular effects associated with the use of the nonspecific MAOIs, phenelzine and tranylcypromine, in the majority of patients treated. Diagnosis does not appear to influence the frequency or severity of effects, nor does age or sex, although the disorders for which MAOIs are most commonly used predominate in females and young and middle-age groups. Frequency and severity of occurrence appear to be dose related. A decrease of dosage may diminish or alleviate side effects. In patients treated with MAOIs alone, these effects do not develop immediately and usually not sooner than 10 to 14 days. Tolerance has not been observed to occur. The time course of development of neuromuscular effects may parallel platelet MAO inhibition (with nonspecific or type B MAOIs) (64), the development of orthostatic hypotension (67), rapid eye movement (REM) sleep suppression (11), and therapeutic action (64).

The phenomenology of the side effects as reported by patients include spontaneous involuntary muscle tension and twitching and jerking movements that involve, in decreasing order of frequency, the lower extremities, upper extremities, truncal, neck, and facial body regions. Also described are clonic movements usually elicited by sudden movements that stretch particularly affected muscles (e.g., gastrocnemius). A frequent associated complaint is muscle or joint pain. These phenomena predominate during rest, sleep onset, and sleep but occur, albeit less often, during wakefulness as well. Frequently, it is the bed partner who reports the occurrence of myoclonic jerks. These sleep movements can be forceful to the extent that the bed partner may suffer physical trauma, e.g., bruises, soreness. Another common anecdote is that told by embarrassed patients whose sudden myoclonic movements while falling asleep in a subway or public area, struck an innocent bystander. Findings on the neurologic examination are postural tremor, nystagmus, diffuse hyperreflexia, including spread in the upper extremities, unsustained ankle clonus, and bilateral tibioadductor responses. Plantar responses are flexor.

We have studied several patients electrophysiologically with all-night sleep recordings, using a 12-channel polysomnagraph with surface electrodes placed over the right and left anterior tibial, right and left medial gastrocnemius, right and left extensor digitorum, and right flexor carpiulnaris muscles, in addition to the standard electroencephalogram (EEG), electrooculogram (EOG), and chin electromyogram (EMG) placement. Recordings were made at standard calibration (50 μV), sensitivity of 100 μV equal to 2 cm, and a paper speed of 15 mm/sec. We found that patients being treated with phenelzine at the time of recording exhibited increased and abnormal neuromuscular activity. Figures 1–7 are of a 42-year-old man receiving phenelzine (75 mg/day). The observed activity included multiple single motor unit discharges, both rhythmic and arrhythmic, repeatedly occurring in various muscle groups throughout the night, in non-REM periods. Occasionally, bursts of 0.5 to 2 sec of duration occurred during non-REM periods. Numerous sustained bursts were seen in both single and multiple muscle groups during REM periods. These bursts of activity were often preceded and/or followed by single motor unit discharges in the involved muscle groups. This muscle activity, both REM and non-REM, was present over 75% of the total sleep time. Additionally, there were numerous sleep arousals associated with tonic muscle activity throughout the night. These findings were markedly distinct from simultaneously run controls (one a nonpatient control, the other a patient with tardive dyskinesia).

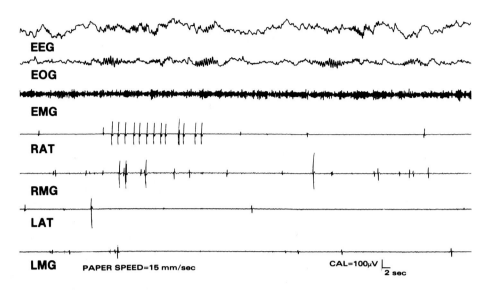

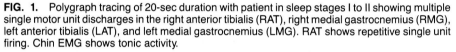

FIG. 1. Polygraph tracing of 20-sec duration with patient in sleep stages I to II showing multiple single motor unit discharges in the right anterior tibialis (RAT), right medial gastrocnemius (RMG), left anterior tibialis (LAT), and left medial gastrocnemius (LMG). RAT shows repetitive single unit firing. Chin EMG shows tonic activity.

Although the myoclonic movements described in MAOI-treated patients in many ways resemble the syndrome of nocturnal myoclonus, there are important differences as well. Coleman et al. (15) have described the periodic movements in sleep (PMS) of so-called nocturnal myoclonus. Movements of PMS are typically stereotyped and repetitive, usually recurring at fixed intervals. The muscle activity and movements of the MAOI-treated patients occurred more often and were random and arrhythmic. The PMS of nocturnal myoclonus are almost entirely confined to non-REM sleep, whereas the muscle activity was more pronounced during REM periods in the MAOI-treated patients. Although insomnia is a feature of depression, the prevalence of nocturnal myoclonus in major affective disorders is extremely low (63).

We attempted to pharmacologically characterize these movements based on the hypothesis that the drug effects were mediated by serotonergic mechanisms. Administering L-tryptophan (3–9 g/day) to patients pretreated with phenelzine aggra-

FIG. 2. Polygraph tracing of 40-sec duration with the patient entering REM sleep followed by a sleep arousal. The chin is atonic; there is repeated burst activity of 0.2-sec duration at 0.6-sec intervals followed by a sustained burst (2 sec duration) in RAT; repetitive bursts of 0.4-sec duration at 0.6-sec intervals in LAT; intermittent single motor unit and burst activity is present in the RMG and LMG. (See Fig. 1 for abbreviations.)

FIG. 3. Polygraph tracing of 32-sec duration with the patient in REM and slow-wave sleep followed by a brief sleep arousal. The chin is atonic. There is tonic activity of 4-sec duration in RAT, RMG, and LAT followed by repeated bursts in RAT and LAT. (See Fig. 1 for abbreviations.)

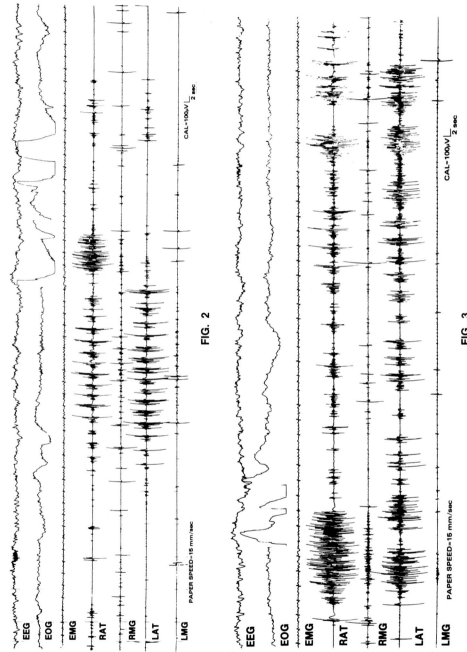

EEG

EOG

EMG

RAT

RMG

LAT

LMG

PAPER SPEED=15 mm/sec

CAL=100μV⌐ 2 sec

FIG. 2

EEG

EOG

EMG

RAT

RMG

LAT

LMG

PAPER SPEED=15 mm/sec

CAL=100μV⌐ 2 sec

FIG. 3

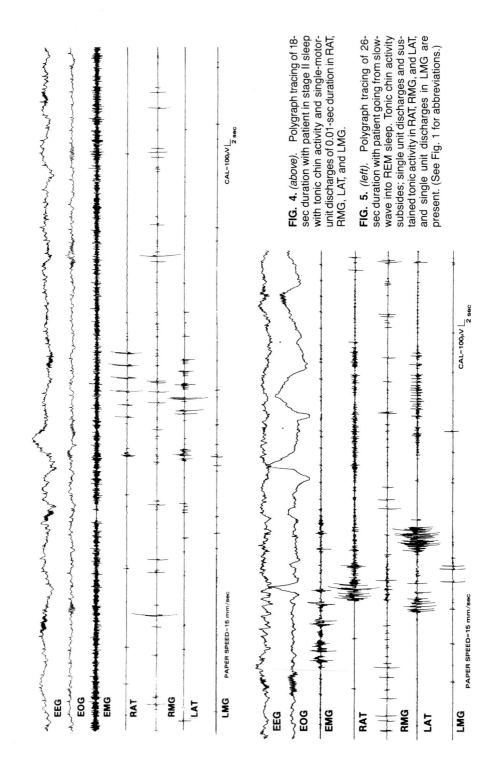

FIG. 4. *(above).* Polygraph tracing of 18-sec duration with patient in stage II sleep with tonic chin activity and single-motor-unit discharges of 0.01-sec duration in RAT, RMG, LAT, and LMG.

FIG. 5. *(left).* Polygraph tracing of 26-sec duration with patient going from slow-wave into REM sleep. Tonic chin activity subsides; single unit discharges and sustained tonic activity in RAT, RMG, and LAT, and single unit discharges in LMG are present. (See Fig. 1 for abbreviations.)

vated the neuromuscular effects and produced additional side effects, including sedation, tremulousness, tachycardia, ataxia, diaphoresis, and flushing. These effects could be antagonized promptly with methysergide or cyproheptadine, putative 5-HT receptor antagonists. When methysergide or cyproheptadine were administered to patients pretreated with phenelzine, the neuromuscular effects were diminished; however, cyproheptadine produced extreme drowsiness as well.

These findings demonstrate that the nonspecific MAOI drugs produce abnormal neuromuscular activity. We suggest that serotonergic systems have a role in their mediation.

NEUROCHEMICAL MECHANISMS

Although not uniform, several lines of evidence suggest that serotonergic mechanisms are involved in the mediation of MAOI-induced neuromuscular effects.

Preclinical Evidence

In laboratory animals, repetitive myoclonic jerking and twitches of the limbs, head, and trunk can be produced by 5-HT precursors [5-hydroxytryptophan (5-HTP), L-tryptophan], receptor agonists (5-HT), dimethyltryptamine (DMT), 5-methoxy-N-N-DMT (5-MeDMT), and releasers (*p*-chloroamphetamine, fenfluramine) (71,72,75–77). This behavior may occur when a 5-HT agonist is given alone but is markedly enhanced by pretreatment with MAOIs, peripheral aromatic amino acid decarboxylase inhibitors, 5-HT uptake inhibitors, or dihydroxylated tryptamines (e.g., 5,-7-DMT), neurotoxins that selectively lesion 5-HT nerve terminals (54,57,71,72,75). This behavioral syndrome produced by manipulations of the 5-HT system often includes fine head and body tremors, postural rigidity, and ataxia and can progress to a generalized tonic–clonic seizure (36). These behaviors can be antagonized with the 5-HT-blocking agents methysergide (42), cyproheptadine (72), and methergoline (80) but not by propanolol, phentolamine, chlorpromazine, or scopolamine (42). These responses appear to be specific for the 5-HT system in that DA agonists, such as apomorphine and L-DOPA, do not produce similar responses, nor does the cholinergic agonist physostigmine (71).

Other evidence suggests that repeated administration of 5-HT antagonists can induce a 5-HT receptor supersensitivity. Klawans et al. (40) induced a myoclonic response to 5-HTP in guinea pigs following repeated administration of methysergide. Stewart et al. (72) were able to induce a myoclonic response to 5-HTP in rats after pretreatment with cyproheptadine but not with methysergide or methergoline.

The importance of the enzyme MAO in limiting the activity of 5-HT is apparent from these research findings. When given alone to neurologically intact rats, 5-HTP will not consistently produce muscle movements, even at high doses which elevate brain 5-HT and 5-hydroxyindoleacetic acid (5-HIAA) levels (71). However, in rats lesioned with 5,7-DMT, 5-HTP administration induces repetitive myoclonic activity (71). In unlesioned rats pretreated with a nonspecific MAOI, 5-HTP and L-tryptophan produce a strong myoclonic response (26). Moreover, Grahame-Smith

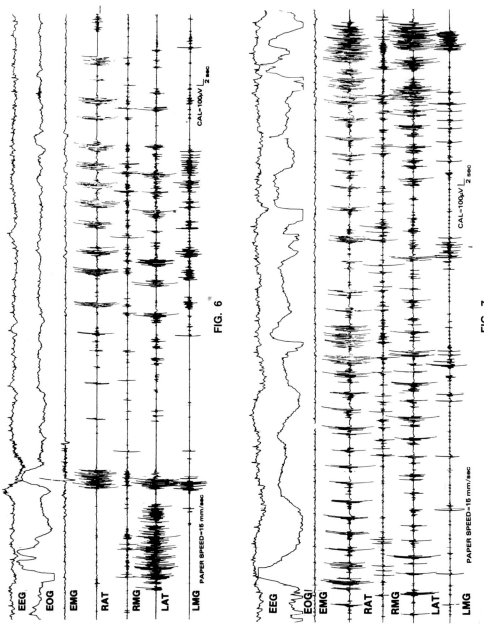

EEG

EOG

EMG

RAT

RMG

LAT

LMG

PAPER SPEED=15 mm/sec

CAL=100μV ⌐ 2 sec

FIG. 6

EEG

EOG

EMG

RAT

RMG

LAT

LMG

PAPER SPEED=15 mm/sec

CAL=100μV ⌐ 2 sec

FIG. 7

and Green (27) reported that in rats pretreated with lithium, the inhibition of MAO produced a syndrome of hyperactivity indistinguishable from that produced by MAOI and 5-HTP. Lithium has been shown to increase 5-HT activity (74). The administration of parachlorophenylalanine (PCPA), a 5-HT synthesis inhibitor, abolishes this hyperactivity-inducing effect (27).

These findings suggest that lesioning, chronic antagonist administration, and MAOI pretreatment all produce a similar condition necessary for 5-HTP-induced myoclonic activity.

Clinical Pharmacologic Evidence

There is evidence for a 5-HT deficiency in posthypoxic intention myoclonus (PHIM) (84). Decreased 5-HIAA levels in the cerebrospinal fluid (CSF) of PHIM patients have been reported (79). L-Tryptophan or 5-HTP alone, and an MAOI and 5-HTP can suppress symptoms of PHIM patients (29,79). Serotonin agonists or precursors exacerbate symptoms in idiopathic, essential, and epileptic myoclonus (30).

Neurohumoral mechanisms may play a role in the pathophysiology of myoclonic symptoms. Coleman (13) reported that 15% of Down's syndrome patients treated with 5-HTP developed infantile spasms, a syndrome characterized by myoclonic jerks. Moreover, increased levels of plasma 5-HT were found in three of five infants with spontaneous infantile spasms (14,45). Another example is the occurrence of shocklike involuntary movements of muscles in children with occult tumors of neural crest origin, e.g., neuroblastoma (42). These tumors produce and secrete various neurochemical substances. The movement disorder associated with the tumor abates when the tumor is removed.

There have been case reports of hyperkinetic movement disorders occurring in patients taking fenfluramine (68); Shoulson and Chase (68) have suggested that its serotonergic effects are responsible. Meyer and Halfin (53) have reported that a syndrome resembling that produced by 5-HT overactivity in animals was caused by the administration of meperidine in a man treated with phenelzine. One effect of meperidine is its potentiation of 5-HT activity by blocking 5-HT reuptake (65).

In the report of a young woman who developed myoclonus and involuntary eye movements while receiving tranylcypromine and L-tryptophan, Baloh et al. (3) pointed out that raphe serotonergic neurons in the brainstem are critical for the production of saccadic eye movements (39). The MAOIs suppress REM sleep (84). Enhancement of 5-HT activity also suppresses REM activity (52). Since the time

---

FIG. 6. Polygraph tracing of 22-sec duration showing a sleep arousal with tonic activity of RAT and LAT from stage III sleep. There are repeated bursts of 0.25-sec duration at 1- to 1.5-sec intervals in RAT and LAT, and of 0.7-sec duration, 1 sec apart, in LMG. The chin is atonic. (See Fig. 1 for abbreviations.)

FIG. 7. Polygraph tracing of 36-sec duration showing dense REM activity, an atonic chin, repeated bursts of 0.1-sec duration at 0.8-sec intervals in RAT, LAT, and RMG, with intermittent single unit discharge and burst activity in LMG. (See Fig. 1 for abbreviations.)

courses of MAOI therapeutic activity, the increase in 5-HT activity, and REM suppression coincide with the development of MAOI-induced neuromuscular effects, it may be inferred that serotonergic mechanisms have a mediating role.

Serotonin Syndrome

Compounds that increase synaptic 5-HT or directly stimulate postsynaptic 5-HT receptors produce in animals a behavioral syndrome comprised of neuromuscular symptoms (myoclonus, tremor, rigidity, head shaking, and hyperactivity) and autonomic nervous system symptoms (salivation, skin flushing, diarrhea, and piloerection) (36). Insel et al. (35) reported two cases in which symptoms analogous to the serotonin syndrome in man were precipitated by one dose of CMI in patients previously treated with clorgyline.

We are aware of two cases in whom similar symptoms developed. A 28-year-old man being treated with phenelzine for depression developed myoclonic jerks, tremor, ataxia, a cardiac tachyarrhythmia, skin flushing, and diaphoresis upon taking 4 g L-tryptophan with pyridoxine. The patient went to an emergency room feeling quite ill; the symptoms were alleviated with methysergide, 4 mg. The second case was a 39-year-old woman being treated for depression with tranylcypromine and L-tryptophan. Due to lack of response, this was stopped and electroconvulsive therapy begun. The day after the first treatment, the patient took CMI, 25 mg, and became restless, diaphoretic, tremulous, ataxic, hyperreflexic, flushed, and tachycardic and exhibited severe muscle twitching. Subjectively, she complained of extreme discomfort, saying she felt as if she were dying. These symptoms were relieved by methysergide, 6 mg.

The previously described cases suggest that MAOI pretreatment renders some patients susceptible to even slight serotonergic stimulation, similar to the cardiovascular response to tyramine ingestion that is well known in MAOI-treated patients. In three of the four cases, the precipitating agent was CMI, a tricyclic antidepressant that preferentially inhibits the uptake of 5-HT synaptically (73). As found in animal models of 5-HTP-induced myoclonus and the serotonin syndrome, there may be a continuum of responses to serotonergic stimulation in humans. The neuromuscular effects of MAOI treatment and the more extreme toxic syndromes described may both be mediated by serotonergic systems with quantitative differences.

Selective MAOI Drugs

Another means to evaluate the role of 5-HT in the neuromuscular effects of MAOIs is to study the selective MAOIs. If the neuromuscular effects are mediated by 5-HT systems, then we would expect to see increased effects caused by the selective MAO-A inhibitor clorgyline. Of three (32,44,82) clinical trials with clorgyline, only one was a comparison with another MAOI. Lipper et al. (44) reported that the side effect profiles of the two drugs in eight patients were not markedly dissimilar in terms of neuromuscular effects (stiffness, tremor, joint discomfort), with the exception of one patient of the clorgyline group who also had muscle twitching. Although the occurrence of the side effects did not appear to differ, the authors' clinical impression was that the severity of the neuromuscular effects was greater with clorgyline (D. Murphy, *personal communication*, 1983). Moreover, the case reports of myoclonus (12) and the serotonin syndrome (35) from this group were of patients treated with clorgyline.

We could find no reports of neuromuscular side effects occurring with L-deprenyl, a selective MAO-B inhibitor, including a trial in which it was combined with L-tryptophan (21,46,47,50,51). It was the clinical impression of several investigators (M. Liebowitz, *personal communication*, 1983; J. Mann, *personal communication*, 1983; F. Quitkin, *personal communication*, 1983) that such side effects were infrequent and less commonly seen than with the commercially available nonspecific MAOIs.

Several points should be made relevant to these findings. The MAO selectivity of pargyline, deprenyl, and clorgyline has been reported to be dose dependent (56,70,85). At high doses, MAO specificity is lost, and crossover inhibition can occur. Moreover, there is no peripheral index of MAO-A as there is for the B form; therefore, one cannot know what degree of MAO-A inhibition has been obtained at a given dose. Examinations of indirect measures, such as monoamine metabolites, are difficult to interpret.

Major et al. (48) examined CSF metabolites of patients treated with clorgyline and pargyline in a crossover design. The authors reported that clorgyline and pargyline decreased homovanillic acid (HVA), with pargyline causing a significantly greater decrease. 3-Methoxy-4-hydroxyphenylglycol (MHPG) and 5-HIAA were reduced comparably by both drugs. These results suggest pargyline produced crossover inhibition of both types of MAO. Linnoila et al. (43) measured concentrations of monoamine metabolites in 24-hr urine samples of four patients treated with low-dose clorgyline. They found marked decreases in MHPG, slight decreases in HVA, and no effect on 5-HIAA.

Additional preclinical evidence complicates the interpretation of selective MAOI response as evidence bearing on the role of 5-HT in MAOI-induced neuromuscular effects (70). Although rats treated with tranylcypromine developed a myoclonic hyperactivity syndrome following a challenge with 5-HTP, the same response did not occur in rats separately pretreated with clorgyline and deprenyl. When both drugs were given in combination, however, the myoclonic behavioral response occurred. These findings suggest that although 5-HT is believed to be normally metabolized by MAO-A, type B may also be relevant to the development of this syndrome (70); they also raise the possibility of other neurotransmitter involvement (28).

DA and 5-HT

Volkman et al. (80) reported that the concomitant administration of haloperidol did not alter the myoclonic activity induced in guinea pigs by tranylcypromine and

5-HTP or 5-MeDMT. However, apomorphine and the novel DA agonist N-n-propyl-N-n-butyl-B(3,4-dihydroxyphenylethylamine) in separate trials suppressed the 5-HTP-induced myoclonus. This DA agonist suppression of 5-HTP-induced myoclonus could in turn be blocked by haloperidol or pimozide. These results suggest that DA activity has an effect in the modulation of 5-HTP-induced myoclonus. A DA pathway is thought to be involved in some way between the point of DA receptor stimulation and the final motor response (8,80). The L-DOPA-induced myoclonic response in humans can be blocked by methysergide (41).

PROPOSED MODEL

Myoclonic neuromuscular activity is produced by the aggregate discharge of motor neurons with increased excitability (31). This can be the result of increased neuronal stimulation or decreased inhibition of the nervous system at almost any level. The form of the symptoms may vary with the extent and level of nervous system involvement (42). The final common pathway of dysregulated motor neuron activity is the anterior horn cells of the spinal cord (1). Serotonin pathways exist between the cortex, brainstem, and cord (49). The behaviors of the serotonin syndrome are mediated by neural mechanisms of the pons, medulla, and spinal cord (37). Bulbospinal 5-HT neurons originate in the medullary raphe nuclei and terminate at the motor neurons in the ventral horn and lateral gray areas (38). Serotonin has been found to modulate the activity of preganglionic sympathetic neurons in the thoracic intermediolateral column and somatic motor neurons in the ventral horn and increase the excitability of neurons, causing them to fire (2,38). Several studies have demonstrated the effects of neurotransmitters on the excitability of the α-motor neuron (17). Increased α-motor neuron excitability as measured by H-reflex recovery curves has been reported in patients with Parkinson's disease, a condition of decreased striatal DA tone (19). Neuroleptic drugs that block DA neurotransmission have been found to augment H-reflex curves, i.e., increase α-motor neuron excitability (25). These findings suggest that DA has an inhibitory influence on α-motor neuron activity. Other studies suggest that 5-HT can have an excitatory effect (1,2). For example, in the "acute spinal cat," 5-HT has been shown to increase α-motor neuron activity (2), whereas methysergide was reported to depress spinal and monosynaptic amplitudes (4).

Grahame-Smith (26) has described the massive activation of 5-HT receptors produced by increased concentrations of ligand that exceed the saturation capacities of binding sites and degradation enzymes leading to the leakage of 5-HT onto adjacent postsynaptic receptor sites as a "spillover effect." This process could result in a loss of the central tonic inhibition of spinal neurons due to an excess of serotonergic activity and, on relative imbalance of DA, 5-HT neuronal systems with a consequent increase in α-motor neuron excitability. These mechanisms could underlie the neuromuscular effects of MAOIs. The polygraph recordings are consistent with such a model. The basal firing rate of single motor units was markedly increased, in no systematic fashion, suggesting a state of heightened neuromuscular excitability. Some single motor unit discharges summated, when sufficient numbers occurred within the necessary temporal proximity in the same muscle group, into bursts, some of which attained the requisite features to be classified as myoclonus.

Cohen et al. (12), observing the association of myoclonus with catalepsy, sleep, and lateral eye movement, suggested that motor pathways normally phasically activated during REM periods or the wakefulness–sleep transition were involved in MAOI-induced myoclonus. During desynchronized sleep, rapid contractions of facial and limb musculature occur synchronously with REM bursts that resemble myoclonic movements of abnormal discharges. Normally during REM sleep, activation is limited to single neurons of the precentral cortex and accompanied by inhibition at the spinal level. The EMG tracings of the MAOI-treated patients (Figures 1–7) show massive muscle activity contrary to what is normally found. Single unit discharges and tonic muscle activity, although present throughout non-REM periods, markedly increased during REM sleep. This could be due to central disinhibition and increased basal levels of spinal motor neuron excitation resulting from MAOI-induced neurochemical changes specifically in 5-HT and DA activities. In this way, MAOIs may have a dysregulatory effect that disturbs the normal patterns of excitation and inhibition that normally occur in the switch from slow-wave to REM sleep (11,12).

The range of severity of symptoms among patients treated might be explained on the basis of quantitative neurotransmitter activity and individual susceptibility. Neurotransmitter activity is determined predominantly by such factors as dose, duration of treatment, and presence of adjunctive medication. Susceptibility is influenced by individual physiologic variables which may be a function of age, sex, primary illness, associated illnesses, and sleep/wake cycle.

SUMMARY

The MAOI class of drugs is known to produce neuromuscular effects at therapeutic and toxic doses when given alone or in combination with other drugs. These effects range from muscle tension and twitches in their mild form to forceful myoclonic jerks. These effects may also be part of a more pervasive toxic syndrome that includes autonomic and mental symptoms as well. There is meager direct and substantial indirect evidence that serotonergic mechanisms play a role in mediating the neuromuscular effects of MAOIs.

We have hypothesized that MAOIs produce a condition of heightened neuromuscular excitability due to a combination of increased serotonergic tone and central disinhibition of α-motor neuron-mediated spinal activity. Further study is needed utilizing objective pharmacologic and neurophysiologic measures.

ACKNOWLEDGMENT

We are grateful to Dr. Charles Pollack who provided advice on the interpretation of the polysomnagraphs.

REFERENCES

1. Anden N, Jukes M, Lundberg A. Spinal reflexes and monoamine liberation. *Nature* 1964;202:1222–3.
2. Anderson EG, Shibuya T. The effects of 5-hydroxytryptophan and L-tryptophan on spinal synaptic activity. *J Pharmacol Exp Ther* 1966;153:352–60.
3. Baloh RW, Dietz J, Spooner JW. Myoclonus and ocular oscillations induced by L-tryptophan. *Ann Neurol* 1982;11:95–7.
4. Banna N, Anderson E. The effects of 5-hydroxytryptamine antagonists on spinal neuronal activity. *J Pharmacol Exp Ther* 1968;162:319–25.
5. Blackwell B. Hypertensive crisis due to monoamine-oxidase inhibition. *Lancet* 1963;2:849–51.
6. Campbell IC, Robinson DS, Lovenberg W, Murphy DL. The effects of chronic regimens of clorgyline and pargyline on monoamine metabolism in the rat brain. *J Neurochem* 1979;32:49–55.
7. Chadwick D, Hallett M, Harris R, Jenner P, Reynolds EH, Marsden CD. Clinical, biochemical and physiological features distinguishing myoclonus responsive to 5-hydroxytryptophan, tryptophan with a monoamine oxidase inhibitor, and clonazepam. *Brain* 1977;100:455–87.
8. Chase TN. Serotonergic mechanisms and extrapyramidal function in man. In: McDowell F, Barbeau A, eds. Advances in neurology. New York: Raven Press, 1974:Vol. 5:31–39.
9. Chase N, Kopin IJ. Drug-induced disorders of movement. In: Goldensohn ES, Appel SH, eds. Scientific approaches to clinical neurology. Philadelphia: Lea & Febiger, 1977.
10. Ciocatto E, Fagiano G, Bava GL. Clinical features and treatment of overdosage of monoamine oxidase inhibitors and their interaction with other psychotropic drugs. *Resuscitation* 1972;1:69–72.
11. Cohen AM, Pickar D, Garnett D, Lipper S, Gillin JC, Murphy DL. REM sleep suppression induced by selective monoamine oxidase inhibitors. *Psychopharmacology* 1982;78:137–40.
12. Cohen RM, Pickar D, Murphy DL. Myoclonus-associated hypomania during MAO-inhibitor treatment. *Am J Psychiatry* 1980;137:105–6.
13. Coleman M. Infantile spasms associated with 5-hydroxytryptophan administration in patients with Down's syndrome. *Neurology (Minneap)* 1971;21:91.
14. Coleman M, Boullin DJ, Davis M. Serotonin abnormalities in the infantile spasm syndrome. *Neurology (Minneap)*, 1971;21:421.
15. Coleman RM, Pollak CP, Weitzman ED. Periodic movements in sleep (nocturnal myoclonus): relation to sleep disorders. *Ann Neurol* 1980;8:416–21.
16. Crane GE. Iproniazid (Marsilid) phosphate, a therapeutic agent for mental disorders and debilitating disease. *Psychiatr Res Rep* 1957;8:142–52.
17. Dahlström A, Fuxe K. Evidence for the existence of monoamine-containing neurons in the central nervous system. I. Demonstration of monoamines in the cell bodies of brain stem neurons. *Acta Physiol Scand [Suppl]* 1964;323:1–55.
18. Dally PJ, Rhode P. Comparison of antidepressant drugs in depressive illnesses. *The Lancet* 1961;1:18–20.
19. Diamantopoulos E, Olsen P. Excitability of spinal motorneuron in normal subjects and patients with spasticity, Parkinsonian rigidity and cerebellar hypotonic. *J Neurol Neurosurg Psychiatry* 1967;30:325–31.
20. Ekstedt B, Magyar K, Knoll J. Does the B form selective monoamine oxidase inhibitor lose selectivity by long term treatment? *Biochem Pharmacol* 1979;28:919–23.
21. Elsworth JD, Glover V, Reynolds GP, et al. Deprenyl administration in man: a selective monoamine oxidase B inhibitor without the "cheese effect." *Psychopharmacology* 1978;57:33–8.
22. Evans DL, Davison J, Raft D. Early and late side effects of phenelzine. *J Clin Psychopharmacol* 1982;2:208–10.
23. Glassman AH, Platman SR. Potentiation of a monoamine oxidase inhibitor by tryptophan. *J Psychiatr Res* 1969;7:83–8.
24. Goldberg LI. Monoamine oxidase inhibitors. Adverse reactions and possible mechanisms. *JAMA* 1964;190:456.
25. Goode D, Meltzer H, Mazura T. Hoffman reflex abnormalities in psychotic patients. *Biol Psychiatry* 1979;14:95–110.
26. Grahame-Smith DG. Studies *in vivo* on the relationship between brain tryptophan, brain 5-HT

synthesis and hyperactivity in rats treated with a monoamine oxidase inhibitors and L-tryptophan. *J Neurochem* 1971;18:1053.

27. Grahame-Smith DG, Green AR. The role of brain 5-hydroxytryptamine in the hyperactivity produced in rats by lithium and monoamine oxidase inhibition. *Br J Pharmacol* 1974;52:19–26.

28. Green AR, Grahame-Smith DG. The role of brain dopamine in the hyperactivity syndrome produced by increased 5-hydroxytryptamine synthesis in rats. *Neuropharmacology* 1974;13:949–59.

29. Growdon JH. Serotonergic mechanisms in myoclonus. *J Neural Transm* 1979;15:209–16.

30. Growdon JH, Young RR, Shahani BT. L-5-hydroxytryptophan in treatment of several different syndromes in which myoclonus is prominent. *Neurology (Minneap)* 1976;26:1135.

31. Halliday AM. The clinical incidence of myoclonus. In: Williams D, ed. Modern trends in neurology, vol. 4. New York: Appleton-Century-Crofts, 1967:69–105.

32. Herd JA. A new antidepressant-M and B9302. A pilot study and a double-blind controlled trial. *Clin Trials* 1969;6:219–25.

34. Howarth E. Possible synergistic effects of the new thymoleptics. *J Ment Sci* 1961;107:100–8.

35. Insel TR, Roy BF, Cohen RM, Murphy DL. Possible development of the serotonin syndrome in man. *Am J Psychiatry* 1982;7:954–5.

36. Jacobs BL. An animal behavioral model for studying central serotonergic synapses. *Life Sci* 1976;19:777.

37. Jacobs BL, Klemfuss H. Brain stem and spinal cord mediation of a serotonergic behavioral syndrome. *Brain Res* 1975;100:450–7.

38. Johannsson O, Hökfelt T, Pernow B, Jeffcoate SL, White N, Steinbusch HWM, Verhofstad AAJ, Emson PC, Spindel E. Immunohistochemical support for three putative transmitters in one neurone: coexistence of 5-hydroxytryptamine, substance P and thyrotropin releasing hormone-like immunoreactivity in medullary neurons projecting to the spinal cord. *Neuroscience* 1981;6:1857–81.

39. Keller EL. Control of saccadic eye movements by midline brain stem neurons. In: Baker R, Berthoz A, eds. Control of gaze by brain stem neurons. Amsterdam: Elsevier, 1977:327–36.

40. Klawans HL, D'Amico DJ, Patel BC. Behavioral supersensitivity to 5-hydroxytryptophan induced by chronic methysergide pretreatment. *Psychopharmacologia (Berl)* 1975;44:297.

41. Klawans HL, Goetz C, Bergen D. Levadopa-induced myoclonus. *Arch Neurol* 1975;32:331.

42. Klawans HL Jr, Goetz C, Weiner WJ. 5-Hydroxytryptophan induced myoclonus in guinea pigs and the possible role of serotonin in infantile myoclonus. *Neurology* 1973;23:1234–40.

43. Linnoila M, Karoum F, Potter WZ. High correlation of norepinephrine and its major metabolite excretion rates. *Arch Gen Psychiatry* 1982;39:521–3.

44. Lipper S, Murphy DL, Slater S, Buchsbaum MS. Comparative behavioral effects of clorgyline and pargyline in man: a preliminary evaluation. *Psychopharmacology* 1979;62:123–8.

45. Lowe NN, Bosma JF, Armstrong MD. Infantile spasms with mental retardation. I. Clinical observations and dietary experiments. *Pediatrics* 1958;22:1153.

46. Mann JJ, Frances A, Kaplan RD, Kocsis J, Peselow ED, Gershon S. The relative efficacy of l-deprenyl, a selective monoamine oxidase type B inhibitor, in endogenous and nonendogenous depression. *J Clin Psychopharmacol* 1981;2:54–7.

47. Mann JJ, Gershon S. L-deprenyl, a selective monoamine oxidase type-B inhibitor in endogenous depression. *Life Sci* 1980;26:877–82.

48. Major LF, Murphy DL, Lippe S, Gordon E. Effects of clorgyline and pargyline on deaminated metabolites of norepinephrine, dopamine and serotonin in human cerebrospinal fluid. *Neurochemistry* 1979;32:229–31.

49. Marsden CA, Bennett GW, Irons J. Localization and release of 5-hydroxytryptamine, thyrotrophin releasing hormone and substance P in rat ventral spinal cord. *Comp Biochem Physiol* 1982;72:263–70.

50. Mendis N, Pare CMB, Sandler M, Glover V, Stern M. Is the failure of L-deprenyl, a selective monoamine oxidase B inhibitor, to alleviate depression related to freedom from the cheese effect? *Psychopharmacology* 1981;73:87–90.

51. Mendlewicz J, Youdim MBH. Anti-depressant potentiation of 5-hydroxytryptophan by L-deprenyl, an MAO "Type B" inhibitor. *J Neural Transm* 1978;43:279–86.

52. Mendelson WB, Gillin JC, Wyatt RJ. *Human sleep and its disorders.* New York: Plenum Press, 1977:21–62.

53. Meyer D, Halfin V. Toxicity secondary to meperidine in patients on monoamine oxidase inhibitors: a case report and critical review. *Brief Rep* 1981;1:319–21.
54. Modigh K. Effects of chlorimipramine and protriptyline on the hyperactivity induced by 5-hydroxytryptophan after peripheral decarboxylase inhibition in mice. *J Neural Trans* 1973;34:101.
55. Murphy DL. The behavioral toxicity of monoamine oxidase inhibiting antidepressants. *Adv Pharmacol Chemother* 1977;14:71–105.
56. Murphy DL, Lipper S, Slater S, Shiling D. Selectivity of clorgyline and pargyline as inhibitors of monoamine oxidases A & B in vivo in man. *Psychopharmacology* 1979;62:129–32.
57. Nakumura M, Fukushima H, Kitagawa S. Effects of amitriptyline and isocarboxazid on 5-hydroxytryptophan induced head twitches in mice. *Psychopharmacology* 1976;48:101.
58. Oates JA, Sjoerdsma A. Neurologic effects of tryptophan in patients receiving a monoamine oxidase inhibitor. *Neurology* 1960;10:1076–8.
59. Pickar D, Murphy DL, Cohen RM, Campbell IC, Lipper S. Selective and nonselective monoamine oxidase inhibitors. *Arch Gen Psychiatry* 1982;39:535–40.
60. Pompeiano O. The generation of rhythmic discharges during bursts of REM. In: Chalazonitis N, Boisson M, eds. Abnormal neuronal discharges. New York: Raven Press, 1978:75–90.
61. Quitkin F, Rifkin A, Klein DF. Monoamine oxidase inhibitors. *Arch Gen Psychiatry* 1979;36:749–60.
62. Ravaris CL, Nies A, Robinson DS, et al. A multiple-dose controlled study of phenelzine in depression-anxiety states. *Arch Gen Psychiatry* 1976;33:347–50.
63. Reynolds CF III, Coble PA, Spiker DG, Neil JF, Holzer BC, Kupfer DJ. Prevalence of sleep apnea and nocturnal myoclonus in major affective disorders: clinical and polysomnographic findings. *J Nerv Ment Dis* 1982;170:565–7.
64. Robinson DS, Nies A, Ravaris L, Ives JO, Bartlett D. Clinical pharmacology of phenelzine. *Arch Gen Psychiatry* 1978;35:629–35.
65. Rogers KJ, Thornton JA. The interaction between MAO inhibitors and narcotic analgesics in mice. *Br J Pharmacol* 1969;36:470–80.
66. Sheehan DV, Ballenger J, Jacobsen G. Treatment of endogenous anxiety with phobic, hysterical and hypochondriacal symptoms. *Arch Gen Psychiatry* 1980;37:51–9.
67. Sheehan DV, Claycomb JB, Kouretas N. Monoamine oxidase inhibitors: prescription and patient management. *Int J Psychiatr Med* 1980–81;10:99–121.
68. Shoulson I, Chase TN. Fenfluramine and dyskinesias. *N Engl J Med* 1974;291:850–1.
69. Soldatos CR, Bixler EO, Kales A, et al. Prevalence of myoclonus nocturnus in chronic insomnia. *Sleep Res* 1976;5:189.
70. Squires RF, Lassen JB. The inhibitor of A and B forms of MAO in the production of a characteristic behavioral syndrome in rats after L-tryptophan loading. *Psychopharmacology (Berlin)* 1975;41:145.
71. Stewart RM, Baldessarini RJ. An animal model of myoclonus related to central serotonergic neurons. In: Hanin I, Usdin E, eds. Animal models in psychiatry and neurology. New York: Pergamon, 1977:431–41.
72. Stewart RM, Campbell A, Sperk G, Baldessarini RJ. Receptor mechanisms in increased sensitivity to serotonin agonists after dihydroxytryptamine shown by electronic monitoring of muscle twitches in the rat. *Psychopharmacology* 1979;60:281–9.
73. Thoren P, Asberg M, Bertilsson L, Mellstrom B, Sjoqvist F, Traskman L. Clomipramine treatment of obsessive-compulsive disorder. *Arch Gen Psychiatry* 1980;37:1289–94.
74. Treiser SL, Cascio CS, O'Donohue TL, Thoa NB, Jacobowitz DM. Lithium increases serotonin release and decreases serotonin receptors in the hippocampus. *Science* 1981;213:1529–31.
75. Trulson ME, Eubanks EE, Jacobs BL. Behavioral evidence for supersensitivity following destruction of central serotonergic nerve terminals by 5,7-dihydroxytryptamine. *J Pharmacol Exp Ther* 1976;198:23–32.
76. Trulson ME, Jacobs BL. Behavioral evidence for the rapid release of CNS serotonin by PCA and florfluoramine. *Eur J Pharmacol* 1976;36:149.
77. Trulson ME, Jacobs BL. Dose-response relationships between systematically administered L-tryptophan or L-5-hydroxytryptophan and raphe unit activity in the rat. *Neuropharmacology* 1976;15:339–44.
78. Tyrer P. Towards rational therapy with monoamine oxidase inhibitors. *Br J Psychiatry* 1976;128:354–60.

79. Van Woert MH, Hwang EC. Myoclonus: biochemical and pharmacological approaches. In: Klawans HL, ed. Clinical neuropharmacology vol. 3. New York: Raven Press, 1978.

80. Volkman PH, Lorens SA, Kindel GH, Ginos JZ. L-5-hydroxytryptophan-induced myoclonus in guinea pigs: a model for the study of central serotonin-dopamine interactions. *Neuropharmacology*, 1978;17:947–55.

81. Weitzman ED, Pollak CP, McGregor P. The polysomnographic evaluation of sleep disorders in man. In: Aminoff MJ, ed. Electrodiagnosis in clinical neurology. New York: Churchill/Livingstone, 1980:496–524.

82. Wheatley D. Comparative trial of a new monoamine oxidase inhibitor in depression. *Br J Psychiatry* 1970;117:573–4.

83. White K, Simpson G. Combined MAOI-tricyclic antidepressant therapy: a reevaluation. *J Clin Psychopharmacol* 1981;1:264–82.

84. Wyatt RJ, Kupfer DJ, Scott J, Robinson DS, Snyder F. Longitudinal studies of the effect of monoamine oxidase inhibitors on sleep in man. *Psychopharmacologia*, 1964;15:233–6.

85. Yang HYT, Neff NH. The monoamine oxidases of brain: selective inhibition with drugs and the consequences for the metabolism of the biogenic amines. *J Pharmacol Exp Ther* 1974;189:733–40.

Advances in Neurology, Vol. 43: Myoclonus,
edited by S. Fahn et al. Raven Press,
New York © 1986.

Drug-Induced Myoclonus

Harold L. Klawans, Paul M. Carvey, Caroline M. Tanner, and
Christopher G. Goetz

*Department of Neurological Sciences, Rush-Presbyterian St. Lukes Medical Center,
Chicago, Illinois 60612*

During the past decade, we have been studying two forms of drug-induced myoclonus both clinically and in our laboratory. These are levodopa-induced myoclonus in patients with Parkinson's disease and tricyclic-antidepressant-induced myoclonus. These two forms form the main body of this chapter.

LEVODOPA-INDUCED MYOCLONUS

Levodopa-induced myoclonus was first described by us in 1975 about 7 years after the use of levodopa became widespread (33). We originally presented 12 patients with Parkinson's disease who developed myoclonus after taking levodopa for at least 12 months. The abnormal movements usually consisted of single, abrupt jerks of the extremities. These movements were usually bilateral and symmetric, involving the arms and legs. When unilateral, the arm and leg on the same side invariably jerked simultaneously. These jerks occurred most frequently during sleep and were observed during sleep in all 12 patients. Although each myoclonic jerk was usually isolated, several instances of repetitive jerks recurring over a period of less than 1 min were observed.

At times, the movements were severe enough to awaken the patient. In those patients not awakened by the sudden movements, the movements were detected because they disturbed the sleep of the spouse or were noted by observation of the sleeping patient. Most of the movements were of this nature and did not overtly disturb the patients. The frequency of these varied from as low as two or three per night to up to 30 or more per night.

The second most frequent time when the movements were noted was during drowsiness. All but two of the patients complained of myoclonic jerks when drowsy and attempting to go to sleep. These jerks would often startle and awaken the patient and prevent him or her from obtaining sleep. Often this was the most distressing result of these abnormal movements. Identical jerks also occurred at rest without apparent drowsiness in most of the patients. The movement, however, rarely occurred during activity. Those that occurred during drowsiness and wakefulness were never associated with loss of consciousness. Overall, the major clinical impact of levodopa-induced myoclonus is to disrupt the drowsiness and sleep of these patients.

TABLE 1. *Effect of pharmacologic manipulations on levodopa-induced myoclonus*

Therapy	No. of patients	Effect on myoclonus	Comments
Increase of levodopa	8	Increased myoclonus in 5 patients	Increased dyskinesias in 4 patients with dyskinesias; precipitated new dyskinesias in 2 other patients
Decrease of levodopa	8	Decreased myoclonus in 8 patients; stopped myoclonus in 6	Increased parkinsonism in 8 patients
Withdrawal of anticholinergics	7	No change	Increased parkinsonism in 3 patients
Addition of anticholinergics	5	No change	Increased parkinsonism in 2 patients
Withdrawal of amantadine	2	No change	Slightly increased parkinsonism in 1 patient
Methysergide	12	Decreased in all 12 patients; stopped myoclonus in 7 patients	No change in parkinsonian signs
Propranolol	6	No change	No change

Seven of the patients also experienced classic levodopa-induced dyskinesias. All seven patients with levodopa-induced dyskinesias had lingual-facial-buccal movements. In four patients, these were the only movements observed, whereas three individuals had truncal and limb movements. The prevalence and distribution of levodopa-induced dyskinesias in this group of 12 patients did not differ substantially from the prevalence and distribution in our entire population being treated with levodopa at that time.

To attempt to elucidate the pharmacology of this form of myoclonus, we carried out a variety of therapeutic maneuvers (Table 1). Levodopa was increased by 250 to 500 mg/day. In four patients with levodopa-induced dyskinesias, these movement abnormalities increased in severity. In four patients without levodopa-induced dyskinesias, the increased dosage of levodopa elicited clinically detectable lingual-facial-buccal dyskinesias in two patients. The myoclonus clearly increased in frequency and severity in five patients when the levodopa dosage was increased. There was no definite change in myoclonus in the other three patients. A reduction in levodopa dosage was also tried in eight patients. This was done by decreasing the daily dosage by 250 mg/day at weekly intervals until symptoms of parkinsonism increased to such a degree that the lower level of levodopa could not be maintained. This resulted in a decrease in the severity and frequency of myoclonus in all eight patients and finally a complete remission in six. There was some increase in parkinsonian signs and symptoms in all eight patients. In seven patients, this worsening required a reinstitution of higher doses of levodopa.

Withdrawal of anticholinergic agents from the seven patients taking such drugs had no effect on the levodopa-induced myoclonus; in another group of parkinsonian patients, such a maneuver reduced levodopa-induced dyskinesias in about one-third. Addition of anticholinergic agents in five other patients not already on these medications also produced no change in the myoclonus, although other dyskinesias were increased by this maneuver in two patients. Withdrawal of amantadine in two patients appeared to have no influence on the myoclonus.

Methysergide, a specific serotonin antagonist, was found to eliminate the levodopa-induced myoclonus in all our patients while having no discernible effect on the other levodopa-induced dyskinesias. All 12 patients, when given methysergide in doses of 2 mg each night at bedtime, noted a decrease in their abnormal movements; in seven patients, the myoclonus stopped completely. Methysergide has been reported previously to have no effect on the tremor, akinesia, and rigidity of Parkinson's disease (34). In our 12 patients, parkinsonian signs and symptoms did not change with the introduction of methysergide; the only effect noted was the decrease in myoclonic movements. All these observations suggest that the pathophysiologic basis of the production of levodopa-induced myoclonus differs from that of levodopa-induced chorea and that it more directly involves a serotonergic mechanism. Propranolol hydrochloride in six patients had no effect on levodopa-induced myoclonus.

Despite this report and the general recognition that levodopa-induced myoclonus is a separate clinical entity, there have been very few studies of this disorder. Nausieda et al (47) have carried out a thorough study of levodopa-induced myoclonus and its relationship to sleep disruptions and hallucinations caused by levodopa. Their survey of 100 parkinsonian patients revealed prominent sleep complaints in 74%. Sleep complaints were unrelated to patient age and the duration of disease but increased in prevalence with longer periods of levodopa therapy. Sleep abnormalities tended to increase in severity with continued treatment, and insomnia tended to be followed by daytime somnolence, altered dream events, and episodic nocturnal vocalization and myoclonus. While dyskinetic side effects and on–off syndrome were encountered in patients with and without sleep complaints, 98% of patients experiencing psychiatric side effects also reported sleep disruption. The authors suggested that sleep-related symptoms constitute an early stage of levodopa-induced dopaminergic psychiatric toxicity in the parkinsonian population, and clinical and experimental observations suggest that serotonergic mechanisms are important in this symptom complex.

Table 2 shows the categories and rating system used by Nausieda et al. (47) in their study, including the severity scale for myoclonus. In this study, there was a relationship between the prevalence of myoclonus and the duration of levodopa therapy (see Fig. 1). In individual patients, there was virtually always a correlation between severity of myoclonus and duration of treatment.

Figure 2 illustrates the pattern of symptom grouping observed in patients with sleep complaints. Sleep fragmentation was the most common symptom overall and the most frequent symptom encountered in isolation. Altered dream events were usually seen in association with sleep fragmentation, whereas myoclonic movements were always accompanied by other sleep-related complaints. Individual analysis

TABLE 2. *Categories and degrees of severity of sleep disruption*

Category	Description
Inability to initiate sleep	Takes more than 30 min to fall asleep
Sleep maintenance	
Mild	Awakens 1–2 times; nocturnal sleep time of 6 hr or more
Moderate	Awakens 2 times a night; sleeps 4–6 hr a night
Severe	Unable to sleep more than 2 hr; total nocturnal sleep less than 4 hr
Excessive daytime sleep	
Mild	Daily naps amounting to less than 1 hr of sleep a day
Moderate	Naps 1–2 hr a day
Severe	Naps more than 2 hr a day
Altered dream events	
Mild	Dreams more vivid than in past
Moderate	Unpleasant dreams with identifiable theme
Severe	Recurring frightening dreams frequently awakening patient, with postawakening confusion
Parasomnias	
Sleep talking	
Mild	Frequent brief episodes of mumbling of soft speech
Moderate	Frequent speaking at conversational amplitude
Severe	Screaming or shouting loud enough to awaken household members
Myoclonus	
Mild	Nightly episodes of involuntary jerking only
Moderate	Involuntary jerking, with flinging arm or leg movements
Severe	Arm, leg, and trunk movements and persistent jerking movements while awake
Sleep walking	Walking in sleep at least once in 3 weeks

revealed an order of symptom appearance that generally followed overall prevalence (Fig. 1), in that sleep fragmentation usually preceded other complaints. It was also noted that restricted (nocturnal) myoclonus always preceded waking myoclonic activity.

Sleep studies confirmed that levodopa-induced myoclonic movements were usually not associated with spontaneous awakening. In addition to their association with various polysomnographic abnormalities and altered dream events, this suggests that myoclonic movements during sleep in parkinsonian patients are probably distinct from those previously reported in other clinical settings.

Myoclonic activity during sleep appeared to be the best predictor of waking hallucinosis. Since myoclonic movements were a relatively late complaint in the study by Nausieda et al. (47), and occurred only in the context of multiple sleep alterations, the authors suggest that their data support the view that hallucinosis is a late event in patients with progressive sleep derangement.

In an attempt to study levodopa-induced myoclonus, we have studied the effect of chronic levodopa treatment on acute 5-hydroxytryptophan (5-HTP)-induced myoclonus in guinea pigs [myoclonic jumping behavior (MJB)].

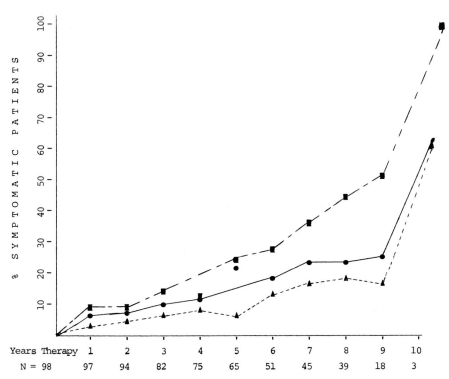

FIG. 1. Symptom prevalence and duration of levodopa therapy at the time sleep complaints appeared. Sleep fragmentation includes complaints of insomnia and excessive daytime sleep. Nocturnal vocalizations are not graphed but have a prevalence similar to that of altered dream events: *(N)*, number of patients in study on levodopa, levodopa/carbidopa for *x* years; (■), sleep fragmentation; (●), altered dream phenomena; (▲) myoclonic movements.

Guinea pigs were given oral levodopa/carbidopa (200/20 mg/kg) daily. After 28 and then 56 days, treatment was interrupted. Forty-eight hours after the last treatment, animals were given 35 mg/kg 5-HTP following further pretreatment with carbidopa. Chronic levodopa was found to produce a statistically significant increase in MJB after both 28 and 56 days of pretreatment ($p < 0.01$) (see Fig. 3). This study lends support to the concept that levodopa-induced myoclonus involves a serotonergic mechanism.

Myoclonus is one of a variety of motor manifestations reported during tricyclic antidepressant overdose. Other manifestations include "seizures," "chorea," and "myoclonic seizures" (7,8,11,58). We have employed the animal model of 5-HTP-induced myoclonus to study this form of myoclonus.

In our first set of experiments, we observed the behavioral effect of subthreshold doses of 5-HTP given alone and in conjunction with 35 mg/kg imipramine. As shown in Table 3, neither imipramine nor subthreshold doses of 5-HTP given alone had an observable behavioral effect on the animals. Imipramine in combination with subthreshold 5-HTP consistently led to myoclonus. While the MJB was neither

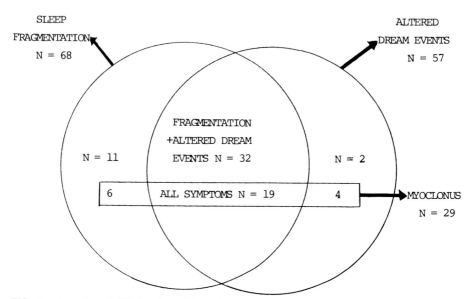

FIG. 2. Symptom distribution in parkinsonian patients with disrupted sleep ($N = 74$). Grouped symptoms: sleep fragmentation includes insomnia and excessive daytime sleep; altered dreaming and vocalizations are combined; all patients with somnambulism are in the group of 19 with all other symptoms.

as rhythmic nor as pronounced as that induced with larger doses of 5-HTP alone, the difference was one of degree rather than kind.

The data were consistent with the hypothesis that imipramine acts as a serotonin agonist, either direct or indirect, to potentiate 5-HTP-induced myoclonus in young guinea pigs. An attempt was made to rule out the possibility that the potentiation of 5-HTP-induced myoclonic seizures by imipramine was due to norepinephrine or some other neurotransmitter, since imipramine has been shown to block the reuptake and thus to increase the available norepinephrine as well as serotonin in the brain. Antagonists of norepinephrine, dopamine, and acetylcholine all failed to block the potentiation of myoclonus with imipramine, suggesting that the imipramine effect is not mediated by these neurotransmitters.

We have recently expanded this study and observed the effects of various doses of two different antidepressants—imipramine and amyltriptiline—on MJB. Imipramine produced a dose-dependent potentiation of MJB, while amyltriptiline, which is said to have less of an effect on serotonin reuptake, did not produce a significant effect (see Fig. 4).

MYOCLONUS PRODUCED BY OTHER AGENTS

Myoclonus has also been reported in humans after exposure to a potpourri of other drugs and toxins. This section briefly reviews these other agents, grouped by drug type.

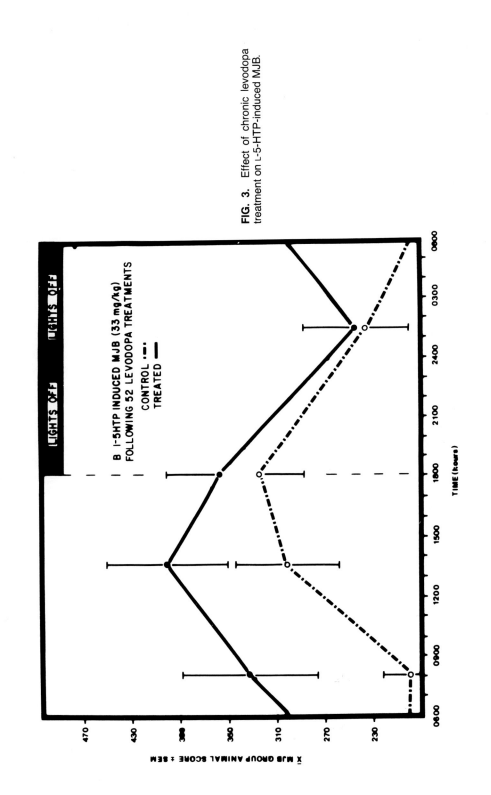

FIG. 3. Effect of chronic levodopa treatment on L-5-HTP-induced MJB.

TABLE 3. *Effect of imipramine and subthreshold 5-HTP on myoclonic activity in guinea pigs*

5-HTP (mg/kg)	Imipramine (mg/kg)	No. of animals	No. of animals with myoclonus
100	0	6	0
0	35	6	0
100	35	6	4
200	0	8	2
200	35	6	6

Antidepressants

Myoclonus has been associated with monoamine oxidase inhibitors (see elsewhere in this volume) and lithium toxicity, as well as with the tricyclic antidepressants. Patients suffering from lithium toxicity commonly exhibit generalized, spontaneous, and stimulus-sensitive myoclonus with associated jerky eye movements as well as severe postural tremor, decreased level of consciousness, and vomiting (16,63). These are usually in association with serum lithium levels several times therapeutic, although one case reports transient myoclonus after lithium levels returned to normal (53). In all cases myoclonus resolves.

Anti-infectious Agents

Penicillin, carbenicillin, ticarcillin, and cephalosporins (5,18,30,38,39) are all associated with a neurotoxic syndrome whose most common symptom is myoclonus. The myoclonus is typically nonrhythmic, asymmetric, and stimulus sensitive, and appears to relate to high drug concentrations in the cerebrospinal fluid (CSF).

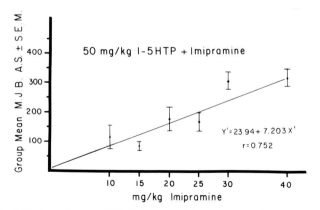

FIG. 4.   Effect of imipramine on L-5-HTP-induced MJB. In analagous studies with amyltriptiline, there was no dose–response relationship ($r = 0.061$).

Patients receiving high-dose continuous infusions, those with renal dysfunction, or those with impaired blood-brain barriers are most vulnerable. In most cases, myoclonus resolves with removal of the drug. Although other symptoms of penicillin toxicity (seizures, hallucinations) may be mediated through the cerebral cortex, the persistence of penicillin-induced myoclonus in a patient with electrocerebral silence on the electroencephalogram (EEG) and absent brainstem reflexes, with resolution of myoclonus after penicillin withdrawal, suggests a more caudal localization of the myoclonus (54).

Piperazine compounds are currently used as anthelmintic agents and have been associated with generalized, asymmetric, nonrhythmic myoclonus coupled with a clinical picture of somnolence, incoordination, headache, confusion, and sometimes generalized seizures, coma, and death (35,45,56). Symptoms are more common in brain-damaged persons or those with renal failure, but the syndrome often occurs at the usual therapeutic doses. In normal children with piperazine myoclonus, EEG changes are limited to generalized 2- to 4-Hz slow waves. Myoclonus does not resolve with anticonvulsant therapy but abates when the drug is removed.

Anesthetics

Various anesthetic drugs have been reported to cause myoclonus. Etomidate, an ultrashort-acting, nonbarbiturate hypnotic, causes transient, generalized, stimulus-sensitive myoclonus in 10 to 66% of all patients (13,15,20,31). The myoclonus is generally limited to the first minute of intravenous infusion. Slower injection time and pretreatment with diazepam or fentanyl (26) may prevent myoclonus. Electrophysiologic studies of this phenomenon have not been reported.

Prolonged maintenance of deep anesthesia using the gaseous anesthetic agent enflurane causes periodic spike–dome complexes alternating with electrical silence on EEG. These are rarely associated with myoclonus, generally in patients with seizure disorders (27,48). The myoclonus is generalized and resolves spontaneously within days. A similar EEG abnormality is produced by high doses of chloralose (10,37). Generalized, asymmetric, stimulus-sensitive myoclonus (which is asynchronous with EEG activity, responds dramatically to intravenous diazepam, and persists up to 12 hr) has been reported in chloralose toxicity.

In contrast to the generalized myoclonus with associated changes in EEG patterns produced by general anesthetics, spinal anesthesia has been reported to cause myoclonus in only one case (19). Transient, bilateral, lower-extremity myoclonus was observed during the recovery period after spinal anesthesia. This responded partially to diazepam and cleared in 24 hr.

Bismuth

Insoluble bismuth salts given orally as a cathartic (40,59), as well as topical preparations containing bismuth (36), produce a characteristic toxic encephalopathy with chronic use. It is characterized by myoclonus which is generalized, asymmetric, action induced, and stimulus sensitive; ataxia; confusion; and, in severe cases, convulsions, coma, and death. Most patients have high blood levels of bismuth. A characteristic EEG pattern of 3- to 5-Hz frontotemporal slow waves, without paroxysmal features, occurs in approximately 75% of patients, but this pattern does not relate either to bismuth blood levels or to clinical myoclonus. Myoclonus clears completely as bismuth levels fall, generally within 3 to 12 weeks. In severe cases, chelation with BAL has effected more rapid recovery (22).

Antineoplastics

Chlorambucil is a slow-acting nitrogen mustard which is used primarily as an antineoplastic agent. In children who have ingested toxic doses (9) or who have poor renal function (3), multifocal myoclonic jerks occur without other neurologic changes. The EEG shows paroxysms of high amplitude spike–wave activity which are not temporally related to the myoclonus. Movement abnormality and EEG changes have resolved completely with cessation of therapy in all reported cases.

Anticonvulsants

Overdoses of the anticonvulsant drugs valproic acid (14), carbamazepine (62), and hydantoin (21) have been associated with myoclonic encephalopathy in a few cases. In one, myoclonus resolved after clonazepam administration. Myoclonus was transient in all cases.

Hypnosedatives

Toxic doses of the sedative-hypnotic methaqualone may produce generalized or asymmetric, stimulus-sensitive myoclonus in association with increased resting tone and brisk deep tendon reflexes, generally accompanied by stupor or coma and sometimes by generalized seizures (1). All symptoms resolve with drug clearance. A similar syndrome has been observed with the chronic use of the sedative-hypnotic bromisovalum (25).

Antihistamines

Overdosages of antihistamines alone (55) or in combination with pseudoephedrine and paracetam (28) have been associated with multifocal, asymmetric, stimulus-sensitive myoclonus in two cases.

Diclofenac

The nonsteroidal antiinflammatory agent diclofenac has caused encephalopathy and myoclonus in patients with renal insufficiency (4) and segmental myoclonus in patients with normal renal function (2).

Marijuana

Marijuana may produce asymmetric, multifocal, action-induced, or stimulus-sensitive myoclonus in some patients without previous brain injury (17).

Saline Emetics

The administration of saline emetics several hours after overdosage with agents that interfere with central emetic centers may result in lethal hypernatremia. In one of these cases, generalized myoclonus preceded coma, convulsions, and death (52).

Benzodiazepine Withdrawal

Withdrawal from benzodiazepines (43,46) may produce myoclonus, but this is rarely a prominent part of the syndrome. Myoclonic jerks are generally nocturnal, are often limited to facial muscles, and always resolve within days or weeks.

Water-Soluble Contrast Media

Iothalamate meglumine (49), iocarmate meglumine (6), angiografin (41), myelografin (61), and metrizamide (29,32) are water-soluble contrast media used in myelography and cisternography. All have been reported to cause segmental myoclonus, generally limited to the lower extremities, often rhythmic and stimulus sensitive, without accompanying EEG changes. Movements are diminished after intravenous diazepam in many cases and resolve spontaneously within hours or days. Myoclonus is more common if high concentrations of contrast media are used, if part of the contrast material is not removed, and if local pathology is present. Any of these agents may also cause generalized seizures if given intracranially.

Accidental Poisonings

Accidental exposure to methyl bromide fumes (23,44) produces stimulus-sensitive and action-provoked myoclonus, which has been observed to correlate directly with EEG spikes. In many cases, myoclonus persists for years.

Accidental poisoning with organic mercury produces a variety of movement abnormalities, including myoclonus (57). The myoclonus is stimulus sensitive, exacerbated by action, and associated with EEG abnormalities. Myoclonus may resolve after chelation, or it may persist.

Poisoning with tetraethyl lead and gasoline vapors via gasoline sniffing can produce bilateral, stimulus-sensitive, action-induced myoclonus with associated behavioral changes. These clear after chelation (24).

Accidental ingestion of the dry cleaning agent dichloroethane (12) has produced myoclonus and somnolence. The myoclonic movements typically resolve within days, but residual ataxia may remain.

Strychnine poisoning and tetanus toxin may also produce stimulus-sensitive myoclonus (60).

Metabolic Disorders

Myoclonus may be a prominent sign in encephalopathic states caused by metabolic derangement, including uremia (50), hypercapnia, and hepatic coma (60). A similar myoclonus has been associated with chronic hemodialysis (42,51) and is presumably the result of aluminum toxicity. In other metabolic encephalopathies with myoclonus, a specific pathogenetic mechanism has not been identified. In all these disorders, myoclonus is multifocal, asymmetric, arrhythmic, and often stimulus sensitive. Jerking of facial and proximal limb muscles predominates. Late in the course, generalized myoclonic jerks and ultimately generalized seizures may occur. The EEG shows paroxysms of symmetric, bifrontal, biphasic, and triphasic waves which do not coincide with myoclonic jerks, as well as slowing of background activity. Recovery is generally dependent on the underlying systemic disorder.

ACKNOWLEDGMENTS

This work was supported in part by grants from the United Parkinson Foundation and the Boothroyd Foundation, Chicago, Illinois.

Dr. Goetz is the recipient of a NINCDS Teacher Investigator Award.

REFERENCES

1. Abboud RT, Freedman MT, Rogers RM, et al. Methaqualone poisoning with muscular hyperactivity necessitating the use of curare. *Chest* 1974;65:204–5.
2. Alcalay M, Thomas P, Reboux JF, et al. Myoclonus during a treatment with diclofenac. *Sem Hop Paris* 1979;55:679–80.
3. Ammenti A, Reitter B, Muller-Wiefel DE. Chlorambucil neurotoxicity: report of two cases. *Helv Paediatr Acta* 1980;35:281–7.
4. Bandelot JB, Mihout B. Myoclonic encephalopathy due to diclofenac. *Nouv Presse Med* 1978;7:1406.
5. Bloomer HA, Barten LJ, Maddock RK. Penicillin-induced encephalopathy in uremic patients. *JAMA* 1967;200:121–3.
6. Bonneau R, Morris JM. Complications of water-soluble contrast lumbar myelography. *Spine* 1978;3:343–5.
7. Brown D, Winsberg BG, Bialer I, et al. Imipramine therapy and seizures: three children treated for hyperactive behavior disorders. *Am J Psychiatry* 1973;130:210–2.
8. Burks J, Walker J, Ott JE, et al. Chorea associated with imipramine poisoning: reversal by physostigmine. *Neurology (Minneap)* 1973;23:393 (Abstr).
9. Byrne TN, Moseley TA, Finer MA. Myoclonic seizures following chlorambucil overdose. *Ann Neurol* 1981;9:191–4.
10. Cornette M, Franck G. Clinical and EEG features of acute drug intoxication with chloralose in eleven recent cases. *Electroencephalogr Clin Neurophysiol* 1981;30:374.
11. Darcourt G, Fadeuihe A, Lavagna J, et al. Trois cas de myoclonics d'action au cours de traitements par l'imipramine et l'amitriptyline. *Rev Neurol* 1970;122:141–2.
12. Dorndorf W, Kresse K, Christain W, et al. Dichloroethane poisoning with myoclonic syndrome, seizures and irreversible cerebral defects. *Arch Psychiatr Nervenkr* 1975;220:373–9.
13. Dubois DJ, Bastenier GJ, Genicot C, Ruoquoi M. A comparative study of etomidate and methohexital as induction agents for analgesia anesthesia. *Acta Anaesthesiol Belg [Suppl]* 1976;27:187–95.
14. Eeg-Olofsson O, Lindskog U. Acute intoxication with valproate. *Lancet* 1982;1(8284):1306.
15. Fameno CE, Odugbesan CO. Further experience with etomidate. *Can Anaesth Soc J* 1978;25:130–2.
16. Favarel-Garrigues B, Favarel-Garrigues JC, Bourgeois M. Two cases of severe poisoning by lithium carbonate. *Ann Med Psychol* 1972;1:253–7.
17. Feeney DM, Spiker M, Weiss GK. Marijuana and epilepsy: activation of symptoms by delta-9-THC. In: Cohen S, Stillman RO, eds. The therapeutic potential of marihuana. New York: Plenum, 1975:343–62.
18. Fossieck B, Parker RH. Neurotoxicity during intravenous infusion of penicillin. A review. *J Clin Pharmacol* 1974;14:504–12.

19. Fox EJ, Villaneuva R, Scutta HS. Myoclonus following spinal anesthesia. *Neurology* 1979;29:379–80.
20. Gooding JM, Corssen G. Etomidate: an ultrashort-acting nonbarbiturate agent for anesthesia induction. *Anesth Analg (Cleve)* 1976;55:286–9.
21. Gottwald W. Transitory healing of psoriasis efflorescences during hydantoin poisoning with unusual central nervous symptoms. *Dermatol Wochenschr* 1968;154:241–51.
22. Goule JP, Husson A, Fondimare A, et al. Encephalopathies aux sels insolubles de bismuth. *Nouv Presse Med* 1975;4:885.
23. Goulon M, Nouailhat F, Escourolle R, et al. Intoxication par le bromure de methyle. *Rev Neurol* 1975;131:445–68.
24. Hansen KS, Shard FR. Gasoline sniffing, lead poisoning and myoclonus. *JAMA* 1978;240:1375–6.
25. Harenko A. Neurologic findings in chronic bromisovalum poisoning. *Ann Med Interne (Paris)* 1967;56:181–8.
26. Helmers JH, Adam AA, Giezen J. Pain and myoclonus during induction with etomidate. *Acta Anaesthesiol Belg* 1981;32:141–7.
27. Hudson R, Ethans CT. Alfathesin and enflurane: synergistic central nervous system excitation? *Can Anaesth Soc J* 1981;28:55–6.
28. Jacquesson M, Saudeau D, Pantin B, et al. Myoclonia caused by a combination of triprolidine, pseudoephedrine and paracetamol. *Nouv Presse Med* 1982;11:2298–9.
29. Junck L, Marshall WH. Neurotoxicity of radiological contrast agents. *Ann Neurol* 1983;13:469–84.
30. Kallay MC, Tabechian H, Riley GR, Chessin LN. Neurotoxicity due to ticarcillin in a patient with renal failure. *Lancet* 1979;1(8116):608–9.
31. Kay B. Some experience of the use of etomidate in children. *Acta Anaesthesiol Belg [Suppl]* 1976;27:86–92.
32. Killebrew K, Whaley RA, Hayward JN. Complications of metrizamide myelography. *Arch Neurol* 1983;40:78–80.
33. Klawans HL, Goetz C, Bergen D. Levodopa induced myoclonus. *Arch Neurol* 1975;32:331–4.
34. Klawans HL, Ringel SP. A clinical trial of methysergide in parkinsonism: evidence against a serotonergic mechanism. *J Neurol Sci* 1973;19:399–405.
35. Kompf D, Neundorfer B. Neurotoxic side effects of piperazine in adults. *Arch Psychiatr Nervenkr* 1974;218:223–33.
36. Kruger G, Thomas DJ, Weinhardt F, et al. Disturbed oxidative metabolism in organic brain syndrome caused by bismuth in skin creams. *Lancet* 1976;1(7984):485–7.
37. Kurtz D, Tempe JD, Weber M, Feverstein J, Reeb M, Mantz JM. Electroclinical aspects of acute intoxication with chloralose. *Electroencephalogr Clin Neurophysiol* 1968;24:489.
38. Kurtzman NA, Rogers PW, Harter HR. Neurotoxic reaction to penicillin and carbenicillin. *JAMA* 1970;214:1320–1.
39. Lerner PI, Smith H, Weinstein L. Penicillin neurotoxicity. *Ann NY Acad Sci* 1967;145:310–8.
40. Loiseau P, Henry P, Jallon P, et al. Iatrogenic myoclonic encephalopathies caused by bismuth salts. *J Neurol Sci* 1976;27:133–43.
41. Loser R, Vogelsang H. Can angiografin be used for lumbar myelography? *Fortschr Geb Rontgenstr Nuklearmed* 1973;118:654–7.
42. Mahurkar SD, Meyers L, Cohen J, et al. Electroencephalographic and radionuclide studies in dialysis dementia. *Kidney Int* 1978;13:306–15.
43. Melcor CS, Jain VK. Diazepam withdrawal syndrome: its prolonged and changing nature. *Can Med Assoc J* 1982;127:1093–6.
44. Mellerio F, Gaultier M, Bismut O. Electroencephalography during acute poisoning by methyl bromide. *Eur J Toxicol* 1974;7:119–32.
45. Miller OG, Carpenter R. Neurotoxic side effects of piperazine. *Lancet* 1967;1(495):895–6.
46. Moore C. Oxazepam withdrawal syndrome. *Med J Aust* 1982;2:220.
47. Nausieda PA, Weiner WJ, Kaplan LR, Weber S, Klawans HL. Sleep disruption in the course of chronic levodopa therapy: an early feature of the levodopa psychosis. *Clin Neuropharmacol* 1982;5:183–94.
48. Ng AT. Prolonged myoclonic contractions after enflurane anesthesia. *Can Anaesth Soc J* 1980;27:502–3.

49. Praestholm J, Lester J. Water-soluble contrast lumbar myelography with meglumine iothalamate (conray). *Br J Radiol* 1970;43:303–8.
50. Raskin NH, Fishman RA. Neurologic disorders in renal failure. *N Engl J Med* 1976;294:143–8; 204–10.
51. Registration Committee of the European Dialysis and Transplant Association. Dialysis dementia in Europe. *Lancet* 1980;2(8187):190–2.
52. Roberts CJ, Noakes MJ. Danger of saline emetics in first aid for poisoning. *Br Med J* 1974;3(5932):683.
53. Rosen PB, Stevens R. Action myoclonus in lithium toxicity. *Ann Neurol* 1983;13:221–2.
54. Sackellares JC, Smith DB. Myoclonus with electrocerebral silence in a patient receiving penicillin. *Arch Neurol* 1979;36:857–8.
55. Schipior PG. An unusual case of antihistamine intoxication. *J Pediatr* 1967;71:589–91.
56. Schuch P, Stephan U, Jacobi G. Neurotoxic side-effects of piperazines. *Lancet* 1966;1:1218.
57. Snyder RD. The involuntary movements of chronic mercury poisoning. *Arch Neurol* 1972;26:379–81.
58. Steel CM, O'Duffey J, Brown SS. Clinical effects and treatment imipramine and amitriptyline poisoning in children. *Br Med J* 1967;3:663–7.
59. Supino-Viterbo V, Sicard O, Risveg-Lvato M, et al. Toxic encephalopathy due to ingestion of bismuth salts: clinical and EEG studies of 45 patients. *J Neurol Neurosurg Psychiatry* 1977;40:748–52.
60. Swanson PD, Luttrell CN, Magladery JW. Myoclonus: a report of 67 cases and review of the literature. *Medicine* 1962;41:339–56.
61. Urso S, Barbuti D. Lumbosacral radiculography with a new water soluble contrast medium: myelografin. *Ital J Orthop Traumatol* 1979;5:321–30.
62. Wendland KL. Myoclonus following doses of carbamazepine. *Nervenzart* 1968;39:231–3.
63. Wilson JH, Donker AJ, Hem GK, et al. Peritoneal dialysis for lithium poisoning. *Br Med J* 1971;2:749–50.

Advances in Neurology, Vol. 43: Myoclonus,
edited by S. Fahn et al. Raven Press,
New York © 1986.

Palatal Myoclonus

J. Lapresle

Service de Neurologie, Centre Hospitalier de Bicêtre, 94270 Le Kremlin Bicêtre, France

In 1886, Spencer (53) employed the term *nystagmus* for a remarkable observation of pharyngeal and laryngeal rhythmic movements, sparing in his case the soft palate but involving the eyes. This nomenclature, widely used afterwards, was criticized by Guillain (21) on the grounds that it presupposes an analogy with the common ocular nystagmus, which is an entirely different phenomenon. Indeed Spencer himself, in a second communication (54), had employed the word *clonus* although he returned later to nystagmus (55). This so-called *nystagmus du voile*, or better named *palatal myoclonus*, has been the subject of numerous studies, especially in France, concerning its clinical and pathological aspects. As already stated in a lecture given at Nagoya in 1978, and published in full elsewhere (34), the main interest of this minor phenomenon, most often ignored by the patient, lies in its demonstration of a transsynaptic degeneration and the discovery of a specific pathway.

CLINICAL DATA

As inspection of the oral cavity shows, palatal myoclonus is characterized by involuntary and usually unconscious movements of the soft palate and pharynx. The soft palate and uvula are drawn upward and backward before returning to rest. At the same time, there is a synchronous closing movement of the pharynx, in which the posterior wall moves forward and the posterior pillars approach each other at the midline. This disorder is most commonly bilateral and symmetric, but it can be unilateral, the palate and uvula then being drawn to one side. The movements are more or less continuous, usually between 100 and 150/min; exceptional rates of 20/min (2) and 600/min (15) have been observed.

It must be stressed that the occurrence of these rhythmic movements is delayed with respect to the occurrence of the causal lesion. This delay is often impossible to ascertain; when known, it is usually of a few weeks' duration but may range from 1 day (8) to 30 months (13). Once established, the rhythmic movements are steady in their intensity and amplitude, interrupted only by voluntary muscle contractions. With the exception of a very few cases (26), they are not affected by sleep (normal or induced by drugs) and persist for the rest of the subject's life. This sets these movements "apart from other movements, normal or abnormal, voluntary or involuntary" (46).

Other movements can be associated with palatal myoclonus. The most unusual is an audible synchronous "clicking" due to the rhythmic involvement of the eustachian tube, which first drew attention to this disorder when described by the 19th century otologists Muller in 1837 and Politzer in 1862 (48). Synchronous movements of the larynx, eyes, and diaphragm are more frequently observed, leading to the syndrome of *myoclonies vélo-pharyngo-laryngo-oculo-diaphragmatiques*, after Guillain and Mollaret (22). The face, the floor of the mouth, and the tongue may also be involved. Finally, these movements may be observed occasionally in skeletal muscles. They are either associated and synchronous with palatal myoclonus or isolated, but they are always rhythmic and prolonged. The clinical limitation of these movements may be more apparent than real. In a case I reported with Garcin and Fardeau (17) of rhythmic skeletal myoclonus limited to the shoulder, which incidentally disappeared during sleep, a rhythmic temporal muscular artifact in the electroencephalogram (EEG) was also noted.

ANATOMIC BASIS

The lesion that is almost always found during autopsy (18,48,52) is a special type of degeneration of the olivary nuclei in the medulla oblongata (the olives). This lesion can be bilateral but is unilateral when the symptom is unilateral, in which case the hypertrophied olive is on the side opposite the myoclonus. The pathological process has been clearly described by Lhermitte and Trelles (40). There is hypertrophy of the olives, often visible on macroscopic examination. The neurons are enlarged, vacuolated, and bizarre in shape; silver impregnation shows that the cell processes are hypertrophic. Astrocytes are increased in size, usually having prominent thick processes. Large, bizarre, multiple nuclei are common, although the increase in the number of these cells has been recently questioned (19). There is severe fibrillary gliosis and demyelination of the white matter around the olives and in their hila. Eventually, sites of lost neurons are marked by empty spaces, or clusters of vacuoles, or by complex argentophilic tangles. These residual glomeruloid structures have been considered by Lhermitte and Trelles (40) to be composed of "paraphytes," i.e., superfluous neoappendices. They are probably "nothing more than hypertrophied pericellular baskets of Cajal" (25), the highly particular dendritic apparatus of the normal olivary cells. These changes explain the persistence of the olivary hypertrophy when the neurons have finally disappeared.

Some ultrastructural studies have been performed. The most constant finding in humans, first demonstrated by Horoupian and Wisniewski (25) and confirmed since (4,31,61), is a proliferation of 100-Å neurofilaments morphologically identical to normal filaments. According to an experimental study in the monkey, these neurofilamentous changes could be reversible (63). A large increase in mitochondria has been noted (61) but not always confirmed (31). Numerous granules within expanded cisternal profiles with derived vacuoles of rough endoplasmic reticulum have been mentioned (4). The histochemical study by Koeppen et al. (32) demonstrated an increased acetylcholinesterase reaction in the neurons of hypertrophied olives. These data together may explain the light microscopic aspects: the hypertrophy of cells and the argyrophilia attributed to the neurofilamentous proliferation (25). They give some indication, at least for a time, of an overworking of the cells, but they do not provide the reason for this surprising pathological process.

This highly peculiar degeneration is considered to be transsynaptic because, with few exceptions, it is associated with a supraolivary causal lesion, predominantly vascular in nature. To a lesser extent, neoplastic, traumatic, and inflammatory processes, malformative or degenerative disorders, and even subacute myeloopticoneuropathy (45), dialysis encephalopathy (51), and herpes zoster (62) have been found. One may assume that, to be causative, this primary lesion must be destructive, a condition that is most readily realized by vascular lesions (34).

The main interest of the primary lesion is its location. Two sites have long been established: the ipsilateral central tegmental tract (14,16,47,57) and the contralateral dentate nucleus (9,30). When the rhythmic myoclonus is unilateral, the causative lesion is on the other side, if in the pons, or on the same side, if in the dentate nucleus. In a first attempt at explanation, Guillain and Mollaret (22) proposed a triangular relationship between the red nucleus and the inferior olive on one side, and the contralateral dentate nucleus. However, no lesion of the olivodentate fibers within the inferior cerebellar peduncle has ever been associated with palatal myoclonus or hypertrophic olivary degeneration. When it became apparent that this side of Guillain and Mollaret's (22) triangle had no significance, Trelles (59,60) postulated a specific pathway from the dentate nucleus to the contralateral inferior olive. Even if it exists, this supposed pathway could not be seen directly in humans, as it would first be part of the superior cerebellar peduncle and then part of the central tegmental tract, turning where these two tracts cross, i.e., in the vicinity of the red nucleus. In order to demonstrate this "most likely" hypothesis (18), Ben Hamida and I (6,38) investigated two possibilities: (a) a topographic relationship between the various structures involved, and (b) a delineation of this hypothetical dentatoolivary pathway in the strategic region of the red nucleus.

A relationship between dentate lesions and a contralateral hypertrophic olivary degeneration is implicit but not discussed in a number of early cases in which lesions of both structures had been noted. Only after a case in which there were small lesions in the dentate nucleus and contralateral olive was this possibility explicitly suggested (28), but this could not be established on the basis of one case alone. Therefore, cases were studied in which a lesion involving only part of the dentate nucleus was associated with a similarly restricted degeneration of the contralateral inferior olive, and where there was a complete absence of lesions in the central tegmental tract. Four cases showed a crossed dentatoolivary somatotopic relationship in the horizontal or ventrodorsal plane (35). To these, the above-noted case of Jonesco-Sisesti and Hornet (28) and a number of earlier cases from the literature in which this somatotopy was implicit may be added (35). Two further cases revealed a crossed dentatoolivary somatotopic relationship in a vertical or orocaudal plane, the first case also confirming the horizontal relationship (36). Eventually, examination of four cases showed a direct homolateral somatotopic relationship between fibers in the superior cerebellar peduncle and their cells of origin in the dentate nucleus (7). These data were largely confirmed by later pathological studies (27,61). Moreover, definite cerebelloolivary connections have been documented in animal studies (1,11,12,43), some clearly indicating a topological arrangement of the dentatoolivary projection in the cat (5,20,58), monkey (10,29), and rat (3). There were some discrepancies concerning the "direct" or "reverse" appearance of these relationships, but human analogies must be drawn cautiously because of the dramatic increase in complexity and development of the structures involved (3).

The finding of a topographic relationship between dentate lesions and olivary degeneration is a persuasive argument in favor of the existence of a pathway linking these two structures, as Trelles (59,60) postulated. This pathway would leave the dentate nucleus, pass through the homolateral superior cerebellar peduncle, and cross the midline in the commissure of Wernekink before joining the central tegmental tract and descending to the contralateral inferior olive. It would thus involve the superior cerebellar peduncle of one side and the central tegmental tract of the other. The critical region of the red nucleus, where the junction of the superior cerebellar peduncle and the central tegmental tract is situated, remains to be discussed. Three cases, in which there was a vascular lesion in the immediate vicinity of the red nucleus associated with ipsilateral olivary degeneration, demonstrated that the dentatoolivary pathway, after crossing the decussation of Wernekink, travels along the internal and then the dorsal surface of the red nucleus before merging with the central tegmental tract at this level (33,37). In addition to these findings, there are some pertinent observations concerning small lesions in the vicinity of the red nucleus (37): olivary hypertrophic degeneration is seen only when such lesions involve the internal and dorsal surfaces of the red nucleus.

MECHANISMS

Palatal myoclonus is due to the involvement of a complex structure linked by a specific pathway (Fig. 1). Several problems remain to be solved. Considering the olivary lesions, assumed to be a transsynaptic degeneration, there is no satisfactory explanation for the hypertrophy of the neurons as well as the astrocytes, a unique phenomenon in the central nervous system. One can only underline the unusual appearance of the normal olive cells, with their extensive dendritic overlap, also unique (50). It is too difficult "to understand why a structure with sources of input as rich and diverse . . . should undergo a transneuronal change . . . when only one of a number of afferent sources, that from the opposite dentate nucleus, has been interrupted" (4). In addition, there have been a few clear cases in which olivary hypertrophy has been definitely isolated, despite complete serial studies (23,39,48).

As to the clinical phenomenon, a brainstem release secondary to a cessation of the olivary cerebellar reticular modulations of motor activity has been suggested (24). It has also been recently postulated that it could be the "manifestation of denervation supersensitivity secondary to lesions involving the dentatorubroolivary system" (44), but this hypothesis has been severely criticized (42); it could explain

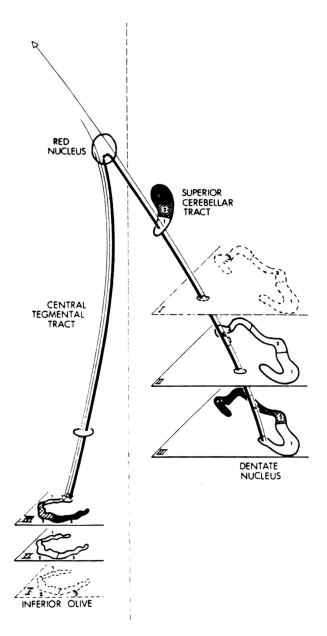

FIG. 1. Dentatoolivary somatotopic relationships in humans are crossed in both horizontal and vertical planes; somatotopic relationships between the dentate nucleus and homolateral superior cerebellar peduncle are direct. The dentatoolivary pathway *(continuous dark line)* passes from the dentate nucleus through the superior cerebellar peduncle and joins the contralateral central tegmental tract on its way to the inferior olive; in the red nucleus region, this pathway *(broken line)* passes by the internal and dorsal surfaces of this structure. (Modified from Lapresle and Ben Hamida, ref. 38.)

the delay following the causal lesion but not the rhythmic frequency. In this respect, an interpretation has been proposed (56,64). The structures involved in palatal myoclonus correspond embryologically to the first five branchial arches, and palatal myoclonus could be the human homologue of a primitive accessory respiratory reflex in gill-breathing vertebrates. With progressive integration of the branchio-meres into the organization of the air-breathing apparatus, there would be a progressive elaboration of the olivodentate system. With the utilization of the gill structure in the further development of the oropharynx, the associated respiratory reflex would be submerged but not lost, becoming apparent if its regulatory system was damaged. Thus the dentatoolivary system would remind us that "through evolution the central nervous system uses everything and forgets nothing" (34).

TREATMENT

Palatal myoclonus is not usually influenced by drugs, which is of little importance for so minor a symptom. Occasionally, however, audible clicking may be a problem. In two such cases, palatal myoclonus has responded to treatment with 5-HTP, the precursor of serotonin (41,62). There has also been a report of palatal myoclonus responding to carbamazepine (49). The relationship of these drugs to the structures involved is not clear.

SUMMARY

This chapter concerns palatal myoclonus. Indeed Spencer's vivid nystagmus is now abandoned in favor of the less ambiguous myoclonus. The clinical data are reviewed: its appearance, rhythmic frequency, delay with respect to the causal lesion, resistance to most external influences, and possible associations. The most frequent lesion associated with this clinical phenomenon is a special type of degeneration with hypertrophy of the olivary nucleus of the medulla oblongata, on the side opposite the myoclonus when it is unilateral. This degeneration is usually secondary to a primary lesion, located either in the ipsilateral (to the hypertrophied olive) central tegmentum tract or in the contralateral dentate nucleus, through a specific dentatoolivary pathway. The probable existence of this pathway is confirmed by the demonstration of a topographic relationship between dentate nucleus and contralateral inferior olive and by its delineation in the vicinity of the red nucleus where the superior cerebellar peduncle crosses the central tegmental tract. The mechanisms of these lesions and their ensuing symptoms are discussed. It is suggested that there is a transsynaptic degeneration probably disclosing an archaic phenomenon. Few drugs influence this steady abnormal movement: 5-HTP and carbamazepine recently have been credited with some success.

REFERENCES

1. Achenbach KE, Goodman DC. Cerebellar projections to pons, medulla and spinal cord in the albino rat. *Brain Behav Evol* 1968; 1:43–57.
2. Alajouanine Th, Thurel R, Wolfromm R. Myoclonies rythmiques du voile, de la glotte et du

diaphragme, survenant par accès périodiques et se traduisant par du hoquet. *Rev Neurol (Paris)* 1944; 76:96–7.

3. Angaut P, Cicirata F. Cerebello-olivary projections in the rat. An autoradiographic study. *Brain Behav Evol* 1982; 21:24–33.

4. Barron KD, Dentinger MP, Koeppen AH. Fine structure of neurons of the hypertrophied human inferior olive. *J Neuropathol Exp Neurol* 1982; 41:186–203.

5. Beitz AJ. The topographical organization of the olivo-dentate and dentato-olivary pathways in the cat. *Brain Res* 1976; 115:311–7.

6. Ben Hamida M. Contribution à l'étude anatomique de couple olivo-dentelé. A propos de 13 observations de dégénérescence hypertrophique des olives. *Thèse de Médecine* Paris, 1965.

7. Ben Hamida M, Lapresle J. Correspondance somatotopique chez l'homme des dégénérescences segmentaires du pédoncule cérébelleux supérieur secondaires à des lésions limitées du noyau dentelé homolatéral. *Rev Neurol (Paris)* 1969; 120:263–7.

8. Bogaert L van. Contribution à l'étude des myoclonies des troubles psychomoteurs et des troubles du sommeil par lésions en foyer du tronc cérébral. *Rev Neurol (Paris)* 1925; II:189–200.

9. Bogaert L van, Bertrand I. Sur les myoclonies associées synchrones et rhythmiques par lésions en foyer du tronc cérébral. Nouvelle observation anatomoclinique. *Rev Neurol (Paris)* 1928; I:203–14.

10. Chan-Palay V. *Cerebellar Dentate Nucleus. Organization, Cytology and Transmitters.* Berlin: Springer-Verlag, 1977:348.

11. Dom R, King JS, Martin GF. Evidence for two direct cerebello-olivary connections. *Brain Res* 1973; 57:498–501.

12. Faull RLM. Descending projections of the superior cerebellar peduncle to the brain stem of the rat. *J Anat* 1976; 121:416.

13. Faure-Beaulieu, Garcin R. Etude anatomique d'un cas de myoclonies vélo-pharyngo-laryngées. *Rev Neurol (Paris)* 1940; 72:734–9.

14. Foix Ch, Chavany J, Hillemand P. Le syndrome myoclonique de la calotte. Etude anatomo-clinique du nystagmus du voile et des myoclonies rythmiques associées, oculaires, faciales, etc. *Rev Neurol (Paris)* 1926; I:942–56.

15. Frank G, Chantraine A, Melon J, Mouchette R. Le syndrome clonique du voile du palais (5 observations). Etude clinique, électromyographique et cinématographique. *Rev Neurol (Paris)* 1965; 113:46–56.

16. Gallet J. Le nystagmus du voile (myoclonie vélo-pharyngo-laryngée), et les myoclonies associées oculaires, faciales, sushyoïdiennes, diaphragmatiques; le syndrome myoclonique de la calotte protubérantielle. *Thèse de Médecine* Paris, 1927.

17. Garcin R, Lapresle J, Fardeau M. Myoclonies squelettiques rythmées sans nystagmus du voile. Etude anatomo-clinique avec présentation d'un film cinématographique. *Rev Neurol (Paris)* 1963; 109:105–14.

18. Gautier JC, Blackwood W. Enlargement of the inferior olivary nucleus in association with lesions of the central tegmental tract or dentate nucleus. *Brain* 1961; 84:341–62.

19. Goto N, Kaneko M. Olivary enlargement: Chronological and morphometric analyses. *Acta Neuropathol (Berl)* 1981; 54:275–82.

20. Graybiel AM, Nauta HJW, Lasek RJ, Nauta WJH. A cerebello-olivary pathway in the cat: an experimental study using autoradiographic tracing techniques. *Brain Res* 1973; 58:205–11.

21. Guillain G. The syndrome of synchronous and rhythmic palato-pharyngo-laryngo-oculo-diaphragmatic myoclonus. *Proc Soc Med* 1938; 31:1031–8.

22. Guillain G, Mollaret P. Deux cas de myoclonies synchrones et rythmées vélo-pharyngo-laryngo-oculo-diaphragmatiques. Le problème anatomique et physiopathologique de ce syndrome. *Rev Neurol (Paris)* 1931; II:545–66.

23. Guillain G, Mollaret P, Bertrand I. Sur la lésion responsable du syndrome myoclonique du tronc cérébral. Etude anatomique d'un cas démonstratif sans lésions focales. *Rev Neurol (Paris)* 1933; II:666–74.

24. Herrmann C Jr, Brown JW. Palatal myoclonus: a reappraisal. *J Neurol Sci* 1967; 5:473–92.

25. Horoupian DS, Wisniewski H. Neurofilamentous hyperplasia in inferior olivary hypertrophy. *J Neuropathol Exp Neurol 1971;* 30:571–82.

26. Jacobs G, Newman RP, Bozian D. Disappearing palatal myoclonus. *Neurology (NY)* 1981; 31:748–51.

27. Jellinger K. Hypertrophy of the inferior olives. Report on 29 cases. *J Neurol* 1973; 205:153–74.

28. Jonesco-Sisesti N, Hornet Th. Le problème du nystagmus vélo-palato-oculaire. Les dégénérescences hypertrophiques systématisées du complexe olivaire bulbaire consécutives aux lésions du noyau dentelé du cervelet. *Rev Otoneuroophthalmol* 1939; 17:481–99.

29. Kalil K. Projections of the cerebellar and dorsal column nuclei upon the inferior olive in the rhesus monkey: an autoradiographic study. *J Comp Neurol* 1979; 188:43–62.

30. Klien H. Zur Pathologie der kontinuerlichen rhythmischen Krämpfe der Schlingmuskulatur (zwei Fälle von Erweichungsherden im Kleinhirn). *Neurol Zentral* 1907; 26:245–54.

31. Koeppen AH, Barron KD, Dentinger MP. Olivary hypertrophy in man. In: Courville et al., eds. The inferior olivary nucleus: anatomy and physiology. New York: Raven Press, 1980:309–14.

32. Koeppen AH, Barron KD, Dentinger MP. Olivary hypertrophy: Histochemical demonstration of hydrolytic enzymes. *Neurology (NY)* 1980; 30:471–80.

33. Lapresle J. Un nouveau cas de dégénérescence hypertrophique de l'olive bulbaire secondaire à un ramollissement limité de la calotte mésencéphalique. *J Neurol Sci* 1971; 12:95–100.

34. Lapresle J. Rhythmic palatal myoclonus and the dentato-olivary pathway. *J Neurol* 1979; 220:223–30.

35. Lapresle J, Ben Hamida M. Correspondance somatotopique, secteur par secteur, des dégénérescences de l'olive bulbaire consécutives à des lésions limitées du noyau dentelé contro-latéral. Etude de 4 observations anatomiques. *Rev Neurol (Paris)* 1965; 113:439–48.

36. Lapresle J, Ben Hamida M. Sur la correspondance somatotopique des dégénérescences de l'olive bulbaire consécutives à des lésions du noyau dentelé controlatéral. *C R Soc Biol (Paris)* 1967; 161:2149–52.

37. Lapresle J, Ben Hamida M. Contribution à la connaissance de la voie dentoolivaire. Etude anatomique de deux cas de dégénérescence hypertrophique de l'olive bulbaire secondaire à un ramollissement limité de la calotte mésencéphalique. *Presse Med* 1968; 76:1226–30.

38. Lapresle J, Ben Hamida M. The dentato-olivary pathway. Somatotopic relationship between the dentate nucleus and the contralateral inferior olive. *Arch Neurol* 1970; 22:135–43.

39. Leestma JE, Noronha A. Pure motor hemiplegia, medullary pyramid lesion, and olivary hypertrophy. *J Neurol Neurosurg Psychiatry* 1976; 39:877–84.

40. Lhermitte J, Trelles JO. L'hypertrophie des olives bulbaires dans la soi-disant pseudo-hypertrophie de l'olive bulbaire. *Rev Neurol (Paris)* 1933; I:495–8.

41. Magnussen I, Dupont E, Prange-Hansen AA, De Fine Olivarius B. Palatal myoclonus treated with 5-hydroxtryptophan and a decarboxylase-inhibitor. *Acta Neurol Scand* 1977; 55:251–3.

42. Marsden CD, Hallett M, Fahn S. The nosology and pathophysiology of myoclonus. In: Marsden CD, Fahn S, eds. Movement disorders. London: Butterworth Scientific, 1982:196–248.

43. Martin GF, Henkel CK, King JS. Cerebello-olivary fibers: their origin, course and distribution in the North American opossum. *Exp Brain Res* 1976; 24:219–36.

44. Matsuo F, Ajax ET. Palatal myoclonus and denervation supersensitivity in the central nervous system. *Ann Neurol* 1979; 5:72–8.

45. Mitsuhashi K, Asakura M, Takayanagi T, Mano T. Palatal myoclonus observed in a case of subacute myelo-optico-neuropathy. *Rinsho Shinkeigaku* 1974; 14:806–10.

46. Nathanson M. Palatal myoclonus. Further clinical and pathophysiological observations. *Arch Neurol Psychiatry* 1956; 75:285–96.

47. Ransohoff A. Uber einen Fall von Erweichung im dorsalen Teil der Brücke. *Arch Psychiat Nervenkr* 1902; 35:403–29.

48. Rondot P, Ben Hamida M. Myoclonies du voile et myoclonies squelettiques. Etude clinique et anatomique. *Rev Neurol (Paris)* 1968; 119:59–83.

49. Sakai T, Shiraishi S, Murakami S. Palatal myoclonus responding to carbamazepine. *Ann Neurol* 1981; 9:199–200.

50. Scheibel ME, Scheibel AB. The inferior olive. A Golgi study. *J Comp Neurol* 1955; 102:77–132.

51. Snider WD, DeMaria AA Jr, Mann JD. Diazepam and dialysis encephalopathy. *Neurology (NY)* 1979; 29:414–45.

52. Sohn D, Levine S. Hypertrophy of the olives: a report on 43 cases. In: Zimmerman HM, ed. Progress in neuropathology vol I. New York: Grune & Stratton, 1971:202–17.

53. Spencer HR. Pharyngeal and laryngeal "nystagmus." *Lancet* 1886; 2:702.

54. Spencer HR. Pharyngeal and laryngeal "nystagmus." *Lancet* 1886; 2:758.

55. Spencer HR. Pharyngeal and laryngeal nystagmus. *Lancet* 1938; 1:227.

56. Stern MM. Rhythmic palatopharyngeal myoclonus. Review, case report and significance. *J Nerv Ment Dis* 1949; 109:48–53.

57. Thomas A. Recherches sur le faisceau longitudinal postérieur et la substance réticulée bulbo-protubérantielle, le faisceau central de la calotte et le faisceau de Helweg. *Rev Neurol (Paris)* 1903; 11:94–6.

58. Tolbert DL, Massopust LC, Murphy MG, Young PA. The anatomical organization of the cerebello-olivary projection in the cat. *J Comp Neurol* 1976; 170:525–44.

59. Trelles JO. Les ramollissements protubérantiels. *Thèse de Médecine* Paris, 1935.

60. Trelles JO. La oliva bulbar. Su estructura, funcion y patologia. *Rev Neuropsiquiatr* 1943; 6:433–521.

61. Vuia O. Aspects morphologiques (optiques et ultrastructuraux) de l'hypertrophie de l'olive bulbaire. *Rev Neurol (Paris)* 1976; 132:51–61.

62. Williams A, Goodenberger D, Calne DB. Palatal myoclonus following herpes zoster ameliorated by 5-hydroxytryptophan and carbidopa. *Neurology (NY)* 1978; 28:358–9.

63. Wisotzkey H, Cole M. Reversible neurofilamentous change with desafferentation of the inferior olive in the monkey. *J Neuropathol Exp Neurol* 1974; 33:187.

64. Yakovlev P. Discussion. *Trans Am Neurol Assoc* 1957; 82:87–8.

Advances in Neurology, Vol. 43: Myoclonus,
edited by S. Fahn et al. Raven Press,
New York © 1986.

Rhythmic Myoclonias Including Spinal Myoclonus

B. P. Silfverskiöld

Department of Neurology, Södersjukhuset, S-100 64 Stockholm, Sweden

Rhythmic myoclonus was common in cases of encephalitis lethargica in some epidemics during the pandemic of the 1920s. The myoclonus could be localized to any muscle or muscle group of the face, limbs, or trunk. It was rather violent in Reimold's (32) series; there was sometimes a synergistic action, and the contractions could produce marked movements of limb segments. The myoclonus often occurred synchronously in the affected muscles in different parts of the body; the frequency was 50 to 70/min, and the rhythm was very stable. It appeared in the acute or chronic stage of the disease and remained in the same muscles. The contractions might persist for months or years, or even permanently.

Krebs (21) and others described a comparatively mild form. This encephalitic myoclonus disappeared or decreased during relaxation. There was a marked increase of the myoclonus during moderate static or postural contraction and a decrease during stronger contraction. In two of Krebs' three cases, the myoclonus decreased or disappeared during movements.

I described (36) a mild form of rhythmic myoclonus in three unrelated girls, all resident in Stockholm, beginning in each case in the early autumn of 1958, suggesting a common infective origin. In two of the patients, there was a peculiar limb myoclonus that occurred at rest. It was synchronous in antagonistic muscles of each limb. The intensity of the individual contractions varied, which tended to mask the rhythm. The rhythmic features were distinctly seen in electromyograms (EMGs). There was a phase difference in the rhythm of the different limbs; only occasionally did the contractions occur simultaneously in two extremities. The frequency was 60 to 80/min. Emotional excitement increased the intensity of the contractions. Certain activities, such as writing, abolished the myoclonus in all the limbs, as recorded in the EMGs. During static muscular contraction (clenching of a fist), the myoclonus persisted. Electroencephalograms showed no cerebral potentials corresponding to the myoclonus.

I compared this type of myoclonus with parkinsonian tremor. Both are increased during emotional excitement. It is a common clinical experience that the tremor contractions in parkinsonism may be temporarily halted during attention and in the initial phase of movements. In some cases, the tremor decreases for prolonged periods during voluntary movements, such as writing.

The influence of motor activity on tremor has been studied in animal experiments. Peterson et al. (30) produced "postural" tremor in monkeys through lesions in the ventral tegmentum of the midbrain; the tremor showed alternating activity between agonists and antagonists, and the rate was that of parkinsonian tremor. The tremor increased during excitement and muscular activity of the static type (in postural adjustment) and disappeared during movements. This difference between static and phasic muscular contraction evidently resembles that found in the presented type of limb myoclonus and in Krebs' cases of encephalitic myoclonus.

Swanson et al. (40) described rhythmic myoclonus in patients (cases 4–6) with a probable virus encephalomyelitis. Case 4 showed repetitive forceful muscular contractions of both eyelids, both arms, and left leg. The involuntary movements in the upper extremities were characterized by strong flexion and external rotation of hand, forearm, and arm. In the leg, they consisted of pronator–extensor spasms. Later these movements spread to involve the tongue, jaw, trunk, and the other leg. They were generally synchronous, with a rate varying between 60 and 100/min. The authors reviewed the experimental data implicating brainstem and spinal cord. Luttrell et al. (24) found that experimentally produced Newcastle disease virus encephalomyelitis in cats is accompanied by strong rhythmic myoclonus in the head, neck, trunk, and limbs. When virus was injected into the cervical spinal cord, the myoclonus developed first in the forelimbs and later in the hindquarters; the mostly rhythmic flexor spasms in forelimbs and hindlimbs were bilaterally synchronous. After inoculation into the lower spinal cord, high thoracic transsection did not alter the hindlimb myoclonus; tongue myoclonus following infection through cranial routes persisted after isolation of the brainstem. Myoclonus, therefore, could result from an effect of virus at either of these levels of the central nervous system.

SPINAL MYOCLONUS

The appearance of segmental myoclonus (15,16) in patients with spinal tumors provides convincing clinical evidence that rhythmic jerks can arise at the spinal cord level. Garcin et al. (12) described a patient with a cervical astrocytoma. Unilateral jerks appeared in shoulder and upper arm muscles. The frequency was about 43/min, and the rhythm was regular. The EMGs showed bursts "relatively" synchronous in antagonistic muscles. A similar patient with bilateral myoclonus was described by Nohl et al. (29). These authors, as well as Frenken et al. (10), reviewed the few cases in which the myoclonus was related to local spinal cord lesions due to tumor.

Recent papers describe a repetitive leg myoclonus, which may be bilaterally synchronous. It is not always rhythmic. Hopkins and Michael (20) reported a patient with rhythmic myoclonus affecting only the lower part of the body. Changes in the cerebrospinal fluid suggested a viral infection. There were continuous rhythmic thrusting movements in the pelvis; jerks of the legs were sometimes bilaterally synchronous. The frequency was 100 to 150/min. Stimulation of one medial popliteal nerve induced myoclonic jerks in both the ipsilateral and contralateral leg with almost identical latencies of about 40 msec, the length of latency suggesting conduction through a spinal pathway with more than one synapse.

Davis et al. (6) found similar electrophysiological abnormalities in a patient with frequent shocklike jerks occurring synchronously in both legs. The jerks were semirhythmic with a rate of 10 to 30/min. They affected predominantly the hip, knee extensors, and plantar flexors. Their amplitude and frequency were increased by a variety of stimuli: conversation, mental arithmetics, sudden loud noises, or tapping a tendon. A spinal cord ischemia was confirmed at autopsy. Another of their patients was considered to have viral neuronitis; she had 6 to 7/sec rhythmic jerks of the glutei and all muscle groups of both lower limbs.

Spinal myoclonus may occur in association with herpes zoster infection (4,18). One such patient (17) developed frequent, jerking thigh movements which were at times synchronous and spread upward to cause massive shocklike movements of the pelvis and lower trunk.

Shivapour and Teasdall (35) observed myoclonic bursts occurring at 20 to 40/min simultaneously in all leg muscles of a patient with tumor compression of the thoracic cord. The autopsy findings showed, in addition, disseminated arteriosclerosis and hypertensive cardiovascular disease.

The myoclonus in all these patients was distinctly related to spinal disease, but, as mentioned by Garcin et al. (12), it is difficult to exclude involvement above the spinal level. In viral or vascular diseases, the lesions may have spread to the brainstem or cerebellum even in the absence of clinical signs of such involvement.

Frenken et al. (10) ascribed "spinal myoclonus" to ischemic myelopathy in one of their cases showing ataxia of gait and extensor plantar reflexes. The patient had synchronous jerks in the legs as shown in EMGs from the right and left anterior tibial muscles. There was a 2.5 to 3/sec rhythm. The jerks increased in amplitude with slight muscle contraction and on standing. They were not visible in walking. Pneumoencephalograms showed cerebral atrophy; there were signs of polyneuropathy in the legs, and some abuse of alcohol had occurred, especially in recent years. The rhythmic 3/sec activity, synchronous in the legs, may be compared with that found in a large series of Swedish alcoholic subjects (see below).

SLOW TREMOR MYOCLONUS

Patterns of Slow Distal Arm Tremor

Holmes (19) suggested that the term tremor be used to denote a clinical phenomenon consisting of the involuntary oscillation of any part of the body around any plane, such oscillations being either regular or irregular in rate and amplitude, and due to the alternate action of groups of muscles and their antagonists. He described several patients with a coarse, slow tremor; in most, the rate was 2.5 to 4/sec. In his two first cases, both with signs ascribed to a vascular lesion in the midbrain, there were adductions–abductions and flexions–extensions of the fingers, the index rubbing against the thumb. Foot flexions–extensions and various movements at the more proximal leg joints were often present. The tremor was generally compound; that is, it was rarely limited to one group of muscles and their antagonists, so that the limb was, as a rule, simultaneously moved at two or more joints. In each case, the influence of gravity on its production and existence was emphasized, "a certain condition of tone of the muscles being essential." The tremor disappeared at rest.

Patterns of Distal Arm Myoclonus

Several French papers, like that of Holmes (19), contain a detailed clinical description and, in some cases, a postmortem examination. Holmes' tremor may be compared with the myoclonus described by Lhermitte and Sigwald (23). Their patient had a left-sided palatal myoclonus at 3/sec, and rhythmic flexions–extensions at 3/sec occurred in the left fingers when, for instance, an ulnar finger was kept in contact with the thumb. The oscillations were never seen at rest. *Myoclonies typiques* appeared when the patient pressed her fingers with moderate force against the examiner's hand; strong pressure could abolish the oscillatory rhythm of this myoclonus. When she leaned against her left hand, rhythmic abductions–adductions of the whole arm were observed. According to the authors, an infarction in the territory of the posterior inferior cerebellar artery had produced a lateral medullary syndrome, but another infarction seemed to have caused some of the complex neurological signs.

Many years ago, Crouzon and Christophe (5) reported a patient with bilateral palatofacial and ocular myoclonus associated with unilateral limb movements, all occurring synchronously and in the same slow rhythm, 100 to 110/min. The movements involved the whole arm; they were more marked distally with extensions–flexions "entirely comparable with a parkinsonian tremor," and were attenuated at complete rest. Similar flexions–extensions were seen in the toes. The application of the term myoclonus to these Parkinson-like oscillations, according to these authors, is rather improper. The similarity in rhythm between the limb oscillations and the palatal myoclonus, however, suggested a common physiopathological process. The authors found that the terminology was a matter of habit; all terms were equally debatable.

It may be added that the word myoclonus simply means muscle jerks (13). Tremor is a shaking movement; prominent authors, such as Brimblecombe and Pinder (3), do not restrict the use of the term tremor to alternating types. "Parkinson-like" tremors, however, are always alternating.

Patterns of Slow Leg Myoclonus

Messimy et al. (26) described patients with *myorhythmies*, another name for skeletal myoclonus. Two of their patients showed 2 to 3/sec leg oscillations with interesting patterns. These patients had lesions in the cerebellar vermis, but the changes were not limited to this structure.

One of the patients (case 2) had an arteriovenous malformation in the left side of the roof of the fourth ventricle. Two to three weeks after extirpation of the malformation, there appeared a "special" 3/sec tremor in the left limbs. The leg oscillations were evidently of the "kicking" type (see below), and they appeared only when the leg was kept flexed in an elevated position. One year later, only sporadic "brusque" adductions of the left leg were noted. The other patient (case 3) had a metastatic tumor in the cerebellar vermis. A week after extirpation of the tumor, clonic adductions of the legs appeared in a 2 to 3/sec rhythm. A week later, muscle jerks or tremors also involved other parts of the leg. Rhythmic movements spread to the right leg and to the pelvis; there were alternating head movements with 2 to 3/sec contractions of the sternocleido muscles. As in case 2, this patient showed upper limb 3/sec pronations–supinations and nystagmus. The clinical description indicates that the patients had alternating limb tremors as well as simple rhythmic jerks, both occurring at a rate of 2 to 3/sec.

The Slow Rhythm

Rondot and Ben Hamida (33) discussed several aspects of rhythmic myoclonus. They found that rhythmic limb myoclonus has much in common with certain tremors. It may appear only in particular postures and could be restricted to a single muscle group, but a similar restriction could be seen in tremors when the muscles were counteracting the weight of a limb. The term postural indicates that the part involved is held still against gravitational forces (3). The limb myoclonus was best characterized by its slow rhythm. The rate was mostly 2 to 3/sec, like that of palatal myoclonus. The frequency was consequently clearly below the 5 to 6/sec characteristic of parkinsonian tremor. One of their patients showed myoclonus of the palate and of the right limbs. According to the EMGs presented, the frequency was 2.5/sec in the palate movements, 3.6/sec in the finger flexion–extensions, and 2.7/sec in the foot flexion–extensions. There was consequently a low frequency at all these levels, but the rate was not identical. A lack of synchrony is also noted in other reports. Tahmoush et al. (41) made polygraphic records in a patient with myoclonus of the palate and face associated with rhythmic ocular and limb movements. The movements occurred at the same rate in all regions. There was a phase difference between the cranial and the limb bursts, however, as seen in the records from submental muscles and wrist extensors. Their clinical description was short; the jerks appeared evidently during maintenance of posture and not at rest.

Garcin et al. (11) described a 74-year-old stroke patient with a left spastic hemiparesis and a paresis of gaze to the left. Two weeks afterward, there appeared a myoclonus with synchronous jerks (with rhythmic rotations of the scapula) in the left arm and the left leg. There was a regular 2 or 3/sec rhythm. No movements of the alternating tremor type were reported. The myoclonus diminished at rest; it disappeared during sleep and reappeared like starting a clock a few moments after awakening. No palatal myoclonus was observed. Ataxia and bilateral sensory changes were additional findings. The patient died after 5 years. Autopsy of the brain showed (a) an extensive infarction in the region of the left dentate nucleus, (b) a marked atrophy of the right inferior olive (the hypertrophic changes were relatively mild), and (c) small vascular lesions of lacunar type in the cerebellum, brainstem, basal ganglia, and internal capsule. No spinal abnormalities were seen. The authors emphasized the infarction in the dentate nucleus area and the olivary changes. The several small infarctions in the brainstem, however, may have been of importance. These produced severe clinical deficits, including the oculomotor abnormalities.

Marked signs of brainstem involvement at various levels are, as a rule, observed in patients with a combined palatal–limb myoclonus [see, for instance, the table of Herrmann and Brown (17)]. Rhythmic limb myoclonus (as well as 2–3/sec tremor) is a rare phenomenon; some unknown factors (anatomic or biochemical) may be responsible for its occurrence in a few of the many patients with various cerebellar-brainstem lesions.

"Rubral" Tremor

Holmes (19) discussed at length the associated clinical signs and the results of postmortem examination in two of his cases. He concluded that tremor in focal cerebral disease may depend on a "lesion of the midbrain, or rather of the cerebello-rubral system." The slow rubral tremor has since been mentioned often in the literature, but the cases are few and only some resemble those originally described by Holmes (19).

Kremer et al. (22) observed 2.5 to 4/sec finger flexions–extensions in two patients from the large Oxford series of head injuries. Severe signs of midbrain injury were reported, and the dominant clinical signs were cerebellar. The authors found a considerable likeness to certain of the tremors studied by Holmes (19).

Connections of the red nucleus have been implicated in the production of postural Parkinson-like tremor in monkeys. Poirier et al. (31) found that the combined interruption of the rubroolivary fibers and the corresponding nigrostriatal fibers are important for the production of postural tremor. Interruption of the rubrooli-vocerebellorubral loop at one point or another is associated with postural tremor only when certain drugs, such as harmaline, are administered to the lesioned monkey causing a pharmacological interruption of the dopaminergic nigrostriatal pathway. The rate of this experimental (alternating) tremor was 4 to 7/sec. The various motor disturbances produced by cerebellar damage (involving the dentate nucleus) evidently did not include myoclonic jerks.

Slow Leg Tremor Myoclonus in Cerebelloolivary Atrophy

The disease is described as "nutritional cerebellar degeneration" by Adams (1). "Cerebelloolivary atrophy" is the name used by Escourolle et al. (8); the essential features are reviewed by Adams (1). Torvik et al. (42) found the characteristic anteromedial cerebellar atrophy in 26.8% of all alcoholics examined postmortem.

The atrophy is consequently a remarkably frequent complication of alcoholism, but only a few of the cases of Torvik et al. (42) had been diagnosed clinically.

The abnormalities of gait and station may be of mild or moderate degree, and they are often neglected or confused with banal alcoholic unsteadiness. Recording of Romberg's test revealed, in our patients and later in a German series, characteristic 3/sec flexions–extensions of the feet (25,37,38). These are difficult to observe at inspection because of complex muscle contractions and leg oscillations. The heel-on-knee position provokes repetitive 3/sec contractions in different proximal muscles of both legs, mainly resulting in synchronous rotations in the hip joints (39); flexions and adductions are added. Amplitude variations contribute to a picture easily confused with completely irregular jerking or ataxia.

Simple single-plane oscillations appeared in appropriate leg postures, and a few new tests were introduced in the standard neurological examination. As a consequence, a marked 3/sec leg tremor was observed at our own and other Swedish hospitals in several hundred patients, mostly advanced alcoholics. Tomographic pneumoencephalograms, made in many of these, showed a typical atrophy of the anterior cerebellar vermis (only a part of this atrophy is seen at computerized tomography). The tests used were reported in a recent paper (34).

Slow rhythmic adductions of the thighs were observed in the supine position with the legs flexed and abducted, feet flat on the couch (Fig. 1). The adductions were constantly bicrural and synchronous, as shown in EMGs (28), and the frequency was always approximately 3/sec. Rhythmic kicking (extension movements) in the 3/sec range appeared when a leg, flexed 90°, was maintained in an elevated position. Rhythmic synchronous leg extensions occurred at the typical 3/sec frequency when the patient was standing with flexed knees. The resulting bobbing of the body could be recorded with an accelerometer attached, for instance, to the head (38).

Some of the patients showed, in addition, a 3 to 5/sec upper limb tremor. This tremor resembled that described by Holmes (19), Adams (1), and others. Synchronous rhythmic leg movements were a typical feature of the 3/sec oscillations seen in our patients. A bicrural synchronism has not been observed in any classic tremor, but the phenomenon has been reported as occurring in both clinical and experimental myoclonus. It may be added that in some of my patients with a marked 3/sec leg tremor, inferior parts of the trunk were involved; there were marked pelvic movements probably resembling those mentioned by Hopkins and Michael (20) and Dhaliwal and McGreal (7) in their descriptions of spinal myoclonus. In a few of my severely affected patients, there appeared, with legs flat on the couch, rhythmic or nonrhythmic contractions in the anterior muscles of the thigh or lower leg. These contractions were distinctly myoclonic within the narrowest definition of the term.

Studies in Animals

Interesting experiments in rhesus monkeys were conducted by Mesulam et al. (27). The animals were subjected to repeated episodes of severe thiamine deficiency

A

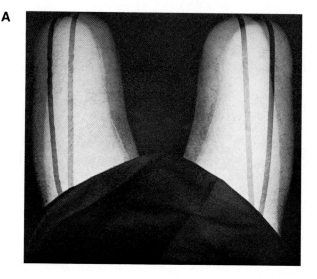

B

Left

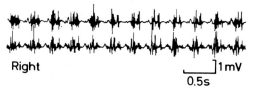

Right   ]1mV
                                    0.5s

No activity in abductor muscles.

Normal needle EMG.

Normal nerve conduction velocities.

Normal H-reflex - no response on

the contralateral side.

FIG. 1A. Position for provocation of rhythmic leg adductions, feet flat on the couch. There is one black stripe on each thigh. (Photo in stroboscopic light made by Istvan Agocs.) **B:** EMG shows bicrurally synchronous 3/sec rhythm in adductor activity. Burst duration ~200 msec. (Electrophysiological studies made by Dr. B. Y. Nilsson.)

during 1 year. Intention tremor appeared in the forelimbs. A coarse leg tremor with increasing amplitude tended to throw the monkey to the floor or against the walls of the cage. According to a personal communication from M. M. Mesulam (1978), these oscillations could be closely related to the body bobbing observed in our patients. It should be added that distinct observation of limb oscillations, demanding the described active maintenance of various postures, cannot be carried out in animals.

At autopsy, the monkeys with a mild ataxia showed a selective degeneration of the granule cells in the anterior cerebellum. More massive changes in the cerebellum and brainstem were found in monkeys with advanced ataxia.

Clonazepam Therapy

I have given clonazepam, 4 to 6 mg/day, to a small series of patients showing a 3/sec slow tremor myoclonus. A marked reduction of oscillation amplitude occurred in two. No other drugs had shown any positive effect in these very chronic cases. Control of treatment compliance is always difficult in alcoholics, especially in long-term therapy; nevertheless, clonazepam therapy should be tried in this group of patients. No increase or decrease of the gait ataxia was observed with the doses used.

RHYTHMIC EYE OSCILLATIONS IN WALLENBERG'S SYNDROME

Nystagmus is one of the standard features of Wallenberg's syndrome. It is often believed that vestibular nuclei in the inferior pontine tegmentum are damaged when nystagmus results from vertebrobasilar ischemia. Fisher et al. (9), however, in their postmortem studies of 16 Wallenberg cases, found that nystagmus could be present when these nuclei were not affected. A cerebellar infarction was observed in only four cases. The typical infarction extended from the lateral medullary surface inward just behind the olive. This is the most typical territory of the inferior posterior cerebellar artery.

We (2) noted a vertical nystagmus with high amplitude in several patients with a Wallenberg syndrome. Recording showed a 1.5 to 2/sec frequency of the prominent vertical eye oscillations in two other Wallenberg patients with complex oculomotor abnormalities (14). Yap et al. (43) recorded 2.5/sec vertical eye oscillations *(ocular bobbing)* in two patients showing nodding of the head and palatofacial myoclonus, both synchronous with the eye bobbing. Their case 2 showed predominantly signs referable to the Wallenberg area, but the brainstem lesions were evidently more widespread in both their patients.

Signs of extension of the lesion to the inferior pons were not found in our patients. Links of little-known mechanisms involved in the production of rhythmic eye movements are located in the Wallenberg area. Our patients had no palatofacial or limb myoclonus, but their marked vertical eye movements occurred at the slow rate observed in most cases of rhythmic myoclonus. There are variations in the extent of Wallenberg infarctions, but they can be strictly bulbar, as seen in one of our patients. The nystagmus as well as the histological lesions were thoroughly studied in this case.

SUMMARY

In rare cases, rhythmic limb movements may appear in association with palatal myoclonus. There is a similar slow rate, below 4/sec. A review by Rondot and Ben Hamida (33) showed that the limb movements had much in common with postural tremors. Lhermitte and Sigwald (23) observed a peculiar pattern of upper limb oscillations in a patient with palatal myoclonus. It resembles a rare type of slow postural tremor, often called rubral tremor, described by Holmes (19).

We found that a large group of alcoholics, showing signs of cerebellar degeneration, exhibit a stereotyped pattern of slow, coarse leg oscillations. There is a stable rhythm, in the 3/sec range, in alternating as well as in nonalternating muscle contractions. Both are in several maintained postures bicrurally synchronous, which is a feature of experimental and clinical myoclonus never observed in classic tremors. A few of these patients have upper limb oscillations, and these are of the kind described by Holmes (19) and Lhermitte and Sigwald (23). The cerebellar degeneration is of the anteromedial type; it is often associated with olivary changes (cerebelloolivary atrophy).

Swanson et al. (40) and others included in the spinal category patients with myoclonus restricted to muscles innervated from one or more spinal cord segments and no recognizable neurological abnormality at higher levels. The most convincing cases of purely spinal origin are those in which segmental jerks are caused by a spinal tumor. These repetitive jerks may sometimes show a slow rhythm.

ACKNOWLEDGMENT

I am indebted to Associate Professor B. Y. Nilsson for the many electrophysiological studies described herein.

REFERENCES

1. Adams RD. Nutritional cerebellar degeneration. In: Vinken PJ, Bruyn GW, eds. Handbook of clinical neurology, vol 28. Amsterdam: North-Holland, 1976:271–83.
2. Bjerver K, Silfverskiöld BP. Lateropulsion and imbalance in Wallenberg's syndrome. *Acta Neurol Scand* 1968;44:91–100.
3. Brimblecombe RW, Pinder RM. *Tremors and tremorogenic agents*. Bristol: Scientechnica, 1972.
4. Castaigne P, Cambier J, Laplane D, Cathala HP, Brunet P, Pierrot-Deseilligny E. Myoclonies rhythmées segmentaires d'origine médullaire: A propos de deux observations. *Rev Otoneuroophthalmol* 1969;41:241–50.
5. Crouzon O, Christophe J. Syndrome pseudo-bulbaire et cérébelleux d'origine protubérantielle avec myoclonies rythmiques et synchrones vélo-pharyngo-facio-laryngées bilatérales et myoclonies oculaires et squelettiques unilatérales. *Rev Neurol (Paris)* 1936;65:76–80.
6. Davis SM, Murray NMF, Diengdoh JV, Galea-Debono A, Kocen RS. Stimulus-sensitive spinal myoclonus. *J Neurol Neurosurg Psychiatry* 1981;44:884–8.
7. Dhaliwal GS, McGreal DA. Spinal myoclonus in association with herpes zoster infection: two case reports. *Can J Neurol Sci* 1974;1:239–41.
8. Escourolle R, Gray F, Hauw JJ. Les atrophies cérébelleuses. *Rev Neurol (Paris)* 1982;138:953–65.
9. Fisher CM, Karnes WE, Kubik CS. Lateral medullary infarction—the pattern of vascular occlusion. *J Neuropathol* 1961;20:323.
10. Frenken CWGM, Notermans SLH, Korten JJ, Horstink MWIM. Myoclonic disorders of spinal origin. *Clin Neurol Neurosurg* 1978;79:107–18.
11. Garcin R, Lapresle J, Fardeau M. Myoclonies squelettiques rhythmées sans nystagmus du voile. Etude anatomo-clinique avec présentation d'un film cinématographique. *Rev Neurol (Paris)* 1963;109:105–14.
12. Garcin R, Rondot P, Guiot G. Rhythmic myoclonus of the right arm as the presenting symptom of a cervical cord tumour. *Brain* 1968;91:75–84.
13. Gastaut H. Les myoclonies. Séméiologie des myoclonies et nosologie analytique des syndromes myocloniques. *Rev Neurol (Paris)* 1968;119:1–30.
14. Hagström L, Hörnsten G, Silfverskiöld BP. Oculostatic and visual phenomena occurring in association with Wallenberg's syndrome. *Acta Neurol Scand* 1969;45:568–82.

15. Halliday AM. The clinical incidence of myoclonus. In: Williams D, ed. Modern trends in neurology, vol. 4. London: Butterworth, 1967:69–105.
16. Halliday AM. The neurophysiology of myoclonic jerking—a reappraisal. In: Charlton MH, ed. Myoclonic seizures. Roche medical monograph series. Amsterdam: Excerpta Medica, 1975:1–29.
17. Herrmann C Jr, Brown JW. Palatal myoclonus: a reappraisal. *J Neurol Sci* 1967;5:473–92.
18. Hoehn MM, Cherington M. Spinal myoclonus. *Neurology (NY)* 1977;27:942–6.
19. Holmes G. On certain tremors in organic cerebral lesions. *Brain* 1904;27:327–75.
20. Hopkins AP, Michael WF. Spinal myoclonus. *J Neurol Neurosurg Psychiatry* 1974;37:1112–5.
21. Krebs E. *Myocolonies et mouvements involontaires de l'encéphalite épidémique.* Doin, Paris, 1929.
22. Kremer M, Russell WR, Smyth GE. A mid-brain syndrome following head injury. *J Neurol Neurosurg Psychiatry* 1947;10:49–60.
23. Lhermitte J, Sigwald J. Myoclonies rhythmées du voile, du pharynx, du larynx et du membre supérieur gauche au cours d'un syndrome latéral du bulbe. *Rev Neurol (Paris)* 1941;73:81–6.
24. Luttrell CN, Bang F, Luxenberg K. Newcastle disease encephalomyelitis in cats. *Arch Neurol Psychiatry* 1959;81:285.
25. Mauritz KH, Dichgans J, Hufschmidt A. Quantitative analysis of stance in late cortical cerebellar atrophy of the anterior lobe and other forms of cerebellar ataxia. *Brain* 1979;102:461–82.
26. Messimy R, Berdet H, Pertuiset B, David M. Myorythmies associées à un syndrome cérébelleux, paraissant consécutives à une lésion des noyaux du cervelet dans deux cas, à une lésion du pédoncule cérébelleux supérieur dans un troisième cas. *Rev Neurol (Paris)* 1963;109:513–28.
27. Mesulam MM, Van Hoesen GW, Butters N. Clinical manifestations of chronic thiamine deficiency in rhesus monkey. *Neurology (NY)* 1977;27:239–45.
28. Nilsson BY, Silfverskiöld BP. Electromyographic recordings of slow leg tremor in chronic alcoholics. *Acta Neurol Scand* 1973;49:227–32.
29. Nohl M, Doose H, Gross-Selbeck G, Jensen HP. Spinal myoclonus. *Eur Neurol* 1978;17:129–35.
30. Peterson EW, Magoun H, McCulloch W, Lindsley D. Production of postural tremor. *J Neurophysiol* 1949;12:371.
31. Poirier LJ, Lafleur J, De Lean J, Guiot G, Larochelle L, Boucher R. Physiopathology of the cerebellum in the monkey. Part 2. Motor disturbances associated with partial and complete destruction of cerebellar structures. *J Neurol Sci* 1974;22:491–509.
32. Reimold W. Uber die myoklonische Form der Encephalitis. *Zbl Ges Neurol Psychiatr* 1925;95:21.
33. Rondot P, Ben Hamida M. Myoclonies du voile et myoclonies squelettiques étude clinique et anatomique. *Rev Neurol (Paris)* 1968;119:59–83.
34. Rosenhamer HJ, Silfverskiöld BP. Slow tremor and delayed brainstem auditory evoked responses in alcoholics. *Arch Neurol* 1980;37:293–6.
35. Shivapour E, Teasdall RD. Spinal myoclonus with vacuolar degeneration of anterior horn cells. *Arch Neurol* 1980;37:451–3.
36. Silfverskiöld BP. Rhythmic myoclonus in three girls. *Acta Neurol Scand* 1962;38:45–59.
37. Silfverskiöld BP. Romberg's test in the cerebellar syndrome occurring in chronic alkoholism. *Acta Neurol Scand* 1969;45:292–302.
38. Silfverskiöld BP. Cortical cerebellar degeneration associated with a specific disorder of standing and locomotion. *Acta Neurol Scand* 1977;55:257–72.
39. Silfverskiöld BP. A 3 c/sec leg tremor in a "cerebellar" syndrome. *Acta Neurol Scand* 1977;55:385–93.
40. Swanson PD, Luttrell CN, Magladery JW. Myoclonus—a report of 67 cases and review of the literature. *Medicine (Baltimore)* 1962;41:339–56.
41. Tahmoush AJ, Brooks JE, Keltner JL. Palatal myoclonus associated with abnormal ocular and extremity movements. A polygraphic study. *Arch Neurol* 1972;27:431–40.
42. Torvik A, Lindboe CF, Rodge S. Brain lesions in alcoholics. A neuropathological study with clinical correlations. *J Neurol Sci* 1982;56:233–48.
43. Yap CB, Mayo C, Carron K. "Ocular bobbing" in palatal myoclonus. *Arch Neurol* 1968;18:304–10.

Advances in Neurology, Vol. 43: Myoclonus,
edited by S. Fahn et al. Raven Press,
New York © 1986.

Essential Myoclonus

Susan Bressman and Stanley Fahn

*Department of Neurology, Columbia University College of Physicians and Surgeons; and
The Neurological Institute of New York, New York, New York 10032*

Essential myoclonus refers to a disorder in which myoclonus occurs as the sole neurological abnormality and etiology is unknown (12). Both hereditary and sporadic varieties have been described.

In their report of a family and review of the literature, Mahloudji and Pikielny (11) proposed criteria for the diagnosis of hereditary essential myoclonus. These included (a) onset of myoclonus before age 20 years, (b) dominant inheritance with variable severity, (c) benign course compatible with an active life of normal span, (d) absence of other neurological deficits, and (e) normal electroencephalogram (EEG). The six affected family members described displayed diffusely distributed myoclonus that was neither rhythmic nor synchronized. In several affected individuals, myoclonus increased with action; in one, it decreased with action. Other familial cases generally conform to this description of arrhythmic, diffusely distributed myoclonus (3,10).

In contrast to this defined inherited condition, sporadic essential myoclonus consists of a larger, more heterogenous group. In Aigner and Mulder's (1) review of 94 patients with myoclonus, 19 had neither seizures nor other neurological deficits, although the EEG was abnormal in six. This group can be considered to have essential myoclonus. Only one patient in this group had a family history of myoclonus. Age at onset varied from 4 to 86 years, with a mean of 20 years. Disability was not progressive, and stimuli, such as movement and bright light, tended to increase myoclonus.

To further characterize the clinical spectrum of essential myoclonus, we reviewed the records of our patients with myoclonus. Our criteria for inclusion were as follows: (a) myoclonus was the sole or primary neurological abnormality; and (b) there was no evidence of any preceding causal event or factor by history or laboratory examination (12). We did not exclude patients in whom we found mild ataxia (one patient) or tremor (two patients). These cases were specifically included in light of previous reports of familial essential myoclonus that described these coexistent abnormalities (3,9). We also did not exclude patients based on the character or distribution of the myoclonus. Thus patients with rhythmic or segmental myoclonus were included if history and examination failed to suggest an etiology.

TABLE 1. *Description of study population[a]*

Patient no.	Sex	Age at onset[b] (years)	Current age[c] (years)
1	F	2	21
2	M	7	9
3	F	14	32
4	F	15	22
5	M	15	26
6	M	18	23
7	F	24	32
8	F	27	28
9	M	28	31
10	M	31	34
11	M	33	35
12	M	46	51
13	M	54	66
14	F	60	61
15	M	64	71

[a]$N = 15$ (9 men, 6 women).
[b]Onset: Mean, 29 years; range, 2–64 years.
[c]Duration: Mean, 7.0 years; range, 1–19 years.

RESULTS

There were 15 patients (nine men and six women) (Table 1). Age at onset ranged from 2 to 64 years, with a mean of 29 years. Duration of illness varied from 1 to 19 years, with a mean of 7 years.

In no case was there marked progression of illness or disability. The course of illness was characterized, in general, by initial worsening followed by a stable or improved state. In nine patients, onset of symptoms occurred over weeks to months. In two, symptoms evolved over several years. In two others, sudden worsening occurred 2 and 15 years after onset. Only two patients had continued steady progression, and in both this was quite mild. All 15 patients were independent in daily activities, and most led fully active lives. One patient had an early retirement, and another was unable to find employment. At the most recent follow-up examination, eight were improved, seven in association with medical therapy. One patient learned to exercise voluntary control over her movements.

Only one patient (case 3) had a family history of myoclonus, which was compatible with autosomal dominant transmission. There was one other patient (case 13) with a family history of tremor affecting his mother and a maternal aunt. The patient himself had an action tremor. The association of tremor and myoclonus, occurring together and separately in members of a single large pedigree, was reported by Korten and colleagues (9). They postulated a single disease allele with phenotypic variation (i.e., tremor or myoclonus, or both) of the involuntary movements; our patient may belong to this same genetic subclass.

Aside from this patient with action tremor, one other patient, without a family history of tremor or myoclonus, also had action tremor. All other patients had normal examinations, except for one young woman (case 1) who displayed mild limb and gait ataxia (Table 2).

Laboratory evaluation was uniformly unrevealing. The EEGs, performed on 13 patients, were normal. Cerebrospinal fluid was examined in 11, and routine studies (protein, glucose, cell count, and VDRL) were normal except for mild elevations of protein (all <57 mg/dl) in four. Ten patients had computerized tomography scans of the head; eight were normal and two showed mild atrophy. Somatosensory evoked responses, measured in seven patients, were unremarkable. Seven patients had electromyogram (EMG) studies. These confirmed or enhanced the clinical assessment of distribution, rhythmicity, and the temporal relationship or synchronicity of widely distributed contractions.

We analyzed the characteristics of the myoclonus according to distribution, rhythmicity, synchrony, presence at rest and with action, stimulus sensitivity, and response to ethanol. Rhythmicity included not only the usual regularly repeating contractions but also oscillatory myoclonus, that is, transient bursts of fairly regular contractions that have waxing and waning amplitude (4). Synchrony was assessed clinically and referred to the simultaneous occurrence of jerks regardless of distribution.

The most frequently involved body regions were the trunk and proximal limbs, then the neck and face (Tables 2 and 3). Distal limbs were infrequently involved. In nine patients, the myoclonus was focal or segmental; involved regions were the right arm in one, both lower extremities in another, cranium in two, and the trunk in five. Occasionally, patients with trunk involvement had spread of myoclonus to the shoulder, neck, or thighs. One patient had neck involvement for 15 years before spread to the trunk. Six had diffuse or multifocal involvement. In two of these patients, onset was segmental with subsequent spread to involve at least both legs and one arm.

Ten patients had synchronized contractions (Table 2). All but one, a patient with diffuse (or generalized) oscillatory myoclonus, had segmental distribution. Synchrony was not absolutely constant; one patient (case 10), with rhythmic synchronized contraction of the tensor velli palatini muscle, had asynchrony between the right and left. Asynchronized contractions occurred in five patients; all were of widespread distribution.

Two patients had rhythmic myoclonus (Table 2). Rhythmicity was not perfect, with contractions varying in frequency from 1 to 3/sec. Rhythmic myoclonus was restricted to cranial and cervical musculature in one patient and an arm in the other. Four patients had oscillatory myoclonus: in two the trunk was involved, in one the neck and trunk, and in one distribution was generalized. The remaining nine patients had arrhythmic myoclonus, although bursts of regularly repeating contractions occurred in three.

The effect of action on myoclonus was quite variable (Table 2). Twelve patients had spontaneous myoclonus. In two of these patients, both of whom had segmental truncal involvement, jerks were more likely to occur when the patient was lying and diminished with standing and walking. Another patient (case 4) found that

TABLE 2. *Characteristics in 15*

Patient no.	Family history	Examination otherwise	Regions affected
1	No	Mild gait + limb ataxia, dysarthria	Arms, legs, trunk (multifocal)
2	No	Normal	Arms, buttocks, legs, face (multifocal)
3	Yes, myoclonus	Normal	Necks, trunk (segmental)
4	No	Normal	Proximal legs, arms, face, trunk (multifocal)
5	No	Normal	Neck, trunk, legs, arms (generalized)
6	No	Normal	Thighs, right arm, trunk (multifocal)
7	No	Normal	Face, legs, trunk, arms (multifocal)
8	No	Normal	Face, neck, rarely shoulders (segmental)
9	No	Postural tremor	Right arm (focal)
10	No	Normal	Tensor velli palatine, palate, pharynx, tongue (segmental)
11	No	Normal	Trunk, shoulder (segmental)
12	No	Normal	Trunk, neck to thighs (segmental)
13	Yes, tremor	Action tremor	Trunk, neck (segmental)
14	No	Normal	Legs (segmental)
15	No	Normal	Trunk (segmental)

complex activity decreased myoclonus. On the other hand, two patients with spontaneous myoclonus had an increase of myoclonus with specific actions. In one case, speaking and writing induced generalized oscillations, and in another, forehead wrinkling produced lower facial and neck contractions. Three patients had myoclonus primarily with action. Two of these patients had oscillatory myoclonus with changes in posture, such as bending or arising from a chair. One woman had arrhythmic myoclonus with intention. In addition to action, other modulators of myoclonus included stretch sensitivity in five patients, painful stimuli in one, and touch in another. Stimulus sensitivity was seen in patients with multifocal and segmental myoclonus as well as in patients with spontaneous and action-induced jerks. Nine patients either drank ethanol or were tested for its effect; five had benefit, and again, this was not related to distribution or the effect of action.

Fourteen patients elected to take medication. Clonazepam was given to 13 in dosages ranging from 1 to 20 mg/day; 10 responded. Two had resolution of symptoms (with dosages of 3.0 mg/day), which has been sustained for 2 and 3 years. Four had moderate improvement (at least 50% reduction), and four had mild improvement (less than 50% reduction). Three had no response with dosages ranging from 2.5 to 12 mg/day. Valproate was given to seven patients. There was *patients with essential myoclonus*

Synchrony	Rhythmicity	Spontaneous/action
No	No	Action (initiation, intention)
No	No	Spontaneous
Yes	Oscillatory	Spontaneous
No	No	Spontaneous; ↓ with action
Yes	Oscillatory	Spontaneous, ↑ with action (activate distant part with writing)
No	No	Spontaneous
No	No	Spontaneous
Yes	No	Spontaneous, ↑ with action (raise eyebrow)
Yes	No	Spontaneous
Asynchrony right and left	Yes	Spontaneous
Yes	No	Spontaneous (positional lying, sitting > standing)
Yes	No	Spontaneous (positional lying, sitting > standing)
Yes	Oscillatory	Action (change in position, squatting)
Yes	No	Spontaneous
Yes	Oscillatory	Action (initiating walking)

no change in five receiving between 1 and 3 g/day. One patient had complete resolution while on 750 mg/day, which has been sustained for 1 year. Other medications were tried in several patients who did not respond to either clonazepam or valproate. These included methysergide, cyproheptadine, trazadone, reserpine, tetrabenazine, baclofen, clonidine, carbamazepine, propranolol, L-tryptophan, and L-5-hydroxytryptophan. None of these produced more than mild improvement,

TABLE 3. *Distribution of myoclonus in 15 patients*

Region	No.
Trunk	9
Legs	8
Arms	5
Neck	5
Face	4
Right arm	2
Buttocks	1
Oral cavity	1

TABLE 4. *Categories of patients with essential myoclonus* [a]

Oscillatory myoclonus	Rhythmic segmental myoclonus
3 Men, 1 woman (2 familial)	2 Men
14, 15, 54, 64 years at onset	28, 31 Years at onset
3 Primarily trunk, 1 generalized	1 Cranial, 1 upper limb
2 Spontaneous; ↑ with action	Not stimulus sensitive
2 Action (posture change)	1 Markedly improved with valproate
2/4 Stretch sensitive	and 1 with clonazepam
3/3 Ethanol responsive	*Nonrhythmic multifocal myoclonus*
1/3 Markedly improved with	2 Men, 3 women
clonazepam	2, 7, 15, 18, 24 Years at onset
Nonrhythmic segmental myoclonus	Asynchronous
2 Men, 2 women	Proximal → distal limbs, trunk, face
27, 33, 46, 60 Years at onset	1/5 Stimulus sensitive
1 Cranial, 2 trunk, 1 thighs,	1/5 ↑ With action, 1/5 ↓ without
synchronous	action
4/4 Spontaneous; 1 ↑ with action and	2/3 Ethanol responsive
2 positional (lying → standing)	1/4 Moderate response to clonazepam
4/4 Stimulus sensitive	
3/4 Improved with clonazepam	

[a]Fractions indicate number of patients with positive finding (numerator) divided by the maximum number of patients tested for this finding (denominator).

although in several instances, dosage or duration of therapy was limited by unacceptable side effects.

DISCUSSION

Our review of 15 patients with essential myoclonus revealed a heterogenous group with respect to age at onset, sex, response to action, sensory stimuli, alcohol, and medication. On review of the salient characteristics of the myoclonus itself, however, we discerned four subcategories (Table 4): (a) oscillatory myoclonus, (b) rhythmic segmental myoclonus, (c) nonrhythmic segmental myoclonus, and (d) nonrhythmic multifocal myoclonus.

There were four patients with oscillatory myoclonus. Myoclonus occurred or increased with specific actions but was not particularly induced by fast movement, as seen in ballistic overflow myoclonus (6). It tended to diminish with ethanol ingestion but was generally resistant to medical therapy, although clonazepam was quite effective in one patient. The two patients with family histories of involuntary movements (myoclonus in one, tremor in another) both had oscillatory myoclonus.

There were two patients, both men, with rhythmic segmental myoclonus. Neither had evidence that suggested an etiology, despite the general assumption that segmental myoclonus (particularly if rhythmic) is symptomatic (2,5,7,8). Both patients had excellent responses to medication (one to valproate and the other to clonazepam).

Four patients had nonrhythmic segmental myoclonus. In two of these patients, however, there were rhythmic bursts of 1 to 3 Hz. All were synchronous and stimulus sensitive. Three responded to clonazepam.

Nonrhythmic multifocal myoclonus occurred in five patients. This group had a younger age at onset; all cases began by age 24 years. Jerks were asynchronous and widespread. Response to action, stretch, touch, and ethanol was quite variable, and only one of four responded to medication. One patient learned to voluntarily control jerks, which had always decreased with complex or fine motor tasks. This last group is similar in several respects to previously reported familial cases; that is, widespread asynchronous myoclonus began in the first two decades of life but did not interfere significantly with an active life.

Despite the emphasis generally placed on familial essential myoclonus, our group of patients with essential myoclonus contained only two individuals with significant family histories. In both cases, myoclonus was not asynchronous and multifocal but oscillatory and restricted in distribution.

We also found that most of our patients had segmental distribution (in two cases rhythmic) despite a careful screen for etiology. Whether segmental arrhythmic myoclonus represents a restricted form of generalized or multifocal essential myoclonus cannot be determined, although there is reason to suggest this is so. Two cases of multifocal myoclonus did appear initially in one region, and in two cases of segmental arrhythmic myoclonus, occasional spread to adjacent regions was seen. Oscillatory myoclonus did occur in both segmental and generalized distributions, and these were grouped together. Furthermore, the sharp distinction drawn between rhythmic and arrhythmic oscillations was not distinctly seen in our patients. In two patients, considered to have arrhythmic contractions, myoclonus was at times quite regular, suggesting a continuum between arrhythmic and rhythmic segmental myoclonus.

Essential myoclonus consists of diverse subgroups of patients, some of clearly genetic origin. Biochemical, pharmacological, and other means have not elucidated the underlying mechanism of myoclonus in these patients. The clinical subcategories described in this chapter may prove, in future studies, to be pathophysiologically distinct.

SUMMARY

The clinical characteristics of 15 patients with essential myoclonus are evaluated. The course of illness was one of initial worsening followed by a stable or improved state. Only two patients had positive family histories of involuntary movements. Nine patients had segmental distribution despite a careful search for etiology; in two of these patients, myoclonus was rhythmic. The trunk and proximal limbs were the most frequently affected body regions. Clonazepam improved myoclonus in 10 of 13 patients, two of whom had complete resolution of symptoms. On review of the salient features of the myoclonus, we discerned four phenomenological subcategories: (a) oscillatory myoclonus, (b) rhythmic segmental myoclonus, (c) nonrhythmic segmental myoclonus, and (d) nonrhythmic multifocal myoclonus.

REFERENCES

1. Aigner BR, Mulder DW. Myoclonus. Clinical significance and an approach to classification. *Arch Neurol* 1960; 2:600–15.
2. Campbell AMG, Garland H. Subacute myoclonic spinal neuronitis. *J Neurol Neurosurg Psychiatry* 1956; 19:268–74.
3. Daube J, Peters HA. Hereditary essential myoclonus. *Arch Neurol (NY)* 1966; 15:587–94.
4. Fahn S, Singh N. An oscillating form of essential myoclonus. *Neurology* 1981; 31:80.
5. Garcin R, Rondot P, Guiot G. Rhythmic myoclonus of the right arm as the presenting symptom of a cervical cord tumour. *Brain* 1968; 91:75–84.
6. Hallett M, Chadwick D, Marsden CD. Ballistic movement overflow myoclonus. A form of essential myoclonus. *Brain* 1977; 100:299–312.
7. Hoehn MM, Cherington M. Spinal myoclonus. *Neurology (NY)* 1977; 27:942–6.
8. Koike H, Yodhino Y. Spinal myoclonus with dermal and retinal changes affected by myelitis. *Arch Neurol* 1977; 34:383–5.
9. Korten JJ, Notermans SLH, Frenken CWGM, Gabreels FJM, Joosten EMG. Familial essential myoclonus. *Brain* 1974; 97:131–8.
10. Lindenmulder FG. Familial myoclonus occurring in three successive generations. *J Nerv Ment Dis* 1933; 77:489–91.
11. Mahloudji M, Pikielny RT. Hereditary essential myoclonus. *Brain* 1967; 90:669–74.
12. Marsden CD, Hallett M, Fahn S. The nosology and pathophysiology of myoclonus. In: Marsden CD, Fahn S, eds. Movements disorders. London: Butterworth, 1982:196–248.

Advances in Neurology, Vol. 43: Myoclonus,
edited by S. Fahn et al. Raven Press,
New York © 1986.

Nocturnal Myoclonus and Restless Legs Syndrome

E. Lugaresi, F. Cirignotta, G. Coccagna, and P. Montagna

Institute of Neurology, University of Bologna, 40123 Bologna, Italy

The term *nocturnal myoclonus* was first introduced by Symonds (37) in a clinical report of five patients affected with "involuntary clonic movements at night." No electromyographic or polygraphic investigations were performed, however, and the author wrongly classified his patients as "epilepsy variants." Symonds' cases varied considerably, but case 4 had familial restless legs syndrome. On the basis of polygraphic and clinical studies in four cases, Oswald (33) rejected Symonds' patients as epileptics and refuted the very existence of a syndrome characterized by nocturnal myoclonus. He concluded that the sudden bodily jerks he recorded in his cases represented physiological phenomena, more or less usual on falling asleep. Retrospectively, however, Oswald's case W. probably had restless legs syndrome.

Nocturnal polygraphic recordings performed from 1965 to 1968 allow us to state the following: (a) Almost all patients affected with restless legs syndrome show periodic movements during sleep which should not be confused with sudden physiological bodily jerks; and (b) similar periodic sleep movements may also occur unassociated with restless legs syndrome. We suggested that besides restless legs syndrome, defined as such by Ekbom (15,16) but described much earlier by Willis (39) and Wittmaack (40), there exists a distinct nosological entity which we have continued to term nocturnal myoclonus in Symonds' honor.

Coleman et al. (11) later reported that nocturnal myoclonus may also occur among normal subjects. To better define the phenomenon, the authors proposed the term *periodic movements in sleep*. More recently, Bixler et al. (4) and Coleman et al. (12) showed that whereas nocturnal myoclonus is a rare finding in young people, it is relatively common in the elderly and thus may not represent an absolutely abnormal finding.

In this chapter, the term nocturnal myoclonus is used throughout for practical purposes, even though we are well aware that, from a purely semantic point of view, the phenomenon cannot be considered a true myoclonus. Furthermore, the term periodic movements in sleep does not account for the fact that the jerks may arise also in wakefulness, as in the restless legs syndrome.

CLINICAL FEATURES OF NOCTURNAL MYOCLONUS

Nocturnal myoclonus is a varied motor phenomenon. In its simplest and most common form, it consists of a dorsiflexion of the big toe and/or the foot. When the phenomenon becomes more intense and diffuse, there appears a flexion of the leg on the thigh and of the thigh on the trunk. Rarely, the forearm may also flex at the elbow.

The contraction of each muscle involved has a mean duration of 1.5 to 2.5 sec, with limits of 0.5 to 5 sec (10). It often begins with a myoclonic jerk, followed, after a short interval, by a tonic contraction. In rare cases, the initial myoclonic jerk is lacking. More often, repeated myoclonic jerks occur at the beginning of each single movement (Fig. 1). Occasionally, repetitive, small-amplitude rhythmic activity may be found in the intervals between episodes of nocturnal myoclonus (7). Overall, the pattern of nocturnal myoclonus resembles that of a triple flexion reflex, even though muscular activity frequently occurs in the sural muscles as well. Nocturnal myoclonus may affect only one or both of the lower limbs; more often, both extremities are involved but usually not symmetrically or simultaneously. Sometimes the phenomenon alternates in each leg (7).

One of the more typical features of nocturnal myoclonus is its spontaneous repetition at periodic intervals; in fact, it tends to recur every 20 to 40 sec with limits of 4 to 90 sec (10), sometimes for many minutes at a time with marked regularity (Fig. 2). By means of complex polygraphic recordings, we have been able to demonstrate that the rhythm of nocturnal myoclonus follows the periodic oscillations that simultaneously involve the electroencephalogram (EEG), heart rate, blood pressure, and breathing activity (25,27). Thus nocturnal myoclonus is usually associated with a K complex on the EEG, an increase in heart rate and blood pressure, and a deepening of breathing. It can therefore be considered as part of a complex arousal phenomenon affecting cortical activity and the motor and autonomic systems at the same time (Figs. 3 and 4). We have tried to elucidate the mechanism of nocturnal myoclonus by means of electrophysiological manipulations. The H reflexes obtained repetitively during sleep in patients showed periodic variations, but these did not have the same timing as nocturnal myoclonus. Direct repetitive electrical stimulation of the peroneal nerve during sleep triggered a tonic contraction similar to nocturnal myoclonus and modified the rhythm of the spontaneously occurring phenomenon. Electrical tactile and noxious stimuli of the foot did not seem to affect nocturnal myoclonus and its rhythm; sometimes, high-intensity noxious stimuli transiently inhibited it. Finally, by back averaging the

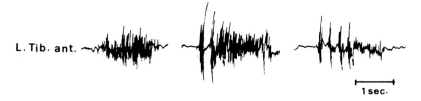

L. Tib. ant.

1 sec.

FIG. 1. Examples of the more usual types of jerks in nocturnal myoclonus as recorded on the left tibialis anterior (L. Tib. ant.) muscle. From left to right: tonic contraction, lasting ∼1.5 sec; myoclonic jerk followed, after a short interval, by a more tonic contraction; polyclonic jerks with a late tonic component.

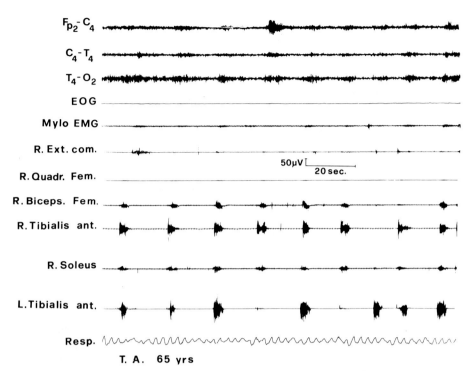

FIG. 2. Nocturnal myoclonus recorded over several leg muscles shows a remarkable periodicity (12–20 sec). It may occur asynchronously in both legs. N-REM sleep. (EOG) electrooculogram; (Mylo EMG) chin muscles EMG; (Ext. com.) extensor digitorum communis; (Quadr. Fem.) quadriceps femoris; (Biceps Fem.) biceps femoris; (Tibialis ant.) tibalis anterior; (Resp.) respirogram.

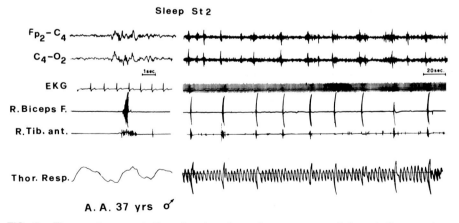

FIG. 3. The spontaneous rhythm of nocturnal myoclonus corresponds to periodic arousals as indicated by K complexes on EEG (*left*, high speed), increased heart rate, and deeper breathing movements (*right*, low speed). Sleep stage 2. (Biceps F.) biceps femoris; (Tib. ant.) tibialis anterior; (Thor. Resp.) thoracic respiration.

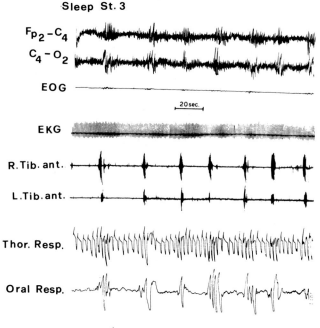

FIG. 4. Nocturnal myoclonus in a patient with sleep apnea. The muscle jerks are associated with EEG activation and tachycardia and occur at resumption of breathing movements after obstructive apneas. Sleep stage 3. (EOG) electrooculogram; (Tib. ant.) tibialis anterior; [Thor. (Oral) Resp.] thoracic (oral) respirogram.

jerks in one case of restless leg syndrome and in two cases of nocturnal myoclonus, we were unable to find any preceding cortical events time-locked to the movements (Fig. 5).

The periodic jerks of nocturnal myoclonus unassociated with restless legs syndrome *(essential nocturnal myoclonus)* arise, with rare exceptions, when the patient is already asleep. They are particularly evident during light sleep (stages 1–2), decrease during deep sleep (stages 3–4), and occur only sporadically or completely disappear during rapid eye movement (REM) sleep. When they persist also during REM sleep, they are attenuated during the bursts of eye movements. On the contrary, in restless legs syndrome, it is a rule to find nocturnal myoclonus when the patient is still awake (Fig. 6), although the pattern of periodic jerks during sleep is the same as that found in nocturnal myoclonus not associated with restless legs syndrome (essential nocturnal myoclonus) (7). Sleep in such patients is extremely disturbed by the repeated and prolonged awakenings caused by the paresthesia and motor agitation (8).

CLASSIFICATION OF NOCTURNAL MYOCLONUS

Essential Nocturnal Myoclonus

Essential nocturnal myoclonus (i.e., nocturnal myoclonus as an isolated finding) represents a sleep phenomenon that is neither the effect nor the origin of any other

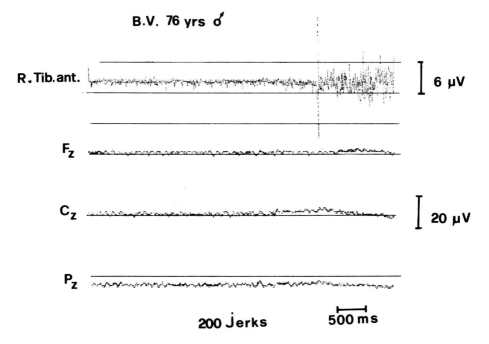

FIG. 5. Back averaging of 200 jerks from the right anterior tibial (R. Tib. ant.) muscle in a 76-year-old patient with nocturnal myoclonus. No related cortical events are seen on EEG in the preceding 4 sec (F_z, C_z, P_z leads referred to linked mastoids; frequency limits, 0.5 Hz–1 kHz).

disturbances, such as insomnia. In fact, its prevalence is similar among insomniacs and normal controls (20). Nocturnal myoclonus is an age-related condition. It is almost absent below the age of 30 years and occurs in 5% of normal subjects aged 30 to 50 years and in 29% of those over 50 years. It seems to affect males slightly more than females (4). Furthermore, in a longitudinal study of 14 patients followed for 1 to 9 years, Coleman et al. (12) demonstrated that nocturnal myoclonus tends to increase with advancing age. These studies diminish the clinical significance of nocturnal myoclonus, but it should be kept in mind that isolated cases may also report nocturnal myoclonus during wakefulness and of such intensity as to hinder falling asleep.

Symptomatic Nocturnal Myoclonus and Restless Legs Syndrome

Restless legs syndrome is characterized by deep, ill-defined paresthesia of the legs, which mainly arises during prolonged muscular rest or when the patient is drowsy and trying to fall asleep. These sensations are relieved by motor agitation and fidgeting movements of the legs or by walking. We have repeatedly underlined the close association between restless legs syndrome and nocturnal myoclonus; there are hardly any patients with restless legs syndrome who present paresthesia and motor agitation alone (7,25). In patients affected with restless legs syndrome, sleep disturbances may be quite severe (8), but it is difficult to ascertain whether

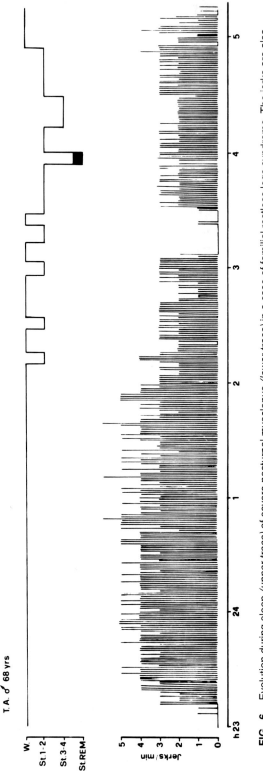

FIG. 6. Evolution during sleep *(upper trace)* of severe nocturnal myoclonus *(lower trace)* in a case of familial restless legs syndrome. The jerks are also present during wakefulness and persist attenuated during light sleep and even during a single episode of REM sleep. The pattern of sleep is grossly disrupted.

insomnia is due only to the motor agitation and the paresthesia or, at least in part, to the particularly intense and persistent myoclonic jerks. Ekbom (15,16) and Coccagna et al. (7) noticed that restless legs syndrome is often a familial disturbance; one case of nocturnal myoclonus reported by Symonds (37) was also familial.

More detailed studies of familial cases of both nocturnal myoclonus and restless legs syndrome (5,29) showed that the disease is transmitted as an autosomal dominant trait, with onset in the second decade and with the tendency to persist for a lifetime. Boghen and Peyronnard (5) also reported that some components of their family did not show restless legs syndrome but only nocturnal myoclonus. Both have been reported associated with chronic myelopathies and peripheral neuropathies (24), anemia (3,31), gastric surgery (2,17), uremia (6), pregnancy (15), chronic pulmonary disease (34), and startle disease (13,23). In the light of recent epidemiological data, it is difficult to say whether these anecdotal reports indicate a causal relationship between restless legs syndrome and these conditions. In this connection, we also found nocturnal myoclonus associated with Isaacs' syndrome (three of three cases) (Fig. 7), stiff-man syndrome (28) (two of two cases), Huntington's chorea (three of four cases), and amyotrophic lateral sclerosis (two of three cases). These are preliminary findings, however, and only systematic investigations will allow us to establish whether other neurological disorders besides restless legs syndrome favor the onset of nocturnal myoclonus.

DIFFERENTIAL DIAGNOSIS OF NOCTURNAL MYOCLONUS

A diagnosis of nocturnal myoclonus can be made confidently only by means of polygraphic recordings performed during sleep. The muscles most commonly involved are the anterior tibial and the peroneal group. The characteristics of the muscular contraction, its distribution pattern, and the periodic jerks make recognition on polygraphic recordings quite simple. There are some physiological phenomena of muscular jerking, however, that have often been confused in past literature and which should be clearly differentiated from nocturnal myoclonus: (a) partial myoclonic jerks, first described by De Lisi in 1932 (14), and (b) massive myoclonic jerks (or sudden bodily jerks or "sleep starts") described by Oswald (33) and by Gastaut and Broughton (18).

Both of these phenomena occur in normal subjects and are devoid of any pathological significance. Partial myoclonic jerks consist of localized muscle jerks of very short duration (10–100 msec) and arise spontaneously and irregularly, especially in the distal muscles. They are particularly evident during light (stage 1) and REM sleep. Massive myoclonic jerks usually consist of sporadic muscle contractions involving simultaneously the axial muscles and the proximal muscles of the limbs but sometimes confined to a single limb.

They last ≥ 1 sec, arise when the subject is falling asleep or during light sleep (stages 1–2), and are favored by a sudden noise. They are associated with intense arousal phenomena, such as feeling a "shock" or "falling into the void," reappearance of the alpha rhythm and/or K complex on the EEG, tachycardia, and marked

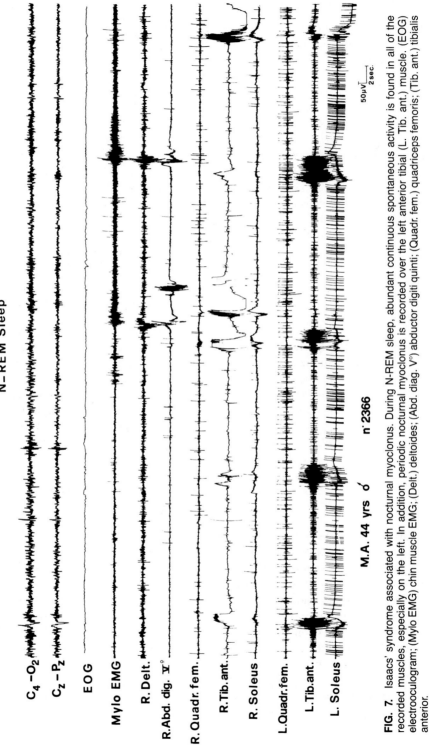

N-REM Sleep

C$_4$-O$_2$

C$_z$-P$_z$

EOG

Mylo EMG

R. Delt.

R. Abd. dig. V°

R. Quadr. fem.

R. Tib. ant.

R. Soleus

L. Quadr. fem.

L. Tib. ant.

L. Soleus

50µV | 2 sec.

M.A. 44 yrs ♂   n° 2366

FIG. 7. Isaacs' syndrome associated with nocturnal myoclonus. During N-REM sleep, abundant continuous spontaneous activity is found in all of the recorded muscles, especially on the left. In addition, periodic nocturnal myoclonus is recorded over the left anterior tibial (L. Tib. ant.) muscle. (EOG) electrooculogram; (Mylo EMG) chin muscle EMG; (Delt.) deltoides; (Abd. diag. V°) abductor digiti quinti; (Quadr. fem.) quadriceps femoris; (Tib. ant.) tibialis anterior.

electrodermal activity. Both clinically and polygraphically, therefore, they are similar to the startle reaction during wakefulness (Fig. 8).

Nocturnal myoclonus should also be differentiated from other clearly abnormal motor phenomena, such as hyperekplexia or startle disease (1,19,36). In cases showing severe startle disease, both Suhren et al. (36) and Gastaut and Villeneuve (19) reported the presence of nocturnal myoclonus. In more recent papers (21), prominent nocturnal myoclonus was considered to be a feature typical of hyperekplexia. This constitutes a confusion in terminology, however, since analysis of the polygraphic recordings obtained during sleep in hyperekplexia shows that the nocturnal jerks are more similar to the massive myoclonic jerks than to nocturnal myoclonus. This does not mean that severe nocturnal myoclonus cannot be found in minor forms of startle disease, and we have described a patient with hyperekplexia associated with nocturnal myoclonus (23).

Another syndrome that should be kept distinct from restless legs syndrome (and nocturnal myoclonus) is the syndrome of "painful legs and moving toes" (35). In this disorder, pain is severe and burning, cannot be relieved by movements of the legs or by walking as in restless legs syndrome, and is not related to the sleep–wake cycle. Furthermore, the spontaneous movements are not periodic and decrease during sleep (30).

The differential diagnosis of nocturnal myoclonus should also take into consideration nocturnal leg cramps, which consist of sporadic, painful, spasmodic contractions, usually limited to the calf muscles or to the small muscles of the sole of the foot. These cramps are brought about by sudden forceful contractions of the lower extremities and are relieved by stretching of the muscles involved (22,38).

Finally, nocturnal myoclonus should be differentiated from the epileptic myoclonias, which can be quite varied and may also occur periodically. However, they usually show an EEG correlate and, while being evident during wakefulness, always decrease or disappear during sleep (26).

PATHOGENESIS OF NOCTURNAL MYOCLONUS

Causative Factors

Nocturnal myoclonus is an age-related paraphysiological phenomenon. In restless legs syndrome, however, it appears very early in the course of the disease and is associated with other disturbances. It is rather prominent and is present also during wakefulness. Thus one may ask whether nocturnal myoclonus, which often represents a quasinormal finding, may not in some cases assume a pathological meaning. The same considerations apply to the startle reaction, which, while often being a physiological reflex phenomenon, may in severe cases be found as a familial disease genetically transmitted. From the same point of view, restless legs syndrome could be interpreted as a pathological variant of nocturnal myoclonus, sometimes genetically determined. The persistence of the muscle jerks during relaxation and their association with paresthesia and motor agitation would mark the onset of an overt disease state.

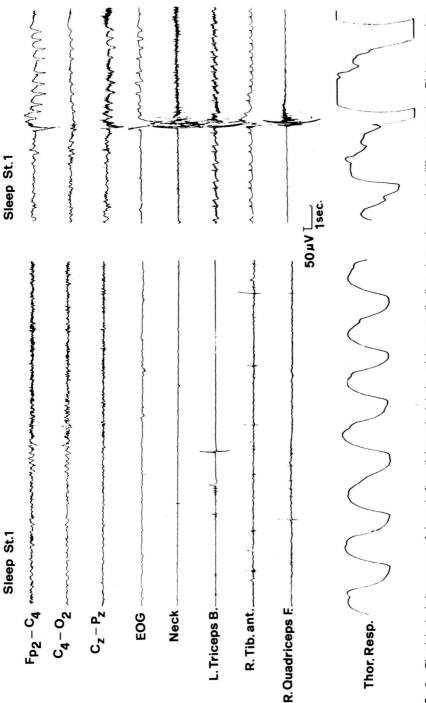

FIG. 8. Physiological phenomena of sleep. *Left*, partial myoclonic jerks, arising sporadically and asynchronously in different muscles. *Right*, a massive myoclonic jerk, or "sleep start," consisting of a sudden contraction of all muscles, lasting about 1 sec and associated with irregular respiration. Sleep stage 1. (EOG) electrooculogram; (Triceps B.) triceps brachii; (Tib. ant.) tibialis anterior; (Quadriceps F.) quadriceps femoris; (Thor. Resp.) thoracic respiration.

Pathogenetic Hypotheses

It is unnecessary to enumerate all the pathogenetic hypotheses that have been proposed as an explanation for nocturnal myoclonus and restless legs syndrome since almost every author has his or her personal views. We mention yet again the oldest and still widely held theory that restless legs syndrome is a psychosomatic disorder simply to underline that the genetically determined cases, the presence of spontaneous jerks during sleep, and the lack of true neurotic traits in many of these patients indicate that it has a clear organic pathogenesis.

With respect to the origin of nocturnal myoclonus, the complex muscular pattern that resembles a flexion reflex and the lack of preceding EEG events on back averaging make a cortical origin improbable. It becomes more difficult to differentiate between a spinal or supraspinal origin. The periodic pattern of the jerks and the demonstration that they occur associated with arousal phenomena involving the cortex and the circulatory and respiratory systems suggest that nocturnal myoclonus is modulated by a pacemaker, which is probably located at the reticular level (25,27). In our opinion, this does not mean that the phenomenon in itself arises at this level. In conclusion, nocturnal myoclonus can be regarded as a subcortical event, probably regulated in its periodicity by reticular discharges but whose level of origin cannot yet be determined with certainty.

TREATMENT

Nocturnal myoclonus per se, in its essential form, does not constitute a clinical problem; it does not disturb the patient, does not disrupt sleep, and therefore does not require treatment. On the other hand, restless legs syndrome does constitute a clinical problem due to its detrimental effects on sleep. Unfortunately, the disease runs a chronic and prolonged course and is scarcely affected by medications (29). A wide number of drugs have been tried by several authors, usually with scant and always transient effects. We found in uncontrolled trials, however, that baclofen and benzodiazepines, in particular diazepam, may prove to be of some help in restless legs syndrome (9), and preliminary uncontrolled trials have demonstrated beneficial effects of clonazepam (32). On the basis of these findings, we recently confirmed the significant effect of this drug in a controlled trial versus placebo. The long-term efficacy of the drug, however, requires further testing.

SUMMARY

Nocturnal myoclonus (or periodic movements in sleep) consists of stereotyped sleep-related movements of the lower limbs and occasionally also upper limbs, ranging from simple dorsiflexion of the big toe and foot to a triple flexion of the entire leg. It is characterized by a typical periodicity, often occurring in association with sleep arousal phenomena. As an isolated finding (essential nocturnal myoclonus), it represents a paraphysiological phenomenon, also found in normal subjects and developing with advancing age. On the other hand, symptomatic nocturnal myoclonus is typically associated with restless legs syndrome; in this condition, it is usually severe and present also during wakefulness.

The exact site of origin of nocturnal myoclonus is unknown. It is almost certainly a subcortical phenomenon, probably modulated in its periodicity by reticular influences. It has frequently been confused with, and should be clearly differentiated from, other normal jerking movements of sleep, such as partial myoclonic jerks and massive myoclonic jerks, or sleep starts. Other abnormal movements that may be confused with nocturnal myoclonus are the startles of hyperekplexia, the syndrome of painful legs and moving toes, nocturnal leg cramps, and the numerous varieties of epileptic myoclonus.

REFERENCES

1. Andermann F, Keene DL, Andermann E, Quesney LF. Startle disease or hyperekplexia. Further delineation of the syndrome. *Brain* 1980;103:985–97.
2. Banerji NK, Hurwitz LJ. Restless legs syndrome, with particular reference to its occurrence after gastric surgery. *Br Med J* 1970;4:774–5.
3. Behrman S. Disturbed relaxation of the limbs. *Br Med J* 1958;1:1454–7.
4. Bixler EO, Kales A, Vela-Bueno A, Jacoby JA, Scarone S, Soldatos CR. Nocturnal myoclonus and nocturnal myoclonic activity in a normal population. *Res Commun Chem Pathol Pharmacol* 1982;36:129–40.
5. Boghen D, Peyronnard JM. Myoclonus in familial restless legs syndrome. *Arch Neurol* 1976;33:368–70.
6. Callaghan N. Restless legs syndrome in uremic neuropathy. *Neurology (NY)* 1966;16:359–61.
7. Coccagna G, Lugaresi E, Tassinari CA, Ambrosetto C. La sindrome delle gambe senza riposo (restless legs). *Omnia Med Ther* 1966;44:619–87.
8. Coccagna G, Lugaresi E. Insomnia in the restless legs syndrome. In: Gastaut H, Lugaresi E, Berti-Ceroni G, Coccagna G, eds. The abnormalities of sleep in man. Bologna: Gaggi Editore, 1968:139–44.
9. Coccagna G, Lugaresi E. Anxietas tibiarum und nächtliche Myokloni. *Z EEG EMG* 1978;9:155–60.
10. Coleman RM. Periodic movements in sleep (nocturnal myoclonus) and the restless legs syndrome. In: Guilleminault C, ed. Sleeping and waking disorders. Indications and techniques. Menlo Park: Addison-Wesley, 1982:265–95.
11. Coleman RM, Pollack CP, Weitzman ED. Periodic movements in sleep (nocturnal myoclonus): relation to sleep disorders. *Ann Neurol* 1980;8:416–21.
12. Coleman RM, Bliwise DL, Sajben N, De Bruyn L, Boomkamp A, Menn ME, Dement WC. Epidemiology of periodic movements during sleep. In: Guilleminault C, Lugaresi E, eds. Sleep/wake disorders: natural history, epidemiology, and long-term evolution. New York: Raven Press, 1983:217–29.
13. De Groen JHM, Kamphuisen HAC. Periodic nocturnal myoclonus in a patient with hyperexplexia (startle disease). *J Neurol Sci* 1978;38:207–213.
14. De Lisi L. Su di un fenomeno motorio costante del sonno normale: le mioclonie ipniche fisiologiche. *Riv Patol Nerv Ment* 1932;39:481–96.
15. Ekbom KA. Restless legs. *Acta Med Scand [Suppl]* 1945;158:4–122.
16. Ekbom KA. Restless legs syndrome. *Neurology (NY)* 1960;10:868–73.
17. Ekbom KA. Restless legs syndrome after partial gastrectomy. *Acta Neurol Scand* 1966;2:79–89.
18. Gastaut H, Broughton R. A clinical and polygraphic study of episodic phenomena during sleep. *Recent Adv Biol Psychiatry* 1965;7:197–221.
19. Gastaut H, Villeneuve A. The startle disease or hyperekplexia. Pathological surprise reaction. *J Neurol Sci* 1967;5:523–42.
20. Kales A, Bixler EO, Soldatos CR, Vela-Bueno A, Caldwell AB, Cadieux RJ. Biopsychobehavioral correlates of insomnia, part 1: role of sleep apnea and nocturnal myoclonus. *Psychosomatics* 1982;23:1–5.
21. Kurczynski TW. Hyperekplexia. *Arch Neurol* 1983;40:246–8.

22. Layzer RB, Rowland LP. Cramps. *N Engl J Med* 1971;285:31–40.
23. Lugaresi E, Gambi D, Berti Ceroni G. Sur un cas clinique de sursauts pathologiques, chutes spontanées et syndrome myoclonique nocturne. *Rev Neurol (Paris)* 1966;115:202–8.
24. Lugaresi E, Coccagna G, Berti Ceroni G, Ambrosetto C. Mioclonie notturne sintomatiche. *Sist Nerv* 1967;19:71–80.
25. Lugaresi E, Coccagna G, Berti Ceroni G, Ambrosetto C. Restless legs syndrome and nocturnal myoclonus. In: Gastaut H, Lugaresi E, Berti Ceroni G, Coccagna G, eds. The abnormalities of sleep in man. Bologna: Gaggi Editore, 1968:285–94.
26. Lugaresi E, Coccagna G, Mantovani M, Berti Ceroni G, Pazzaglia P, Tassinari CA. The evolution of different types of myoclonus during sleep. A polygraphic study. *Eur Neurol* 1970;4:321–31.
27. Lugaresi E, Coccagna G, Mantovani M, Lebrun R. Some periodic phenomena arising during drowsiness and sleep in man. *Electroencephalogr Clin Neurophysiol* 1972;32:701–5.
28. Martinelli P, Pazzaglia P, Montagna P, Coccagna G, Rizzuto N, Simonati S, Lugaresi E. Stiff-man syndrome associated with nocturnal myoclonus and epilepsy. *J Neurol Neurosurg Psychiatry* 1978;41:458–62.
29. Montagna P, Coccagna G, Cirignotta F, Lugaresi E. Familial restless legs syndrome: Long-term follow-up. In: Guilleminault C, Lugaresi E, eds. Sleep/wake disorders: natural history, epidemiology, and long-term evolution. New York: Raven Press, 1983:231–5.
30. Montagna P, Cirignotta F, Sacquegna T, Martinelli P, Ambrosetto G, Lugaresi E. "Painful legs and moving toes" associated with polyneuropathy. *J Neurol Neurosurg Psychiatry* 1983;46:399–403.
31. Nordlander NB. Therapy in restless legs. *Acta Med Scand* 1953;145:453–7.
32. Oshtory MA, Vijayan N. Clonazepam treatment of insomnia due to sleep myoclonus. *Arch Neurol* 1980;37:119–20.
33. Oswald I. Sudden bodily jerks on falling asleep. *Brain* 1959;82:92–103.
34. Spillane JD. Restless legs syndrome in chronic pulmonary disease. *Br Med J* 1970;4:796–8.
35. Spillane JD, Nathan PW, Kelly RE, Marsden CD. Painful legs and moving toes. *Brain* 1971;94:541–56.
36. Suhren O, Bruyn GW, Tuynman JA. Hyperexplexia. A hereditary startle syndrome. *J Neurol Sci* 1966;3:577–605.
37. Symonds CP. Nocturnal myoclonus. *J Neurol Neurosurg Psychiatry* 1953;16:166–71.
38. Weiner IH, Weiner HL. Nocturnal leg muscle cramps. *JAMA* 1980;244:2332–3.
39. Willis T. *The London Practice of Physick*. London: Basset T and Crooke W, 1685.
40. Wittmaack T. *Pathologie und Therapie der Sensibilität Neurosen*. Leipzig: Schäfer, 1861.

Advances in Neurology, Vol. 43: Myoclonus,
edited by S. Fahn et al. Raven Press,
New York © 1986.

Dominantly Inherited Restless Legs with Myoclonus and Periodic Movements of Sleep: A Syndrome Related to the Endogenous Opiates?

*Arthur Walters, *Wayne Hening, *†Lucien Côté,
and *Stanley Fahn

Departments of *Neurology and †Rehabilitation Medicine, Columbia University College of
Physicians and Surgeons, New York, New York 10032

We have recently studied a patient who is severely incapacitated by dominantly inherited restless legs and dysesthesias (3,11–13), with myoclonus while awake (2) and periodic movements of sleep with sleep disturbance (Lugaresi et al., *this volume*; 23,25,26). This patient serendipitously discovered that her symptoms were totally abolished by relatively small doses of opiates. We are following a second patient who likewise has dominantly inherited restless legs and insomnia due to nocturnal dyskinesias. He, too, has found that opiates abolish his symptoms.

We have investigated these two patients while off all medications and while on an opiate. Our results indicate that opiates specifically suppress their symptoms, the improvement is reversed by naloxone, suggesting that the endogenous opiate system is involved in this syndrome.

CASE 1

A 67-year-old nurse began to note evening restlessness associated with discomfort in her legs, more severe on the left side, when she was 19 years old. To relieve these symptoms, the patient moved her legs, got out of bed, and walked around the house. In the ensuing years, she developed involuntary, rapid flexion jerks (myoclonus) of the hips and knees, which were also most prominent in the evening while awake. Over the years, both the restlessness of the legs and myoclonus progressed in severity to the point where she could not sit for more than a few minutes in the evening, and she had extreme difficulty in falling asleep. She also experienced frequent nighttime awakenings because of involuntary movements of her legs. Despite the gradual worsening of her condition, there were fluctuations in her symptoms. For instance, her symptoms were worse during both pregnancies but cleared completely for 3 months after delivery of her first child.

In the past, she tried many drugs without relief, including valproate and clonazepam, which are often useful for myoclonus. She also tried diazepam, phenobarbital, chlorpromazine, cyproheptadine, phenytoin, ethanol, meprobamate, calcium, carbamazepine, carisoprodol, nitroglycerin, vitamin preparations, cyclobenzaprine hydrochloride, and propranolol. She tried bromocriptine but stopped taking it after two 2.5-mg doses because of severe side effects. Acupuncture, biofeedback, diathermy, and transcutaneous nerve stimulation provided no benefit.

The patient received oxycodone (Percodan) 20 years ago for an unrelated shoulder disorder and discovered that it attenuated all features of her movement disorder and permitted much more restful and long-lasting sleep. She reports that propoxyphene (Darvon) was at one time beneficial, but it lost its effectiveness with time. Subsequently she responded to other opiates, including methadone (Dolophin) and pentazocine (Talwin). She responded best to methadone, which eliminated all her symptoms for almost 24 hr; her response to oxycodone, on the other hand, was partial and lasted only 3 to 5 hr. Her response to pentazocine was brief (1 to 2 hr) and incomplete. For varied reasons, on a few occasions she took other opiates, such as codeine, and meperidine (Demerol) in relatively low amounts and for only one or two doses. She noted no beneficial effect on her movement disorder from these medications.

Her two children, a son and a daughter, both have a milder form of the syndrome, which is intermittent and occurs only under stress with sleep deprivation and fatigue. Their symptoms do not prevent them from sleeping or functioning normally.

The patient's general medical history is notable only for hypertension, a mild nephropathy of unknown etiology, and an atrial tachyarrythmia not requiring medication. Her neurological and general physical examinations are normal except for her movement disorder.

CASE 2

A 62-year-old priest had a transient left hemiparesis at age 16 years following a head injury. One night 2 years later, he noted involuntary movements of the left leg, which aroused him from sleep. He had no further movements until age 30 years when they recurred. From that time, they increased in severity, spreading in the last few years to involve all limbs but remaining most severe in the left leg. These movements usually occurred at night, were associated with restlessness, and have recently become manifest when he is awake and asleep. He has tried several medicines for this problem, including clonazepam, but only propoxyphene (Darvon) or codeine suppressed his movements and permitted longer, more restful sleep. He also reported that diazepam (Valium) taken alone allowed him to sleep. His symptoms have been controlled for 5 years on stable doses of propoxyphene. For the past few years, he has noted some clumsiness and stiffness of his right hand associated with a tremor. A diagnosis of parkinsonism has been made. His general medical history is remarkable for prostate carcinoma.

The patient's mother lives in the Ukraine and has movements that awaken her at night. She was not examined by us.

Neurological examination discloses intermittent cogwheeling of the right upper extremity; an infrequent, slight resting tremor; masked facies; a positive glabellar reflex (Myerson's sign); and left-sided hyperreflexia. The remainder of the neurological examination is unremarkable except for his movement disorder.

METHODS

The first patient (case 1) was observed for 6 days in the hospital, 3 days on and 3 days off methadone, with serial all-night sleep monitoring and an 8-hr period of daytime monitoring. She was monitored with standard sleep-study electroencephalogram (EEG) leads, electrooculogram (EOG) leads, electrocardiogram (EKG), and a nasal thermistor to monitor respiration. Electromyogram (EMG) leads were applied to both quadriceps, the left hamstrings, and the left tibialis anterior. An accelerometer was secured to the dorsum of the left foot. Continuous videotaping of the patient was performed and correlated to the polygraphic records obtained with the other monitors. During the daytime study, a split-screen videotape simultaneously recorded the patient and the polygraph records. The other patient (case 2) was hospitalized twice. During the second admission, he was intensively monitored in the hospital for 2 days off and 2 days on opiates.

Both patients were subjected to naloxone challenge while on opiates. The first patient, while on 20 mg/day methadone, was given an intravenous infusion of naloxone in a dose of 0.64 mg over 30 min while being monitored. While on methadone, she was also given an intravenous infusion of a placebo, which she believed to be naloxone. The second patient, while on propoxyphene, 195 to 260 mg at bedtime, was given intramuscular or intravenous naloxone prior to going to bed at night. While on propoxyphene, he was given naloxone placebo on a separate night. In addition, he was challenged with intramuscular naloxone while off opiates. We reviewed both patients' videotape and electrophysiological records for their entire hospitalizations. We enumerated all dyskinesias during two full nights' recording, one night on and one night off medication. Dyskinesias were identified on EMG by their unique configuration. Periodic movements of sleep were enumerated as such only if five movements occurred in succession (7).

RESULTS

While off methadone, the first patient had severe insomnia and slept only for several brief "snatches" in 3 days. During this time, she had severe, fluctuating restlessness that was worst in the evenings. She also described a deep aching sensation in her left hip. She complained of an irresistible urge to move. She paced about and marched in place; she often shifted her legs and rubbed one foot on the other. While awake, the patient had myoclonus of the legs, which also occurred most frequently during the evening hours. There were 992 myoclonic jerks while she was fully awake on a representative night's recording. These consisted of abrupt, often repetitive flexions at the hips, knees, and ankles. They occurred most often while she was lying quietly. Sometimes repetitive adduction and abduction occurred with internal rotation. Some of her movements terminated in a slow flexion phase that included pronounced dorsiflexion of the left foot and extension of the great toe. Her myoclonic movements often occurred in clusters, with the individual movements recurring at regular intervals of between 2 and 20 sec. When the patient extended her legs fully, the myoclonus increased dramatically in frequency and intensity. In this position, the myoclonus recurred consistently, with a median period of approximately 5 sec (Fig. 1). While lying supine, she often voluntarily flexed her legs at the hips and knees and crossed her legs at the ankles. In this position, the frequency of myoclonus was markedly reduced. Between movements, she sometimes kept her left foot dorsiflexed and inverted and her left great toe extended.

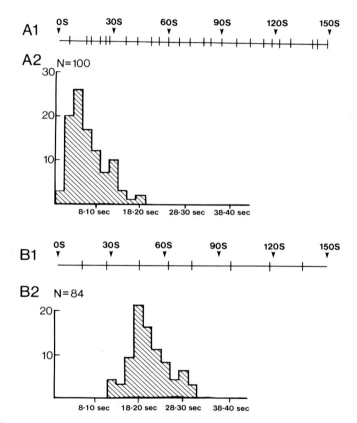

FIG. 1.   Differences between the periodicity of the myoclonus while awake **(A1)** and that of periodic movements of sleep **(B1)**. The myoclonus while awake ($N = 100$ consecutive movement intervals) and the periodic movements of sleep ($N = 84$ consecutive movement intervals) occurred during long periods of constant condition. During the myoclonus while awake, the patient was supine with legs extended. During the periodic movements of sleep, the patient was in stage I and stage II sleep.   **A1** and **B1**: 150-sec duration time lines (taken from the beginning of each sample) in which each vertical line indicates the occurrence of a dyskinesia. Time is indicated by arrows.   **A2** and **B2**: Histograms that show the distribution of intermovement intervals. The myoclonus while awake has a significantly shorter interval ($p < 0.001$) and a larger coefficient of variation (53.3 versus 20.2%) than periodic movements of sleep, indicating its shorter period and greater proportional irregularity in period.

On the few occasions when she did manage to sleep briefly, she continued to have involuntary movements. These took the form of periodic movements of sleep (7), which quickly aroused and awakened her. The movements were sometimes initiated by a jerk but invariably were characterized by slow, monophasic flexions of the lower extremities, lasting up to several seconds, most marked at the knees and most prominent on the left. The periods between movements varied but were usually about 20 sec. These movements were in contrast to the invariably abrupt, less periodic myoclonic jerks that occurred when she was awake (Fig. 1). However, both types of movements had the same distribution and direction: they were seen only in the legs, especially on the left, and consisted mainly of flexion movements.

On 20 mg methadone given as a single oral morning dose, the patient had almost complete suppression of all the cardinal features of her syndrome, without any side effects. On a representative night's recording, there were only four myoclonic jerks while awake. She manifested no other signs of her syndrome. This permitted a full and restful night's sleep. While the patient was awake and on methadone, an intravenous naloxone challenge reactivated the myoclonus after she received 0.16 mg. The myoclonic movements increased in frequency for 16 min until they blended into a generalized motor restlessness that lasted for 30 min after the naloxone was stopped. On a separate day and while the patient was on methadone, she received a placebo, which she believed to be naloxone; this did not reactivate the myoclonus.

The EMG while the patient was awake and having myoclonic movements (Fig. 2) showed 400- to 1,000-msec complexes, each composed of a series of two to five bursts. These complexes had an abrupt and simultaneous onset in all muscles monitored. The EEG tracing often showed desynchronization, with a predominance of low-voltage activity at the time of the movements (Fig. 2). When she fell asleep, the patient passed into sleep stages I and II with normal vertex waves and sleep spindles. During this time, her periodic movements of sleep were accompanied by EMG complexes of 1 to 4 sec in duration (Fig. 3). These, like the EMG activity associated with her myoclonus while awake, were distributed synchronously to all muscles monitored. The EEG demonstrated signs of arousal or awakening following a series of these movements (Fig. 3).

The patient has remained symptom free since initiation of a stable single morning dose of 20 mg methadone 1½ years ago. There have been no side effects from the medication.

The second patient (case 2) had involuntary movements while awake and asleep. When awake, the movements ranged in speed from sustained (dystonic) to shocklike (myoclonic), and the patient experienced an associated restlessness in his legs. While the patient was asleep, the movements took the form of periodic movements of sleep. The dyskinesias of our second patient, unlike those of our first, were similar in periodicity and frequency while he was awake and asleep. While off propoxyphene, he had a total of 458 dyskinesias awake and asleep during one night's recording. These movements were suppressed and his restlessness alleviated by propoxyphene (195–260 mg) at bedtime while under observation. While on this

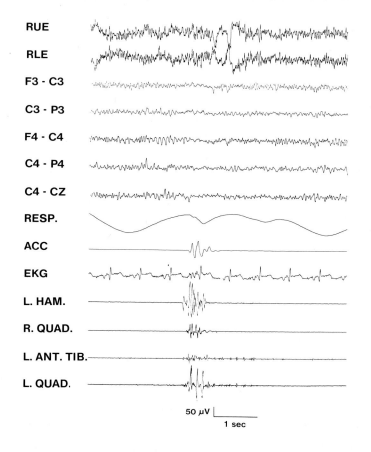

RUE

RLE

F3 - C3

C3 - P3

F4 - C4

C4 - P4

C4 - CZ

RESP.

ACC

EKG

L. HAM.

R. QUAD.

L. ANT. TIB.

L. QUAD.

50 µV

1 sec

FIG. 2. EMG and EEG changes associated with myoclonus while awake. The EMG recording shows a complex of several bursts associated with jerking recorded by an accelerometer placed on the dorsum of the left foot. The EEG is desynchronized and of lower voltage during the movement. RUE, RLE: EEG leads above and below the right eye referenced to the right ear; Resp, respirometer: Acc, accelerometer; L. Ham., left hamstrings; R. Quad., right quadriceps; L. Ant. Tib., left anterior tibial; L. Quad., left quadriceps.

dose of medication, he had only 97 dyskinesias awake and asleep during a subsequent night's recording. These were all primarily in the early part of the evening, which permitted him a restful night's sleep. He experienced no side effects from the medication. While the patient was on propoxyphene, the movements were reactivated when naloxone was given intramuscularly prior to sleep. These movements subsequently awakened the patient. While he was on propoxyphene, naloxone placebo had no effect. When naloxone was given without the patient having received propoxyphene, the involuntary movements were not 'exacerbated. The patient's involuntary movements were reduced by methadone, but he did not tolerate a full dose. The patient has been mostly symptom free on a stable dose of propoxyphene, 130 to 260 mg at bedtime, for the last 5 years without side effects.

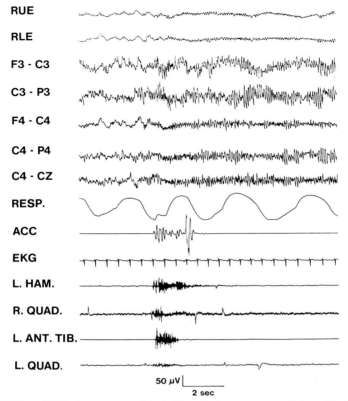

FIG. 3. EMG and EEG changes associated with periodic movements of sleep. The EMG shows brief and sustained superimposed bursts forming 1- to 2-second complexes associated with accelerometer activity. The EEG shows stage II sleep interrupted by arousal. After this movement, the patient awakened. Labels as in Fig. 2.

DISCUSSION

Both these patients appear to have a dominantly inherited syndrome of restless legs. As previously described in this syndrome (3,11–13), patients have periodic movements of sleep which may awaken them (Lugaresi et al., *this volume*; 23,25,26) and myoclonus while awake (2; Lugaresi et al., *this volume*). The other affected members of their families show a milder version of the syndrome, indicating the variable expressivity of the syndrome. Affected individuals may manifest the complete syndrome or only one or two of the elements (2).

This syndrome of restless legs with dyskinesias, unlike almost all other involuntary movement disorders, is a disorder associated with repose, evening, and sleep, suggesting that circadian modulation of neural activity is involved in its pathogenesis. One possibility is that there is an abnormal neural generator in these patients which produces involuntary movements when influenced by circadian variations in neural activity. On the other hand, there may be an abnormality in circadian variation which drives normal motor circuits to become generators of abnormal movements. Since we have observed that the four sensorimotor elements of the syndrome (restless legs, dysesthesias, periodic movements of sleep, and myoclonus while awake) covary under a number of different influences (e.g., time of day, state of activity, pregnancy, pharmacotherapy), it is likely that they share a common pathophysiology. Like periodic movements of sleep, spinal myoclonus is often rhythmic (4,15,19,33), can have prolonged EMG bursts (5,8), and may persist in sleep (8,9,15,20,24). This observed similarity between spinal myoclonus and periodic movements of sleep, plus the fact that the dyskinesias rarely if ever involve the face in the restless legs syndrome, raises the question of whether the generator for at least the periodic movements of sleep is located in the spinal cord.

The findings we report here provide additional evidence linking opiates to disorders of the motor system and of sleep (14). Opiate therapy in our two patients alleviated all elements of the syndrome, while naloxone, an opiate antagonist, blocked the benefits of opiate therapy. This observation indicates that the therapeutic effect is specific for the opiate receptor. The fact that the movements did not increase in severity or number when naloxone was given to the second patient in the absence of opiates is not surprising since naloxone given alone has few physiological effects (21).

There are a number of experimental and clinical observations that relate myoclonus to the opiate receptor (16,18,22,28,31). Among the various subtypes (29), the mu opiate receptor is the leading candidate for a specific subtype whose activation is able to suppress myoclonus. This candidacy is supported by the following observations. Mu opiate receptors are widely distributed throughout motor regions of the brain and spinal cord (30). All the opiates that we used successfully in this study were strong mu receptor agonists (17,34). In one study, which examined the role of opiate receptor subtypes in experimentally induced myoclonus, a delta receptor agonist (enkephalin analogue) produced myoclonus, while a mu receptor agonist effectively blocked it (10). These results together with our findings support the idea that the endogenous opiate system (e.g., enkephalins, endorphins), the opiate receptor, and the mu opiate receptor, in particular, are implicated in the pathogenesis of the restless legs syndrome.

The treatment of restless legs and related nocturnal dyskinesias has not been very successful (6,7). In recent years, clonazepam, because of its efficacy in treating various myoclonias, has been tried with partial success for the treatment of restless legs and periodic movements of sleep (27,32). Other benzodiazepines, such as diazepam, to which our second patient apparently responded, may help to reduce symptoms in some patients. A few investigators have anecdotally noted that the syndrome of restless legs may respond to opiates (1,11–13,35), but most have disparaged this type of treatment, and none have systematically examined the therapeutic response. Although we cannot say whether all patients will respond, the striking beneficial response of our patients to opiates indicates that this is a potentially important therapeutic avenue. This might be particularly true of patients who are severely affected and unresponsive to other medications. Further studies are now needed to establish what percentage of all such patients will respond. It is particularly gratifying to us that neither of our two patients (on propoxyphene or methadone) has suffered any of the worrisome and dysfunctional side effects of opiate medications. In particular, they have shown neither addictive behavior nor tolerance, and have been maintained on a stable dose for years. Among the medications to which our patients responded, Tylenol with codeine and propoxyphene have the advantage of being milder and more readily available, and methadone for more severely affected patients has the advantage of having an extremely long half-life (up to 15 hr) (21).

SUMMARY

The restless legs syndrome is a sensory and motor disorder of evening, repose, and sleep. The cardinal features include (a) restlessness, which is frequently associated with (b) dysesthesias, (c) myoclonic jerks and other dyskinesias while awake, (d) periodic movements of sleep, and (e) sleep disturbances. We have recently had the opportunity to study two patients severely affected by this syndrome whose family histories are consistent with dominant inheritance. Both patients serendipitously discovered that their symptoms responded uniquely well to opiate medication. Both patients were studied extensively with electrophysiological and videotape monitoring, and their movements were characterized. In both patients, all elements of the syndrome responded to opiates, with marked relief of symptoms and without any significant side effects. The specific opiate antagonist naloxone blocked the therapeutic benefit of the opiates. Our findings support the involvement of the endogenous opiate system in the pathogenesis of restless legs and related dyskinesias and suggest that opiate therapy may be a potentially valuable treatment for this sometimes disabling syndrome.

ADDENDUM

Since the writing of this chapter, we have confirmed our results with three additional patients who have the restless legs syndrome and one with periodic movements of sleep alone. These results will be reported elsewhere.

ACKNOWLEDGMENTS

Dr. Arthur Walters was supported in part by a grant from the Parkinson's Disease Foundation and by a Peggy Engl Fellowship. Dr. Wayne Hening was supported by the Dystonia Medical Research Foundation. We express our thanks to Dr. Timothy Pedley and Dr. Eli Goldensohn and to Ms. Alberta Domalakes of the Columbia Presbyterian EEG Department for their assistance in these studies.

REFERENCES

1. Akpinar S. Treatment of restless legs syndrome with levodopa plus benserazide. *Arch Neurol* 1982;39:739.

2. Boghen D, Peyronnard JM. Myoclonus in familial restless legs syndrome. *Arch Neurol* 1976;33:368–70.
3. Bornstein B. Restless legs. *Psychiatr Neurol* 1961;141:165–201.
4. Campbell AMG and Garland H. Subacute myoclonic spinal neuronitis. *J Neurol Neurosurg Psychiatry* 1956;19:268–74.
5. Castaigne P, Cambier J, Laplane D. Myoclonies rhythmées segmentaires d'origine médullaire. *Rev Otoneuroophthalmol* 1969;41:241–50.
6. Coleman RM. Periodic movements in sleep (nocturnal myoclonus) and restless legs syndrome. In: Guilleminault G, ed. Sleeping and waking disorders: indications and techniques. Menlo Park: Addison-Wesley, 1982:265–95.
7. Coleman RM, Pollak CP, Weitzmann ED. Periodic movements in sleep (nocturnal myoclonus): relation to sleep disorders. *Ann Neurol* 1980;8:416–21.
8. Davis SM, Murray NMF, Diengdoh JV, Galea-Debono A, Kocen RS. Stimulus-sensitive spinal myoclonus. *J Neurol Neurosurg Psychiatry* 1981;44:884–8.
9. Dhaliwal GS, McGreal DA. Spinal myoclonus in association with herpes zoster infection: two case reports. *Can J Neurol Sci* 1974;1:239–41.
10. Dzoljic MR, vd Poel Heisterkamp AL. Delta opiate receptors are involved in the endopiod-induced myoclonic contractions. *Brain Res Bull* 1982;8:1–6.
11. Ekbom KA. Restless legs: a clinical study. *Acta Med Scand* 1945;158:1–123.
12. Ekbom KA. Restless legs. A report of 70 new cases. *Acta Med Scand* 1950;246:64–8.
13. Ekbom KA. Restless legs syndrome. *Neurology* 1960;10:868–73.
14. Fry JM, Pressman, MR. The treatment of narcolepsy with codeine. *Neurology (NY)* 1983;33(2):176.
15. Garcin R, Rondot P, Guiot G. Rhythmic myoclonus of the right arm as the presenting symptom of a cervical cord tumor. *Brain* 1968;91:75–84.
16. Helmers JH, Adam AA, Giezen J. Pain and myoclonus during induction with etomidate. *Acta Anaesthesiol Belg* 1981;2:141–7.
17. Herling S, Woods JH. Discriminative stimulus effects of narcotics: evidence for multiple receptor-mediated actions. *Life Sci* 1981;28:1571–84.
18. Herzlinger RA, Kandall, SR, Vaughan HG Jr. Neonatal seizures associated with narcotic withdrawal. *J Pediatr* 1977;91:638–41.
19. Hoehn MM, Cherington M. Spinal myoclonus. *Neurology (NY)* 1977;27:942–6.
20. Hopkins AP, Michael WF. Spinal myoclonus. *J Neurol Neurosurg Psychiatry* 1974;37:1112–5.
21. Jaffe JH, Martin WR. Narcotic analgesics and antagonists. In: Goodman LS, Gilman A, eds. The pharmacological basis of therapeutics. New York: MacMillan, 1975:268–9; 273.
22. Kaiko RF, Foley KM, Grabinski PY, Heidrich G, Rogers AG, Inturrisi CE, Reidenberg MM. Central nervous system excitatory effects of meperidine in cancer patients. *Ann Neurol* 1983;13:180–5.
23. Lugaresi E, Cirignotta F, Montagna P, Coccagna G. Myoclonus and related phenomena during sleep. In: Chase M, Weitzman ED, eds. Sleep disorders: basic and clinical research. New York: Spectrum, 1983:123–7.
24. Lugaresi E, Coccagna G, Mantovani M, Berti Ceroni G, Pazzaglia P, Tassinari CA. The evolutions of different types of myoclonus during sleep. *Eur Neurol* 1970;4:321–31.
25. Lugaresi E, Coccagna G, Tassinari CA, Ambrosetto C. Rilievi poligrafici sui fenomeni motori nella sindrome delle gambe sense riposo. *Riv Neurol* 1965;35:550–61.
26. Lugaresi E, Tassinari C, Coccagna G, Ambrosetto C. Particularités cliniques et polygraphiques du syndrome d'impatience des membres inférieurs. *Rev Neurol (Paris)* 1965;113:545–55.
27. Matthews WB. Treatment of restless legs syndrome with clonazepam. *Br Med J* 1979;i:751.
28. Meldrum BS, Menini CH, Stutzmann JM, Nanquet R. Effects of opiate-like peptides, morphine and naloxone in the photosensitive baboon, *Papio Papio. Brain Res* 1979;170:333–48.
29. Miller RJ. Multiple opiate receptors for multiple opioid peptides. *Med Biol* 1982;60:1–6.
30. Ninkovic M, Hunt SP, Emson PC, Iversen LL. The distribution of multiple opiate receptors in bovine brain. *Brain Res* 1981;214:163–7.
31. Nistico G, Stephenson JD, Montanini S, Marmo E. Behavioral and electrocortical effects of beta endorphin after intracerebral infusion in rats. *J Med* 1981;12(6):463–74.
32. Oshtory MA, Vijayan N. Clonazepam treatment of insomnia due to sleep myoclonus. *Arch Neurol* 1980;37:119–20.
33. Patrikos MJ. Sur un cas d'automatisme moteur particulier des membres supérieurs après traumatisme de la moelle cirvicale. *Rev Neurol (Paris)* 1938;69:179–88.

34. Pert CB. The opiate receptor. In: Bassett EG, Beers RF Jr., eds. Cell membrane receptors for viruses, antigens, and antibodies, polypeptide hormones, and small molecules. New York: Raven Press, 1976:435–50.
35. Willis T. *The London Practice of Physick*, 1st ed. London: Thomas Bassett and William Crooke, 1685:404.

Advances in Neurology, Vol. 43: Myoclonus,
edited by S. Fahn et al. Raven Press,
New York © 1986.

Excessive Startle Syndromes: Startle Disease, Jumping, and Startle Epilepsy

Frederick Andermann and Eva Andermann

Montreal Neurological Hospital and Institute, Montreal, Quebec, Canada H3A 2B4

Startle, a basic alerting reaction common to all mammals, is a rapid reflex not amenable to voluntary control. It was studied extensively by Strauss in 1929 (45) and is the subject of a monograph by Landis and Hunt (35) and a more recent study by Gogan (24). In the human adult, except for minor interpersonal variations, a stereotyped motor pattern is seen consisting of eye blinking, facial grimacing, flexion of the head, elevation of the shoulders, and flexion of the elbows, trunk, and knees. With repeated stimulation, the intensity of the surprise reaction decreases but never completely disappears. Tension, fatigue, and heightened expectation of the stimulus enhance it. The intensity is greater in infancy, where it appears at the same time as the Moro reflex (an extensor response to sudden stimuli). However, startle becomes more noticeable in time, while the Moro reflex disappears (25). This reflex, so basic to humans, can be present in a pathologically exaggerated form, which is embarrassing, sometimes interferes with normal activities, and occasionally may be dangerous.

Abnormal, excessive startle is a feature of three distinct conditions: startle disease or hyperekplexia, jumping (the jumping Frenchmen of Maine), and startle epilepsy.

STARTLE DISEASE

More than 15 years ago, a mother brought her two girls, who had been diagnosed and treated for epilepsy, complaining that the older girl was falling when startled. Both girls had a mechanical, broad-based gait, which suggested cerebellar dysfunction, but they were not ataxic; they were hyperreflexic. Since extensive questioning did not solve the problem, a kidney basin was dropped to the stone floor and the older girl fell forward like a log, hit her head on the foot of the metal examining table, and began to cry. This response was far greater than anticipated. The patient, the family, and the examiner were quite mortified, and the girl has always been wary in her neurologist's presence since.

Kirstein and Silfverskiöld (29) first described startle disease in 1958. Two sisters, their father, and the daughter of one of the sisters suffered from sudden violent falls precipitated by stress, fright, or surprise. Three of these family members also had nocturnal myoclonus. The authors cautiously considered the disorder to represent an unusual, genetically determined form of drop seizures.

In a letter to *Lancet* in 1962, Kok and Bruyn (31) drew attention to a hereditary disease affecting 29 individuals in six generations of a German-Dutch family with 127 members (Fig. 1). In 1966, Suhren (née Kok) et al. (46) described this family in greater detail. The affected individuals had a strikingly excessive response to startle elicited by visual, auditory, and proprioceptive stimuli that failed to produce a startle response in most normal individuals. The disorder occurred in two forms: a minor form, in which the response was quantitatively different from normal (that is, the startle response was more violent), and a major form, in which there were also additional clinical symptoms. In the major form, patients when startled experienced momentary generalized muscular stiffness with loss of voluntary postural control causing them to fall, as if frozen, with their arms at their sides, unable to carry out protective movements. As soon as they hit the ground, muscle tone and control of voluntary movements returned, and there was never evidence of loss of consciousness. Kirstein and Silfverskiöld (29) did describe brief loss of consciousness in association with these falls, but this was probably related to concussion. Urinary incontinence may occur and is probably due to increased intraabdominal pressure associated with the extensor spasm. This abnormal response was always present from the time the affected child first attempted to walk. It was increased by emotional tension, nervousness, fatigue, and the expectation of being frightened, while alcohol, phenobarbital, and chlordiazepoxide lessened its intensity to some degree.

In the major form, there was also transient generalized hypertonia during infancy. As babies, when awakened or handled, affected individuals had an immediate increase in muscle tone in flexion, which disappeared during sleep. This abnormality diminished as spontaneous activity increased during the first year of life. Around the time of its disappearance, frequent violent and often repetitive jerks of the limbs were described as the child fell asleep. The jerks could lift the child off the bed.

The neonatal form of this condition was redescribed by Klein et al. (30) as a "familial congenital disorder resembling Stiff-Man Syndrome" occurring in 10 individuals from three generations of a family. The family stressed the onset of stiffness within 4 or 5 hr after birth, the absence of crawling (with the children scooting about in a seated position propelling themselves with their arms), and some delay in walking. Stiffness disappeared during sleep. Difficulty swallowing and frequent choking were also described. The infants had hard, tense shoulder girdle muscles and faces set in a somewhat unhappy and inappropriate expression. Lingam et al. (36), in a second report on the hereditary stiff-baby syndrome, suggested the identity of this condition with startle disease. The infants have a high incidence of umbilical and other hernias, previously noted by Suhren et al. (46), and probably related to their hypertonicity. Apnea due to spasm of respiratory muscles may also occur; and in a patient mentioned by Kurczynski (34), this led to the child's death.

The major and minor forms of startle disease can occur in the same family, as illustrated by the large family reported by Suhren et al. (46) (Fig. 1) and that

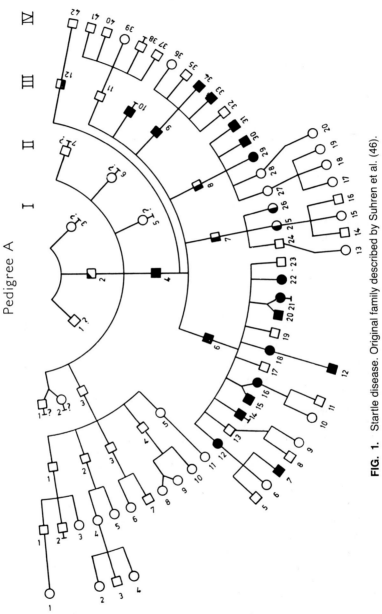

Pedigree A

FIG. 1. Startle disease. Original family described by Suhren et al. (46).

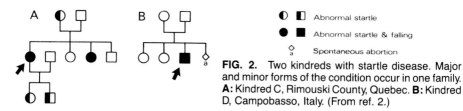

FIG. 2. Two kindreds with startle disease. Major and minor forms of the condition occur in one family. **A:** Kindred C, Rimouski County, Quebec. **B:** Kindred D, Campobasso, Italy. (From ref. 2.)

reported by Andermann et al. (2) (Fig. 2). The minor form of the disease consists only of excessive startle. A parent with the minor form can have children with the major form, and vice versa, but siblings tend to be affected to the same degree. Therefore it is likely, as Suhren et al. (46) have suggested, that these two forms represent different phenotypic expressions of the same autosomal dominant gene.

A positive family history may be difficult to elicit in this condition because of this phenotypic variation. In the family we described, the disorder was obvious in the proband and her sister. Only the minor form was present in the proband's children and only when they were ill. For years, it was impossible to obtain a history of abnormal startle from either of the proband's parents. Eventually it became clear that, in the years leading up to the mother's divorce from her alcoholic husband, she startled excessively and literally jumped off her chair when the telephone rang. Thus autosomal dominant inheritance with variable expressivity was again confirmed. In the second family reported by us, however, no other member was found to be affected by either the major or the minor form, even on intensive questioning. This may be explained by a new mutation in the proband or by lack of penetrance of the gene in other family members. A sporadic patient with this disease was also described by Boudouresques et al. (12) in 1964.

In 1967, Gastaut and Villeneuve (20) presented in detail 12 patients with sporadic startle disease. The authors also stressed the psychogenic precipitation of startle and falling. Eleven of their patients had falling attacks, and in at least one these were, according to their description, identical to those occurring in familial cases. The incidence of mild retardation or low intelligence was higher than expected and similar to that noticed by Andermann et al. (2) and Suhren et al. (46). Nine had nocturnal jerking of the legs. Andermann et al. (2) felt that their patients were different from those described by Suhren et al. (46), although it seems likely that at least some of their patients had the same disorder but without an obvious family history.

There is no good evidence that the patients with sporadic startle disease differ from the familial cases described by Suhren et al. (46), as Gastaut and Villeneuve (20) have suggested. Our own cases, familial or sporadic, appear to have the same syndrome. These two forms would thus appear to represent a single genetically determined disorder.

Suhren et al. (46) and Gastaut and Villeneuve (20) suggested that, since jerking of the legs occurred only at night, it presumably represented an exaggerated form of hypnagogic myoclonus. Two of our patients had such attacks in the daytime as well, and all limbs were involved, although the legs always more than the arms.

When the attacks occurred at night, the patients woke with a feeling described as unsteadiness, similar to their diurnal state when unexpected stimuli would be particularly likely to provoke a fall. The jerking would begin later, lasting for several minutes. There were no electrographic features to suggest an epileptic etiology. Clinically, these attacks resembled spontaneous generalized clonus. De Groen and Kamphuisen (16) studied the periodic nocturnal myoclonic jerks of one of the patients of Suhren et al. (46). They concluded that these are due to spontaneous arousal reactions, caused mainly by excitability increase of motor neurons, hyperexcitability of the brainstem arousal system, and markedly increased influence of respiratory variables on reticular hyperexcitability.

The electroencephalogram (EEG) correlates of startle were similar in the patients reported by Gastaut and Villeneuve (20), Suhren et al. (46), and Andermann et al. (2). The EEG response consisted of an initial spike recorded from the centroparietal vertex followed by a short-lasting train of slow waves and then by desynchronization of background activity lasting 2 to 3 sec (Fig. 3). The response was abolished by intravenous diazepam (Fig. 4). This complex discharge, the most consistent electrographic correlate of excessive startle, may represent an evoked response to various sensory stimuli. Averaged somatosensory, visual, and brainstem auditory evoked responses, however, have shown no significant abnormality in patients with the major form of startle disease, according to B. Rosenblatt and A. Majnemer *(personal communication,* 1983).

The electromyogram (EMG) changes were well described by Gastaut and Villeneuve (20): isolated or grouped volleys of 10 to 12 elements with a latency of 10 to 40 msec (starting from the frontal muscles and going to those of the leg). According to the number of motor units recruited, the amplitude varied from 1 to 10 mV, while the duration was of 20 to 60 msec. Activity of interferential type followed, sometimes after an interval of approximately 20 msec, and lasted from a fraction of a second to several seconds, thus lengthening the initial jerk. These muscle potentials were generalized to the agonist and antagonist muscular systems without reciprocal innervation. Their amplitude decreased from the head and neck to the trunk, from the root of the limbs to their extremities, and from the upper to the lower limbs.

Other polygraphic features were sudden lowering of skin resistance, variable but often persistent tachycardia, rise of arterial blood pressure (mainly systolic), and a fall in systolic peripheral blood flow. Frequently, the most intense stimuli induced, after the early muscular potential, an interferential muscular activity sufficient to engender a tonic spasm lasting several seconds. The spasm was accompanied by a vegetative discharge bringing on an apnea lasting several seconds and a heart rate accelerated by 100% (20).

Suhren et al. (46) considered the disorder to be nonepileptic. They believed the abnormality in these patients probably resulted from retarded maturation of control of brainstem centers by higher inhibitory mechanisms, particularly by the rhombomesencephalic reticular formation. Epileptogenic EEG abnormalities were found in several of their patients who fell, and many had excessive slow activity, which

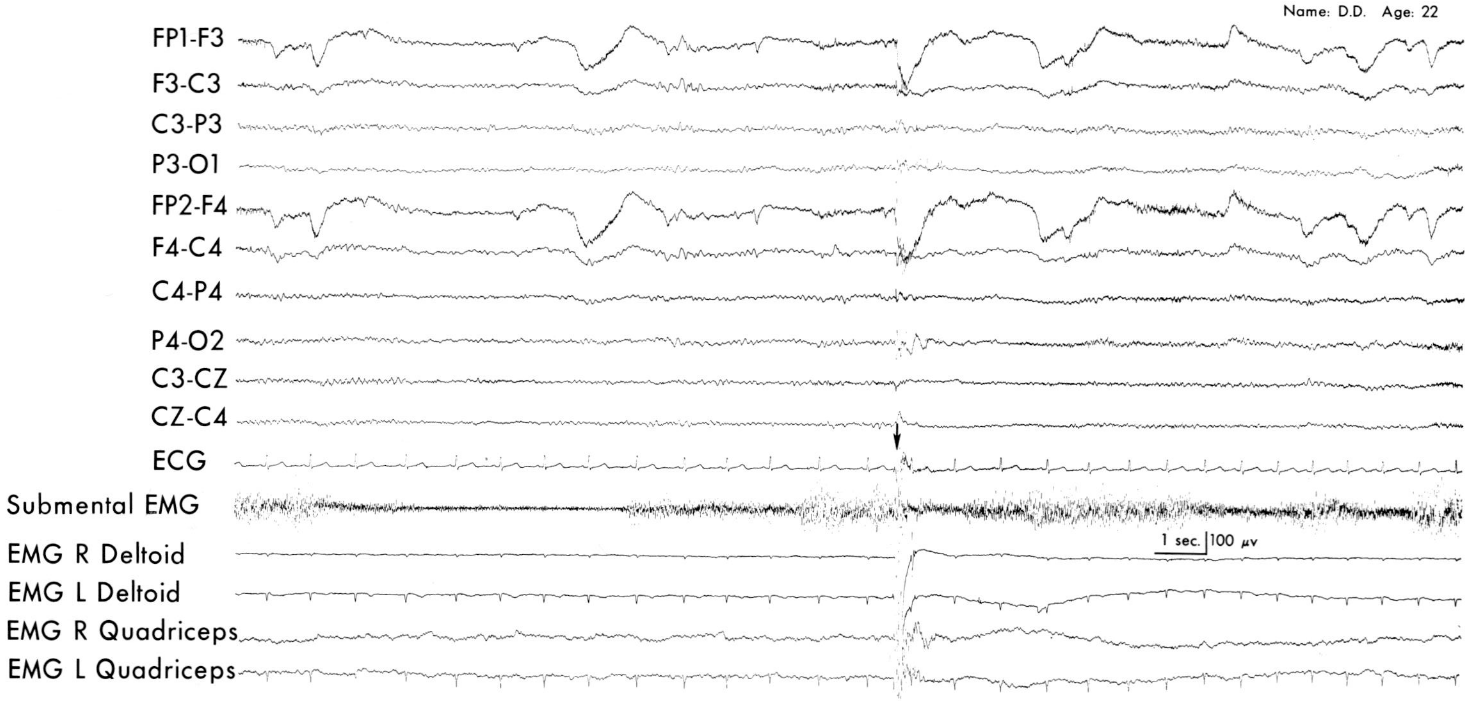

FIG. 3. Effect of a sudden stimulus in a 22-year-old patient with startle disease, before diazepam administration. *Arrow* indicates start of stimulus. (From ref. 2.)

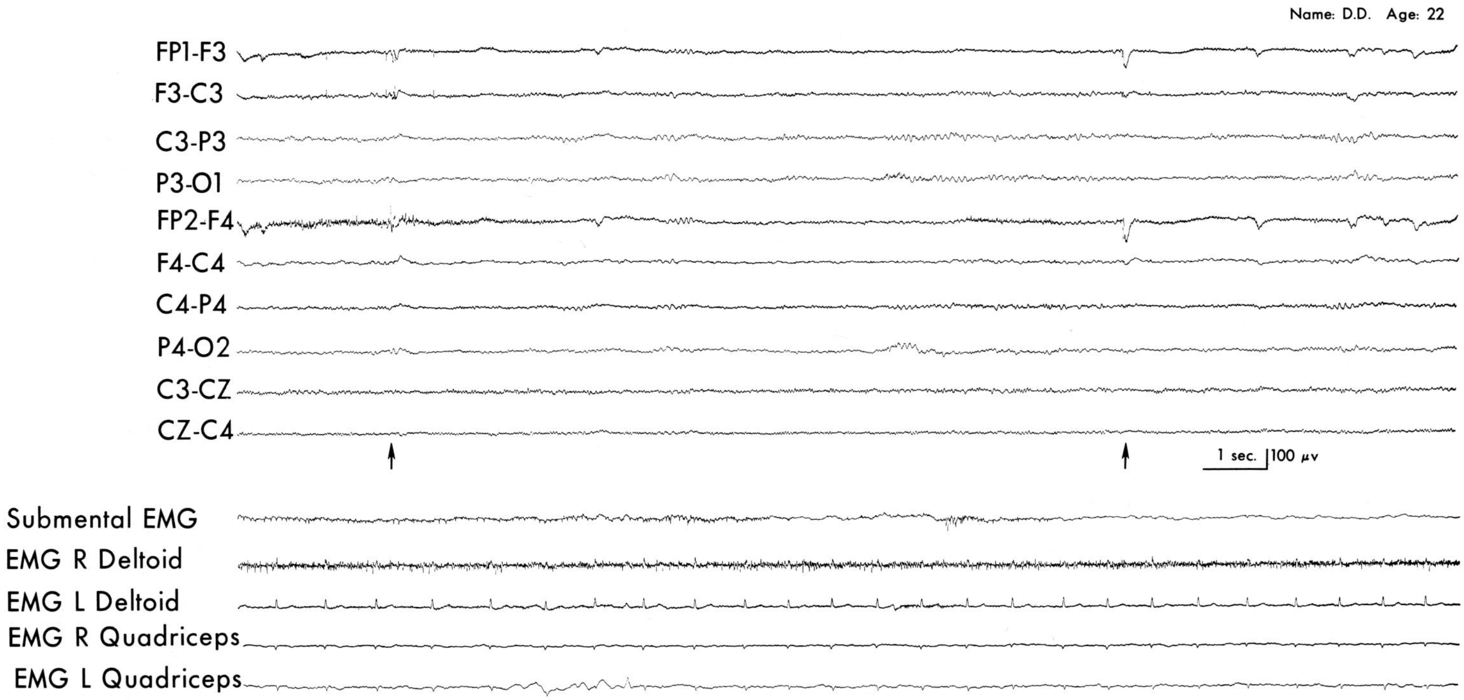

FIG. 4. Effect of startle is temporarily abolished 10 min after administration of 5 mg i.v. diazepam. Same patient as in Fig. 3. *Arrow* indicates start of stimulus. (From ref. 2.)

the authors attributed to the repeated head injuries. Some patients display evidence of more widespread cerebral dysfunction not explainable by a maturational defect in a specific system alone and unlikely to be due merely to the repeated falls. One of the patients of Andermann et al. (2) had an active generalized spike–wave discharge, and another had a parietal sharp wave focus, although neither had epileptic seizures or episodes other than the specific clinical phenomena just described. Indeed, the spike–wave discharge was blocked by startle (Fig. 5). Several of the patients reported by Gastaut and Villeneuve (20) had a low convulsive threshold, and one had seizures as well. Four of their patients had or were suspected to have mild mental retardation. Low average intelligence was also encountered in two of the three patients of Andermann et al. (2) with the major form, suggesting diffuse cerebral dysfunction. The hypertonicity and hyperreflexia implied an abnormality of the pyramidal system. No pathological studies of individuals with this condition are available.

The diagnosis of startle disease should not be difficult if one is aware of this syndrome. The condition is probably rare, and one would suspect that it is commonly misdiagnosed as epilepsy, as it was at first in most patients. Hypertonia in infancy is easily misinterpreted as spastic quadriplegia, as it was in the cases of Andermann et al. (2), where its disappearance was quite baffling. The most puzzling symptom is the unsteady gait, which the physician may attribute to a cerebellar disorder instead of the uncertainty and fear of falling that actually causes it.

The course of the condition is variable (13). Some patients with early onset eventually improve, whereas in others the symptoms only arise or increase later in life. In our patients, there has been little change over the years, although on the whole the manifestations were more severe in childhood, when the hypertonicity was striking and the falls frequent. The disorder is not entirely benign considering the risk of sudden death in infancy attributable to spasm of respiratory muscles and the possible complications of hernias. Later, patients may suffer multiple fractures, including skull fractures, as well as repeated lacerations and cerebral concussions.

At present, clonazepam, a benzodiazepine and potent serotonin agonist, appears to be the drug of choice in the treatment of this condition. In small doses (0.1 mg/kg), it abolishes the falling attacks and greatly reduces the episodic jerking. There is a remarkable disappearance of the uncertainty of the gait, and the patients walk more freely, no longer holding hands or continuously touching the wall. Although clonazepam does not cause the startle response to return to normal, its effect is greater than that of diazepam and appears to be sustained. Excessive head retraction on forehead or nose tapping persists and appears to represent residual reticular reflex myoclonus. Under conditions of exceptional emotional stress, falling or nocturnal leg jerking occasionally recur. The effect of clonazepam suggests that a serotonergic mechanism may be involved. Alcohol, phenobarbital, phenytoin, primidone, and chlordiazepoxide—although they have some effect on the falling attacks, startle, and repetitive jerks—are not the drugs of choice for treatment of this disorder.

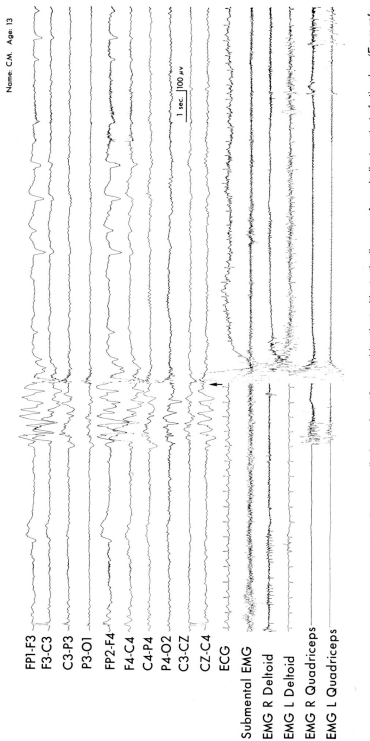

FIG. 5. Startle blocks the asymptomatic spike–wave discharge in a 13-year-old patient with startle disease. *Arrow* indicates start of stimulus. (From ref. 2.)

JUMPING

It is difficult to improve on Dr. George Beard's (7,8) original descriptions made more than a century ago of the jumpers of Maine, and it is worth quoting them *in extenso*:

About two years ago my attention was directed by my friend Mr. W. A. Croffut to the fact that, in the northern part of Maine, especially in the region of Moosehead Lake, there were to be found a class of people who presented most incredible nervous phenomena. These people were called in the language of that region "Jumpers" or "Jumping Frenchmen." It was claimed that all, or most of them, were of French descent and of Canadian birth, and that their occupation was mainly that of lumbering in the Maine woods. Mr. Croffut introduced me to D. W. Craig, Esq., a gentleman who had spent much time in that portion of Maine, and who had amused himself with watching and playing with these unfortunates.

I found two of the Jumpers employed about the hotel. With one of them, a young man twenty-seven years of age, I made the following experiments:

1. While sitting in a chair, with a knife in his hand, with which he was about to cut his tobacco, he was struck sharply on the shoulder, and told to "throw it." Almost as quick as the explosion of a pistol, he threw the knife, and it stuck in a beam opposite; at the same time he repeated the order "throw it" with a certain cry as of terror or alarm.
2. A moment after, while filling his pipe with tobacco, he was again slapped on the shoulder and told to "throw it." He threw the tobacco and the pipe on the grass, at least a rod away, with the same cry and the same suddenness and explosiveness of movement.
3. When standing near one of the employees of the house he was told to "strike," and he struck him violently on the cheek. I took this person into the quiet of my own room, only my friend being with me, in order that the experiments might be made without interruption or disturbance. I sat down by him, explained to him the object of my visit, conversed with him in regard to his family history and his own personal experience and observation of his peculiarity, and every now and then, during the conversation, I struck him without warning on the shoulder or on the back, or mildly kicked him; and every time he was so struck he moved his shoulders upward slightly, sometimes moving both the shoulders and the arms, with or without the peculiar cry. He knew that I was studying his case; he knew that the kicks and strokes came from me, and yet he could not avoid making a slight jump or motion, as though startled.

When the two Jumpers were close together, they were commanded to "strike:" each struck the other simultaneously—not mild or polite, but severe and painful blows. I took one of these men to my room and quietly conversed with him, and made the same experiments with him as with the other case. I found him much less irritable than the other, and he needed usually stronger excitation to produce the phenomena.

I experimented with him in the phenomenon of repeating language that was addressed to him. When the command was uttered in a quick, loud voice, he repeated the order as he heard it, at the same time that he executed it. When told to strike, he said "Strike" at the same time that he struck; when told to throw it, he said "Throw it" at the same time that he threw whatever was in his hand. It made no difference what language was used. I tried him with the first part of the first line of Homer's "Iliad," and with the first part of Virgil's "Aeneid," languages, of course, of which he knew nothing, and he repeated quickly, almost violently, the sound as it was uttered—"Menin Aida," the first part of the first line of the "Iliad," and "Arma-vi," the first part of the first line of Virgil. In order to have it repeated, it was necessary that the command should be very short, as well as quickly and strongly uttered. He would not repeat a whole line, or even half a line, but simply a word or two.

Some, if not all, of the Jumpers, are ticklish—exceedingly so—and are easily irritated by touching them in sensitive parts of the body.

Thus the features of this condition are excessive startle, echolalia, and automatic obedience. Echopraxia also occurs.

Beard (7,8) was aware of the hereditary nature of the disorder. Among 50 affected people he studied, there were 14 affected members in four families:

Before I visited Moosehead Lake, while I knew only those facts that were obtained at second or third hand, I felt quite sure that this disease would be likely to be a family inheritance. This deductive reasoning was confirmed by inductive observation. It is fully as hereditary as insanity, or epilepsy, or hay-fever, although it has no special relation to any of those forms of disease. In the family of one of those with whom I experimented there were five Jumpers, the father, two sons, and two grandchildren of the respective ages of four and seven years. In the family of another with whom I experimented there were four, all brothers. In the family of another of whom I obtained information, but did not study, there were three cases, an uncle, a mother, and a brother. In another family there were two boys, both Jumpers. Here, then, were fourteen cases in four families. By the study of these cases, it was possible to trace the malady back at least half a century.

Despite the genetic evidence, Beard did not believe that the condition represented a "pathological nervous disease;" instead he considered it to be "a fixed psychological state" and "a remarkable illustration of the involuntary life." He thought that after the day's work the loggers engaged in mutual tickling, punching, and startling of the fearful, and that this repeated horseplay eventually resulted in the condition he described: "Jumping is probably an evolution of tickling." Thus Beard is responsible not only for superlative observations and field studies of the condition; he also sowed the seeds of its interpretation as a social, behavioral, or learned form of activity, an interpretation that is still occasionally invoked today.

Beard (7,8) was also remarkably farsighted in his view of the ultimate fundamental nature of the disorder:

Far out of the range of the aided senses, far beyond the reach of the microscope, or perhaps of the spectroscope, there may be molecular changes or disturbances which manifest themselves in these jumpings and strikings and throwings as a result and correlative. But for the present, possibly for all time, we can only study this subject psychologically; we can only approach it satisfactorily from the psychological side.

Apparently Beard planned further studies of the disorder, but he died soon afterward. After an initial flurry of interest in jumping, there ensued a period of silence lasting more than half a century.

In 1944, Thorne (47) described four young people with a condition identical to that of the jumpers, but his paper is not generally known to neurologists. In 1964, Stevens presented and later published (43) an account of three jumping patients. The first was a French-Canadian male whose father came from northern Maine. He startled excessively, and, if startled when standing, he might be thrown off balance and fall. The second, a Scottish-Irish-German woman from Carolina, startled excessively and showed echolalia, repeating the final words of statements or commands. Her 20-year-old niece was similarly affected. Stevens (44) discusses the relationship of jumping to Gilles de la Tourette's *tic convulsif*; indeed, this relationship has been debated since the original descriptions were published.

Familial excessive startle and falling occurring in five siblings were observed by Fitch (17) in an Acadian family from Wedgport, Nova Scotia. Whether members of this family suffered from startle disease or jumping is unclear.

The next opinion regarding the nature of jumping came from Rabinovitch (40), who was raised in rural Quebec. He again propounded the concept of a culturally determined learned behavior originating from the pranks and horseplay practised in remote, isolated logging camps, but such an interpretation is not convincing and in particular fails to account for the genetic aspects of the disorder.

Dr. Charles Kunkle (32,33), working in Maine, has had the largest recent experience with jumpers. In 1965 (32) and 1967 (33), he reported on 19 patients of various national backgrounds (French-Canadian, Irish, and Italian). Of 15 jumpers examined, 13 were male, and in 12 the condition began in childhood. Automatic obedience on some occasions was noted in seven, and echolalia in two. An involuntary, aggressive gesture directed to the nearest bystander was present in 11. Kunkle states that men with the latter propensity are known as "killer jumpers." Four were known to have been unusually ticklish from childhood, and one was remarkably intolerant of being touched on the torso; even with adequate warning, he became indescribably tense from such contact. Tickle as a form of sensation is related to pain, and there is considerable genetically determined variability in its intensity. Although probably also modulated by cultural and social factors, it is not merely a pattern of acquired social response.

In four adults, Kunkle (32,33) found that jumping developed as a well-defined chronic sequel to a physical illness. The patients were tense and depressed. There is a striking similarity between this "secondary jumping" and the triggering of tics by a physical illness or their precipitation and aggravation by tension and emotion. Kunkle's neurological examination of all 19 jumpers, including the four with the secondary form, was normal.

Dr. Kunkle kindly drew our attention to a recent column entitled "Are the jumping frenchmen of Maine goosey?" by Joseph Hardison (28), who provides an excellent description:

> I was raised in a small southern rural community. I was 17 years old when my girlfriend confided to me that her mother was goosey. I was astonished that this reserved, kind, intelligent woman responded when startled or tickled by jumping in the air and shouting curse words that I had not thought possible for her to utter.
>
> To my further amazement, she responded to sudden loud commands by repeating the command while performing the order. If, for instance, she was suddenly told: "Stir your tea with your finger," she would shout: "Stir your tea with your finger," while stirring her tea with her finger. She appeared to be normal in every other way, but she could not prevent these remarkable responses when poked or startled. Her daughter was not goosey.

Hardison concludes that "jumping" and "goosey" are identical and provides further evidence that the condition is not confined to the French-Canadian group who settled in northern Maine. The increased incidence in that population and area may be explained by the population migration patterns of the region. The Beauce, a district of Quebec south of Quebec City along the Chaudière river, was settled in the 17th century by a relatively small French founding population. From this area, the lumbermen migrated to the Moosehead Lake region of Maine to which the Beauce is linked by a direct road. Recently, Dr. Jean Marc Saint-Hilaire and his daughter Dr. Marie-Hélène Saint-Hilaire (*personal communication*, 1979) videotaped interviews with several jumpers living in the Beauce region, confirming the continued existence of the disorder in that region. Considering the small number of original settlers, a founder effect may explain the large number of affected people in the area. Awareness of the condition would then lead to its ready recognition when it occurs in members of other national groups in Maine and elsewhere.

The heredity of the condition suggests autosomal dominant inheritance with variable expressivity. It is not compatible with mere intrafamily imitation and is similar to the genetic pattern of tics. The stereotypy and the range of the clinical manifestations, the absence of neurological abnormalities, the involuntary nature, and the relationship to tension and anxiety are all features supporting the diagnosis of an unusual and specific tic syndrome. It is evidently quite different in its manifestations from the usual continuum of childhood tics that culminate in Tourette's syndrome of *tic convulsif*. It should be noted, however, that excessive startle is also a feature of tic disease or Tourette's syndrome, where it occurs in 20% of patients (37). According to Shapiro et al. (41), echopraxia and echolalia are also seen in 20% of patients with this condition. Tics themselves, however, are not induced by startle, although they are similarly subject to precipitation by tension or fatigue and may be triggered by illness.

As in tic disease, the basic pathophysiological mechanism of jumping is still unclear. By analogy with tic disease, treatment with antidopaminergic agents, such as haloperidol or pimozide, certainly seems worth trying in people whose jumping constitutes a social disability. In view of the effect of the potent serotonergic agent clonazepam in startle disease and to a lesser extent in Tourette's syndrome (26), this substance should also be tried in the treatment of jumping.

Jumping, Latah, and Myriachit: Culturally Determined Variability of an Identical Neurological Disorder?

Beard (7,8) was aware of latah (ticklish), a Malay disorder featuring echopraxia, excessive startle, and swearing. Georges Gilles de la Tourette (21) translated Beard's writings and discussed the relationship of jumping to latah and to myriachit (to act foolishly), a condition encountered in Siberia and other parts of Asia and Africa. The latter had been reported by Hammond (27), then Professor of Diseases of the Mind and of the Nervous System in the New York Postgraduate Medical School and Hospital. Hammond quoted from an account of a Siberian journey made by Lieutenant Buckingham and Ensigns Foulk and McLean of the United States Navy. The condition was demonstrated to them by a Russian general-staff captain, who stated that it was not uncommon in Siberia, particularly around Yakutsk, and that it was more common in women. People with myriachit also display echopraxia, echolalia, and excessive startle as prominent features.

In 1952, Yap (48) published a long and searching article on the latah reaction based on his observation of seven cases made during a voyage to Malaysia. The three severe cases he described showed echolalia, echopraxia, and automatic obedience. Excessive startle was alluded to in some patients, and coprolalia was often a feature. At least one of the subjects was very ticklish. These clinical features are quite similar to those of jumping. It is difficult to understand the significance of the long duration of some of the attacks of latah Yap described. As far as we know, such long-lasting attacks have not been described in jumpers.

Simons (42), in a recent study of latah, distinguishes three phases: first is the immediate response, corresponding to excessive startle and expletive. Second is the attention capture, which corresponds to echopraxia and automatic obedience, requiring "framed and forceful presentation of commands and models" occurring particularly in a state of "arousal determined narrowing of attention." This effectiveness of brief forceful commands for automatic obedience and echopraxia has already been stressed in jumping by Beard (7,8). The third component is "role latah," consisting of an elaboration of some of the responses into intentionally amusing performances. This may be an important component of this disorder in Imu, the Ainu equivalent of latah, where affected individuals attend special functions expecting to "perform." This readiness or willingness to perform is not a feature in jumping, which is considered a handicap and a disability in North American society.

Simons (42) considers the Burmese Jauns, Thai Bah-Tsche, Phillipine Mali Mali or Silok, Siberian Ikota or Amurakh, Ainu Imu, Lapp panic, and the Bantu or South West African disorder to represent the same condition as jumping, latah, and myriachit. In an attempt to find this disorder or behavioral pattern in American society, Simons advertised in local newspapers for easily startled persons. Reactions found among the 12 respondents included, in addition to violent startle, a loud cry, expletive swearing or coprolalia, dropping objects, or a fighting posture. This condition, then, represents an exaggeration of the physiological reaction relating to normal startle, as cataplexy relates to getting "weak with anger" or "buck fever," and Lachschlag relates to getting "weak kneed with laughter." Studies of emotional, genetic, and neurophysiological aspects in severely and mildly affected individuals with this disorder will provide further clarification.

From these accounts, it seems that jumping, myriachit, and latah may represent the same basic pathophysiological disorder of the nervous system since excessive startle, echolalia, echopraxia, and automatic obedience are present in all three. It is also clear that there is a considerable and variable cultural overlay to these conditions in the different populations in which they occur. This culturally determined behavioral variation makes accurate comparison among the three conditions difficult. Clearer observations of the biological core of the disorders in these different populations should enable us to decide whether or not they represent the same process.

STARTLE EPILEPSY

Alajouanine and Gastaut (1) describe two types of abnormal startle associated with seizures occurring in individuals with infantile hemiparesis or quadriparesis and diffuse cerebral dysfunction: (a) startle synkinesis, consisting of a 5- to 10-sec tonic contraction of the affected side without other clinical or electrographic evidence of epileptic discharge, and (b) startle epilepsy, where, in addition to this excessive response, there are other clinical or electrographic epileptic manifestations. The distinction between these two types may be somewhat artificial, since surface epileptic discharges may not be striking or obvious in some patients, as subsquently shown by Bancaud et al. (5,6).

Cases of startle-induced epileptic manifestations in patients with secondary generalized corticoreticular epilepsy have been described by Gastaut and Villeneuve (20) and by Ohtahara et al. (39). Startle epilepsy has also been described in association with Sturge–Weber syndrome (38) and Down's syndrome (23), and cases of startle epilepsy with impressive clinical histories but without good electrographic correlation continue to be presented in the literature (4,9,10). Activation by startle is relatively common in patients with partial epilepsy, particulary in those whose symptoms and signs suggest involvement of the postcentral area.

Implanted electrode studies were carried out by Bancaud et al. (5) in a patient with hemiplegia and startle epilepsy. The authors demonstrated the origin of the seizures to be in the supplementary motor area, in the interhemispheric fissure. A second patient studied by Bancaud and his group (6) had excessive startle at times without clear additional epileptic manifestations; at other times, startle was clearly associated with other epileptic features. The area of epileptogenic abnormality involved mesiofrontal structures in the vicinity of the paracentral lobule. The authors concluded that the startle reflex may be responsible through a feedback mechanism for triggering the epileptic focus. Surgical treatment and removal of the epileptogenic area in their first patient led to complete cessation of seizures and startle phenomena during a 3-year follow-up.

A third study from this group by Chauvel et al. (14) reviewed 11 patients with a perinatal lesion. Onset of startle seizures occurred at an average age of 9 years, and proprioceptive stimuli (stumbling), as well as noise or touch, were effective. They began as an intense startle reaction, followed by a complex partial motor seizure. Polygraphic studies showed that this startle pattern was asymmetric, predominant or limited to the hemiplegic side, focused on one muscle, and subject to habituation. The seizure itself, either tonic or tonic–clonic, started precisely in the limb (or muscle) first involved by the startle reflex and propagated to the corresponding contralateral limb as well as to the ipsilateral side. Depth electrode recordings showed that the transition between the two successive parts of the seizures originated in an abnormal part of the motor area of the cerebral cortex.

Reduction in startle seizures or myoclonus was also found following anterior callosal section in one patient (3). The operation initially led to a reduction of nonstartle-related epileptic events. The addition of clonazepam proved to be more effective than it had been prior to callosotomy in reducing the startle-dependent attacks.

Activation of a diffusely abnormal cortex by the startle reflex can lead to the generalized spike–wave discharges accompanied by a massive myoclonic jerk described by Gastaut and Villeneuve (20), Gastaut and Tassinari (19), and in some of their patients by Gimenez-Roldan and Martin (22). This illustrates that startle-induced epileptic events can occasionally be a feature of secondary generalized epilepsy, just as startle can activate partial cortical epileptic discharge.

In summary, in patients with cerebral dysfunction, startle may activate either focal or generalized epileptic discharges, although the former have been much better studied than the latter. The startle response itself may be abnormal or excessive in these patients; on the other hand, there may be focal or diffuse cortical hyperexcitability to the startle reflex. Finally, in some patients, diffuse encephalopathies may affect the same neuronal systems and lead to similar clinical manifestations as are found in genetically determined startle disease. Occurrence of such nonepileptic abnormal startle in patients with diffuse encephalopathy has been suggested by Gastaut and Villeneuve (20).

According to Gastaut and Broughton (18), conventional anticonvulsant drug therapy is of little value in the treatment of startle epilepsy. Booker et al. (11) suggested that extinction techniques may be useful in treatment of this condition, but this approach has met with little acceptance. Chlordiazepoxide was found effective in the treatment of a patient with startle epilepsy as early as 1961 (15). Recently, Gimenez-Roldan and Martin (22) have shown the effectiveness of clonazepam in treating startle-induced seizures in children. Two patients with hemiparesis who had startle seizures as the only epileptic manifestation remained permanently controlled after a mean of 34 months of continuous therapy. Startle-induced seizures recurred after 1 and 4 years, respectively, in two patients with the Lennox–Gastaut syndrome. The authors postulate that clonazepam inhibits abnormal brainstem mechanisms mediating pathologically enhanced startle reactions in these patients, thus avoiding activation of a discharging focus in the vicinity of the supplementary motor area. The reported effect of clonazepam further supports the concept of a common pathway in the pathophysiology of startle disorders. In our experience, however, clonazepam was ineffective in controlling startle epilepsy in three young adults with this disorder.

ACKNOWLEDGMENTS

We thank Dr. Victoria Lees for editorial assistance, Geneviève Limoges for secretarial help, and Drs. Marie-Hélène and Jean-Marc St-Hilaire for the loan of the videotape showing interviews with jumpers presented at the myoclonus workshop. We are grateful to the Seiden family for their support of the workshop, and to Dr. Stanley Fahn for his stimulation to carry out this review.

REFERENCES

1. Alajouanine T, Gastaut H. La syncinésie-sursaut et l'épilepsie-sursaut à déclanchement sensoriel ou sensitif inopiné. *Rev. Neurol (Paris)* 1955; 93:29–41.
2. Andermann F, Keene DL, Andermann E, Quesney LF. Startle disease or hyperekplexia: further delineation of the syndrome. *Brain* 1980; 103:985–97.
3. Avila JO, Radvany J, Huck FR, Pires de Camargo CH, Marino R, Jr, Ragazzo PC, Riva D. Anterior callosotomy as a substitute for hemispherectomy. *Acta Neurochir [Suppl] (Wien)* 1980; 30:137–43.
4. Baier WK. The startle disease in brain-damaged patients: report of a case. *Neuropaediatrie* 1980; 11:72–5.
5. Bancaud J, Talairach J, Bonis A. Physiopathogénie des épilepsies-sursaut: a propos d'une épilepsie de l'aire motrice supplémentaire. *Rev Neurol (Paris)* 1967;117:441–53.
6. Bancaud J, Talairach J, Lamarche M, Bonis A, Trottier S. Hypothèses neurophysiopathologiques sur l'épilepsie-sursaut chez l'homme. *Rev Neurol (Paris)* 1975;131:559–71.
7. Beard GM. Remarks on jumpers or jumping frenchmen. *J Nerv Ment Dis* 1878; 5:526.
8. Beard GM. Experiments with the jumpers of Maine. *Pop Sci Monthly* 1880;18:170–8.
9. Bermejo PF, Peraita AMR, Picornell DI. Epilepsia sobresalto. A proposito de un caso. *Arch Neurobiol (Madr)* 1975;38:247–59.
10. Bhandari B, Gupta BM, Garg AR. Touch epilepsy. *Indian J Pediatr* 1973;40:111–3.
11. Booker HE, Forster FM, Klove H. Extinction factors in startle (acousticomotor) seizures. *Neurology (NY)* 1965;15:1095–103.
12. Boudouresques J, Roger J, Tassinari CA, Régis H, Salamon G, Chiarelli R. Reflexions à propos d'un sursaut pathologique. *Rev Neurol (Paris)* 1964;111:561–70.
13. Bruyn GW. Hyperekplexia (startle disease). In: Vinken PJ, Bruyn GW, eds. Handbook of clinical neurology, vol. 42. Amsterdam: North Holland, 1981:228–9.
14. Chauvel P, Liegeois C, Chodkiewicz JP, Bancaud J, Talairach J. Startle epilepsy with infantile hemiplegia: the physiopathological data leading to surgical therapy. Abstracts of the 15th epilepsy international symposium, 1983:180.
15. Cohen NH, McAuliffe M, Aird R. Startle epilepsy treated with chlordiazepoxide (Librium). *Dis Nerv Syst* 1961;22:20–7.
16. De Groen JHM, Kamphuisen HAC. Periodic nocturnal myoclonus in a patient with hyperexplexia (startle disease). *J Neurol Sci* 1978;38:207–13.
17. Fitch TP, quoted by Stevens H. *Arch Neurol* 1965;12:311–4.
18. Gastaut H, Broughton R. Epileptic seizures. Clinical and electrographic features. Diagnosis and treatment. Springfield, Illinois: Charles C Thomas, 1972:153–5.
19. Gastaut H, Tassinari CA. Triggering mechanisms in epilepsy: the electroclinical point of view. *Epilepsia*, 1966;7:85–135.
20. Gastaut H, Villeneuve A. The startle disease or hyperekplexia: pathological surprise reaction. *J Neurol Sci* 1967;5:523–42.
21. Gilles de la Tourette G. Jumping, latah, myriachit. *Arch Neurol* 1884;8:68–74.
22. Gimenez-Roldan S, Martin M. Effectiveness of clonazepam in startle-induced seizures. *Epilepsia* 1979;20:555–61.
23. Gimenez-Roldan S, Martin M. Startle epilepsy complicating Down syndrome during adulthood. *Ann Neurol* 1980;7:78–80.
24. Gogan P. The startle and orienting reactions in man: a study of their characteristics and habituation. *Brain Res* 1970;18:117–35.
25. Goldstein K, Landis C, Hunt WA, Clarke FM. Moro reflex and startle pattern. *Arch Neurol Psychiatry* 1938;40:322–77.
26. Gonce M, Barbeau A. Seven cases of Gilles de la Tourette's syndrome. Partial relief with clonazepam. A pilot study. *Can J Neurol Sci* 1977;4:279–83.
27. Hammond W. Miryachit; a newly described disease of the nervous system: and its analogues. *NY Med J* 1884;39:191–2.
28. Hardison J. Are the jumping frenchmen of Maine goosey? *JAMA* 1980;244:70.
29. Kirstein L, Silfverskiöld B. A family with emotionally precipitated drop seizures. *Acta Psychiatr Scand* 1958;33:471–6.
30. Klein R, Haddow JE, De Luca C. Familial congenital disorder resembling stiff-man syndrome. *Am J Dis Child* 1972;124:730–1.

31. Kok O, Bruyn GW. An unidentified hereditary disease. *Lancet* 1962;1359.
32. Kunkle EC. The jumpers of Maine: past history and present status. *J Maine Med Assoc* 1965;56:191–3.
33. Kunkle EC. The jumpers of Maine: a reappraisal. *Arch Intern Med* 1967;119:355–8.
34. Kurczynski TW. Hyperekplexia. *Arch Neurol* 1983;40:246–8.
35. Landis C, Hunt WA. The startle pattern. New York: Farrar and Rinehart, 1939.
36. Lingam S, Wilson J, Hart EW. Hereditary stiff-baby syndrome. *Am J Dis Child* 1981;135:909–11.
37. Murray TJ. Tourette's syndrome: a treatable tic. *Can Med Assoc J* 1978;118:1407–10.
38. Nakamura M, Kanai H, Miyamoto Y, Kadobayashi I, Ukida G, Kato N. A case of Sturge-Weber syndrome with startle epilepsy. *No To Shinkei* 1975;27:325–31.
39. Ohtahara S, Oka E, Ban T, Yamatogi Y, Inoue H. Startle epilepsy with the Lennox syndrome. *Rinsho Shinkeigaku* 1971;11:201–7.
40. Rabinovitch R. An exaggerated startle reflex resembling a kicking horse. *Can Med Assoc J* 1965;93:130.
41. Shapiro AK, Shapiro ES, Bruun RD, Sweet RD. Gilles de la Tourette syndrome. New York: Raven Press, 1978.
42. Simons RC. Resolution of the Latah paradox. *J Nerv Ment Dis* 1980;168:195–206.
43. Stevens H. Jumping frenchmen of Maine. *Arch Neurol* 1965;12:311–4.
44. Stevens H. Jumping frenchmen of Maine (myriachit). In: Vinken PJ, Bruyn GW, eds. Handbook of clinical neurology, vol 42. Amsterdam: North Holland, 1981:231–3.
45. Strauss H. Das zusammenschrecken. Experimentell-kinematographische studie zur physiologie und pathophysiologie der reaktivbewegungen. *J Psych Neurol* 1929;39:111–231.
46. Suhren O, Bruyn GW, Tuynman JA. Hyperexplexia: a hereditary startle syndrome. *J Neurol Sci* 1966;3:577–605.
47. Thorne FC. Startle neurosis. *Am J Psychiatry* 1944;101:105–9.
48. Yap PM. The latah reaction: its pathodynamics and nosological position. *J Ment Sci* 1952;98:515–64.

Advances in Neurology, Vol. 43: Myoclonus,
edited by S. Fahn et al. Raven Press,
New York © 1986.

Evolving Ideas on the Neurophysiology of Myoclonus

A. M. Halliday

Medical Research Council, Institute of Neurology, National Hospital for Nervous Diseases, London WC1N 3BG, United Kingdom

The association between myoclonic jerking and electrical activity recorded from the scalp was noted by some of the earliest electroencephalographers. Gibbs et al. (16) in 1935 found that patients with spike-and-wave discharges in their EEG might occasionally show jerking at the same rate, and similar observations were made by Jasper and Andrews in 1938 (27). In the same year, Grinker et al. (17) appear to have been the first to record polyspike discharges, closely associated with the myoclonic jerking, in a family with progressive myoclonic epilepsy. They recorded two channel EEGs, with a frontal and occipital derivation, in three unaffected and two affected members (Figs. 1, 2). The two patients with myoclonus, who were related as aunt and niece, both showed sharp wave discharges in the EEG (see Fig. 1B). When the younger patient was hospitalized and phenobarbital treatment was stopped for 2 or 3 days, bursts of polyspikes appeared in the frontal record (see Fig. 1C, where they are marked with an X).

Off medication, this patient showed a very characteristic cycle in her myoclonic jerking. This gradually increased in severity over 2 to 4 days, culminating in a major fit. At first, the twitchings were limited to the face, but they gradually became more frequent and violent and spread to the limbs. After a major fit, the jerking would disappear for a few hours and then begin again, gradually increasing over the next few days, to end in a further fit. This cycle repeated itself indefinitely as long as the patient was off drugs. Figure 2 shows the bursts of polyspikes characteristically seen in both frontal and occipital leads during the preictal phase (A) and their absence immediately after a major seizure, when the myoclonus also disappeared, the record being dominated at this stage by slow-wave activity (B). In Fig. 2C, the simultaneous record of EEG and EMG demonstrates the close association between the cerebral spikes and the muscle bursts.

EARLY ANIMAL EXPERIMENTS

One year after this pioneering study, Adrian and Moruzzi (1) discovered by chance, while experimenting on the sensory nuclei in the medulla of the cat, that they could record from the fibers of the pyramidal tract with a wire electrode and that, where these closely packed fibers spread out in the motor decussation, it was

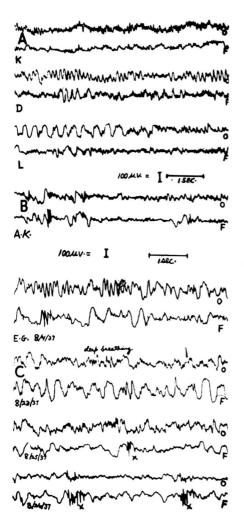

FIG. 1. Two channel EEG recordings with frontal (F) and occipital (O) derivations, recorded from three unaffected members of the family **(A)**, the mother (K), son (D), and eclamptic sister (L) of the younger of the two affected patients. **B:** Records from two of the affected members of the family, the propositus (E. G.) and her aunt (A. K.), both of whom suffered from myoclonic jerking and fits. **C:** Recordings of E. G. in hospital on phenobarbital medication (8/23/37) and 2 and 3 days after coming off medication (8/25/37 and 8/26/37, respectively). X marks the clusters of spikes observed at this time. (From Grinker et al., ref. 17, with permission.)

possible to isolate single-unit discharges originating in the motor cortex. Among the anesthetics they used in these experiments on the cat was chloralose, and they were thus able to observe and give a detailed description of the stimulus-sensitive myoclonic jerking characteristic of this drug.

To quote from the account of Adrian and Moruzzi (1, pp. 170–171):

> Sensory stimulation gives a much more constant and striking effect when the animal is under chloralose (35 mg/kg). The familiar effect of this drug is to produce a combination of deep anaesthesia with increased responsiveness to an abrupt stimulus such as a light tap on one of the feet or even on the table near the animal. This evokes a sudden movement, sometimes restricted to the limb which was touched, but often a convulsive jerk involving all four limbs and the trunk as well. . . . The convulsive response to a touch is a cortical reaction. We find that destruction of both motor

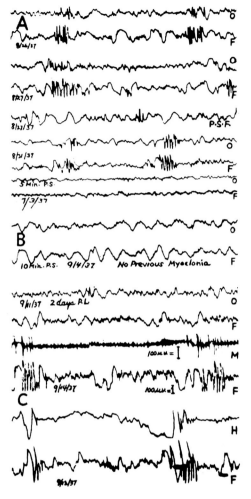

FIG. 2. Further recordings taken on Grinker and co-workers' hospitalized patient off medication. **A:** the occipital spiking has become more marked than in Fig. 1C (8/26/37); recorded on 8/27/37 3 hours before a major seizure, there are large bursts of spikes synchronous in the two channels; 30 min after an attack (8/27/37, P.S.F.), the single tracing shows large slow-waves and only occasional spikes, but 4 days after the seizure (8/31/37), the clusters of large spikes have recurred. **B:** The first record shows the flattened EEG 5 min after a major seizure (5 min P.S., 7/3/37); 10 min after the seizure on 9/4/37, there are large slow-waves with no accompanying jerking, whereas the record on 9/11/37 shows the relative reduction in spiking following 2 days on phenobarbital. **C:** A simultaneous EMG (M) and frontal EEG (F) shows the association between the cortical spikes and the muscle jerks. (From Grinker et al., ref. 17, with permission.)

areas abolishes the response, leaving only some increase in the limb reflexes, and that temporary occlusion of the carotids produces a temporary failure; also, whenever the jerking movement occurs there is an abrupt potential wave in the motor area and a corresponding discharge of impulses in the pyramidal tract. The frequency of the impulses in this discharge can vary widely. In some preparations there are not more than two or three impulses in each unit at intervals of 1/50 sec or more; in others the number may be higher and the intervals less, and we have twice found the discharge changing gradually into the characteristic high-frequency type to be described later as the result of convulsant drugs. Evidently chloralose has some of the properties of a convulsant besides those of an anaesthetic.

Adrian and Moruzzi (1) measured the latency of the ascending volley in the cuneate nucleus produced by a tactile stimulus to the forefoot and compared it with the resulting descending volley in the pyramidal decussation. They found that the latencies were remarkably constant from one animal to another, but that after the time required for the afferent volley to travel to and from the cortex had been taken into account, there still appeared to be about 10 msec unaccounted for. Similar results were obtained from stimulation of the hind limb, although here the latency could occasionally be much longer. The delay could also be increased if stimulation was repeated at very short intervals, although it was necessary to stimulate as often as six times a second in order to cause an appreciable increase in latency.

Both the cortical diphasic wave and the pyramidal discharge were still evoked in deep chloralose anesthesia, although no accompanying muscular movement was then seen. This demonstrated that the descending pyramidal discharge was not in itself sufficient to cause the jerk. In lighter anesthesia, where the primary discharge was accompanied by a jerk, there was often a secondary cortical discharge exhibiting a longer burst of impulses in the pyramidal fibers. This was more vulnerable to ischemia and fatigue than was the primary discharge. This work by Adrian and Moruzzi (1) marks the beginning of a long series of animal studies that have helped to throw light on the neurophysiology of clinical myoclonus (2–5,7,7a,b,12,34,35).

FURTHER CLINICAL STUDIES

In 1946 and 1947 Dawson (8–10) produced three papers that brought a new degree of scientific precision to the clinical studies. In the first (8), he studied the relationship between the EEG spikes and the muscle jerks in two nonfamilial myoclonic subjects, who, like the patients studied by Grinker et al. (17), showed a gradual buildup of generalized, irregular myoclonic jerking culminating in a grand mal attack, although the period over which this increase occurred was much shorter than in the earlier cases.

Dawson (8) pointed out the frequent occurrence of recruitment in the muscle jerks, suggesting that the train of cortical spikes, which had a frequency of about 8 to 13 per second, had to build up a state of excitability in the intervening pathways by repetitive firing. He also noted that the flexors tended to begin firing one or two beats before the extensors and that they showed evidence of more prolonged facilitation following a burst of spikes, in that they were more easily fired when a second discharge followed after a short gap (Figs. 3,4). In the jerk, there was a failure in the reciprocal innervation of flexors and extensors, since they both fired within 5 to 10 msec of each other. In the fully developed syndrome, a tendon tap would induce a generalized myoclonic jerk of the same type as those occurring

---

FIG. 3. Illustration of the close temporal relationship between the EEG spikes and the muscle action potentials. The muscle discharge recruits throughout the EEG spike discharge, starting earlier in the flexor than in the extensor groups of muscles. A brief silent period follows the spike burst in the EEG. The records in **b, c, d,** and **e** are from a continuous recording, with 8-sec intervals between them, showing corresponding increases in the number of EEG and muscle discharges. (From Dawson, ref. 8, with permission.)

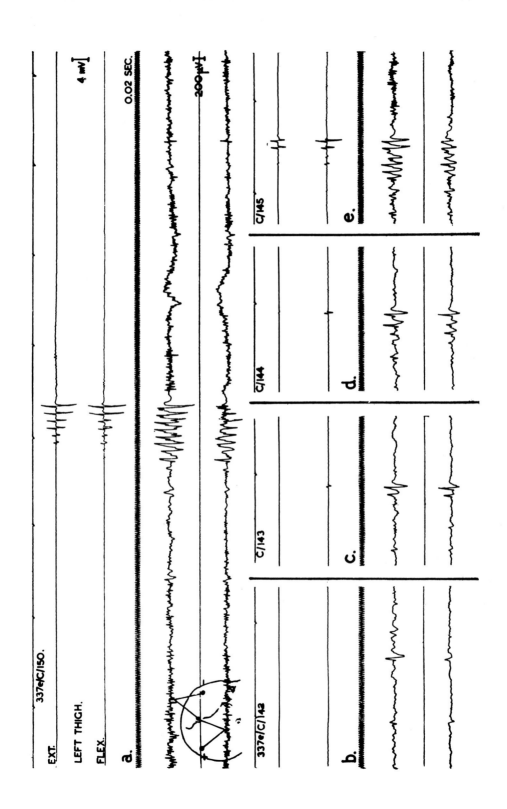

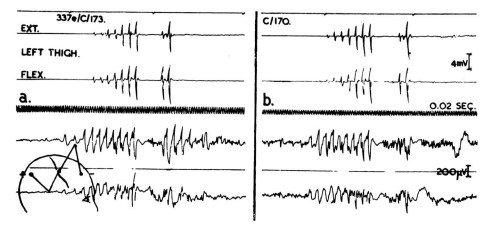

FIG. 4. Following a break in the EEG discharge, the muscle action potentials restart, with the size of those in the flexor groups reduced less than those in the extensor groups. (From Dawson, ref. 8, with permission.)

spontaneously, and such jerks could also be provoked by a sudden unexpected noise.

In the same study, Dawson (8) also recorded a third epileptic patient with grand mal fits who was also subject to mild attacks of muscular jerking lasting for up to 48 hr, associated with continuous spike-and-wave discharges in the EEG. For the first 5 or 6 hr of these attacks there was a slight clouding of consciousness, with diffuse and irregular twitchings of the muscles all over the body accompanied by continuous irregular spikes intermixed with slow waves in the EEG. After some hours, the clouding of consciousness would disappear, and the jerkings would become regular and synchronous in all parts of the body at about 3 per second. At this time, the EEG showed regular 2.5 to 3-per-second spike-and-wave discharges. The jerks were clearly related to the spikes, but the latency relationship was much looser in this patient than in the other two, and the jerks could even precede the earliest recognizable phase of the EEG spike. Furthermore, the EMG of the jerks was usually of an altogether less simple form than in the two other cases, being both longer and having more phases.

Two further papers by Dawson (9,10), published in 1947, proved to be landmarks in the history of clinical neurophysiology. In them he demonstrated for the first time that the somatosensory evoked potential (SEP) could be recorded from the scalp electrodes situated over the rolandic cortex in awake, conscious man (9) and that the normal response could be enlarged some five to ten times in certain myoclonic patients (10). The patient on whom this finding was established, however, was very different clinically from the other three studied by Dawson (8) in his 1946 paper. This was a case not of generalized, irregular jerking of the muscles of the face, limbs, and occasionally trunk, associated with the preictal phase of a grand mal fit, but of a 42-year-old man with an 18-month history of severe and violent jerking attacks, usually starting in the right leg. Superimposed on the jerking, there were attacks in which the limb became dystonic. The patient had also had a number of grand mal fits in association with the jerking.

Dawson (10) found that the spontaneous jerks were related in time to the occurrence of a fast focal sinusoidal discharge, picked up by an electrode over the central cortex and that the same afterdischarge could be evoked by a tendon tap on the affected limb (Figs. 5,6). The cerebral discharge was associated with a negative shift in the cortical potential. The myoclonic jerking attack was independent of the size of the tendon jerk itself and could occur in its absence (Fig. 6B) but was not seen if the focal cortical afterdischarge and its accompanying negative shift failed to appear (Fig. 5C, D), even though the primary cortical response was still evident.

Dawson (10) demonstrated that his patient had abnormally large cortical somatosensory responses to electrical stimulation of the lateral popliteal nerve in the leg or the ulnar nerve in the arm. The primary SEP had a contralateral maximum, related to the representation of the hand and foot areas in the rolandic cortex, but the myoclonic response was some 3 to 4 cm anterior to that in the healthy subject, suggesting that it might come from the motor strip rather than the primary sensory area. The electrical stimulus to the peripheral nerve, like the tendon jerk, could produce the same type of focal afterdischarge and accompanying myoclonic jerking, but stimulation of the ulnar nerve at the wrist was associated with a delay of 150 to 200 msec longer between the stimulus and the jerks, compared with a tap to the patellar tendon and the accompanying jerk in the thigh muscles or a tap to the

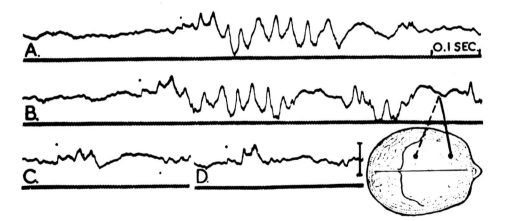

FIG. 5. The record, made with a cathode ray oscillograph, shows the form of the EEG discharge following a tap on a tendon. The black dots indicate the contact of the hammer with the skin. This is followed by a pair of waves, during which the back electrode on the head became positive with respect to the front one. In **A** and **B**, the back electrode then became negative, and a train of spikes followed that was accompanied by a myoclonic jerk. In **C** and **D**, no negative deflection occurred, and no train of spikes or myoclonic jerking followed. The calibration mark in **D** shows 100 μV. (From Dawson, ref. 10, with permission.)

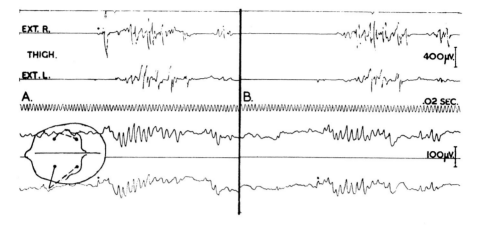

FIG. 6. The records show the results of taps applied to the right **(A)** and the left **(B)** patellar tendon. Though the knee-jerk action potential following the tap on the left side is hardly perceptible, the following myoclonic jerk is as large as that which followed a much stronger knee jerk on the right side. (The black dot under the records indicates the artifact produced electrically by the contact of the tendon hammer with the skin). (From Dawson, ref. 10, with permission.)

tendon of the biceps muscle in the arm and the following jerk in the anterior tibial muscles. It was not clear whether this curious difference was related to the type or site of stimulation or had some other explanation.

It is perhaps worth mentioning that not all patients showing a fast focal afterdischarge associated with jerking attacks have shown large accompanying somatosensory responses. Halliday (21,24) has described a patient with the same type of attack (Fig. 7), who had a somatosensory evoked response the amplitude of which was within the normal range (Fig. 8).

Dawson's (10) patient showed evidence of an excitability cycle, with regard to both the amplitude of the primary cerebral response to paired stimulation at different intervals and the driving of the focal afterdischarges in the EEG. Stimulating the ulnar nerve at frequencies between 4 and 30 per second, the amplitude of the focal sinusoidal waves became particularly large at a stimulus frequency of 30 per second (corresponding to that of the spontaneous rhythm), and this was accompanied by especially violent myoclonic jerking. The cortical discharge tended to organize itself into bursts at intervals of 0.3 to 0.4 (Fig. 9). By comparing the response to the second of a pair of stimuli at different intervals, Dawson (10) demonstrated clearly that there was a marked reduction in the size of the second response at intervals between 10 and 30 msec, followed by a period of facilitation between 60 and 100 msec and a second period of depression and delay of the response at longer intervals (Fig. 10). This "refractoriness" or inhibition lasted

FIG. 7. Simultaneous EEG and EMG of a 32-year-old man with jerking attacks of the left leg associated with a fast focal sinusoidal discharge in the EEG with a maximum near the vertex. Note the tendency to 3-per-second periodicity in the bursts of abnormal discharges in the clang-evoked jerking attack **(right)**. (From Halliday, ref. 24, with permission.)

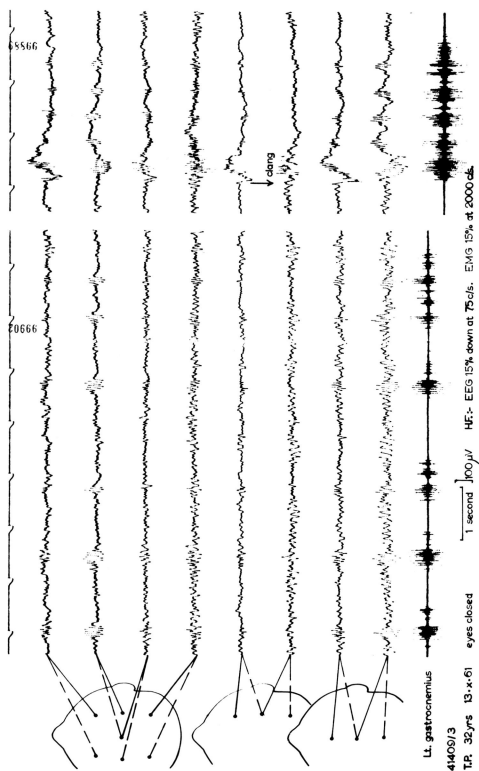

clang

99903

99906

Lt. gastrocnemius

41409/3

T.P. 32yrs 13·x·61 eyes closed

1 second]100μV HF:- EEG 15% down at 75c/s. EMG 15% at 2000 c/s.

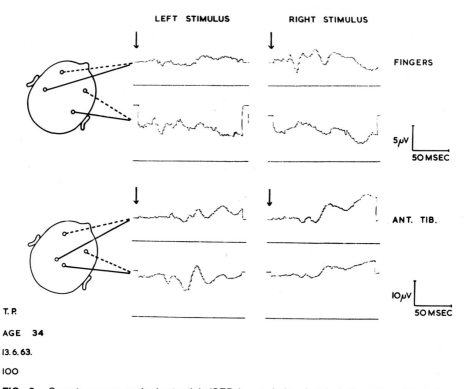

FIG. 8. Somatosensory evoked potentials (SEPs) recorded to electrical stimulation of the index and middle fingers of each hand and of the anterior tibial nerves at each ankle in the same myoclonic patient whose records are shown in Fig. 7. Note the normal amplitude of the SEPs, in contrast to the findings on the patient reported by Dawson (10).

until approximately 300 msec, and the latter interval corresponded to the frequency at which groups of high-voltage discharges tended to occur in the frequency-following experiments. There was thus evidence of a clear excitability cycle, which looked as if it was underlying the 3-per-second periodicity in the EEG.

There is such a wealth of observation in these few early papers that one might be excused for feeling that relatively little of importance has been added since, although many of these original findings have been confirmed in other studies. In one respect, however, the whole picture has changed. We know now that at least some of these types of myoclonus can survive decortication or high brainstem section. This is not to say that the cortex is not playing a role in the production of the jerking in the intact nervous system; it is simply to recognize that a very similar type of jerking can occur in the absence of the cortex under certain circumstances. This goes against the original observation of Adrian and Moruzzi (1), but it is established by a number of studies, including those of Alvord and Whitlock (3), Ascher et al. (5), Denny-Brown (12), Van Woert and Chung (34), and Zuckerman

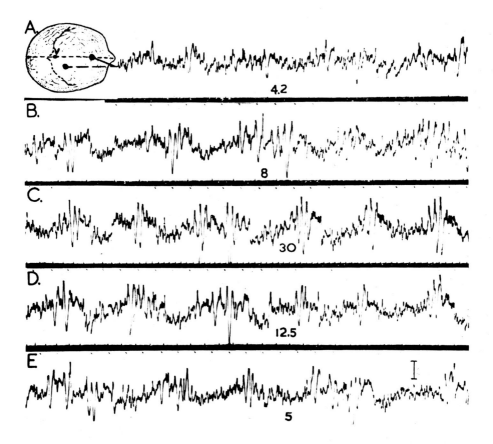

FIG. 9. EEG during stimulation of the left ulnar nerve at frequencies from 4 to 30 per second. The rate of stimulation is shown at the center of each record, and the spikes at the bottom of the record show the position of the stimulus. At a rate of 30 per second, the stimuli provoked large bursts of oscillations at intervals of 0.3 to 0.4 sec and with a frequency of 30 per second. These outbursts were accompanied by particularly violent myoclonic jerkings. The marks at the tops of the records indicate intervals of 0.1 sec, and the calibration mark in **E** represents the deflection due to 50 μV. (From Dawson, ref. 10, with permission.)

and Glaser (35). Ascher et al. (5) have also shown that experimental myoclonus will survive lesions of the pyramidal tracts at medullary level. This evidence has been reviewed in some detail by the author elsewhere (22,24).

MYOCLONUS INDUCED BY DECORTICATION IN THE MONKEY

Denny-Brown (12) has demonstrated that in the monkey irregular, brief, stimulus-sensitive myoclonic jerking actually develops 3 or 4 weeks after ablation of either the postcentral or precentral cortex, and that when it does so, removal of the cerebellum increases its severity, so that neither cortex nor cerebellum are necessary for its production. It can, however, be abolished by a small transverse cut some 2

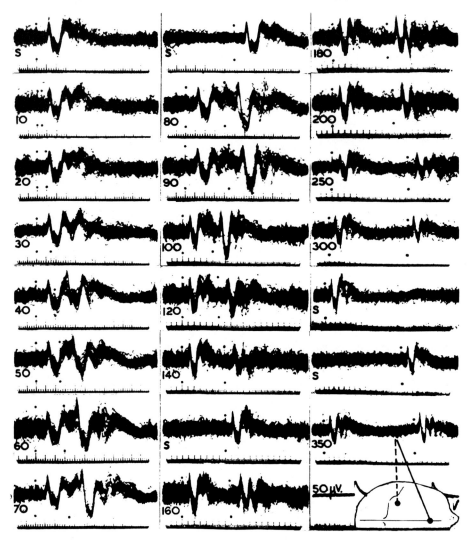

FIG. 10. Records from Dawson's (10) patient showing the response to a pair of shocks separated by intervals of from 10 to 350 msec. S indicates single control stimuli, and in each record 50 single shocks or pairs of shocks at the separation marked on the record were applied at 1-sec intervals. The black dots indicate the stimulus markers in the time scale and the stimulus artifacts in the cerebral response. The response to the second shock of the pair is depressed at a separation of the shocks of 10 to 30 msec, it is facilitated from 60 to 100 msec, depressed and delayed at 140 msec, and has almost returned to normal at 300 to 350 msec. The time scales indicate 5- and 20-msec intervals. (From Dawson, ref. 10, with permission.)

mm from the midline at the level of the obex, penetrating in depth as far as the pyramid, a lesion that is known to abolish the spinobulbar spinal reflex by interrupting the reticulospinal pathway on one side while leaving most of the other descending tracts untouched. Unilateral section leads to abolition of both the reflex and the myoclonus on the ipsilateral side. As Brodal (6) points out, this descending pathway, which originates in the medullary and pontine rectircular formations, both of which receive a dense projection from the pyramidal fibers of the contralateral rolandic cortex, forms an alternative motor pathway from cortex to muscle. This efferent pathway is distinguished from the corticospinal pathway by the fact that it is not somatotopically organized.

There is experimental evidence incriminating the medullary reticular formation in the production of myoclonic jerking. Studies on the myoclonic state induced by local cobalt implantation by Cesa-Bianchi et al. (7) and by intravenous infusion of urea by Zuckerman and Glaser (35) have both shown the importance of this area, and particularly the nucleus gigantocellularis, in generating the abnormal epileptic discharge responsible for some forms of myoclonic jerking. DDT-induced myoclonus, more recently studied by Van Woert and Chung (34; Chung and Van Woert, *this volume*), appears to have a similar origin.

However, it is well to remember that the reticular formation is not the sole origin of all forms of myoclonic jerking. It is quite clear from the experimental evidence reported by Ascher (4,5) that the somatotopically organized transcortical pathway exerts an important and powerful action on the reticular formation when it is present. The wide variety of clinical settings in which myoclonic jerking occurs includes instances of cortical reflex myoclonus (19,22), as well as reticular myoclonus (18), and these two types of jerking may well coexist in the same case. The rolandic cortex can, in any case, initiate a muscular discharge by an efferent volley traveling either by the somatotopically organized corticospinal system or the nonsomatotopically organized corticoreticulospinal route.

LARGE SEPs IN MYOCLONUS

The abnormally large SEPs typically seen in progressive myoclonic epilepsy are not invariably found in myoclonic patients. Even in familial progressive myoclonic epilepsy, where they are particularly characteristic, they are encountered only at the time when the patients are exhibiting clinical jerks and may revert to a normal size if the jerking is well controlled by medication (13,15,20,26,29). Furthermore, they are not seen in benign essential myoclonus, although the muscle jerks themselves are not obviously very different in the two conditions (26). In general, the large SEPs go hand in hand with the characteristic EEG abnormalities of myoclonic epilepsy; these include the bilaterally synchronous polyspike–slow-wave complexes so often seen in this condition, as well as the more diffuse and less stereotyped central spike discharges without accompanying slow waves. Those patients with focal jerking of the type originally observed by Dawson in his 1947 paper (9) may show a large SEP, as Dawson's patient did, or not, as in the case reported by the author. Normal SEPs and EEG are the rule in patients with the "dancing eyes" syndrome of infantile myoclonus and also of the rhythmical segmental myoclonus associated with tumors or viral infections (21,24). The same applies to palatal myoclonus.

CLINICAL FEATURES

There are a number of easily recognized clinical features of myoclonus that must be significant pointers to the involvement of different generator mechanisms. The first of these is the distinction between action myoclonus and myoclonus at rest. The latter is a relatively rare syndrome but is absolutely characteristic when one encounters it. Curiously, the original patient with paramyoclonus multiplex described by Friedreich in 1881 (14) was of this rare variety, and the present author has seen another similar case in a 22-year-old woman with benign essential myoclonus, which appeared to have been inherited in her family as a dominant trait (21). She suffered from the jerking only when in a situation of enforced rest, for instance, when sitting in the audience at a concert or on some other formal social occasion, when she was under some social restraint to remain still. The jerking was at once abolished if the patient could get up and move around. The distinction between action myoclonus, which is relatively common, and the rare myoclonus at rest is so striking and so closely reminiscent of the familiar clinical distinction between intention tremor and tremor at rest that it must have some direct bearing on the mechanisms producing the two types of myoclonus (23).

A second important clinical distinction seems to be between generalized and focalized myoclonus, i.e., between the type of jerking seen in epilepsia partialis continua, which clearly has a constant primary focal distribution (even if it may spread from the focus by a jacksonian march), and the generalized diffuse myoclonus that is so characteristic of many of the progressive myoclonic epileptic patients. It seems plausible to relate these two types of syndrome to the organization of the pathways in the central nervous system (24,25). Both the neuroanatomical and neurophysiological evidence shows that there are two sensorimotor pathways able to produce stimulus-sensitive jerking in the muscles under conditions of abnormally heightened excitability, such as with chloralose. On the one hand, there is a nonsomatotopically organized system relaying in the bulbar reticular formation, served on its afferent side by the spinoreticular fibers, which travel up in the anterolateral columns mixed with the spinothalamic fibers, and served on its efferent side by the reticulospinal tract, which passes down ipsilaterally to innervate the body musculature at all levels. Superimposed on this nonsomatotopically organized system and integrated with it by the projections from the sensorimotor cortex to the pontine and medullary reticular formation is the somatotopically organized classical pathway, subserved by the dorsal column–medial lemniscus on its afferent side and the corticospinal tract on its efferent side. The pyramidal tract contains fibers originating in the central cortex, which are destined for both the spinal motoneurons and the neurons of the reticular formation (in particular, the cells of the nucleus gigantocellularis in the medulla). There is a good deal of converging evidence that both of these systems are involved to a greater or lesser extent in the production of myoclonic syndromes.

The author has already drawn attention to a third important clinical distinction, that between the irregular, lightning-like muscular jerking of many clinical syndromes and the rhythmical myoclonus characteristic of segmental myoclonus, whether owing to local viral infection, trauma, or a local neoplasm (22,24). Apart from their rhythmicity, these types of jerking are characteristically rather insensitive to outside influences and typically persist during sleep. These features are shared by palatal myoclonus. Periodic burst discharges, associated with myoclonic jerking, are also characteristic of various viral and subviral encephalitides (21,22,24).

IS MYOCLONUS A FORM OF EPILEPSY?

There has been much discussion in the literature as to whether myoclonus should or should not be regarded as epileptic. In a sense, this question is now settled, although the answer depends to some extent on what one arbitrarily decides to call epileptic. It is now clear that the same type of paroxysmal depolarization shift and accompanying superimposed burst discharge is seen in the neurons of the nucleus gigantocellularis of the bulbar reticular formation in the genesis of urea-induced myoclonus as is seen in the cortical neurons in association with classical jacksonian attacks (35). Recent work on cell membrane physiology in isolated hippocampal slices is leading to new insights into this fundamental epileptic phenomenon (28,32,33).

Work along the same lines has also offered an explanation for the mechanism underlying the rhythmical or periodic bursts underlying rhythmical myoclonus in viral infections. Traub and Pedley (31) have pointed out that in subacute spongiform encephalopathy the earliest changes detected under electron microscopy consist of swelling of neuronal processes, followed by breaks in plasma membranes and fusion and vacuolation of nerve cell processes. They suggest that this may lead to abnormal electrotonic coupling between cells, resulting in large neuronal aggregates discharging in synchrony. This hypothesis would appear to fit in well with the earlier evidence of similar spontaneous periodic burst discharges recorded by Dampsher et al. (11) in the rat sympathetic ganglia infected with pseudorabies virus, which appeared to originate in the presynaptic nerve terminals or postsynaptic dendrites.

SUMMARY

Early observations, made between 1935 and 1947, on the EEG discharges associated with myoclonic jerking are reviewed, together with the contemporary findings on the stimulus-sensitive myoclonus produced in cats under chloralose anesthesia. The accumulating evidence on the relative roles of cortex, brainstem, and cerebellum in producing this type of myoclonus is briefly summarized. The significance of large SEPs and their presence and absence in various clinical types of myoclonus is considered.

Three distinctions are drawn with regard to the clinical features of myoclonic jerking: between action myoclonus and myoclonus at rest; between focal and generalized jerking; and between the lightning-like, irregular, stimulus-sensitive jerks of myoclonic epilepsy and the rhythmical, stimulus-insensitive jerking of segmental myoclonus. Some findings bearing on the possible mechanisms of the abnormal discharges responsible at cell membrane level are mentioned.

REFERENCES

1. Adrian ED, Moruzzi G. Impulses in the pyramidal tract. *J Physiol (Lond)* 1939;97:153–99.
2. Alvord EC, Fuortes MGF. A comparison of generalized reflex myoclonic reactions elicitable in cats under chloralose anaesthesia and under strychnine. *Am J Physiol* 1954;176:253–61.
3. Alvord EC, Whitlock DG. Role of brainstem in generalised reflex myoclonic reactions in cats under chloralose anaesthesia. *Fed Proc* 1954;13:2–4.
4. Ascher P. Lemniscal influences on motor responses of extralemniscal origin. *Brain Res* 1966;2:233–53.
5. Ascher P, Jassik-Gerschenfeld D, Buser P. Participation des aires corticales sensorielles á l'élaboration de réponses motrices extrapyramidales. *Electroencephalogr Clin Neurophysiol* 1963;15:246–64.
6. Brodal A. *Neurological anatomy in relation to clinical medicine*. New York: Oxford University Press, 1981.
7. Cesa-Bianchi MG, Mancia M, Mutani R. Experimental epilepsy induced by cobalt powder in lower brainstem and thalamic structures. *Electroencephalogr Clin Neurophysiol* 1967;22:525–36.
7a. Chung E, Van Woert MH. DDT myoclonus: sites and mechanism of action. *Exp Neurol* 1984:273–82.
7b. Chung E, Yocca F, Van Woert MH. Urea-induced myoclonus: medullary glycine antagonism as mechanism of action. *Life Sci* 1985;36:1051–58.
8. Dawson GD. The relation between the electroencephalogram and muscle action potentials in certain convulsive states. *J Neurol Neurosurg Psychiatry* 1946;9:5–22.
9. Dawson GD. Cerebral response to electrical stimulation of peripheral nerve in man. *J Neurol Neurosurg Psychiatry* 1947;10:134–40.
10. Dawson GD. Investigations on a patient subject to myoclonic seizures after sensory stimulation. *J Neurol Neurosurg Psychiatry* 1947;10:141–62.
11. Dempsher J, Larrabee MG, Bang FB, Bodian F. Physiological changes in sympathetic ganglia infected with pseudorabies virus. *Am J Physiol* 1955;182:203–16.
12. Denny-Brown D. Quelques aspects physiologiques des myoclonies. In: Bonduelle M, Gastaut H, eds. Les myoclonies. Paris: Masson, 1968:121–29.
13. Ebe M, Meier-Ewert KH, Broughton R. Effects of intravenous diazepam (Valium) upon evoked potentials of photosensitive epileptic and normal subjects. *Electroencephalogr Clin Neurophysiol* 1969;27:429–35.
14. Friedreich N. Paramyoklonus multiplex. *Virchows Arch [Pathol Anat]* 1881;86:421–30.
15. Gath I. Effect of drugs on the somatosensory evoked potentials in myoclonic epilepsy. *Arch Neurol* 1969;20:354–7.
16. Gibbs FA, Davis H, Lennox WG. The electro-encephalogram in epilepsy and in conditions of impaired consciousness. *Arch Neurol Psychiatry* 1935;34:1133–48.
17. Grinker RR, Serota H, Stein SI. Myoclonic epilepsy. *Arch Neurol Psychiatry* 1938;40:968–80.
18. Hallett M, Chadwick D, Adam J, Marsden CD. Reticular reflex myoclonus. *Arch Neurol Psychiatry* 1977;40:253–64.
19. Hallett M, Chadwick D, Marsden CD. Cortical reflex myoclonus. *Neurology* 1979;29:1107–25.
20. Halliday AM. Cerebral evoked potentials in familial progressive myoclonic epilepsy. *J R Coll Physicians Lond* 1967;1:123–34.
21. Halliday AM. The clinical incidence of myoclonus. In: Williams D, ed. Modern Trends in neurology 4. London: Butterworth, 1967:69–105.
22. Halliday AM. The electrophysiological study of myoclonus in man. *Brain* 1967; 90:241–84.
23. Halliday AM. Les différent types de myoclonies. *Rev Neurol (Paris)* 1968;119:135–8.
24. Halliday AM. The neurophysiology of myoclonic jerking—a reappraisal. In: Charlton MH, ed. *Myoclonic seizures*. Amsterdam: Excerpta Medica, 1975:1–30.
25. Halliday AM. Clinical and neurophysiological aspects of the relationship between myoclonic jerking and the tonic-clonic convulsion in epilepsy. In: Speckmann EJ, Elger CE, eds. *Epilepsy and motor system*. Munich: Urban and Schwarzenberg, 1983:272–86.
26. Halliday AM, Halliday E. Cerebral somatosensory and visual evoked potentials in different clinical forms of myoclonus. In: Desmedt JE, ed. *Clinical uses of cerebral brainstem and spinal somatosensory evoked potentials*. Basel: Karger, 1980:292–310. (Progress in Clinical Neurophysiology, vol 7).

27. Jasper HH, Andrews HL. Brain potentials and voluntary muscle activity in man. *J Neurophysiol* 1938;1:87–100.
28. Klee MR, Lux HD, Speckmann EJ. *Physiology and pharmacology of epileptogenic phenomena.* New York: Raven Press, 1982.
29. Sutton GG, Mayer RF. Focal reflex myoclonus. *J Neurol Neurosurg Psychiatry* 1974;37:207–17.
30. Traub RD, Knowles WD, Miles R, Wong RKS, Linsker R. Synchronised after discharges in the hippocampus: simulation studies of the cellular mechanism. *Neuroscience* 1984;12:1191–200.
31. Traub RD, Knowles WD, Miles R, Wong RKS. Synchronized after discharges in the hippocampus: simulation studies of the celulimp mechanism. *Neuroscience* 1984;12:1191–200.
32. Traub RD, Wong RKS. Cellular mechanism of neuronal synchronization in epilepsy. *Science* 1982;216:745–7.
33. Traub RD, Wong RKS. Synaptic mechanisms underlying interictal spike initiation in hippocampal network. *Neurology* 1983;33:257–66.
34. Van Woert MH, Chung E. Stimulus-sensitive myoclonus: hyper-excitable medullary reticular neurons. San Antonio: Raven Press, 1983. (in press) (Workshop on Neurotransmitters in Epilepsy).
35. Zuckermann EG, Glaser GH. Urea-induced myoclonic seizures. *Arch Neurol* 1972;27:14–28.

Advances in Neurology, Vol. 43: Myoclonus,
edited by S. Fahn et al. Raven Press,
New York © 1986.

Electroencephalographic Correlates
of Myoclonus

*Hiroshi Shibasaki, **Yoriaki Yamashita, *†Shozo Tobimatsu, and
*Ryuji Neshige

*Department of Internal Medicine, Saga Medical School, Saga City, 840-01;
**Department of Neurology, University of Occupational and Environmental Health,
Kitakyushu, 817; and *†Department of Neurology, Neurological Institute, Faculty of
Medicine, Kyushu University, Fukuoka, 812, Japan

In 1938, Grinker et al. (7) found small bursts of rapid spikes in the electroen-cephalograms (EEGs), accompanied by myoclonic twitchings, in two familial pa-tients with myoclonic epilepsy. Since then, the relationship between myoclonus and EEG activities has been studied by many investigators, using EEG and electro-myogram (EMG) polygraph or cathode-ray oscillograph recordings (1,3,4,6,8,12–16,18–21,23,24,30,31). By the conventional polygraphic technique, however, it has often been difficult to study the temporal or topographic relationship between myoclonic discharges and paroxysmal EEG activities.

Shibasaki and Kuroiwa (25) in 1975, by using a back-averaging technique time-locked to the myoclonic EMG discharge, recorded the EEG correlates of myoclonus that were not recognizable on the routine polygraphic recordings. Since then, the technique of jerk-locked or back averaging has been found useful by several investigators (2,5,9–11,17,26,27). This chapter reports the EEG correlates of myo-clonus thus studied and discusses the current view of its underlying mechanism.

SUBJECTS AND METHODS

Fifty-five consecutive cases of myoclonus due to various etiologies, 29 men and 26 women, were the subjects for the present study (Table 1). Their ages ranged from 8 to 70 years. Three of the four cases of cherry-red-spot myoclonus syndrome (lipidosis) had sialidase and β-galactosidase deficiency, and one had sialidase de-ficiency. PME group in this paper is composed of progressive myoclonic epilepsy (PME), lipidosis, Lafora body disease, neuronal ceroid lipofuscinosis and posthy-poxic myoclonus. Of 27 cases of PME group, generalized convulsions were present in 21. Myoclonus in this group was usually postural and/or action myoclonus.

In addition to conventional EEG, polygraphic recordings of EEG and EMG were carried out by using surface electrodes and electroencephalographs. To further investigate EEG correlates of spontaneous myoclonus, back-averaging was per-formed in 30 cases. EEG was recorded by multiple surface electrodes, either in

TABLE 1. *Clinical diagnosis of the subjects in the present study*

Diagnosis	Number of cases
Progressive myoclonic epilepsy (PME)	19
Cherry-red-spot myoclonus syndrome (lipidosis)	4
Lafora body disease	1
Neuronal ceroid lipofuscinosis	1
Posthypoxic myoclonus	2
Subacute sclerosing panencephalitis (SSPE)	1
Creutzfeldt–Jakob disease (CJD)	3
Epilepsy with myoclonus	7
Essential myoclonus	5
Oculopalatal–somatic myoclonus	2
Others	10
Total	55

reference to the ipsilateral ear electrode or bipolarly by using a band-pass filter of 1 to 250 or to 2,000 Hz. EMG was recorded by a pair of surface electrodes placed over a muscle that was showing frequent myoclonic jerks, and was rectified. The EEG and the rectified EMG were averaged by an opisthochronic averaging program time-locked to the EMG onset pulse.

Somatosensory evoked potential (SEP) was recorded by stimulating the median nerve at wrist by electric pulse of 0.1-msec duration (stimulus strength 10 to 20% above the motor threshold). In most cases, the same electrode placement as used for the back-averaging was used for the SEP. To record the long-latency reflex, or C reflex (terminology of Sutton and Mayer, ref. 28), the EMG was usually recorded from the thenar muscle of the stimulated side, but in some cases it was recorded from other muscles. The EMG was rectified, and then averaged, together with the EEG, time-locked to the stimulus pulse.

In order to compare characteristics of the myoclonus-related cortical spike, which was detected by back-averaging, with those of the giant SEP, the scalp topography of both potentials was investigated by multichannel simultaneous recordings and an evoked potential mapping program in some cases of PME group. The time interval from the cortical spike to myoclonus was compared with that from the giant SEP to C reflex. In a few cases, cortical excitability following the myoclonus-related EEG activities was evaluated by stimulation of the median nerve at the onset of or variable intervals after the myoclonic jerk (jerk-locked–SEP paradigm) and was compared with SEPs following a paired electric stimulation of the median nerve (paired-stimulation SEP paradigm). Effects of various drugs on the myoclonus-related spike and on the giant SEP were studied in some subjects.

RESULTS

PME Group

Paroxysmal EEG Activities and Myoclonus by Polygraphy

Spike-and-wave bursts or complexes were recognized in 20 of 27 cases of PME group. In most cases showing spike and waves, those bursts or complexes were occasionally associated with myoclonus, but the temporal or topographic relationship between the spike and myoclonus varied (Fig. 1). In two patients with lipidosis and in one with PME, short runs of rhythmic fast activities or rhythmic spikes at approximately 20 Hz were seen in the central region, frequently in association with myoclonic EMG discharges (Fig. 2). The EEG spikes, when accompanied by myoclonic discharges, were usually predominant over the contralateral hemisphere (Fig. 2). In a patient with PME, however, the spikes were symmetric, and the myoclonus involved proximal muscles bilaterally and synchronously (Fig. 3). In some cases, EEG responded to various kinds of stimuli, such as tendon tap, by showing spike-and-wave complex or central rhythmic fast activities.

EEG

C3–A1

C4–A2

O1–A1

O2–A2

EMG

Lt biceps br.

Rt biceps br.

Lt quadriceps fem.

Rt quadriceps fem.   100μV
                                                                                       1 sec

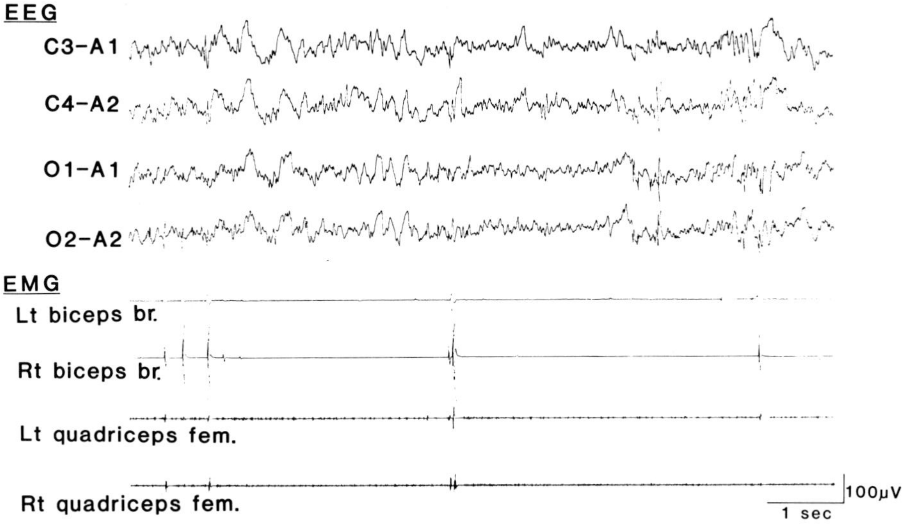

FIG. 1. Polygraphic records in a patient with PME, showing variable relationship between EEG spikes and myoclonus.

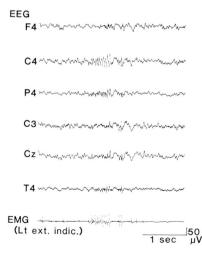

EEG

F4

C4

P4

C3

Cz

T4

EMG
(Lt ext. indic.)   50
                      1 sec   μV

FIG. 2. Polygraphic records in a patient with sialidase deficiency. Fast rhythmic spikes at 20 Hz are localized to the right central region in association with myoclonic discharges of the left index finger extensor muscle.

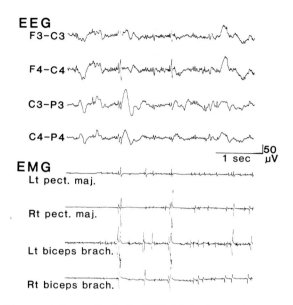

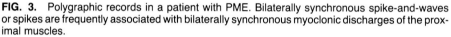

FIG. 3. Polygraphic records in a patient with PME. Bilaterally synchronous spike-and-waves or spikes are frequently associated with bilaterally synchronous myoclonic discharges of the proximal muscles.

Myoclonus-Related Cortical Spike by Back-Averaging

Of 17 cases of PME group, in whom the back-averaging technique was applicable, positive–negative, biphasic sharp EEG activities time-locked to the myoclonic jerks were demonstrated in 15 (Table 2). An example is shown in Fig. 4. Five of these 15 cases had no recognizable spikes on the routine EEG. In 12 cases, the spike was maximal at the central region contralateral to the myoclonus of an upper extremity (Fig. 5). It was maximal at the vertex when the myoclonus was recorded from a lower extremity (Fig. 5). In two cases of PME showing bilaterally synchronous myoclonus of proximal upper limb muscles, the spike was maximal close to the vertex.

The early positive peak of the cortical spike preceded the onset of myoclonic EMG discharge of an upper extremity by 6 to 22 msec. The more proximal the muscle that myoclonus was recorded from, the shorter was the time interval, and vice versa (Fig. 5).

Relationship Between Myoclonus-Related Cortical Spike and Giant SEP

Of 26 cases in whom the median nerve SEP was studied, 23 cases showed the extremely large $\overline{P25}$-$\overline{N33}$ components. In 21 of them, the giant SEP was accompanied by an enhanced C reflex, which corresponded to the evoked myoclonus as clinically observed. As shown in Table 3, the giant SEP was observed regardless of the presence or absence of myoclonus-related cortical spike demonstrated by back-averaging. In six cases, back-averaging was inapplicable because of rare

TABLE 2. *Myoclonus-related cortical activities by back–averaging (number of cases)*

Diagnosis	Spike	Sharp wave	None	Total
PME	10	0	0	10
Lipidosis	4	0	0	4
Ceroid LF	0	0	1	1
Posthypoxic	1	0	1	2
CJD	0	3	0	3
Essential	0	0	4	4
Palatal	0	0	2	2
Others	1	1	2	4
Total	16	4	10	30

PME, progressive myoclonic epilepsy; LF, lipofuscinosis; CJD, Creutzfeldt-Jakob disease.

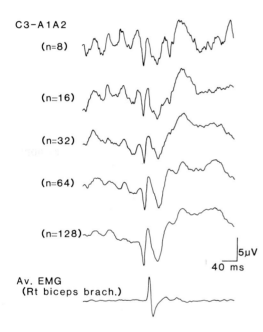

FIG. 4. Results of back-averaging in a patient with PME. Potentials time-locked to the myoclonic EMG discharge are better visualized as the number of sweeps increases.

occurrence of myoclonus, but all of them showed the giant SEP. In two cases, in which myoclonus involved bilateral proximal muscles synchronously, the myoclonus-related spike was maximal near the vertex, and there was no giant SEP.

In those cases showing both the myoclonus-related spike and the giant SEP, the wave form of the spike frequently resembled that of the $\overline{P25}$-$\overline{N33}$ components of the giant SEP (Fig. 6), although the amplitude of the SEP components was usually larger than that of the spike. The scalp topography of the myoclonus-related spike was quite similar to that of the giant SEP components, both being maximal at the central region contralateral to the myoclonus or stimulation (Fig. 7). The giant

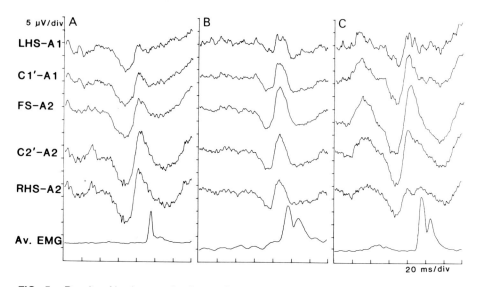

FIG. 5. Results of back-averaging in a patient with PME. Cortical spike related to myoclonus of (**A**) the left thenar muscle is maximal at the right hand sensory (RHS) and C2′ electrodes ($n = 52$), that of the left quadriceps femoris muscle at the foot sensory (FS) electrode (**C**, $n = 50$), and that of the left biceps brachii muscle in between (**B**, $n = 100$). The positive peak of the spike precedes the myoclonus onset of the thenar muscle by 22 msec, that of the biceps brachii by 14 msec, and that of the quadriceps femoris by 22 msec. C1′ and C2′, halfway between LHS (left-hand sensory) and FS and between FS and RHS, respectively.

TABLE 3. *Myoclonus-related cortical spike in relation to giant SEP in PME group (including PME, lipidosis, ceroid LF and posthypoxic myoclonus)*

Myoclonus-related cortical spike by back-averaging	Giant $\overline{P25}$-$\overline{N33}$		
	Present	Absent	Total
Present	13	2	15
Absent	1	1	2
Unable to test due to rare occurrence of myoclonus	6	0	6
Not tested	3	0	3
Total	23[a]	3	26

[a]Accompanied by enhanced C reflex in 21 cases. SEP, somatosensory evoked potential; PME, progressive myoclonic epilepsy; LF, lipofuscinosis.

SEP components showed a wider scalp distribution compared with the myoclonus-related spike (Fig. 7).

Comparison of the time interval from the positive peak of the myoclonus-related spike to the onset of the myoclonic jerk with that from the $\overline{P25}$ peak of the giant SEP to the onset of the C reflex in each individual case is shown in Fig. 8. The interval from spike to myoclonus was almost identical to or slightly shorter than

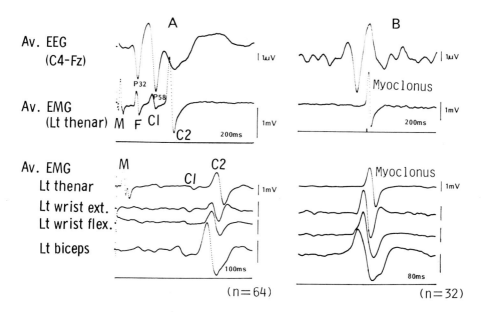

Av. EEG (C4-Fz)

P32

P58

Av. EMG (Lt thenar) M F Cl

C2 200ms

1mV

1μV

A

B

Myoclonus

200ms 1mV

1μV

Av. EMG

Lt thenar

Lt wrist ext.

Lt wrist flex.

Lt biceps

M Cl C2

1mV 100ms

(n=64)

Myoclonus

1mV 80ms

(n=32)

FIG. 6. SEP **(A)** and back-averaging **(B)** in a patient with PME, showing the similar wave form of the $\overline{P25}$ component of giant SEP and the myoclonus-related cortical spike on the top tracings. **Bottom:** The C reflex or evoked myoclonus and the spontaneous myoclonus show the same pattern of spread from proximal to distal muscles of an upper extremity.

FIG. 7. Scalp topography of **(left)** the $\overline{P25}$ component of giant SEP (left median nerve stimulation) and **(right)** of the myoclonus-related spike (myoclonus from left thenar muscle) by evoked potential mapping program in a patient with PME. Both potentials are maximal at C4 electrode. The giant SEP shows wider scalp distribution than does the myoclonus-related spike.

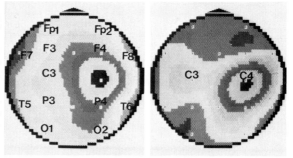

that from SEP to C reflex. In some cases, the myoclonic jerks consistently showed a spread from proximal to distal muscles of an upper extremity. In those cases, the spontaneous myoclonus and C reflex showed the same pattern of spread (Fig. 6).

In a jerk-locked–SEP paradigm, the high-amplitude $\overline{P25}$-$\overline{N33}$ components of the median nerve SEP were generally attenuated after the onset of spontaneous myoclonus, but there was a relative enhancement during a 20-msec postmyoclonus period (Figs. 9, 10). During this postmyoclonus period, the giant SEP was clearly recognized also on the hemisphere ipsilateral to the stimulation, with a latency difference of 9.6 msec, and the C reflex was also enhanced (Fig. 9). In a paired-stimulation SEP paradigm, the $\overline{P25}$-$\overline{N33}$ components in response to the second stimulus were especially enhanced, with an interstimulus interval of 35 to 55 msec,

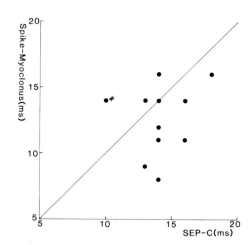

FIG. 8. Time interval from the giant SEP to C reflex versus that from the cortical spike to myoclonus in 11 cases of PME group. The latter interval is almost identical to or slightly shorter than the former; (#) C reflex recorded from wrist extensor.

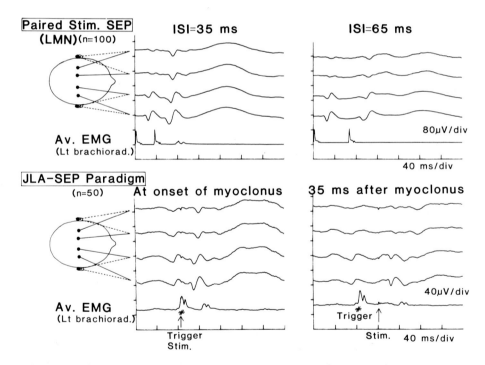

FIG. 9. Cortical excitability following electrical stimulation versus myoclonus in a patient with PME. In the paired-stimulation SEP paradigm **(top)**, the $\overline{\text{P25}}$-$\overline{\text{N33}}$ components in response to the second stimulus are enhanced, being accompanied by an enhanced C reflex, with an interstimulus interval (ISI) of 35 msec, but not with 65 msec. In the back-averaging (JLA)–SEP paradigm **(bottom)**, the SEP components are enhanced with prominent conduction to the opposite hemisphere and with enhanced C reflex when the stimulus is delivered just at the onset of myoclonus, but not 35 msec after the myoclonus. LMN, left median nerve.

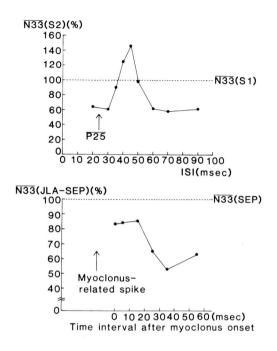

FIG. 10. Cortical excitability following electrical stimulation versus myoclonus in a patient with PME (the same case as in Fig. 9). There seems to be a period of cortical enhancement of approximately 20 msec duration following both stimulation and myoclonus, although it is impossible to stimulate before the myoclonus in the back-averaging (JLA)–SEP paradigm.

accompanied by a similarly enhanced response on the hemisphere ipsilateral to the stimulation with a latency difference of 10 msec, and by an appearance of C reflex (Figs. 9, 10). C reflex was not recognized with an interstimulus interval of longer than 55 msec (Fig. 9).

Intravenous infusion of 100 mg 5-hydroxytryptophan (5-HTP) in a patient with PME markedly suppressed the frequency of myoclonus and EEG spikes. The amplitude of the $\overline{P25}$ component of the median nerve SEP decreased from 24.5 to 17.6 μV and that of the $\overline{N33}$ component from 47.5 to 34.0 μV (Fig. 11). The myoclonus-related cortical spike demonstrated by back-averaging also decreased in its amplitude from 11.8 to 6.4 μV (Fig. 11). Similar results were observed in another patient on clonazepam.

Creutzfeldt-Jakob Disease

Paroxysmal EEG Activities and Myoclonus by Polygraphy

In two cases, the typical periodic synchronous discharge (PSD) was seen in frequent association with myoclonus. In one of them, myoclonus predominantly involved the right upper extremity, whereas PSD was predominant over the left hemisphere (Fig. 12). This patient showed repetitive, jerky, conjugate eye movements toward the left, which occurred synchronously with the myoclonic jerks of the right upper extremity as well as with PSD (Fig. 12). In a third patient, autopsy-verified PSD was not recognized in spite of repeated EEG examinations.

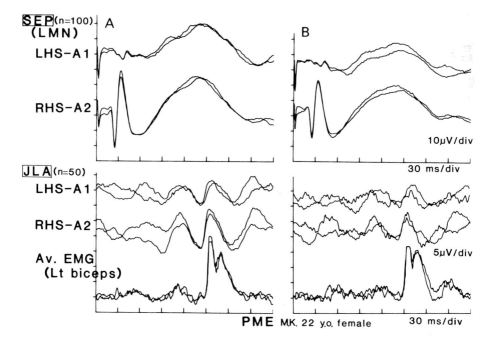

FIG. 11. Effects of 5-hydroxytryptophan (5-HTP), 100 mg, i.v., on the giant SEP and on the myoclonus-related cortical spike in a patient with PME. Both potentials are attenuated by the drug, being associated with reduction of myoclonus frequency and EEG spikes. **A:** Before 5-HTP. **B:** During 5-HTP i.v. infusion. LHS, left hand sensory; RHS, right hand sensory.

Myoclonus-related Cortical Activities by Back-Averaging

Back-averaging demonstrated a sharp wave time-locked to the myoclonus in all three cases, including a case without PSD on the routine EEG (Table 2). The sharp wave was predominant over the hemisphere contralateral to the myoclonus (Fig. 13), and its onset preceded the onset of myoclonus by 50 to 85 msec.

Cortical Excitability and Myoclonus by Jerk-locked–SEP Paradigm

In a patient with Creutzfeldt-Jakob disease (CJD) manifesting rhythmic myoclonic jerks of the right upper extremity in association with PSD over the left hemisphere (Figs. 12, 13), the $\overline{P25}$ component of the right median nerve SEP recorded from the left-hand somatosensory area became attenuated at 75 msec post-myoclonus, most attenuated at 200 to 350 msec post-myoclonus, and returned to normal at about 400 msec post-myoclonus (Fig. 14). PSDs in this patient occurred at an approximate rate of every 570 msec.

Essential Myoclonus

None of five cases in this group showed paroxysmal EEG activities. Back-averaging performed in four cases did not demonstrate any EEG activity time-locked to the myoclonus.

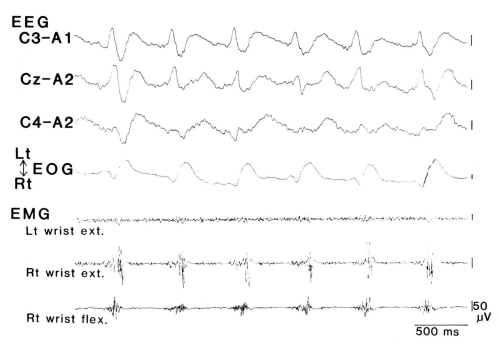

FIG. 12. Polygraphic records in a patient with CJD. PSDs predominant over the left hemisphere are associated with the rhythmic myoclonic jerks of the right upper extremity as well as the jerky ocular movements to left.

Oculopalatal-Somatic Myoclonus

There was no paroxysmal EEG abnormality in two cases of this group. Back-averaging did not demonstrate any EEG activity time-locked to the myoclonus of either facial or hand muscles.

DISCUSSION

The present study confirmed our previous findings (25–27) and usefulness of the technique of jerk-locked back-averaging, not only for detecting EEG correlates of myoclonus, which are not recognizable on the routine polygraphic recordings, but also for investigating the temporal and topographic relationship between EEG activities and myoclonus.

Many cases of the present PME group showed both the myoclonus-related cortical spike demonstrated by back-averaging and the typical giant SEP accompanied by enhanced C reflex. Myoclonus in these cases was usually postural and/or action myoclonus. The EEG spike preceded the myoclonus of an upper extremity by 6 to 22 msec and was localized to the contralateral central area corresponding to the muscle from which the myoclonus was recorded. These features are compatible with those of "pyramidal myoclonus" by Halliday (12,13) or of "cortical reflex myoclonus" by Hallett et al. (11).

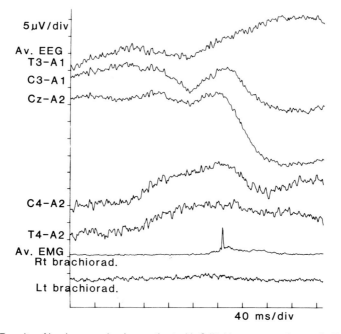

FIG. 13. Results of back-averaging in a patient with CJD (the same patient as in Fig. 12). Myoclonus of the right brachioradialis muscle is associated with a sharp wave at the C3 and Cz electrodes, preceding the myoclonus onset by 55 msec.

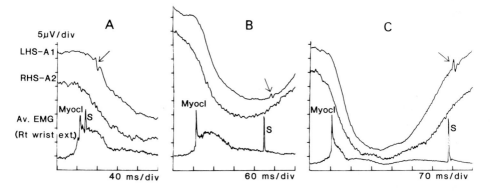

FIG. 14. Cortical excitability after myoclonus in a patient with CJD (the same case as in Figs. 12 and 13). The $\overline{P25}$ component of the median nerve SEP is 4.6 μV when stimulated 10 msec after the myoclonus onset (**A**), attenuates to 1.3 μV when stimulated 200 msec after it (**B**), and returns to 4.6 μV when stimulated 400 msec after it (**C**): *(Myocl)* myoclonus; *(LHS)* left-hand sensory; *(RHS)* right-hand sensory.

Shibasaki et al. (27) in 1978 reported, in cases of "cortical reflex myoclonus," similarity of the myoclonus-related cortical spike to the $\overline{P25}$-$\overline{N33}$ components of the giant SEP in terms of the wave form, scalp topography, and temporal relationship. The present study seems to provide more evidence to support the previous findings. The wave form was similar, although the giant SEP components were usually larger than the myoclonus-related spike. The scalp topography was also similar, although the giant SEP components were more widely distributed over the scalp than the myoclonus-related spike. The time interval from the myoclonus-related spike to myoclonus was almost identical to or slightly shorter than that from the giant SEP to C reflex, probably because the C reflex in most cases was recorded from the thenar muscle, whereas the spontaneous myoclonus was frequently recorded from the more proximal muscles. In addition, the spontaneous myoclonus and the C reflex showed the same pattern of spread from proximal to distal muscles.

The cortical excitability following the spontaneous myoclonus, studied in a patient with PME by electrical stimulation of the median nerve at variable intervals from the myoclonus onset (jerk-locked–SEP paradigm), was enhanced during 20-msec postmyoclonus period, or between 12 and 32 msec after the positive peak of the myoclonus-related cortical spike (the positive peak of the spike preceded the myoclonus onset of the brachioradialis muscle by 12 msec in this patient). In a paired-stimulation SEP paradigm studied in the same patient, enhancement of the cortical excitability was observed with an interstimulus interval of 35 to 55 msec, as reported by Sutton and Mayer (28) in 1974. This period of enhancement actually started at 11 msec after the $\overline{P25}$ peak and ended at 31 msec after the peak (the peak latency of $\overline{P25}$ was 24 msec). These findings suggest the presence of similar cortical enhancement of 20 msec duration starting about 10 msec after the myoclonus-related spike and after the giant SEP. The inhibitory effect of 5-HTP was also similar on both the myoclonus-related spike and the giant SEP. It is concluded from these findings that the myoclonus-related cortical spike and the giant SEP seen in those cases of "cortical reflex myoclonus" have common physiological mechanisms, although they may not be identical.

In two cases of PME, the SEP was not large, and the EEG spike time-locked to the myoclonus of an upper extremity was localized near the vertex. Myoclonus in these cases was also postural and/or action myoclonus, and it frequently involved proximal muscles bilaterally and synchronously. This type of myoclonus is similar to the "reticular reflex myoclonus" of Hallett et al. (9) in some respects, but they did not find any myoclonus-related cortical spike by back-averaging in their cases. The significance of this subgroup remains to be established.

Several cases of the present PME group showed the typical giant SEP accompanied by an enhanced C reflex, but back-averaging either did not show any EEG activity time-locked to the myoclonus or was inapplicable because of only rare occurrence of myoclonus. These cases had generalized convulsions and spike-and-waves in the EEG, but myoclonus itself was less frequent and less severe than in cases of "cortical reflex myoclonus." The discrepancy between the spontaneous myoclonus and the evoked myoclonus in these cases suggests that the myoclonus-related cortical spike and the giant SEP, as seen in cases of "cortical reflex myoclonus," may not be exactly identical in terms of their physiological mechanism.

As previously reported by the authors (26), myoclonus seen in cases of CJD is closely associated with a sharp wave that is predominant over the contralateral hemisphere. This sharp wave, demonstrated by the back-averaging, seems to correspond to the PSD because the two activities are quite similar in terms of the wave form, scalp topography, and time relationship. In contrast with the myoclonus-related cortical spike demonstrated in the PME group, the sharp wave or PSD precedes the myoclonus by 50 to 85 msec, which is too long for the impulse conduction from the cerebral cortex to an upper extremity muscle by any fast-conducting neuronal pathway (22). Both PSD and myoclonus in CJD, therefore, seem to be results of a discharging focus in the deep cerebral structures. The fact that the jerky eye movement to the left was synchronously associated with the PSD on the left hemisphere and with the myoclonus of the right upper extremity in one of the present cases also appears to be in favor of subcortical origin of the myoclonus.

In a patient with CJD, the $\overline{P25}$ component of the median nerve SEP was shown to be attenuated during the period from 75 msec post-myoclonus to 400 msec post-myoclonus. Since the PSDs occurred every 570 msec in that particular patient, this period of depressed excitability corresponds to the interval between PSDs. Umezaki et al. (29) in 1977, by recording SEP at variable intervals following each PSD, found a relative cortical refractory period of approximately 500 msec duration between PSDs. The present findings by the jerk-locked–SEP paradigm seem to be in conformity with their results, although different methods of triggering were used.

In essential myoclonus and oculopalatal-somatic myoclonus, there is neither myoclonus-related cortical activity nor a giant SEP. This type of myoclonus seems to be subcortical in its origin, not stimulus-sensitive. Oculopalatal-somatic myoclonus, however, is clearly different from essential myoclonus, since the former shows the EMG discharge of longer duration and is rhythmic.

SUMMARY

Fifty-five consecutive cases of myoclonus owing to various etiologies were studied by conventional EEG–EMG polygraphic recordings and/or jerk-locked or back averaging. The technique of back-averaging was shown to be useful not only for detecting EEG correlates of myoclonus that are not recognizable on the routine polygraph but also for investigating the temporal and topographic relationship between the EEG activities and myoclonus.

Thirteen of 17 cases of PME and related disorders, in whom back-averaging and SEP were studied, were shown to have both a myoclonus-related cortical spike over the contralateral central area, preceding the myoclonus of an upper extremity by 6 to 22 msec, and a giant SEP accompanied by an enhanced C reflex. In these cases of "cortical reflex myoclonus," the myoclonus-related spike was similar to the $\overline{P25}$-$\overline{N33}$ components of the giant SEP in its wave form, scalp topography, temporal relationship to myoclonus or to C reflex, succeeding cortical excitability, and drug effect. All of this suggests participation of common physiological mechanisms in those two activities.

In two cases of PME, in which myoclonus involved bilateral proximal muscles synchronously, the myoclonus-related spike was maximal near the vertex, and there was no giant SEP. The significance of this subgroup remains undetermined.

In six cases of the PME group, back-averaging was inapplicable because of rare occurrence of myoclonus, but they showed a typical giant SEP accompanied by an enhanced C reflex.

In CJD, back-averaging demonstrated a sharp wave or PSD over the contralateral hemisphere, preceding the myoclonus by 50 to 85 msec. This form of myoclonus seems to be subcortical in origin.

In essential myoclonus and oculopalatal-somatic myoclonus, there was neither myoclonus-related cortical spike nor giant SEP. Electrical stimulation of the peripheral nerve at variable intervals after the myoclonus onset (jerk-locked–SEP paradigm) was shown to be useful for investigating the influence of myoclonus on cortical excitability.

REFERENCES

1. Bradshaw JPP. A study of myoclonus. *Brain* 1954;77:138–57.
2. Chadwick D, Hallett M, Harris R, Jenner P, Reynolds EH, Marsden CD. Clinical, biochemical, and physiological features distinguishing myoclonus responsive to 5-hydroxytryptophan, tryptophan with a monoamine oxidase inhibitor, and clonazepam. *Brain* 1977;100:455–87.
3. Dawson GD. The relation between the electroencephalogram and muscle action potentials in certain convulsive states. *J Neurol Neurosurg Psychiatry* 1946;9:5–22.
4. Engel J Jr, Rapin I, Giblin DR. Electrophysiological studies in two patients with cherry red spot-myoclonus syndrome. *Epilepsia* 1977;18:73–87.
5. Franceschetti S, Uziel G, Di Donato S, Caimi L, Avanzini G. Cherry-red spot myoclonus syndrome and α-neuraminidase deficiency: neurophysiological, pharmacological and biochemical study in an adult. *J Neurol Neurosurg Psychiatry* 1980;43:934–40.
6. Gastaut H, Rémond A. Étude électroencéphalographique des myoclonies. *Rev Neurol (Paris)* 1952;86:596–609.
7. Grinker RR, Serota H, Stein SI. Myoclonic epilepsy. *Arch Neurol Psychiatry* 1938;40:968–80.
8. Haguenau J, Christophe J, Rémond A, Pecker J. Epilepsie myoclonique progressive généralisée. Étude clinique et bioélectrique. *Rev Neurol (Paris)* 1950;82:116–22.
9. Hallett M, Chadwick D, Adam J, Marsden CD. Reticular reflex myoclonus: a physiological type of human post-hypoxic myoclonus. *J Neurol Neurosurg Psychiatry* 1977;40:253–64.
10. Hallett M, Chadwick D, Marsden CD. Ballistic movement overflow myoclonus. A form of essential myoclonus. *Brain* 1977;100:299–312.
11. Hallett M, Chadwick D, Marsden CD. Cortical reflex myoclonus. *Neurology* 1979;29:1107–25.
12. Halliday AM. The clinical incidence of myoclonus. In: Williams D, ed. Modern trends in neurology. 4th ed. London: Butterworths, 1967:69–105.
13. Halliday AM. The electrophysiological study of myoclonus in man. *Brain* 1967;90:241–84.
14. Halliday AM. The neurophysiology of myoclonic jerking—a reappraisal. In: Charlton MH, ed. Myoclonic seizures. Amsterdam: Excerpta Medica, 1975:1–29.
15. Hambert O, Petersén I. Clinical, electroencephalographical and neuropharmacological studies in syndromes of progressive myoclonus epilepsy. *Acta Neurol Scand* 1970;46:149–86.
16. Harriman DGF, Millar JHD. Progressive familial myoclonic epilepsy in three families: its clinical features and pathological bases. *Brain* 1955;78:325–49.
17. Janzen RWC. Myoklonus—motorisches Elementarphänomen bei gestörter zentraler Erregbarkeit.

In: Mertens HG, Przuntek H, eds. Pathologische Erregbarkeit des Nervensystems und ihre Behandlung. Berlin: Springer-Verlag, 1980:40–65.

18. Kelly JJ Jr, Sharbrough FW, Westmoreland BF. Movement-activated central fast rhythms: an EEG finding in action myoclonus. *Neurology* 1978;28:1037–40.

19. V. Koschitzky H, Zschocke S, Rohr W, Janzen RWC. Entwicklung abnormer Erregbarkeit im Akutverlauf bei Jacob-Creutzfeldtscher Erkrankung. In: Mertens HG, Przuntek H, eds. Pathologische Erregbarkeit des Nervensystems und ihre Behandlung. Berlin: Springer-Verlag, 1980:443–6.

20. Lance JW, Adams RD. The syndrome of intention or action myoclonus as a sequel˜to hypoxic encephalopathy. *Brain* 1963;86:111–36.

21. Lhermitte F, Talairach J, Buser P, Gautier J-C, Bancaud J, Gras R, Truelle J-L. Myoclonies d'intention et d'action post-anoxiques. Étude stéréotaxique et destruction du noyau ventral latéral du thalamus. *Rev Neurol (Paris)* 1971;124:5–20.

22. Pagni CA, Ettorre G, Infuso L, Marossero F. EMG responses to capsular stimulation in the human. *Experientia* 1964;20:691–2.

23. Rosén I, Fehling C, Sedgwick M, Elmqvist D. Focal reflex epilepsy with myoclonus; electrophysiological investigation and therapeutic implications. *Electroencephalogr Clin Neurophysiol* 1977;42:95–106.

24. Shibasaki H, Logothetis JA, Torres F. Intention myoclonus: a case report. *Neurology* 1971;21:655–8.

25. Shibasaki H, Kuroiwa Y. Electroencephalographic correlates of myoclonus. *Electroencephalogr Clin Neurophysiol* 1975;39:455–63.

26. Shibasaki H, Motomura S, Yamashita Y, Shii H, Kuroiwa Y. Periodic synchronous discharge and myoclonus in Creutzfeldt-Jakob disease: diagnostic application of jerk-locked averaging method. *Ann Neurol* 1981;9:150–6.

27. Shibasaki H, Yamashita Y, Kuroiwa Y. Electroencephalographic studies of myoclonus. Myoclonus-related cortical spike and high amplitude somatosensory evoked potentials. *Brain* 1978;101:447–60.

28. Sutton GG, Mayer RF. Focal reflex myoclonus. *J Neurol Neurosurg Psychiatry* 1974;37:207–17.

29. Umezaki H, Goto K, Suetsugu M, Noda S. Studies on pathophysiology of periodic synchronous discharge (PSD) in Creutzfeldt-Jakob disease (CJD). *Electroencephalogr Clin Neurophysiol* 1977;43:486.

30. Van Bogaert L, Radermecker J, Titeca J. Les syndromes myocloniques. *Folia Psychiatr Neurol Neurochirurg Neerland* 1950;53:650–90.

31. Watson CW, Denny-Brown D. Studies of the mechanism of stimulus-sensitive myoclonous in man. *Electroencephalogr Clin Neurophysiol* 1955;7:341–56.

Advances in Neurology, Vol. 43: Myoclonus,
edited by S. Fahn et al. Raven Press,
New York © 1986.

Somatosensory Evoked Potentials in Myoclonus

*J. A. Obeso, J. C. Rothwell, and C. D. Marsden

*University Department of Neurology, Institute of Psychiatry, and King's College Hospital Medical School, London SE5, United Kingdom; and *Movement Disorders Unit, Department of Neurology, Clinica Universitaria, University of Navarra Medical School, Pamplona, Spain*

Pathological enhancement of cortical responses following sensory stimulation of one limb was first described by Dawson (3). Indeed, such observation led Dawson to discover somatosensory evoked potentials (SEPs) in normal subjects (2).

Although SEPs of large amplitude have been recorded in a few patients with brainstem, third-ventricle, or parietal lesions (10,12), greatly enhanced (>20-μV) SEPs are most commonly seen in some types of myoclonus (10). Not all patients with myoclonus have enlarged SEPs. However, in those who do, myoclonic jerking is usually evoked by the same stimulus that produces the "giant" SEP. The time interval between the initial cortical components of the enhanced SEP and the muscle jerks is the same as the latency of the muscle contraction produced by direct motor cortex stimulation (18). This type of myoclonus is called cortical reflex myoclonus. Cortical motoneurons also may discharge spontaneously. In such cases of spontaneous cortical myoclonus, back-averaging the EEG activity preceding the spontaneous muscle discharge reveals a simple brain wave preceding the myoclonus by roughly the same latency as the time interval between the large SEP and the myoclonus. In many such patients, a mixed form of reflex and spontaneous myoclonus is found.

The size of the SEP generally is correlated with the intensity of myoclonic activity. Thus, enlarged SEPs may be recorded in some patients only from the contralateral hemisphere and while jerking (8,9), and usually there is a reduction in the amplitude of the averaged SEPs when adequate therapeutic control of the myoclonus is achieved (10,17). Such findings may suggest that the giant SEPs are causally linked with the origin of the myoclonus. In this chapter we shall review the characteristics and origin of pathological SEPs in patients with myoclonus, as well as the clinical significance of such abnormality.

NOMENCLATURE AND TECHNICAL CONSIDERATIONS

In most studies, SEPs have been evoked by electrical stimulation of digital nerves or by motor threshold stimulation of the trunk of mixed nerves. In our laboratory, muscle stretching and touch also have been regularly used to study stimulus-sensitive myoclonus.

In a normal SEP following electrical stimulation, three main components can be distinguished. Initially, there are short-latency subcortical potentials. Subsequently, there is a primary triphasic complex, which represents the initial cortical response to the afferent volley. Finally, there are long-latency, more variable cortical waves occurring within 50 to 300 msec after the stimulus. At present, many authors label evoked potential components according to the polarity and latency of each wave. However, important variations in the components of the SEP can be observed even when analyzing normal data. The exact timing and morphology of cortical evoked potentials change according to the site of peripheral stimulation, size of the subject, and positioning of electrodes used as references. In patients with giant SEPs, there is no guarantee that the pathologically large waves are homologous with any counterparts of the normal SEP. Accordingly, in the study of patients with myoclonus we have opted to designate the first cortical negative wave at approximately 20 msec as N1, the following positive potential at approximately 25 to 32 msec as P1, and the subsequent negative wave at approximately 33 to 40 msec as N2 (see Rothwell et al., *this volume*, Fig. 1).

We also would like to pay attention to a possible source of error in studying evoked potentials in myoclonus. Patients with focal jerks may have large SEPs only while actually jerking. We also have observed that SEPs may be larger when the stimulus is given randomly than when the stimulus is given between jerks (Fig. 1). The decrease in amplitude of SEPs with intercalated stimulation could be due to an interaction between the electrically evoked response and the afferent input from the jerking limb. Another explanation could be that the electrically evoked afferent volley impinges on the cortex at a time of decreased excitability following the motor discharge that gave rise to the preceding spontaneous muscle jerk.

ETIOLOGY OF MYOCLONUS IN PATIENTS WITH ENLARGED ABNORMAL SEPs

The normal amplitude of the component of the N1–P1–N2 complex in the SEP to digital nerve stimulation, measured peak-to-peak, usually ranges between 1 to 3.5 μV. We have never recorded this component of the SEP larger than 7 μV in a normal volunteer or a patient without myoclonus.

There is no specific relationship between enlarged SEPs and the etiology of myoclonic jerking. In many cases of focal myoclonus with enlarged SEPs, the cause has never been determined (10,11,19). However, cases of multifocal and/or generalized myoclonus with giant SEPs may have a variety of different pathologies. Among children and adolescents with myoclonus, giant SEPs are seen in infantile GM_2 gangliosidosis (Tay–Sachs disease) (by some, but not all, investigators), juvenile Gaucher's disease, cherry-red-spot myoclonus syndrome (sialidosis), late infantile and juvenile ceroid lipofuscinosis, Lafora body disease, and Ramsay Hunt syndrome (10; Rothwell, Obeso, and Marsden *this volume*). Some of these condi-

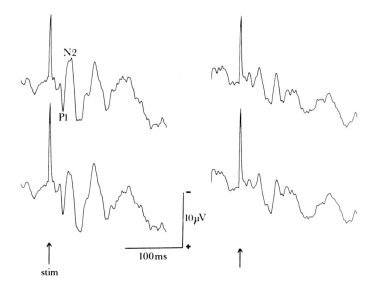

FIG. 1. The influence of stimulus timing on the size of the evoked potential in a patient with regular spontaneous jerking of the right flexor carpi ulnaris. **Left:** electrical stimuli (stim) were given to the digital nerves of the right hand at random intervals between 1 and 2 sec. **Right:** the stimuli were given 50 msec after the end of each jerk. In this case, the size of the P1–N2 component was much reduced. Each record is the average of 128 trials. The electrodes were positioned over C3 **(top)** and the sensorimotor area of the right hand **(bottom)** (7 cm lateral on a line joining the external auditory meatus to a point 2 cm behind the vertex), referred to a linked mastoid reference.

tions also may present in adult life, including sialidosis, adult ceroid lipofuscinosis, and Ramsay Hunt syndrome. In addition, adults may develop myoclonus with giant SEPs due to cerebral anoxia, head injury, vascular disease, and other focal cortical lesions. On the other hand, there are a few conditions in which enhanced SEPs are not encountered. These include myoclonus induced by L-DOPA in Parkinson's disease (15), familial essential myoclonus (6), the myoclonic jerking present in some patients with idiopathic torsion dystonia (16), and uremic myoclonus (*unpublished observations*). SEPs also are of normal amplitude in a particular type of myoclonus named "reticular reflex myoclonus" by Hallett et al. (1,5,13,14), which has been well documented in a few patients with postanoxic myoclonus and in two patients suffering from a nonspecific type of encephalomyelitis (15). To our knowledge, the SEPs in children with myoclonus and epilepsy have not been investigated in detail.

CHARACTERISTICS OF ENHANCED SEPs IN MYOCLONUS

Short-latency subcortical potentials and the initial cortical wave (N1) following somaesthetic stimulation of a limb usually are of normal amplitude in patients with myoclonus (17,20). It is mainly the P1–N2 wave that is increased in size. The

amplitude of this wave is maximal in electrodes placed over the primary sensorimotor area (Fig. 2) in most, but not all, cases.

Such enhanced SEPs, associated with myoclonus, can be divided into three
categories (Fig. 3):

1. Unilaterally enlarged SEPs in focal limb myoclonus. The myoclonus usually
consists of a combination of stimulus-sensitive (reflex) and spontaneous jerking,
made worse by action. Electrical stimulation of the affected limb results in a giant
SEP, which usually is followed by a reflex muscle jerk. The physiological abnormality appears to be limited to the intrinsic neuronal machinery of a small area of
cortex.

2. Bilaterally enlarged SEPs in multifocal or generalized myoclonus. The myoclonus usually is provoked by action but also may occur spontaneously or in
response to external stimuli. Electrical stimulation of either side of the body
produces giant contralateral SEPs, which may be followed by a muscle jerk localized to the stimulated limb or by a generalized whole-body jerk. Such enlargement
of the SEP may be due to generalized encephalopathy or to a loss of inhibitory
influences on the cortex from other centers. For example, most of our patients with

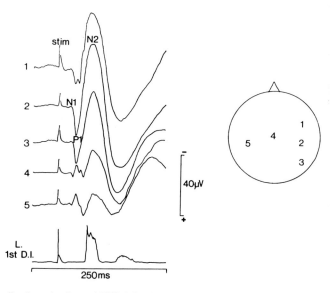

FIG. 2. Localization of enlarged SEP following electrical stimulation (stim) of the digital nerves
of the left forefinger in a patient (P. M.) with epilepsia partialis continua and focal reflex myoclonus
of the left arm. The **top** five channels are an average of 128 monopolar EEG records referred to
a linked mastoid reference. The **bottom** trace is the average rectified EMG response from the
left first dorsal interosseus muscle (1st D.I.). Electrode 4 is at the vertex and electrodes 2 and 5
over the sensorimotor hand areas. Electrodes 1 and 3 are 4 cm anterior and posterior to electrode
2. Details of this patient given by Rothwell et al. *(this volume)*.

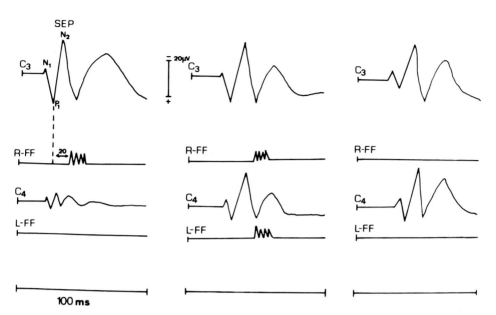

FIG. 3. Diagrammatic summary showing three types of commonly encountered associations between enhanced SEPs and reflex myoclonic jerking. In each column, the traces should be read in pairs. The **top** pair in each column represents the average evoked response recorded unipolarly from a C3 scalp electrode, and the corresponding average rectified EMG from the contralateral (right) finger and wrist flexor muscles (R-FF). The **bottom** pair shows the evoked response from C4, and EMG response from the left finger and wrist flexors (L-FF). The electrical stimulus to the digital nerves is indicated at the start of each sweep. **Left column:** Features observed in patients with unilaterally enlarged SEPs and focal limb myoclonus. Stimulation of the right side evokes a large contralateral SEP and a focal reflex muscle jerk **(upper traces)**, whereas stimulation of the left side **(lower traces)** produces a normal SEP with no accompanying muscle jerk. **Middle column:** Features of patients with bilaterally enlarged SEPs and multifocal or generalized myoclonus. Stimulation of either side evokes a large contralateral SEP and reflex muscle jerk. **Right column:** Features of patients with bilaterally enlarged SEPs and no myoclonus. Stimulation of either side evokes giant contralateral SEPs without any reflex jerks.

bilaterally enlarged SEPs presented with cerebellar ataxia in addition to myoclonus, suggesting a loss of cerebellar inhibition on the sensorimotor cortex.

3. Enlarged SEPs without reflex myoclonus. We have seen a number of patients whose main complaint was action myoclonus accompanied by bilaterally enlarged SEPs. In such cases, the electrical stimulus did not provoke a reflex muscle jerk. We regard them as examples of dissociation between the size of the SEP and muscle jerking (see below).

Finally, it must be pointed out that enlarged SEPs may not be recorded in all patients with cortical myoclonus. There is now substantial experimental evidence indicating that cortical motoneurons situated in layer V may discharge so as to produce focal muscle jerking without any detectable potential being recorded from surface electrodes or even from epidural electrodes (4).

SIGNIFICANCE OF ENLARGED SEPs IN MYOCLONUS

In patients with spontaneous and reflex cortical myoclonus, the EEG activity time-locked to the jerks and the SEPs share the same morphology, topography, and time relation to the myoclonic jerking (7,18,19) (Fig. 4). Accordingly, it has been proposed that the giant SEP and the EEG cortical wave preceding the reflex-evoked and spontaneous myoclonus, respectively, represent the same pathophysiological mechanism. Many authors have suggested that there may be a direct causal link between giant SEPs and EMG discharges responsible for the visible reflex myoclonus. In other words, the giant SEP might represent the discharge of those cortical neurons responsible for activating the anterior horn cells innervating the jerking muscles. However, there are a number of objections to this proposal.

Dissociation Between the Size of the SEP and Reflex Muscle Jerk

First of all, it must be emphasized that giant SEPs are not followed by reflex muscle jerking in all patients. Even in those who show large SEPs and associated reflex myoclonus, examining the correlation between SEP amplitude and size of the evoked EMG discharge on single sweeps reveals an enormous variation from one stimulus to the following (Fig. 5B). Yet, a positive correlation is found on averaged records (Fig. 5A). Halliday (8) has suggested that such occasional lack of correlation on individual runs might be due to a transitory refractory state of the spinal cord motoneurons. However, we have observed important variations in the size of the SEPs and EMG discharges producing the myoclonus without change in the amplitude of the H wave recorded from the same muscle evoked by the same

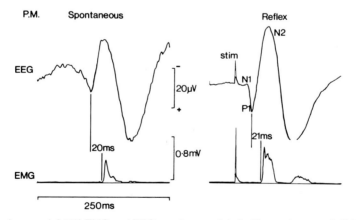

FIG. 4. Average (of 128) EMG and EEG events associated with spontaneous **(left traces)** and reflex-evoked **(right traces)** myoclonus in patient P. M. The EEG during spontaneous jerks was back-averaged from a trigger point on the rectified EMG record. Reflex jerks were elicited by giving electrical stimuli (stim) to the left forefinger, 50 msec after the start of the recording sweep. The time interval between the large P1 positive wave in the EEG and the start of the myoclonic EMG burst is indicated. EMGs taken from left first dorsal interosseus; EEG records from the contralateral sensorimotor hand area, referred to a linked mastoid reference. (From Rothwell et al., ref. 17, with permission.)

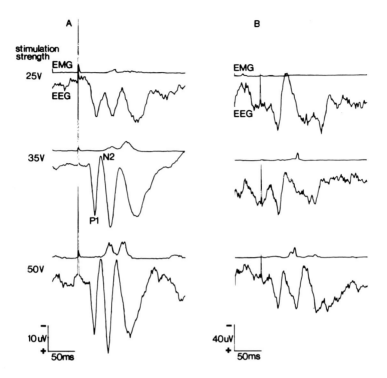

FIG. 5. The relationship between the size of the P1–N2 component of the SEP and the size of the reflex-evoked myoclonic EMG burst in one patient with focal myoclonus of the right arm (J. B.). **A:** The traces are the *average* of 128 sweeps and show how the size of both the EEG and EMG event increase together as the intensity of finger stimulation changes from 25–50 V (200-μsec pulse width). **B:** Three pairs of *single* records, each made at a stimulation intensity of 35 V. In *single* sweeps there is frequently a discrepancy between the size of the P1–N2 wave and the reflex EMG burst. EEG records from the sensorimotor hand area, referred to a linked mastoid reference, EMG from flexor carpi radialis. Details of patient are given in Rothwell et al. *(this volume)*. (From Rothwell et al., ref. 17, with permission.)

stimulus that provoked the long-latency muscle jerk (Fig. 6). These findings suggest that the dissociation in amplitude between SEPs and reflex myoclonus may not depend entirely on changes in the excitability of spinal cord motoneurons.

Drug Dissociation of SEPs and Reflex Myoclonus

Recently, we have had the opportunity to document a marked dissocation between the size of SEP and reflex myoclonus. In five patients with cortical myoclonus, the acute administration of lisuride (0.1–0.15 mg, i.v.) reduced the amplitude and incidence of myoclonus, while at the same time the amplitude of the giant SEP (P1–N2) often was increased (Fig. 7; Table 1). Similar results were obtained in two patients after i.v. administration of clonazepam (1 mg) and in one case following a 90-min i.v. infusion of 5-hydroxytryptophan (5-HTP) (180 mg) plus oral carbidopa (75 mg) (Table 2).

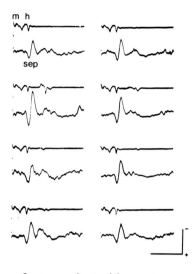

FIG. 6. Series of consecutive pairs of records of EMG **(upper trace)** from flexor carpi radialis; and EEG **(lower trace)** from contralateral sensorimotor hand area (referred to linked mastoids) from a patient with reflex myoclonus due to olivoponto-cerebellar atrophy. A single electrical shock was given to the median nerve in the cubital fossa at the start of each sweep. This produced a direct muscle twitch (m) and a spinal latency monosynaptic H reflex (h), which are of the same amplitude in each record. However, the size of the evoked cortical response (sep) and the longer-latency reflex muscle jerk (r) change considerably. In particular, note that despite spinal cord excitability remaining constant, the relationship between cortical potential and reflex size varies. Calibration: 40 μV and 50 msec.

In one patient with spontaneous and reflex myoclonus affecting the right forearm muscles, the injection of clonazepam (1 mg, i.v.) reduced the amplitude of the spontaneous myoclonus and cortical potential preceding it. Reflex myoclonus induced by electrical stimulation of the digital nerves of the right forefinger also was reduced or abolished by clonazepam, but the abnormal SEP preceding the jerks was increased in size (Fig. 8). In this patient, there was no change after clonazepam in the recruitment curves of the M and H waves recorded from the left forearm muscles, suggesting that the drug was not producing a generalized inhibition of spinal motoneurons.

There are three main possibilities that could explain the observed dissociation between SEP and reflex muscle jerking:

1. If the giant SEP does represent the discharge of motor cortex pyramidal tract neurons, then the dissociation between the cortical event and muscle jerk could occur at spinal level. However, in both spontaneous and drug-induced dissociations, the excitability of spinal cord motoneurons, as tested with H reflexes, was unchanged. The possibility remains that pathways other than the direct monosynaptic corticospinal tract are involved in the production of corticospinal myoclonus. If this is so, then inhibitory changes at the interneuronal level might explain the observed dissociation. Nevertheless, such mechanisms would not easily account for drug-induced enhancement of the SEP.

2. The giant SEP might arise in the motor cortex, but the final output could be conditioned by the level of activity in local inhibitory interneurons.

3. The source of the abnormal SEP might not lie in the neurons of the motor cortex itself. Indeed, in most patients, there is no clinical evidence to suggest direct impairment of cortical motor functions, as judged by the absence of muscle weakness or incoordination of fine manual motor tasks. Furthermore, giant SEPs may be localized either anterior (3) or posterior *(unpublished observations)* to the central

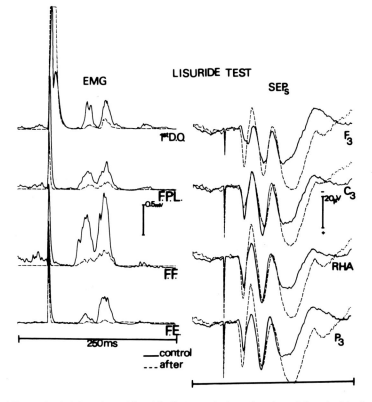

FIG. 7. Effect of administration of lisuride (0.1 mg, i.v.) on the size of the electrically evoked EMG response **(left)** and the cortical SEPs **(right)** in patient J. B. The stimulus was given to the index finger of the right hand and rectified surface EMGs recorded from the first dorsal interosseus (1st D.O.), flexor pollicis longus (F.P.L.), flexor carpi radialis (F.F.), and extensor digitorum communis (F.E.). The SEPs were recorded from the left side of the scalp at F₃, C₃, and P₃ and from the sensorimotor hand area of the right hand (RHA) referred to linked mastoid reference. Average of 128 trials before and after lisuride. —, control records taken before administration of lisuride; --- records taken 30 min after i.v. administration of lisuride. Note how administration of lisuride reduces the reflex muscle jerk yet enhances the cortical evoked potential.

sulcus, suggesting that abnormal function of a distant area could drive pyramidal tract neurons in motor cortex to produce myoclonic jerks. In this case, it is possible to see why there may be dissociations between the size of the SEP and muscle jerk. Random or drug-induced changes in excitability could influence the interconnection between the two areas.

In conclusion, we suggest that giant SEPs do not necessarily represent the discharge of cortical neurons directly responsible for the muscle jerk.

CELLULAR MECHANISM OF GIANT SEPs

In normal subjects, the $\overline{N20}$, $\overline{P25\text{-}32}$, $\overline{N33\text{-}40}$ complex is thought to arise by sequential activation of cortical neurons within the primary sensorimotor cortex.

TABLE 1. *Effect of lisuride (0.1–0.15 mg, i.v.) on the amplitude of SEPs and reflex myoclonus*

Patient	Sex	Age	Diagnosis	Clinical response of spontaneous and reflex myoclonus	Amplitude of SEP (P1–N2 in µV)		Amplitude of myoclonic EMG burst (µV·sec)	
					Control	Drug	Control	Drug
E. A.	F	56	Post-traumatic	Dramatic	12	18	2.3	1.8
C. G.	F	52	Unknown	Moderate	25	32	6.4	1.0
J. B.	F	34	Unknown	Dramatic	30	42	4.2	1.8
P. M.	M	19	Unknown	Moderate	45	43	10.0	0.5
J. D.	F	15	Ramsay Hunt syndrome	Dramatic	42	68	2.0	0.0

TABLE 2. *Effect of clonazepam and 5-HTP on the amplitude of SEPs and reflex myoclonus*

Patient	Drug	Clinical response of spontaneous and reflex myoclonus	Amplitude of SEP (P1–N2 in µV)		Amplitude of myoclonic EMG burst (µV·sec)	
			Control	Drug	Control	Drug
C. G.	Clonazepam (1 mg, i.v.)	Moderate	25	33	6.2	1.3
J. B.		Dramatic	30	44	4.2	0.2
J. D.	5-HTP + carbidopa[a]	Dramatic	44	55	2.3	0.1

[a]180 mg 5-HTP was given over a 90-min period. The patient had been pretreated with 75 mg carbidopa 1 hr before the infusion.

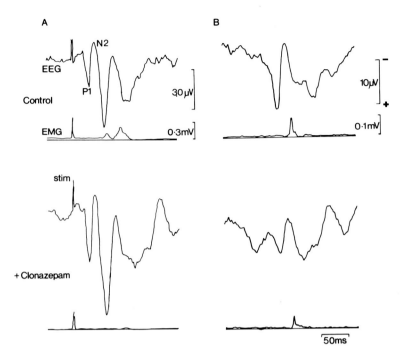

FIG. 8. The effect of clonazepam on the size of the EMG and EEG events in reflex **(A)** and spontaneous **(B)** myoclonic jerks in patient J. B. The top two traces show averaged records (128 sweeps in **A**, 64 sweeps in **B**) before clonazepam. The two **bottom traces** show the averaged records 10–20 min after injection (1 mg, i.v.) of clonazepam. Reflex myoclonus and SEPs were provoked by electrical stimulation of the index finger of the right hand by ring electrodes at twice sensory threshold (stim). The cerebral activity preceding spontaneous myoclonus was recorded by back-averaging the ongoing EEG from the onset of the EMG of the jerks. After clonazepam, reflex EMG jerks are almost abolished, but the SEP (P1–N2) is increased in size. In contrast, clonazepam reduced the size of both EMG jerks and the preceding EEG event in spontaneous jerking. EEG recorded monopolarly from the contralateral sensorimotor hand area, referred to a linked mastoid reference. Rectified surface EMG from right flexor carpi radialis. (From Rothwell et al., ref. 17, with permission.)

An increment in amplitude of the abnormal P1–N2 might be due to synchronous depolarization of a large group of neurons in deep layers of the sensorimotor cortex. However, the cellular events leading to the generation of enlarged SEPs are not known in detail. By analogy with the electrical activity recorded from a cortical focus in experimental epilepsy, the P1–N2 wave may be due to a paroxysmal depolarization shift arising from the summed excitatory postsynaptic potentials (EPSPs) from discharging neurons in deep cortical layers.

Such abnormal potentials could arise because of enhanced afferent input to the cortex. Although animal studies indicate that such mechanism is possible (A. Angel, *this volume*), in human studies, the primary N1 ($\overline{N20}$) component of the SEP has rarely been reported to be grossly enlarged, especially when compared with the later P1–N2 response. An alternative explanation would be a primary disorder of cortical inhibitory interneurons or a secondary failure of inhibitory influences from other subcortical structures.

CONCLUSIONS

The available data suggest that giant SEPs do not necessarily represent abnormal function of cortical pyramidal tract motoneurons. Increased excitability of cortical areas may generate enlarged SEPs, which then drive the motor cortical output. For this to occur, we suggest either a disorder of inhibitory interneurons in the affected area of cortex or a disorder of inhibitory inputs from subcortical areas into the cerebral cortex.

REFERENCES

1. Chadwick D, Hallett M, Harris R, et al. Clinical, biochemical and physiological factors distinguishing myoclonus responsive to 5-hydroxytryptophan, tryptophan plus a monoamine oxidase inhibitor and clonazepam. *Brain* 1977;100:455–87.
2. Dawson GD. Cerebral responses to electrical stimulation of peripheral nerve in man. *J Neurol Neurosurg Psychiatry* 1947;10:137–40.
3. Dawson GD, Investigations on a patient subject to myoclonic seizures after sensory stimulation. *J Neurol Neurosurg Psychiatry* 1947;10:141–62.
4. Elger CE, Speckman EJ. Focal interictal epileptiform discharges (FIED) in the epicortical EEG and their relations to spinal field potentials in the rat. *Electroencephalogr Clin Neurophysiol* 1980;48:447–60.
5. Hallett M, Chadwick D, Adam J, et al. Reticular reflex myoclonus: a physiological type of human post-hypoxic myoclonus. *J Neurol Neurosurg Psychiatry* 1977;40:253–64.
6. Hallett M, Chadwick D, Marsden CD. Ballistic movement overflow myoclonus. A form of essential myoclonus. *Brain* 1977;100:299–312.
7. Hallett M, Chadwick D, Marsden, CD. Cortical reflex myoclonus. *Neurology* 1979;29:1107–25.
8. Halliday AM. The electrophysiological study of myoclonus in man. *Brain* 1967;90:241–84.
9. Halliday AM. The neurophysiology of myoclonic jerking—a reappraisal. In: Charlton MH, ed. Myoclonic seizures. Amsterdam: Excerpta Medica, 1975:1–29.
10. Halliday AM. Cerebral somatosensory and visual evoked potentials in different clinical forms of myoclonus. In: Desmedt JE, ed. Clinical uses of cerebral, brainstem and spinal somatosensory evoked potential. Basel: Karger, 1980:292–310.
11. Kugelberg E, Widen L. Epilepsia partialis continua. *Electroencephalogr Clin Neurophysiol* 1954;6:503–6.
12. Laget P, Mamo H, Houdart R. De l'interet des potentials evoquées somesthetiques dans l'étude du lobe parietale de l'homme. *Neurochirgie* 1967;13:841–53.
13. Leigh DN, Rothwell JC, Traub MM, et al. A patient with reflex myoclonus and muscle rigidity: jerking stiff-man syndrome. *J Neurol Neurosurg Psychiatry* 1980;43:1125–31.
14. Marsden CD, Hallett M, Fahn S. The nosology and pathophysiology of myoclonus. In: Marsden CD, Fahn S, eds. Movement disorders. London: Butterworths, 1982:196–248.
15. Obeso A, Quinn N, Rothwell JC, et al. Myoclonus in Parkinson's disease. VII International Symposium on Parkinson's Disease, Frankfurt. 1982:58.
16. Obeso JA, Rothwell JC, Lang AM. Myoclonic dystonia. *Neurology* 1983;33:825–30.
17. Rothwell JC, Obeso JA, Marsden CD. On the significance of giant somatosensory evoked potentials. *J Neurol Neurosurg Psychiatry* 1984;47:33–42.
18. Shibasaki H, Yamashita Y, Kuroiwa Y. Electroencephalographic studies of myoclonus. Myoclonus-related cortical spikes and high amplitude somatosensory evoked potentials. *Brain* 1978;101:447–60.
19. Sutton GG, Meyer RF. Focal reflex myoclonus. *J Neurol Neurosurg Psychiatry* 1974;37:207–17.
20. Young RR, Shahani BT. Clinical neurophysiological aspects of post-hypoxic intention myoclonus. In: Fahn S, et al. eds. Advances in neurology; vol. 6. New York: Raven Press, 1979;85–105.

Advances in Neurology, Vol. 43: Myoclonus,
edited by S. Fahn et al. Raven Press,
New York © 1986.

Electrophysiology of Somatosensory Reflex Myoclonus

J. C. Rothwell, J. A. Obeso, and C. D. Marsden

Department of Neurology, Institute of Psychiatry, London SE5 8AF, United Kingdom

No one pathophysiological mechanism can account for all of the types of myoclonus seen in clinical practice. In some patients, the jerks occur while the subject is at rest *(spontaneous myoclonus)*. In others, they appear only during attempted voluntary movement *(action myoclonus)*, or they may be triggered by appropriate sensory stimuli *(reflex myoclonus)*. Patients may exhibit any one or a combination of these three categories of myoclonus (13,14,19,24). In this chapter, some of the possible physiological mechanisms responsible for the reflex myoclonic response to somatosensory stimuli will be examined.

Reflex myoclonus itself may be caused by various different mechanisms. The jerks that are evoked may differ in their latency, duration, the range of muscles involved, and the order of activation of muscles in each jerk. The specific stimulus may be cutaneous, muscle-afferent, or both. The EEG may or may not show time-locked changes in activity preceding each muscle jerk. All of these features may provide clues as to the pathophysiological origin of the myoclonic response in individual patients (19,24).

CORTICAL REFLEX MYOCLONUS

Cortical reflex myoclonus is one of the commonest forms of reflex myoclonus and was first documented in detail by Dawson in 1947 (7). Its characteristics are as follows: (a) a focal sensitive area, commonly on the hand and forearm, stimulation of which evokes the myoclonic jerk; (b) a focal muscle jerk limited to a few muscles in the same part of the body; (c) a short burst of EMG activity (10–30 msec), which may occur synchronously in antagonist muscles; (d) if the myoclonus involves many muscles, they are activated in a sequence passing down the brainstem and spinal cord; (e) an enlarged somatosensory evoked potential (SEP) frequently can be recorded over the cortex contralateral to the stimulus site; (f) if the patient also has spontaneous or action myoclonus, a cortical event can be recorded time-locked to the myoclonic jerks that has the characteristics of the enlarged SEPs; (g) the latency of the large SEP (upper limb, 18–25 msec; lower limb, 30–35 msec) is approximately half that of the latency of the reflex muscle jerk (upper limb, 36–50 msec; lower limb, 60–70 msec).

Figure 1 shows some of these features in the records from a patient (J. B.) who had reflex jerking in the right hand in response to light touch of the fingers. In order to study the electrophysiology of this myoclonus, ring electrodes were applied around the index finger and the patient was stimulated every 2 to 3 sec by electrical shocks at twice sensory threshold intensity. EEG events recorded from over the contralateral somatosensory hand area and EMG events from finger and wrist flexors and extensors and from the first dorsal interosseus muscle were recorded and averaged by computer over a number of trials. The EMG records show that the stimulus evoked a synchronous burst of activity in all three muscles recorded on the right side, with a latency of 45 to 50 msec. This was followed by another burst some 30 msec later. The evoked cortical response recorded from the scalp over the contralateral hand area showed two grossly enlarged positive waves (P1 and P2) with a latency to peak of 30 msec and 70 msec, respectively. These were separated by a large negative wave (N2). Stimulation of the normal (left) side evoked SEPs of normal amplitude. Figure 2 illustrates bipolar recording of the same potentials and shows that these responses were localized over the contralateral somatosensory cortex. (In this chapter, we refer to these components of the SEP according to their polarity and sequence. We do not employ the convention of labeling the different peaks by their normal latency, for there is no reason to guarantee that the abnormal peaks in patients with myoclonus are similar to normal responses.)

Figure 3 shows the SEPs in more detail. Stimulation of the normal side gave rise to the usual complex of negative potentials recorded over the cervical cord with a peak latency of 13 msec (5). The N1 deflection was the first major peak recorded at the scalp. Its latency and time course suggest that it is analogous in these patients to the N20 response of normal individuals. It probably signals the arrival of the afferent volley at the cortex (9). Comparison of these responses with those produced after stimulation of the right hand shows that both the cervical potentials and the N1 cortical potential are of normal size. The abnormal response appears to begin with the P1 component. A similar phenomenon has been reported in a patient studied by Young and Shahani (34). If we assume that the sizes of the primary evoked responses in the cervical cord and the N1 component of the cortical response are proportional to the size of the afferent signal that generates them, then it would seem that, in this subject, the afferent volley that reaches the somatosensory cortex is the same size whether the left or right hand is stimulated. The abnormality in this patient is due to either the subsequent processing of the afferent input or the later arrival of an enlarged slowly conducting afferent input, which generates the large P1 response in the left hemisphere.

The muscle jerk in the first dorsal interosseus follows onset of the P1 and P2 responses by 22 msec, which is the latency of activation of the same muscle following direct electrical stimulation of the human motor cortex (26; *unpublished observations*). It is suggested, therefore, that the myoclonus is the result of abnormal activity in a cortical loop reflex (12,20,29,32). The anatomical pathway for this reflex would involve rapid conduction up to the sensory cortex via the dorsal

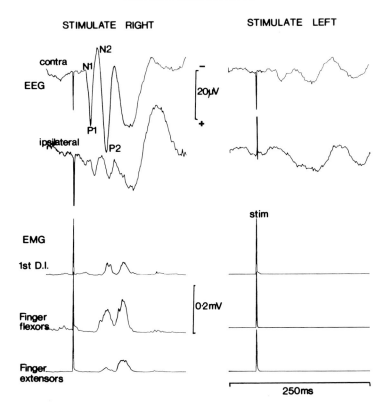

FIG. 1. Average of 128 scalp-recorded somatosensory evoked responses (EEG) and rectified EMG responses following electrical stimulation of the index finger on the right or left hand at twice the sensory threshold intensity in a patient (J. B.) with reflex myoclonus affecting the right hand and forearm. EEG records **(top two traces)** were recorded monopolarly to a linked mastoid reference from electrodes placed over the sensorimotor hand area (7 cm lateral on a line joining the external auditory meatus to a point 2 cm posterior to the vertex) contralateral **(first trace)** and ipsilateral **(second trace)** to the stimulated finger. EMG records were taken from surface electrodes placed over the first dorsal interosseus (1st D.I.), finger/wrist flexors, and finger/wrist extensors on the stimulated side. The timing of the stimulation is evident from the electrical artifact (stim). The apparent response in the ipsilateral cortex after stimulation of the right hand is due to activity in the contralateral hemisphere being picked up by the mastoid reference (see Fig. 2 for localization of response). In this and all subsequent figures, negative EEG potentials are represented by an upward deflection. J. B., a 34-year-old woman, had an undiagnosed left-hemisphere lesion. For some 6 years she had experienced rare grand mal seizures but continuous flexor jerking of the right hand and forearm while awake. These jerks occurred spontaneously, on action, or in response to touch of the fingers or a tap with a tendon hammer. On examination, apart from the focal myoclonus of the right hand, there were no other neurological signs. CT scans repeatedly were normal, as were a left arteriogram and CSF examination. Routine EEG showed a focal abnormality over the region of the left sensorimotor area, with spike–sharp-wave discharges.

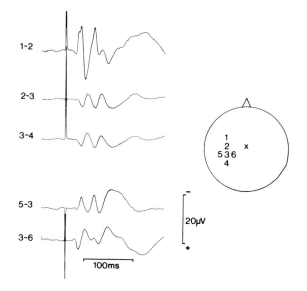

FIG. 2. Localization of the enlarged SEP response to electrical stimulation of the right index finger in the patient (J. B.) illustrated in Fig. 1. The bipolar EEG records show a phase reversal about electrode 3, placed over the left sensorimotor hand area. Traces are the average of 128 responses. Stimulus, shown by artifact, 50 msec after start of sweep. Electrode spacing: 2 cm.

column–medial lemniscal and thalamocortical systems, transmission in cortico-cortical pathways to the motor cortex, and rapid conduction of the motor volley in corticospinal pathways to the spinal α-motoneurons (28) (Fig. 4). This idea is particularly attractive since cortical "long loop" reflexes have been demonstrated in normal human subjects by a number of authors (8,17,20,21). Thus, stretch of an actively contracting human muscle (especially those of the forearm and hand) evokes both a spinal-latency (M1) and a long-latency (M2) reflex EMG response. The latency of the M2 response is approximately 40 msec, and it is abolished by lesions of the dorsal columns, internal capsule, and sensorimotor cortices, all of which lie at points on the long-loop pathway (22,23). In the same way, electrical stimulation of the cutaneous nerves of the fingers can evoke multiple EMG responses in contracting muscles of the hand and forearm. These consist of an early small peak of excitation (E1) at a latency similar to that of the tendon jerk, followed by inhibition (I1) and a later, large excitation (E2) that has a latency of 50 to 60 msec in the first dorsal interosseus. The E2 response also is abolished by lesions in the long-loop pathway (2,17).

There has been some debate over whether the M2 stretch reflex response and the E2 cutaneous reflex response are mediated by such long-loop pathways, or whether they are, in fact, polysynaptic spinal events that are influenced by descending pathways. However, the study of patients with cortical reflex myoclonus provides further evidence that such transcortical pathways do exist in man, and it is

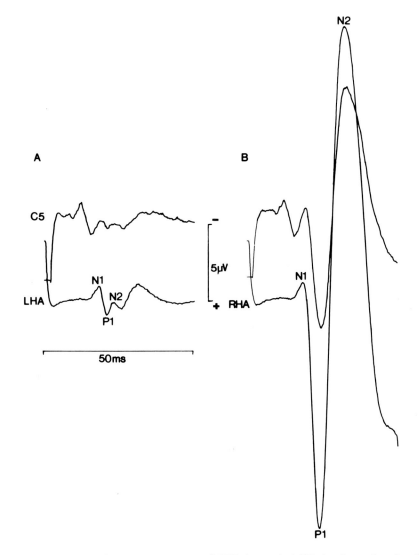

FIG. 3. Detail of short-latency components of SEPs in cervical (C5; **top traces**) and cortical hand area of the left and right hands. (LHA, RHA; **bottom traces**) following electrical stimulation of the index finger of the left **(A)** and right **(B)** hand in the patient (J. B.) illustrated in Figs. 1 and 2. The early cervical potentials, with a peak latency of 13 msec, and the first major cortical response (N1), with a latency of 20 msec, are the same size on both sides. The later components are much enlarged after right hand stimulation **(B)**. Traces are the average of 999 sweeps, with the stimulation given at the beginning of the sweep. Electrodes referred to a reference at Fz. The apparent large late responses recorded at the cervical electrode in **B** are due to activity at the Fz reference.

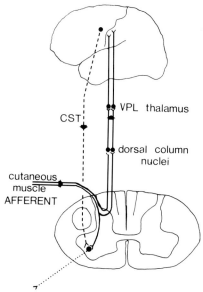

FIG. 4. Diagrammatic summary of afferent *(—)* and efferent *(---)* pathways involved in the production of "long loop" transcortical reflexes. Cutaneous and muscle afferents traverse the dorsal column–medial lemniscal pathway to the ventral-posterolateral thalamus and sensory cortex. Pyramidal tract cells in the motor cortex conduct impulses via the corticospinal tract (CST) to the α-motoneurons in the ventral horn of the spinal cord. Other polysynaptic pathways from cortex to cord, which may be involved, are not shown. The possible connection at cortical level between afferent input and motor output has been left vague in view of the controversy surrounding direct lemniscal input to the motor cortex (10). At spinal cord level, the monosynaptic connection between muscle afferents and α-motoneurons also is shown.

our thesis that overactivity in these pathways is responsible for this form of myoclonus.

The specific sensory stimulus needed to produce reflex muscle jerks may be, in different patients, either purely cutaneous, muscle-afferent, or both. The patient described by Sutton and Mayer (31,32) was sensitive only to cutaneous stimuli. Muscle stretch, applied when the skin was anesthetized, was insufficient to produce jerking. In contrast, Dawson's (7) original patient was sensitive only to muscle stretch and not cutaneous stimuli. An example of another patient (P. M.) in whom myoclonic jerks could be evoked by both sorts of stimulation is shown in Fig. 5. In the intact state, electrical stimulation of the cutaneous nerves of the thumb and rapid stretch of the flexor pollicis longus muscle both evoked myoclonic jerks in the first dorsal interosseus. (In the normal subject, electrical stimulation of the cutaneous nerves of the thumb causes a very much smaller response in the first dorsal interosseus muscle, and extension of the top joint of the thumb with the proximal phalanx clamped has no effect on that muscle.) In P. M., anesthetizing the thumb with a digital nerve block abolished the cutaneous response, while leaving the myoclonic response to muscle stretch in the first dorsal interosseus virtually intact. Since movement of the long flexor muscle under the intact skin of the forearm produces little or no sensation in normal subjects, we conclude that in this patient, both cutaneous and muscle-afferent stimuli were alone sufficient to evoke myoclonic jerking.

On the basis of the long-loop theory outlined above, the pathology of the cortical reflex myoclonus must be capable of differentially affecting transmission in either cutaneous or muscle reflex pathways. Since both types of afferent input project to

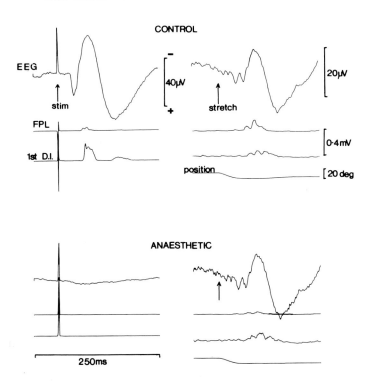

FIG. 5. Average of 64 EEG and EMG responses to electrical stimulation of the digital nerves of the thumb **(left)** or to rapid stretch of flexor pollicis longus **(right)** before **(top traces)** and after **(bottom traces)** anesthesia of the thumb by digital nerve block (2 ml plain lignocaine) in a patient (P. M.) with reflex jerking of the left hand. The EEG record is taken from a monopolar electrode placed over the contralateral sensorimotor hand area referred to a linked mastoid reference. EMG is rectified and taken from surface electrodes over the flexor pollicis longus (FPL) and first dorsal interosseus (1st D.I.). **Right:** A fourth channel shows the excursion of the interphalangeal joint of the thumb responsible for the stretch of FPL. Thumb extension produced downward deflection of the trace. Both stretch and electrical stimuli were given 50 msec after the start of the sweep. Anesthesia abolished the response to electrical stimulation in both muscles and in the EEG. It had no effect on the EEG or the myoclonic EMG response of 1st D.I. to muscle stretch. Note, however, the reduction in size of the FPL stretch reflex, although it was not abolished. Anesthesia normally reduces the size of the long-latency stretch reflex in the FPL of control subjects (21). P. M., a 19-year-old man had suffered epilepsy since the age of 11 years, consisting of focal jacksonian seizures in the left arm, often progressing to generalized grand mal attacks. In addition, there were spontaneous jerks of the fingers of the left hand that got worse on movement and that also could be triggered by touch or a tendon tap to the hand. On examination, there was a reduction in appreciation of passive movement and of two-point discrimination in the left hand. There was no weakness, and the rest of the neurological examination was normal. The cause of the epilepsy was not clear. There was no definite history of birth injury or of head trauma. A CT scan showed slight dilation of the right lateral ventricle, but a right carotid arteriogram was normal, as was CSF examination. A positron emission tomogram utilizing [¹¹C]deoxyglucose revealed an area of decreased metabolism in the region of the right parietal lobe posterior to the central sulcus. There also was a focal abnormality in the routine EEG over the same region, consisting of spikes/sharp waves.

different portions of the ventrobasal thalamic nuclei and to different areas of sensorimotor cortex (10), there is ample scope for such an effect. Unfortunately, detailed pathology of these patients is rarely known. In some cases it may involve the cerebellum, suggesting that the myoclonus arises from a loss of cerebellar inhibitory influence on cortical mechanisms; in others, there is no obvious pathological correlate at all (20; J. A. Obeso et al., *this volume*).

Finally, it should be mentioned that some cases of cortical reflex myoclonus may exhibit slightly different features from those described above. For example, some patients have an enhanced N1 response in the SEP, which may indicate that the afferent volley reaching the cortex is enlarged. In such a case, abnormal "gating" of incoming somatosensory input at the thalamus or dorsal column nuclei could be the site of the primary pathology. Alternatively, some patients may not have any enlargement of the SEP at all. This may be because the orientation of the dipole in the focus is so anteroposterior (e.g., in the bank of the central sulcus) that it is not detected on the surface of the scalp. In such a case, electrocorticography (33) or positron emission tomography may be the only way to prove definite cortical involvement in the jerks.

RETICULAR REFLEX MYOCLONUS

Although cortical reflex myoclonus has the most distinctive electrophysiological features of all forms of reflex-sensitive jerking, reticular reflex myoclonus (11,19,24) also may be identified quite regularly in a number of patients who have generalized, whole-body jerks in response to a single somatosensory stimulus. The features are as follows: (a) generalized muscle jerks; (b) brief EMG bursts of activity (30–50 msec); (c) no enlargement of the SEP components that occur prior to the EMG bursts; (d) if the patient also has spontaneous or action myoclonus, no cortical event can be recorded time-locked to and in advance of the myoclonic jerks; (e) the order of muscle activation is up the brainstem and down the spinal cord.

Some of these features are illustrated in the records of Fig. 6 taken from a patient (A. A. M.), who had generalized jerks in response to tendon taps applied to the leg, arm, and facial muscles or to electrical stimulation of peripheral nerves. The early components of the SEP were not enlarged in this patient. Large and generalized later components are evident but are difficult to dissociate from movement artifact produced in the EEG record by the evoked myoclonic jerk. The major distinguishing feature of this type of reflex myoclonus is the order of activation of the cranial nerve musculature in each jerk. The jerk began in the sternocleidomastoid (nerve XI), and was followed by the orbicularis oculi (nerve VII) and the masseter (V nerve). These characteristics suggest an origin for the reflex jerks nearest the nucleus of the XIth nerve. This patient has not been described in detail before, and it is of interest to compare the electrophysiological features with that of the patient reported by Hallett et al. (11).

Details of the time relationships between all muscles for tendon tap stimuli applied to the head and limbs are shown in Table 1. Figure 7 shows how these

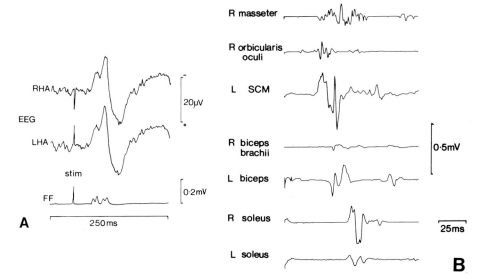

FIG. 6. A: Average of 128 EEG and EMG responses to electrical stimulation (stim) of the index finger of the right hand in a patient (A. A. M.) with reticular reflex myoclonus. EEG recorded monopolarly from over the sensorimotor hand area (RHA, right-hand area; LHA, left-hand area) referred to a linked mastoid reference. Rectified EMG from surface electrodes placed over the flexor carpi radialis (FF). No enlargement of the EEG response is evident preceding the myoclonic muscle jerk. The bilateral late response probably is produced by movement artifact from the generalized muscle jerk. **B:** Order of muscle activation on a single generalized myoclonic jerk in the same patient, produced by a light tap with a tendon hammer to the forehead at the start of the sweep. The jerk begins in the sternocleidomastoid (SCM) and travels up the cranial nerves and down the spinal cord. A. A. M., a 41-year-old man, developed increasing generalized muscle stiffness and jerks over a period of about 1 year. Eventually, he became bedridden with severe rigidity but remained alert and, according to his relatives, suitably responsive. On examination, although alert, he was severely dysarthric, and he could not move voluntarily. His limbs were held in flexion and exhibited extreme rigidity. Tendon reflexes were brisk, and the plantar responses were flexor. Any stimulus, including visual menace, load noise, light touch, or a tap with a tendon hammer, evoked massive generalized muscle jerking. All investigations failed to reveal a pathological diagnosis, although clinically it was suspected that he had a diffuse encephalomyelitis.

timings can be used to calculate the afferent and efferent conduction velocities of the reflex pathway, assuming an origin in the brainstem. The difference between EMG latencies when stimuli are given to the knee and forearm allows an estimate of the afferent conduction time in spinal cord pathways if the efferent (motor) latencies are assumed to remain unchanged. Thus, for the sternocleidomastoid, biceps brachii, triceps femoris, and triceps surae, the average time difference between jerks elicited by taps to the forearm and knee was 14.5 msec. The time taken for the afferent volley to reach the reflex center is given by $T_f + T_{cr}$ for the forearm, and $T_k + T_{cr} + T_{lc}$ for the knee. The difference between these values, $(T_k + T_{cr} + T_{lc}) - (T_f + T_{cr}) = T_k - T_f + T_{lc}$ (Fig. 7), gives the difference in latency between the times of arrival of the afferent volley and hence is equal to the difference in latency between the muscle jerks evoked by stimulation at the two sites. The patient had normal peripheral nerve conduction velocities. Estimating

TABLE 1. *Latencies of reflex muscle jerks in a patient with reticular reflex myoclonus following brisk taps with a tendon hammer given to various parts of the body*[a]

Muscle	Site of stimulation			
	Forehead ($N = 12$)	Chin ($N = 10$)	Forearm ($N = 4$)	Knee ($N = 6$)
Sternocleidomastoid	32.0 ± 0.8	27.5 ± 1.0	38.5 ± 2	49.4 ± 1.5
Orbicularis oculi	34.8 ± 0.8	—	—	—
Masseter	42.4 ± 0.6	—	—	—
Biceps brachii	44.4 ± 0.6	35.6 ± 0.5	33.0 ± 2	55.5 ± 2.6
Biceps femoris	—	51.7 ± 2.1	48.0 ± 3	61.5 ± 1.4
Triceps surae	62.2 ± 0.6	55 ± 1.3	51.2 ± 1.5	62.0 ± 1.5

[a]Average latencies to onset of the EMG response given in milliseconds ± 1 SE.

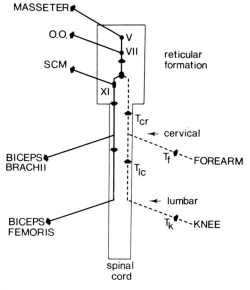

FIG. 7. Diagrammatic summary of afferent *(---)* and efferent *(—)* pathways involved in reticular reflex myoclonus. Hypothetical reflex "center" shown by large dot in middle of reticular formation; fifth and seventh cranial nerve nuclei shown as smaller dots above, the spinal nucleus of the eleventh nerve as bar below. The motor fibers of the sternocleidomastoid (SCM) are believed to arise from cervical segments C2 and C3. T_f, afferent conduction time from forearm to cervical spinal cord; T_k, conduction time from knee to lumbar cord; T_{lc}, conduction time from lumbar to cervical spinal cord; T_{cr}, conduction time from cervical cord to reflex "center." O.O., orbicularis oculi.

the peripheral conduction time to the spinal cord gave values for T_f of about 11 msec for the forearm, and for T_k of about 14 msec for the knee. In our patient, $T_k - T_f + T_{lc} = 14.5$ msec, and therefore the spinal conduction time from lumbar to cervical cord was approximately $14.5 - (14 - 11) = 11.5$ msec. This is very similar to the value calculated by Hallett et al. (11) in their original description of a patient with this form of myoclonus. It is almost twice the latency of the fastest-conducting spinal afferent pathways, as recorded with evoked potential techniques, and presumably represents transmission in a slowly conducting ascending pathway.

The efferent conduction velocity in the cord may be estimated in the same way. In our patient, the latency difference between EMG onset in biceps brachii and biceps femoris was 16 msec when stimuli were given to the head, 15 msec when given to the arm, and 6 msec when given to the leg. We have no explanation of this difference in timings, unless different mechanisms are responsible for producing jerks recorded after stimulation of the leg. Nevertheless, the efferent spinal conduction velocity is of the same order as that in the afferent pathway. This slow efferent conduction velocity is in contrast to the much faster spinal pathway reported in the patient of Hallett et al. (11).

Finally, it is possible also to estimate the speed of conduction of the efferent volley up the brainstem, if we presume (a) an origin in the brainstem, above the spinal nucleus of the eleventh cranial nerve, and (b) the same conduction time from cranial nerve nucleus to periphery for each of the three muscles examined. In the present patient, it took 7.6 msec for the efferent volley to travel from the seventh to the fifth nucleus, which is somewhat faster than the value of 9 msec quoted by Hallett et al. (11). These differences between the efferent conduction velocities in both spinal and brainstem pathways suggest that there may be more than one form of reticular reflex myoclonus. Indeed, Leigh et al. (18) have reported a case of "jerking stiff man syndrome" in which reflex jerks with a probable origin in the brainstem could be recorded after stimuli applied to the head. In this patient, the brainstem conduction time was extremely rapid (1.0 msec from seventh-nerve to fifth-nerve activation).

There may therefore be various subtypes of reticular reflex myoclonus, all with the common feature of an origin for the jerks in the brainstem. Whether this represents overactivity of some reflex pathway that exists in normal man, like cortical reflex myoclonus, is unknown. It is tempting to compare this type of reflex myoclonus with the spino-bulbo-spinal reflex (25,30). However, that reflex is characterized by a fast afferent spinal conduction velocity and slow efferent pathway, a combination that we have never seen in any of our patients. Chadwick and French (4) have described a similar form of reticular myoclonus, although without detailed electrophysiological findings, in patients with uremia and hyponatremia. They believe that this form of jerking, arising in the brainstem, may be one of the commonest forms of symptomatic metabolic myoclonus.

Experimentally, this is the type of myoclonus described by Zuckerman and Glaser after urea infusions in the cat (35). Electrophysiological recording demonstrated this to be generated by discharges in the region of the nucleus reticularis gigantocellularis. It is also related to the myoclonus produced by focal injections of cobalt into the brainstem (3). Thus, both clinical and experimental evidence exists to suggest that this is a fundamental form of myoclonus arising from a brainstem discharge provoked by afferent sensory input.

OTHER FORMS OF SUBCORTICAL MYOCLONUS

Cortical reflex and reticular reflex myoclonus are the two clearest forms of somatosensory reflex myoclonus that we have seen in human patients. However, it must be pointed out that both cortical and reticular reflex myoclonus may occur in the same patient, as in some cases of posthypoxic or metabolic myoclonus. Thus,

Dawson's 1947 (7) patient showed a focal limb jerk following an enlarged SEP to a single tendon tap and generalized jerks (reticular?) with generalized EEG spikes with a series of taps. It also seems highly probable that a cortical discharge might provoke a brainstem reticular discharge, which could cause a generalized myoclonic jerk (see also ref. 14). However, we have not yet encountered a convincing example of this pathophysiological mechanism in humans.

STIMULUS-SENSITIVE SPINAL MYOCLONUS

In spinal myoclonus, jerks occur spontaneously and synchronously in the muscles innervated by affected spinal cord segments (14–16). The frequency of contractions may vary from 2 to 600 per minute, and they usually persist during sleep. In these respects, this type of myoclonus is very similar to that of palatal myoclonus. In the latter, synchronous rhythmic contractions occur at 100 to 180 per minute in the muscle of the soft palate and pharynx. Rarely, muscles of the larynx, diaphragm, neck, and face also may be involved. Palatal myoclonus is unaffected by voluntary movement, external stimuli, sleep, or even barbiturate anesthesia (1,27). Spinal myoclonus is believed to be due to some disturbance of normal inhibitory inter-neuronal function in the cord (14). Spinal myoclonus usually is uninfluenced by external stimuli, but occasionally patients with spinal myoclonus also exhibit stimulus-sensitive jerking (6). The latency of the EMG responses is short and appropriate for spinal cord conduction times. They appear in all affected muscles, even when both sides of the body are involved (Fig. 8).

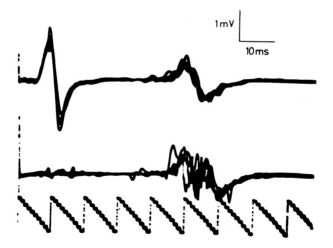

1mV

10ms

FIG. 8. Superimposed surface EMG records from right **(upper)** and left **(lower)** gastrocnemius muscles following stimulation of the right posterior tibial nerve at the start of the sweep. Stimulation evokes a direct M wave in the right side and a bilateral reflex response at 44 msec. Stimulus-sensitive myoclonus in a 75-year-old man with jerking of both legs of 8 days duration; shown at necropsy to be associated with spinal cord ischemia. (From Davis et al., ref. 6, with permission.)

CONCLUSIONS

Despite considerable experimental and clinical neurophysiological study, understanding of the pathophysiology of the many varieties of reflex-sensitive myoclonus encountered in clinical practice is not complete. Careful investigation of each patient commonly reveals unsuspected and little-understood abnormalities that cannot always be explained by the mechanisms reviewed here. However, we put this classification forward as a working approach to the physiological understanding of myoclonus.

REFERENCES

1. Alajouanine T, Hornet T. Myoclonies de desafferentation olivaire. In: Bondelle M, Gastout M, eds. Les myoclonies. Paris; Massion, 1968:143–6.
2. Caccia HR, McComas AS, Upton ARM, Blogg T. Cutaneous reflexes in small muscles of the hand. *J Neurol Neurosurg Psychiatry* 1973;36:960–77.
3. Cesa-Bianchi MG, Mancia M, Mutani R. Experimental epilepsy induced by cobalt powder in lower brainstem and thalamic structures. *Electroencephalogr Clin Neurophysiol* 1967;22:525–536.
4. Chadwick D, French AT. Uraemic myoclonus: an example of reticular reflex myoclonus? *J Neurol Neurosurg Psychiatry* 1979;42:52–55.
5. Chiappa KH, Ropper AM. Evoked potentials in clinical medicine (part II). *New Engl J Med* 1982;306:1205–11.
6. Davis SM, Murray NMF, Diengdoh JV, Calea-Debono A, Kochen RS. Stimulus sensitive spinal myoclonus. *J Neurol Neurosurg Psychiatry* 1981;44:884–8.
7. Dawson AD. Investigations on a patient subject to myoclonic seizures after sensory stimulation. *J Neurol Neurosurg Psychiatry* 1947;10:141–62.
8. Desmedt JE, ed. *Progress in clinical neurophysiology; Vol. 8.* Basel: Karger, 1978.
9. Desmedt JE, Cheron G. Non-cephalic reference recording of early somatosensory potentials to finger stimulation in adult or aging normal man: differentiation of widespread N18 and contralateral N20 from the prerolandic P22 and N30 components. *Electroencephalogr Clin Neurophysiol* 1981;52:553–70.
10. Friedman DP, Jones EG. Thalamic input to areas 3a and 2 in monkeys. *J Neurophysiol* 1981;45:59–85.
11. Hallett M, Chadwick D, Adam J, Marsden CD. Reticular reflex myoclonus: a physiological type of human post hypoxic myoclonus. *J Neurol Neurosurg Psychiatry* 1977;40:253–64.
12. Hallett M, Chadwick D, Marsden CD. Cortical reflex myoclonus. *Neurology* 1979;29:1107–25.
13. Halliday AM. The electrophysiological study of myoclonus in man. *Brain* 1967;90:241–84.
14. Halliday AM. The neurophysiology of myoclonic jerking—a reappraisal. In: Charlton HH, ed. Myoclonic seizures. Amsterdam: Excerpta Medical, 1975:1–29.
15. Hoen MM, Cherington M. Spinal myoclonus. *Neurology* 1977;27:942–6.
16. Hopkins AP, Michael WF. Spinal myoclonus. *J Neurol Neurosurg Psychiatry* 1974;37:1112–5.
17. Jenner JR, Stephens JA. Cutaneous reflex responses and their central nervous pathways studied in man. London: *J Physiol* 1982;333:405–19.
18. Leigh PN, Rothwell JC, Traub MM, Marsden CD. A patient with reflex myoclonus and muscle rigidity: jerking stiffman syndrome. *J Neurol Neurosurg Psychiatry* 1980;43:1125–31.
19. Marsden CD, Hallett M, Fahn S. The nosology and pathophysiology of myoclonus. In: Marsden CD, Fahn S, ed. Movement disorders. London: Butterworth Scientific, 1981:196–248.
20. Marsden CD, Merton PA, Morton HB. Is the human stretch reflex cortical rather than spinal? *Lancet* 1973;1:759–61.
21. Marsden CD, Merton PA, Morton HB. Servo action in the human thumb. London: *J Physiol* 1976:197;257:1–44.
22. Marsden CD, Merton PA, Morton HB, Adam J. The effect of posterior column lesions on servo responses from the human long thumb flexor. *Brain* 1977;100:185–200.
23. Marsden CD, Merton PA, Morton HB, Adam J. The effect of lesions of the sensorimotor cortex and the capsular pathways on servo responses from the long thumb flexor. *Brain* 1977;100:503–26.

24. Marsden CD, Obeso JA, Rothwell JC. The clinical neurophysiology of muscle jerks: myoclonus, chorea and tics. In: Desmedt JE, ed. Brain and spinal mechanisms of movement control in man. New York: Raven Press, 1983 (in press).
25. Meier-Ewert K, Himme U, Dahn J. New evidence favouring long loop reflexes in man. *Archiv für Psychiatrie und Nervenkrankheiten* 1972;215:121–8.
26. Merton PA, Morton HB, Hill DK, Marsden CD. Scope of a technique for electrical stimulation of human brain, spinal cord and muscle. *Lancet* 1982;1:597–600.
27. Nathanson M. Palatal myoclonus: further clinical and pathophysiological observations. *Arch Neurol* 1956;75:285–96.
28. Pagni CA, Marossero F, Cabrini G, Ettore A, Infuso L. Pathophysiology of stimulus sensitive myoclonus: a stereo-EEG study. *Electroencephalogr Clin Neurophysiol* 1971;31:176.
29. Shibasaki H, Yamashita Y, Kuroiwa Y. Electroencephalographic studies of myoclonus. Myoclonus-related cortical spikes and high amplitude somatosensory evoked potentials. *Brain* 1978;101:447–60.
30. Shimamura M, Mori S, Matsushima S, Fujimori B. On the spino-bulbo spinal reflex in dogs, monkeys and man. *Jpn J Physiol* 1964;14:411–21.
31. Sutton CA. Receptors in focal reflex myoclonus. *J Neurol Neurosurg Psychiatry* 1975;38:505–7.
32. Sutton CG, Mayer RF. Focal reflex myoclonus. *J Neurol Neurosurg Psychiatry* 1974;37:207–17.
33. Thomas JE, Reagan TJ, Klass DW. Epilepsia partialis continua. A review of 32 cases. *Arch Neurol* 1977;34:266–75.
34. Young RR, Shahani BT. Clinical neurophysiological aspects of post hypotic intention myoclonus. In: Fahn, S et al. ed. Advances in neurology, vol. 26. New York: Raven Press, 1979;85–105.
35. Zuckerman EG, Glaser GH. Urea-induced myoclonic seizures. *Arch Neurol* 1972;27:14–28.

Advances in Neurology, Vol. 43: Myoclonus,
edited by S. Fahn et al. Raven Press,
New York © 1986.

Myoclonus in Alzheimer's Disease and Minipolymyoclonus

Mark Hallett and Dennis E. Wilkins

*Section of Neurology, Department of Medicine, Brigham and Women's Hospital and
Harvard Medical School, Boston, Massachusetts 02115*

The physiologic classification of the different types of myoclonus has value in establishing an etiologic diagnosis and identifying appropriate therapy. Since different physiological types often have similar clinical appearance, it is frequently necessary to turn to electrophysiological techniques to make distinctions. Valuable information can be produced by EEG or EMG alone or by the correlation of EEG with EMG.

The first step in the analysis of a case is to examine the EMG correlation of the myoclonic jerk (2). An EMG burst duration of greater than 200 msec can be seen in dystonic myoclonus and subacute sclerosing panencephalitis (SSPE). Burst durations of 50 to 150 msec are seen in ballistic movement overflow myoclonus (4), a type of essential myoclonus, "hysterical" myoclonus, and tic. EMG bursts of 30 to 60 msec, frequently synchronous in antagonist muscles and difficult to mimic voluntarily, characterize several types of myoclonus. Two types with these short EMG bursts of probable cortical origin are cortical reflex myoclonus (5), which can be seen after anoxia and in certain epileptic states, and myoclonus of subacute spongiform encephalopathy (Creutzfeldt–Jakob disease) (7). Another type, reticular reflex myoclonus (3), has probable brainstem origin, and this type also may be seen after anoxia or with uremia. Physiological separation of these types requires EEG correlation. In cortical reflex myoclonus, the muscle jerking may be associated with a central beta rhythm; with myoclonus of subacute spongiform encephalopathy, there may be a periodic record; and with reticular reflex myoclonus, there may be associated generalized spikes. The most powerful method of separating these types of myoclonus, however, is to correlate the EMG with the EEG by jerk-locked back averaging of the EEG, as demonstrated by Shibasaki and Kuroiwa (6). In cortical reflex myoclonus, there is a focal, contralateral negativity, with onset 10 to 20 msec prior to the jerk and a duration of 15 to 40 msec. In the myoclonus associated with subacute spongiform encephalopathy, there is a widespread contralateral negativity, with onset 50 to 80 msec prior to the jerk and a duration of 100 to 160 msec. There is no time-locked EEG event yet demonstrated in reticular reflex myoclonus. In this chapter we will summarize the characteristics of two additional physiological types of myoclonus that we have recently described (9–11).

MYOCLONUS OF ALZHEIMER'S DISEASE

Myoclonus is not usually described as a frequent concomitant of Alzheimer's disease, but this is because most physicians see patients with Alzheimer's disease only in the early stage. In the later stage, myoclonus is common, and we easily identified seven Alzheimer's patients with myoclonus in a hospital for chronic disease. Our study included also three patients with trisomy 21 (Down's syndrome) who were older than 45 years and therefore should have had Alzheimer's changes in the brain (1). We thought that the characterization of Alzheimer's myoclonus would be useful, at least to help distinguish between Alzheimer's disease and subacute spongiform encephalopathy in adults presenting with dementia and myoclonus.

Clinically, the myoclonus in Alzheimer's disease had the appearance of small multifocal distal muscle jerks. A whole limb might be involved, and rarely the whole body might be involved. The frequency was variable. Myoclonus occurred at rest and might be provoked by stimulation or voluntary movement.

EMG findings showed bursts of 20 to 80 msec in individual muscles, with synchrony of antagonist muscles when they were involved. EEG was slow, often with some epileptic activity that could not be readily correlated with the jerks. The EEG activity time-locked to the myoclonus was a focal contralateral central negativity (Fig. 1), with onset 20 to 40 msec prior to the jerk and a duration of 40 to 80 msec. The focal nature and polarity of the EEG correlate is similar to that in cortical reflex myoclonus, but both onset time and duration are longer. The event differs from that in subacute spongiform encephalopathy in being more focal and shorter in onset time and duration. In two patients, a bifrontal negativity preceded the myoclonic jerk, and this phenomenon will be discussed more fully below.

In all nine patients who were studied, the myoclonus could be produced in arm muscles by stimulating the ipsilateral median nerve (C reflex) at latencies varying between 35 and 75 msec. In three of these patients, the somatosensory evoked potential to this stimulus was enhanced. These features do not provide definite further differentiation of Alzheimer's disease and subacute spongiform encephalopathy.

The findings in the majority of the patients with Alzheimer's disease are indicative of a type of cortical myoclonus electrophysiologically distinguishable from those previously described.

MINIPOLYMYOCLONUS OF CENTRAL ORIGIN

The term *minipolymyoclonus* was coined several years ago to describe a certain type of tremulousness of the outstretched hands in patients with motoneuron disease (8). Presumably, this is due to having only a few large motor units in a muscle, which is therefore not able to generate a smooth contraction. We have seen a similar clinical phenomenon in which central nervous system disease seems responsible. The nine patients whom we have studied include four with Lennox–Gastaut syn-

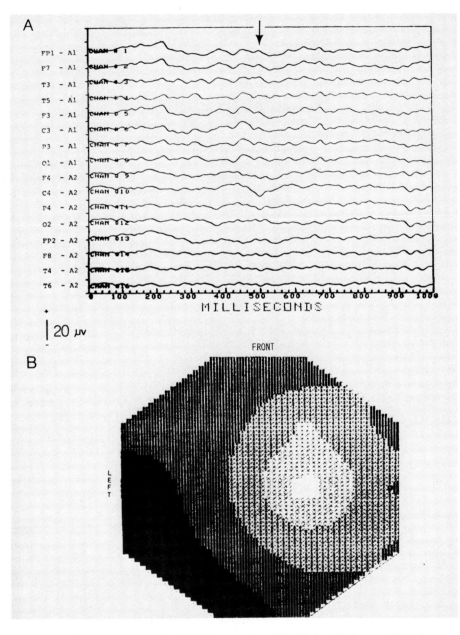

FIG. 1. EEG correlate of myoclonic jerks in a patient with Alzheimer's disease; this is the most common pattern of a contralateral central negativity. **A:** EEG activity collected before and after myoclonic jerks that occurred in the left wrist extensor at 500 msec. Traces are averages of 32 events. **B:** Topographic display of the maximal negativity of the EEG at the time of the arrow in **A**. (The topographic display is derived from the voltage values in the 16 EEG channels. Light areas, negative; dark areas, positive.) (From Wilkins et al., ref. 10, with permission.)

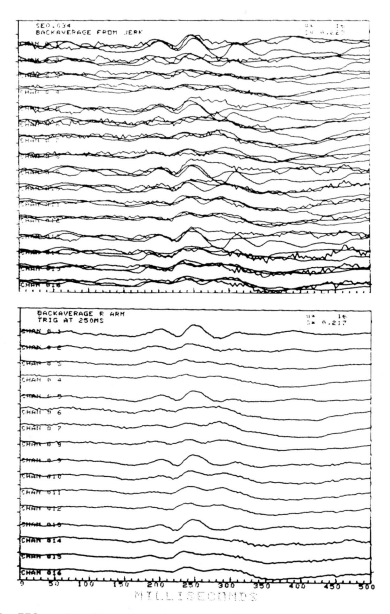

FIG. 2. EEG correlate of myoclonic jerks in a patient with an encephalopathy of unknown type. **Top:** EEG activity collected before and after the jerks, which occurred in the right wrist flexors at 250 msec. There are three superimposed traces, each of which is the average of 16 events. **Bottom:** the grand average of the three traces in the top half. The montage is the same as for Fig. 1.

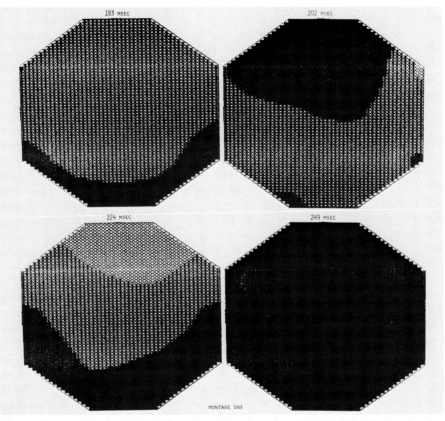

FIG. 3. Topographic display of EEG activity at four times from the potentials displayed on the bottom half of Fig. 2. Note that the bifrontal negativity 25 msec before the jerk is preceded by a bifrontal positivity.

drome, two with cerebral palsy, two with Alzheimer's disease (as noted above), and one with an unknown degenerative syndrome.

Clinically, the myoclonus in these patients consisted of small distal muscle jerks, frequently leading only to tiny individual finger movements. Less commonly, more of the limb was involved. Jerks were present at rest and were sometimes enhanced by voluntary movement.

The EMG correlate of the myoclonus was 20- to 50-msec bursts in individual muscles or simultaneously in antagonist pairs. Interestingly, jerks could be seen synchronously in right and left hands. This observation, which is impossible to make clinically, would seem to be valuable in differentiating minipolymyoclonus of peripheral and central origin.

The EEG was markedly abnormal in all cases with prominent bifrontal delta activity seen in seven cases. Atypical spike–wave paroxysms were common. With the back-averaging technique, a bifrontal negative slow wave was found in seven patients, preceding the jerk by 20 to 500 msec and having a duration of 150 to 250 msec. Each of three patients had a bifrontal negative sharp wave (one patient showed both types of waves in different recordings) preceding the jerk by 40 to 70 msec, with a duration of 30 to 80 msec (Figs. 2 and 3). The same bifrontal event could be identified when back-averaging from either hand. The sharper the negativity, the more precisely time-locked was the myoclonus to the EEG event.

The duration of the bifrontal negative event often could be correlated with the frequency of the bifrontal delta activity in the spontaneous EEG. In one remarkable case, the bifrontal activity was an 8-Hz rhythm, and several cycles of the rhythm could be identified in the back-averaged event.

The physiology of this phenomenon is not clear. What is observed is a bifrontal negativity in the EEG associated with an increased excitability of distal hand muscles, leading at times to synchronous jerks in the two hands. This would seem to be more consistent with a subcortical generator than with a cortical generator.

SUMMARY

The typical electrophysiological correlates of myoclonus in Alzheimer's disease are similar to those of cortical reflex myoclonus, with a focal, contralateral negativity in the EEG preceding the myoclonic jerk. One difference from cortical reflex myoclonus is that the duration of the negativity is longer and its onset before the jerk earlier. The features differ from those described for subacute spongiform encephalopathy and should be helpful for differential diagnosis. The electrophysiological correlate of minipolymyoclonus that can be seen in Alzheimer's disease and in other pathological states is a bifrontal negativity in the EEG that precedes the myoclonic jerk. This new type of electrophysiological correlate of myoclonus may reflect activity of a subcortical generator.

REFERENCES

1. Ellis WG, McCulloch JR, Corley CL. Presenile dementia in Down's syndrome. *Neurology* 1974;24:101–6.
2. Hallett M. Analysis of abnormal voluntary and involuntary movements with surface EMG. In: Desmedt JE, ed. Motor mechanisms in health and disease. New York: Raven Press, 1983.
3. Hallett M, Chadwick D, Adam J, Marsden CD. Reticular reflex myoclonus; a physiological type of human post-anoxic myoclonus. *J Neurol Neurosurg Psychiatry* 1977;40:253–64.
4. Hallett M, Chadwick D, Marsden CD. Ballistic movement overflow myoclonus. *Brain* 1977;100:299–312.
5. Hallett M, Chadwick D, Marsden CD. Cortical reflex myoclonus. *Neurology* 1979;29:1107–25.
6. Shibasaki H, Kuroiwa Y. Electroencephalographic correlates of myoclonus. *Electroencephalogr Clin Neurophysiol* 1975;39:455–63.
7. Shibasaki H, Motomura S, Yamashita Y, Shii H, Kuroiwa Y. Periodic synchronous discharge and myoclonus in Creutzfeldt–Jacob disease; diagnostic application of jerk-locked averaging method. *Ann Neurol* 1981;9:150–6.
8. Spiro AJ. Minipolymyoclonus: a neglected sign in childhood spinal muscular atrophy. *Neurology* 1970;20:1124–6.

9. Wilkins DE, Hallett M, Berardelli A, Walshe T, Alvarez N. Physiological analysis of the myoclonus of Alzheimer disease. *Neurology* 1982;32(2):A72.
10. Wilkins DE, Hallett M, Berardelli A, Walshe T, Alvarez N. Physiological analysis of the myoclonus of Alzheimer disease. *Neurology (Cleveland)* 1984;34:898–903.
11. Wilkins DE, Hallett M, Erba G, Alvarez N. Minipolymyoclonus of central origin. *Neurology* 1983;33(Suppl 2):225.

Note Added in Proof

Since the conference on which this volume is based was held, our thinking on this subject has changed. The reader is referred to D. E. Wilkins, M. Hallett, and G. Erba, Primary generalized epileptic myoclonus: A frequent manifestation of minipolymyoclonus of central origin, *J. Neurol. Neurosurg. Psychiatry*, 48:506–516 (1985).

Advances in Neurology, Vol. 43: Myoclonus,
edited by S. Fahn et al. Raven Press,
New York © 1986.

The Primate Serotonergic System: A Review of Human and Animal Studies and a Report on *Macaca fascicularis*[1]

*Efrain C. Azmitia and †Patrick J. Gannon

*Department of Biology, New York University, New York, New York 10003;
and †Department of Otolaryngology, Mount Sinai School of Medicine,
New York, New York 10021

The serotonin-producing neurons of the mammalian brain comprise the most expansive chemical circuitry known (for a preview, see Fig. 51).

Serotonergic cells are phylogenetically ancient and have been identified in every nervous system from aplysia to human. Ontogenetically, these cells are among the first to differentiate. The cell bodies are largely confined to the brainstem, that part of the neuroaxis that is the oldest area of the CNS, and are a component of the reticular formation, the most primitive nuclear arrangement. The most significant characteristic of this small collection of neurons, numbering in the tens of thousands, is that they innervate nearly every area of the brain. The extent of this anatomical distribution is difficult to comprehend when it is noted that the brain contains neurons numbering in the thousands of billions (10^{15}). Yet functional studies confirm this expansive nature of the serotonergic system. Alterations in the CNS serotonin neurons have produced changes in sleep, eating behavior, sexual activity, memory, learning, pain, aggression, locomotor activity, sensory processing, motor reflexes, adrenocorticotropic hormone (ACTH), prolactin, growth-hormone and luteinizing-hormone release, diurnal rhythms, vasodilation, and temperature regulation, and they have been implicated in human disorders such as myoclonus, Down's syndrome, Parkinson's disease, Huntington's chorea, depression, insomnia, autism, suicide, schizophrenia, and epilepsy.

This chapter provides both morphological and biochemical data on the anatomical distribution of the serotonergic system in the primate brain. A great deal has been published on human postmortem brain tissue, and almost all of these studies deal with the biochemical measurement of serotonin levels. The histochemical fluorescent study by Nobin and Bjorklund (63) of the monoaminergic systems in the fetal brain provides the only morphological data on the human serotonergic system. However, the use of fetal tissue is not sufficient to understand the adult system. The study of nonhuman primates is therefore needed to fill the gap between

---

[1] This article is dedicated to Morris B. Bender, M.D.

biochemistry and anatomy, since these two disciplines must be joined before the function of the system can be appreciated.

Numerous anatomical studies of the serotonergic system in the nonhuman primate have been published. The majority of these have been limited to a description of the nuclear organization in the brainstem. Although these data are useful, the general pattern appears to resemble that described in lower mammals—cat, rat, mouse, rabbit—and more detail is needed to understand the unique characteristics of the primate system.

The serotonergic distribution in the Old World monkeys, *Macaca fascicularis*, is described in this chapter, using immunocytochemistry, radioautography, and biochemistry. The emphasis will be on those aspects of the primate brain that are different from lower mammals. Furthermore, special attention will be given to the cortical distribution of serotonergic fibers, since the tremendous expansion of this brain area is a special characteristic of primates. New insights into how the primate brainstem 5-hydroxytryptamine (5-HT) system maintains its influence during this expansion will be presented. However, the basic description of nuclear organization and subcortical distribution is also included, so that the reader can appreciate that, despite the upward expansion, the basic infrastructure remains essentially unchanged.

MATERIALS AND METHODS

Monkeys, *M fascicularis* (female, 3.3–3.5 kg, purchased from Charles River Breeders, Boston), were injected with ketamine. The animals were decapitated and the brain removed and placed in ice-cold Ringer's bicarbonate solution containing pargyline (10^{-4}M), ascorbic acid (10^{-3}M), and dextrose (10^{-2}M) within 5 to 10 min after death. Selected areas were dissected, using standard topographic boundaries (Figs. 1–6). The structures were prepared for measurement and localization of [^{3}H]5-HT reuptake in synaptosomes and slices, respectively. Two animals were pretreated with pargyline (Sigma, St. Louis, 50 mg/kg) 30 min before an intraperitoneal injection of L-tryptophan (50 mg/kg). One hour later the animals were perfused through the ascending aorta with 4% paraformaldehyde, 0.2% glutaraldehyde, and 0.1% $MgSO_4$ in 0.1 M phosphate buffer (pH, 7.4) for 10 min and continued without glutaraldehyde (total volume was 1.5 liters) for 20 min. The brains were postfixed for at least 4 hr (5°C) and then processed for immunocytochemistry.

[^{3}H]5-HT Reuptake into Synaptosomes

Structures were homogenized in 10 vol of 0.32 M sucrose (5°C), and the tissue centrifuged at 800 G (15 min) to remove unbroken cells and other heavy contaminants (P1). The supernatant was centrifuged at 14,000 G for 15 min, and the P2 pellet resuspended in Ringer's solution. The incubations were performed in triplicate or quadruplicate in multiwelled plates (Linbro 76-002-04) in a total volume of

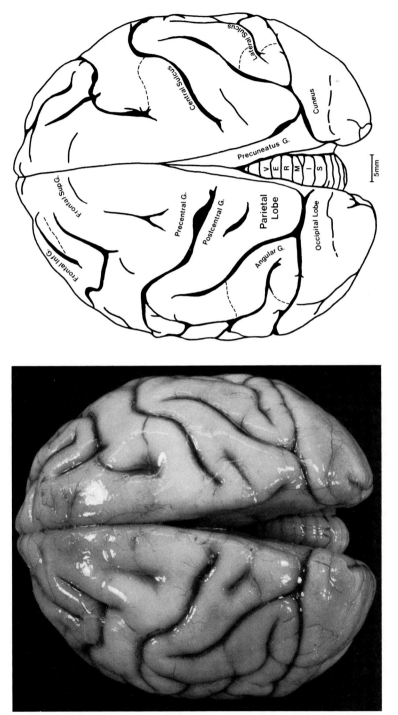

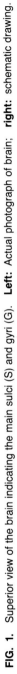

FIG. 1. Superior view of the brain indicating the main sulci (S) and gyri (G). **Left:** Actual photograph of brain; **right:** schematic drawing.

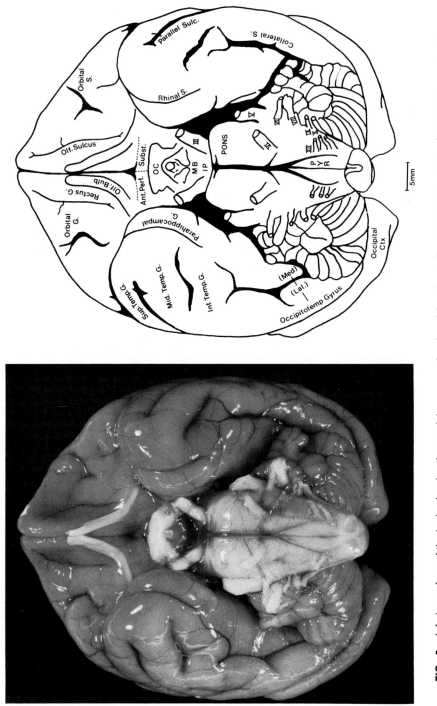

FIG. 2. Inferior surface of the brain showing the cranial nerves and main sulci and gyri. (See List of Abbreviations Used in Illustrations.)

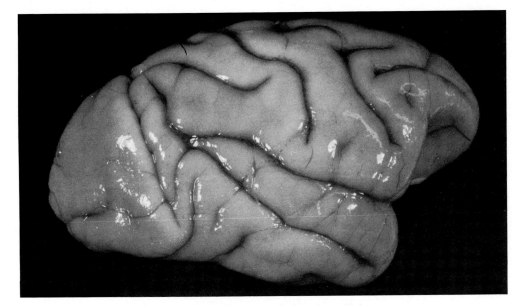

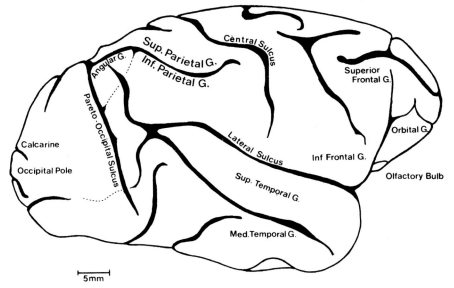

FIG. 3. Lateral surface of the brain showing main sulci and gyri. Actual photograph is dorsal to the schematic drawing.

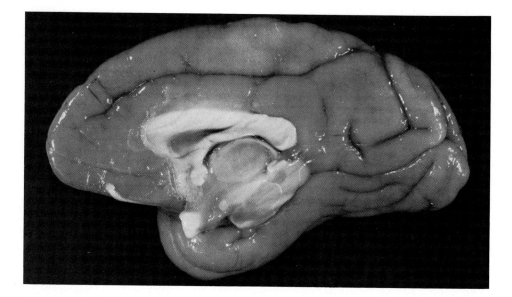

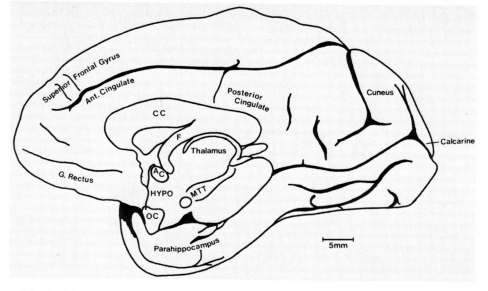

FIG. 4. Medial surface of the brain with hemisection of diencephalon showing the main sulci and gyri. Fiber systems marked are anterior commissure (AC), corpus callosum (CC), fornix (F), mammillothalamic tract (MTT), and optic chiasm (OC).

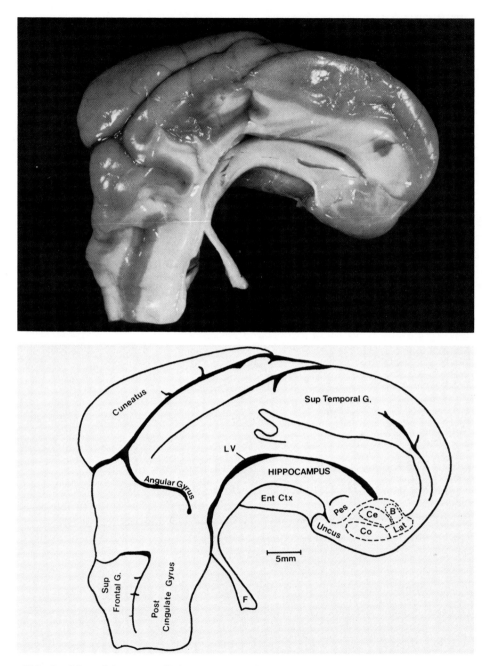

FIG. 5. View of the temporal lobe in the mediodorsal surface of the brain following removal of the diencephalon and all other cortical lobes. The hippocampus is exposed deep in the temporal lobe. The amygdaloid nuclei in the parahippocampal gyrus internal to the uncus are shown: cortical (Co), central (Ce), basal (B), and lateral (Lat). Ent Ctx, entorhinal cortex; LV, lateroventral.

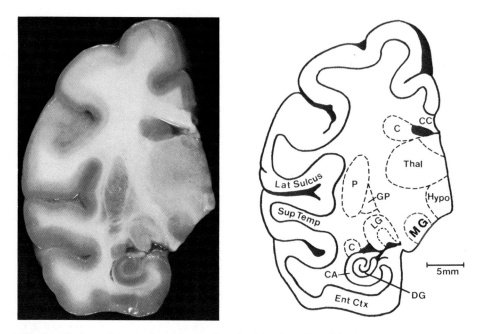

FIG. 6. Photograph and schematic drawing of a frontal section of the brain at the level of the lateral geniculate body. In this section, the portions of all components of the basal ganglion are present: C, caudate; GP, globus pallidus; P, putamen. The medial and lateral geniculate body (MG and LG) are dorsal to the hippocampal complex (cornu Ammonis, CA; dentate gyrus, DG). Ent Ctx, entorhinal cortex.

300 μl containing 15 μl of the P_2 suspension (for details of the reaction and isolation steps, see ref. 6).

Radioautography after [³H]5-HT Reuptake into Slices

Thin slices (0.5 mm) were incubated with 5×10^{-8} of [³H]5-HT (New England Nuclear, Boston, 25.1 Ci/mM) in 10 ml of the Ringer's solution for 12 min in a shaking water bath (37°C). Control slices were treated similarly except 10^{-5} M of unlabeled 5-HT was added to the media. The slices were then processed for light and electron microscopy (for details, see refs. 4,9,12).

Immunocytochemistry with a 5-Hydroxytryptamine Antibody

The tissue for immunocytochemistry was cut into small blocks (approximately 1 cm³) and sectioned on a vibratome (Oxford). Brainstem areas were cut at 100 μm for light-microscopic analysis, and hypothalamus at 20 μm for electron-microscopic analysis. The sections were extensively rinsed and incubated in 5-HT antiserum (generous gift of Dr. Jean Lauder) overnight at 5°C, followed by 2 hr at 20°C. The 5-HT antiserum (1:1,500 dilution) was in 0.1 M TRIS-buffered saline (pH, 7.2) with 1% normal sleep serum (Antibodies Inc.) and 0.3% Triton detergent for light microscopy and 0.1% Triton detergent for electron microscopy. The sections were then processed using the peroxidase–antiperoxidase technique as previously described for light-microscopic (41) and electron-microscopic (10) immunocytochemistry.

FINDINGS

Cell Bodies

The 5-HT–immunoreactive (IR) cell bodies in the monkey brain can be divided into rostral (Figs. 7–16) and caudal (Figs. 16–35) brainstem groups. The rostral group essentially consists of three main nuclei: the nucleus centralis superior (B_5, B_7, and B_8), the nucleus dorsal raphe (B_6 and B_7), and the nucleus prosupralemniscus (B_9). The caudal group consists of four main nuclei: the nucleus raphe obscurus (NRO) (B_2), the nucleus raphe pallidus (NRPa) (B_1), the nucleus raphe magnus (NRM) (B_3), and a group of 5-HT–IR cells in the nuclei reticular lateralis (LRN) and paragigantocellularis lateralis (NPGL).

With regard to the rostral group, one of the main features of our classification is that the nucleus annularis (nucleus interfascicularis), located between the medial longitudinal fasciculi (MLF), is combined with the nucleus centralis superior (NCS) instead of the nucleus raphe dorsalis (NRD). This classification is consistent with that of the human brainstem atlas by Olszewski and Baxter (64). Normally, this large collection of serotonergic neurons is associated with B_7, the designation devised by Dahlstrom and Fuxe (33) and is generally regarded as synonymous with NRD. However, there is both historical and anatomical justification for including this group with NCS. First, this group of cells is morphologically distinct from the cells seen more dorsal in the central gray because the cells are spindle shaped and oriented in a perpendicular plane. These neurons have been labeled as the NCS dorsalis by Olszewski and Baxter (64), the nucleus annularis by Felten et al. (39) and Taber et al. (76), and the interfascicular nucleus by Azmitia (3) and Zhou and Azmitia (83). Furthermore, in their fluorescent studies in the squirrel monkey, Hubbard and DiCarlo (48), based on cytological characteristics, also proposed that B_6, situated dorsal and lateral to the MLF, was part of the NCS dorsalis. However, we have chosen to assign this latter group (B_6) to the NRD because the cells in the lateral wings of this nucleus extend caudally as far as the nucleus locus ceruleus. Second, in the caudal midbrain, behind the superior cerebellar decussation, the cells of NCS dorsalis merge caudally with B_5 and ventrally with B_8 (NCS ventralis). The cells of NRD, on the other hand, merge caudally with B_6. Finally, the ascending projections of the NCS dorsalis closely overlie the cells of NCS medialis. In the rat, both groups project to the dorsal hippocampus (3,83), whereas in the monkey, they both project to the cingulate and prefrontal cortex (67).

With regard to the caudal group, several points should be emphasized. The 5-HT–IR cells in the NRO extend into the spinal cord, where they are associated with the descending MLF, the central canal (lamina X), and the motoneurons

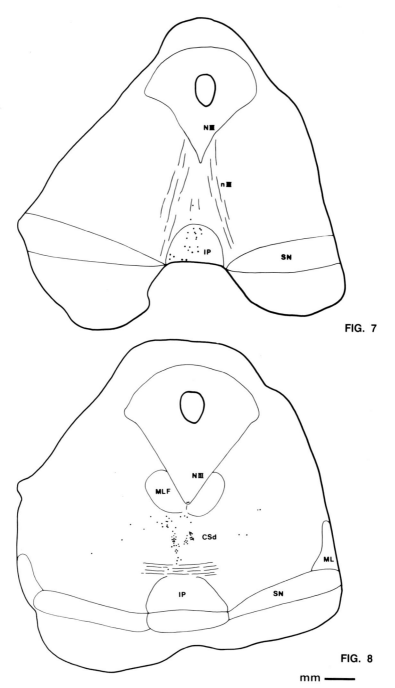

FIG. 7

FIG. 8

mm ━━━

FIGS. 7–33. The brainstem of *M fascicularis* was coronally sectioned at 100 μm on a vibratome (Oxford) and reacted with an antibody raised against serotonin conjugated to hemocyanine. The antibody was visualized using the peroxidase–antiperoxidase method. Every fifth section was drawn using a camera lucida, and each 5-HT-immunoreactive (IR) cell was drawn as a filled circle. These 5-HT-IR cells are seen first within the interpeduncular nucleus (IP) in Fig. 7 and are seen last within the anterior horn (AH) and central gray (CG) near the central canal (CC) of the cervical spinal cord in Fig. 33. (See List of Abbreviations Used in Illustrations). A description of the main serotonergic nuclei is presented in the text.

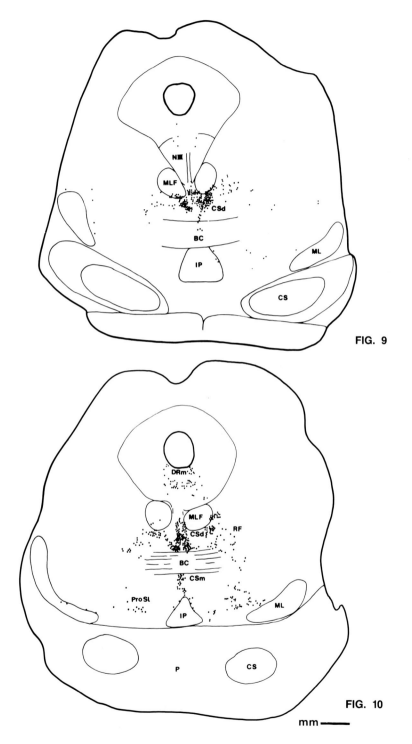

FIG. 9

FIG. 10

mm ——

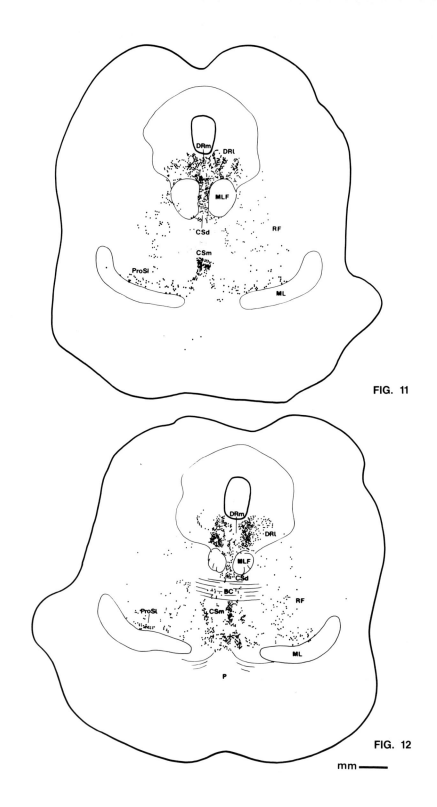

FIG. 11

FIG. 12

mm ——

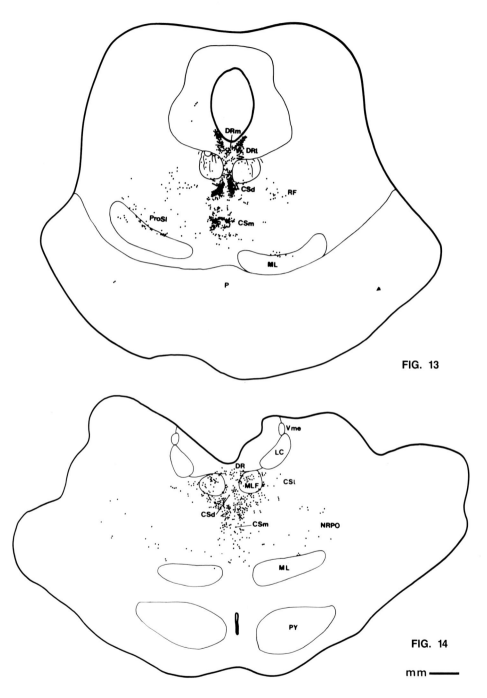

FIG. 13

FIG. 14

mm ━━━

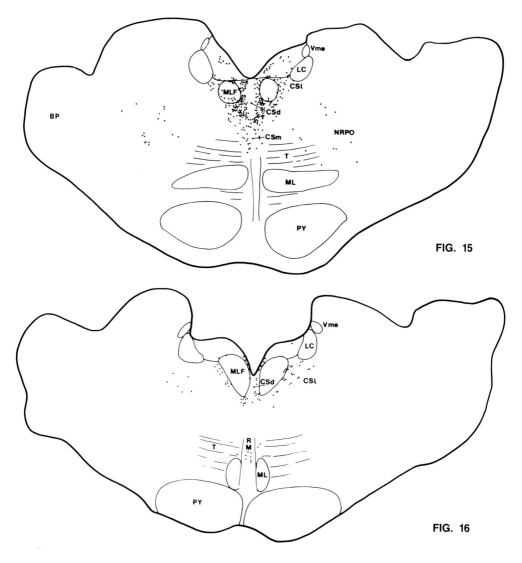

FIG. 15

FIG. 16

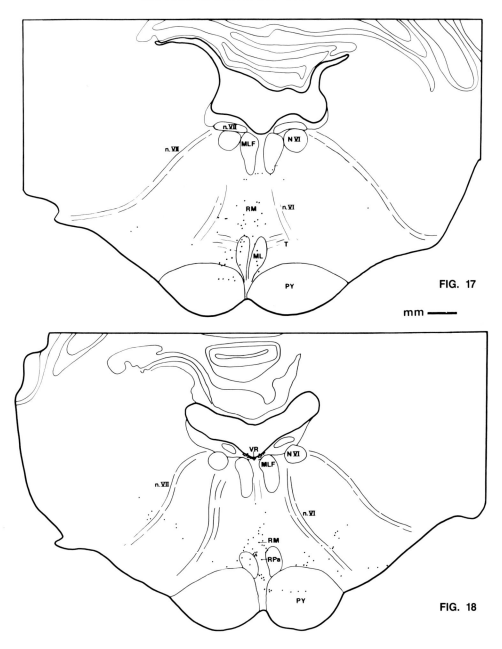

FIG. 17

mm ▬▬

FIG. 18

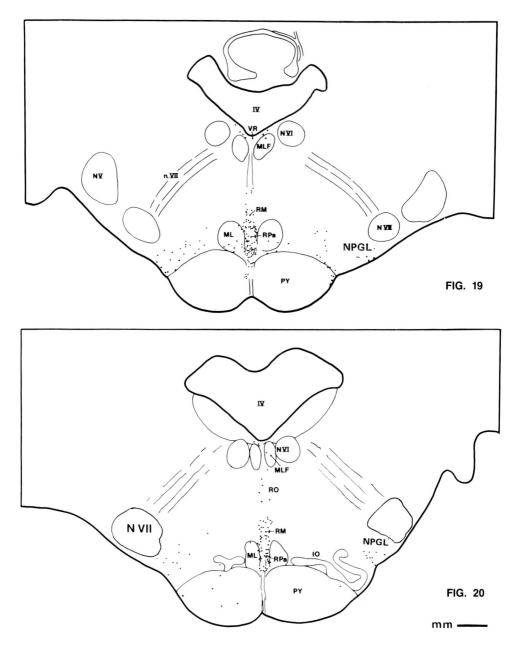

FIG. 19

FIG. 20

mm ——

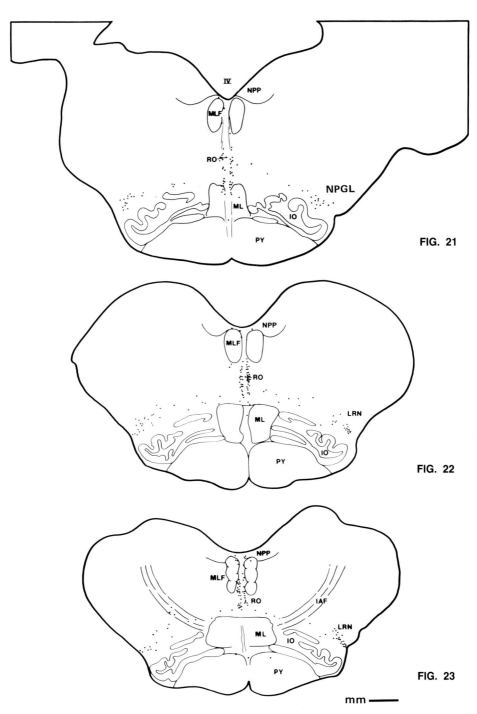

FIG. 21

FIG. 22

FIG. 23

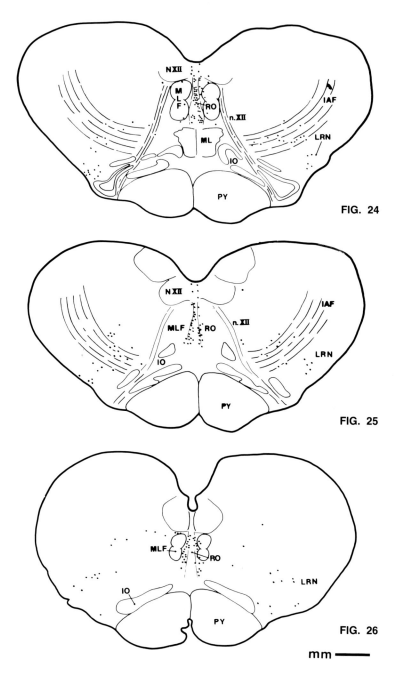

FIG. 24

FIG. 25

FIG. 26

mm ——

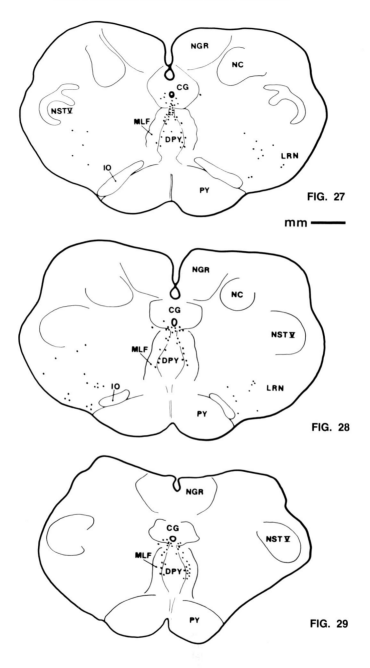

FIG. 27

mm ▬▬

FIG. 28

FIG. 29

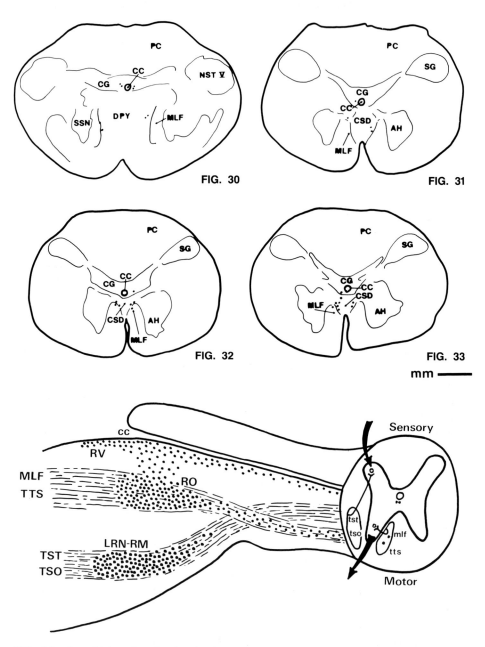

FIG. 34. A sagittal section showing the descending projections of the medial longitudinal fasciculus (MLF) [this tract called *faisceau longitudinal posterieur* by Cajal (23)]. The serotonergic cells in nucleus raphe magnus (RM) and lateral reticular nucleus (LRN), ventricular raphe (RV), and in obscurus (RO) are shown (as filled circles) giving rise to two descending projections. It should be noted that the NRM and LRN project along the tracti spinal thalamicus (TST) and spinal olivaris (TSO) arcuate fibers (IAF), whereas the NRO projects ventrally along the MLF. The RMST projects via a lateral descending route to innervate the substantia gelatinosa, and the ROST projects via a ventromedial descending route to innervate the motoneurons of the anterior horn. (Modified from Cajal, ref. 23, p. 913, Fig. 409.)

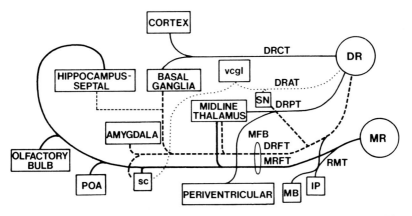

FIG. 35. Main ascending tracts from the dorsal raphe (DR) and median raphe (MR) nuclei, determined by the autoradiographic tracing technique following injection of [³H]proline. The six pathways found are DRCT, DR cortical tract; DRAT, DR arcuate tract; DRPT, DR periventricular tract; DRFT, DR forebrain tract; MRFT, MR forebrain tract; RMT, raphe medial tract. IP, interpeduncular nucleus; MB, mammillary body; MFB, medial forebrain bundle; POA, preoptic area, sc, suprachiasmatic nucleus; SN, substantia nigra; vcgl, ventrolateral geniculate nucleus. (Modified from Azmitia, ref. 2, Fig. 4.)

(lamina IX). This group divides into two clusters rostrally. The dorsal one is below the fourth ventricle and at this point is called the nucleus raphe ventricularis. A second point is the existence of a large cluster of neurons on the ventrolateral floor of the medulla oblongata. These cells are located in the LRN and more rostrally in the NPGL. Thus, the ventrolateral medullary 5-HT–IR cell group extends from the emergence of the sixth nerve to that of the twelfth. In this ventral position, the cells are often associated with blood vessels entering the brain at this level. In the rat, the cells have been termed the nucleus paragigantocellularis lateralis by Andrezik et al. (1) and nucleus reticularis paragigantocellularis by Lidov and Molliver (57). This group of cells has been identified in the cat by Wiklund et al. (81) and by Jacobs et al. (50). The final point is the existence of small 5-HT–IR cells in the area postrema. These cells were seen in the monkey after pretreatment with pargyline (a monoamine oxidase inhibitor) and L-tryptophan (the amino acid precursor of serotonin biosynthesis).

Both the rostral and caudal groups of 5-HT–IR neurons are closely associated with major motor and sensory pathways. The cells of NCS, NRD, and NRO are all near or intermingled with the MLF. This pathway interconnects the oculomotor nuclei, the spinal motoneurons, and the vestibular nuclei. The cells of prosupralemniscus nucleus (ProSL) and NRM lie adjacent to the medial lemniscal tract. This is the major ascending sensory pathway conveying proprioceptive information from the spinal cord via the dorsal column nuclei. The cells of NRM are associated with the trapezoid body. This pathway is involved in auditory transmission to the midbrain. The cells of the NRPa are around, and sometimes indented within, the pyramidal tract. Finally, the lateral 5-HT–IR cells in the LRN and NPGL are associated with the tractus spinal olivaris and tractus spinal thalamicus. These two pathways convey sensory information from the spinal cord to the brainstem.

Various 5-HT–IR cells are closely positioned to key brainstem nuclei. The cells of NCS surround the interpeduncular nucleus. Cells from this serotonergic nucleus also extend laterally into the central reticular formation of the midbrain and pons. Cells from NRM and NRPa extend into the inferior olive and also into the reticular formation. The cells in the ventrolateral medulla are associated with the lateral reticular and lateral paragigantocellular nuclei. Finally, the cells of NRD and NRO mix with the cells in the central gray from the midbrain to the spinal cord.

Associations also are seen with nonneuronal cell types. Neurons in the NRD and NCS have been shown to be in apposition to oligodendrocytes (2,36). 5-HT–IR cells from the NRD are also apposed to the ependymal cells of the cerebral aqueduct and the fourth ventricle. A small group of 5-HT–IR cells separated caudally from NRD also was seen to be in close proximity to the ependymal cells of the fourth ventricle. We term these cells nucleus raphe ventricularis (NRV). We have even observed the rare ependymal cells that were immunoreactive to our 5-HT antibody. Bundles of raphe neuronal dendrites and ventricular tanycytes have been previously reported (40). Finally, 5-HT–IR cells often are associated with large blood vessels. This is most striking in the NCS medialis and in the NPGL. A final observation we have made is the existence of very small 5-HT–IR cells in the area postrema. These cells are visible in our pretreated monkey, as they are in pretreated rats (33).

The widespread distribution of the 5-HT–IR cells in the primate brainstem attest to the crucial role played by serotonin in a variety of brainstem functions. The association of the serotonergic cells with known fiber pathways and brainstem nuclei provide a means for direct 5-HT modulation of both sensory and motor functions. The varied contacts with nonneuronal cells emphasize that more generalized mental states (e.g., depression, euphoria), possibly hormonal in nature, can also be influenced by serotonergic neurons.

Rostral Brainstem Group

NCS

Using the division proposed by Olszewski and Baxter (64), NCS (B_8, B_5, and part of B_7) can be divided into three components: dorsalis, medialis, and lateralis (Figs. 7–16). The dorsal component lies between the MLF. This group is continuous with B_5 [nucleus raphe pontis oralis (NRPo)] in the pons and extends as far rostrally as the oculomotor nuclei.

The medialis component is generally considered to be B_8. It is a paramedian and median cluster of cells. The group has a rostrocaudal oblique orientation as previously described in the rat (3,57). The cells of the medialis component remain ventral to the decussation of the superior cerebellar peduncle. Rostrally, the cells from this group end around and within the interpeduncular nucleus. The cells are mainly seen dorsal and lateral to this nucleus. Caudally, the ventral border of this group is the trapezoid body. The final cluster of cells of NCS is the lateralis group, which is seen ventrolateral to the MLF. A large number of cells extend from this group into the midbrain reticular formation. These cells are widely scattered and seem to form a ring around the NRPO (Figs. 14 and 15). A similar arrangement has been noted in the cat (50).

Nucleus raphe pontis (B_5)

A small paramedian cluster of 5-HT–IR cells (Fig. 15), with a few cells lying directly on the midline, form the caudal border of the nucleus centralis superior dorsalis (B_8). The cells are located just medial and ventral to the MLF and extend caudally to the level of the abducens nucleus. Some of the cells and many dendrites are situated within the MLF. At the very caudal portion of this group, the cells are situated dorsal to the raphe magnus cells. In the rat, this group was described as being continuous with the median raphe nucleus (57).

NRD

The dorsal raphe nucleus (B_7 and B_6) (Figs. 10–13) is divided into a medial and a lateral component. The medial component is in the central gray just below the cerebral aqueduct. These cells extend caudally to merge with B_6 in the pons. The cells extend rostrally to the caudal border of the oculomotor nuclei.

The lateral component forms the larger division of NRD and extends as far rostrally as the oculomotor nuclei. This pair of laterally situated 5-HT–IR cells (Fig. 15) can be seen in the central gray of the pons just ventral to the fourth ventricle. The cells lie between the MLF and the locus ceruleus and some of the cells penetrate into the boundaries of these two areas. The serotonergic cells in the nucleus of the locus ceruleus were first described by Sladek and Walker (75) in the brains of stump-tailed macaques. The cells comprising the B_6 groups are first seen at the level of the motor nucleus of V and become continuous rostrally with the lateral wings of NRD. This continuity also was seen in the developing rat brain (57).

ProSL nucleus (B_9)

The last group to be described in the rostral brainstem is located along the dorsal surface of the medial lemniscus from the rostral border of the inferior olive to the level of the red nucleus (Figs. 9–15). These cells are occasionally continuous with the paramedian cells of the medial component of the NCS. The similar cytological and fluorescent characteristics of the cells in NCS and ProSL were first noted in the brainstem of the squirrel monkey by Hubbard and DiCarlo (48). These findings extended the observation of similarity between these two nuclei made in the rat by Dahlstrom and Fuxe (33).

Caudal Brainstem Group

NRO

The largest collection of 5-HT–IR neurons in the caudal brainstem lie in a symmetrical paramedian cluster. NRO (B_2) (Figs. 20–33) extends caudally from the border of the pons to the cervical spinal cord. In the spinal cord, the cells are scattered in the central gray area just ventral to the central canal of the spinal cord and on the medial border of the ventral horn. The majority of these neurons are associated with the fibers of the MLF and the tractus tectospinalis (TTS) as these tracts move from their superior position in the medulla to an inferior position in the spinal cord. The cells in the spinal cord lying below the central canal have been described previously by Lamotte et al. (56). NRO extends rostrally up to the level of the exit of nerve VI. At these anterior levels, a smaller number of 5-HT–IR cells have split from the main cluster and are designated NRV.

NRPa (B_1)

A midline cluster of cells located ventrally in the medulla oblongata extends from nerve XII to the rostral pole of the inferior olive (Figs. 17–23). The cells lie mainly between the pyramidal tract both dorsally and ventrally. The dorsal border is continuous with the raphe magnus rostrally. The dorsal group forms two paramedian clusters and some cells are actually located directly on the midline. Cells extend caudally along the medial border of the medial lemniscus.

NRM (B_3)

This group of large cells is more random and extends much more laterally into the nucleus reticularis gigantocellularis (Figs. 16–20). The group extends rostrocaudally from the emergence of nerve roots to the rostral inferior olive. Its location overlaps the trapezoid body and the dorsal border of the medial lemniscus. It is continuous with both B_1 and B_2.

Nucleus reticularis paragigantocellularis lateralis

Neurons from this group extend laterally along the trapezoid, medial leminiscal, and pyramidal fibers. These 5-HT–IR cells are located in the reticular formation of the ventrolateral medulla. Rostrally they appear to be in the NPGL and caudally in the ventral part of the LRN (Figs. 17–28). This substantial group of cells extends from the emergence of the roots of the sixth nerve to the caudal part of the inferior olivary nucleus. This lateral group was described by Schofield and Dixon (71) in the common marmoset and called the nucleus reticularis paragigantocellularis lateralis (1,28). In the developing rat brain, this group was attributed to a lateral wing of B_1 by Lidov and Molliver (57). The original classification proposed by Dahlstrom and Fuxe (33) in the adult rat assigned the cells to both B_1 and B_3. In the cat, these cells were described as reaching the floor of the medulla (50,81). In our preparations, the cells also reached the ventral pia and in certain cases were associated with the large blood vessels entering the medulla.

NRV (B₄)

A group of 5-HT–IR cells was seen just ventral to the fourth ventricle at the level of the genu of nerve VII and extended caudally to join the NRO (Figs. 18–20). The cells were small and located on the midline. This group was not previously described in the primate brain and may have been visible in our preparation because the animals were pretreated with pargyline and tryptophan. In the rat, B_4 has been described as being continuous with B_7 (the superior medial component) (57). In our preparation, the ventricular raphe group appears distinct from B_7, but is continuous with B_3.

Ultrastructure of Cell Bodies

Two types of neuronal cell bodies were seen in the raphe nuclei of the monkey; the first type received numerous axosomatic synapses and the second type received few neuronal synapses (40). This second type of raphe cell, which was the most prevalent, had prominent oligodendroglial contacts. The oligodendroglial raphe–neuron association has been previously described in the rat (2,36). The serotonergic nature of neurons contacting oligodendroglia was confirmed by the chromium tagging technique (40) in the monkey. In the rat, we have observed 5-HT–IR neurons in contact with oligodendrocytes *(unpublished observations)* and Descarries and his co-workers (36) have observed this by using [³H]5-HT labeling to identify their neurons.

The cytoplasm of 5-HT–IR cells in the dorsal raphe of the monkey had numerous rough endoplasmic reticulum (RER) cisternae and mitochondria and a well-formed Golgi body (55). The immunoreactivity was present in RER and in dense-core vesicles. 5-HT–IR myelinated and unmyelinated axons were found by this group within the midbrain raphe area. Evidence for serotonergic endings on serotonergic soma was observed, indicating some form of chemical autoregulation.

A detailed electron-microscopic radioautographic study was also performed in the NPGL of the rhesus monkey (28). Cells labeled with [³H]5-HT had extensive RER and an elaborate Golgi apparatus. The nucleus was also labeled, which is consistent with studies in the rat (36). Myelinated and unmyelinated fibers were seen in the NPGL of the monkey. Here again, evidence for serotonergic endings on serotonergic soma was observed. The [³H]5-HT was believed to be highly localized to the dense-core vesicles that were seen in the cytoplasm of 5-HT neurons.

Pathways

Descending Projection to Spinal Cord

Pathways and terminals

There is abundant evidence that serotonin modulates both motor and sensory processing at the level of the spinal cord. In the monkey spinal cord, a dense plexus of 5-HT–IR fibers is present in the substantia gelatinosa and around the motoneurons in the ventral horn. Serotonergic endings have been shown to make direct contact with the neurons in the dorsal horn that give rise to the spinothalamic tract. This projection is believed to be important in the transmission of nociceptive information in humans and monkeys (44) and is believed to originate in the raphe magnus.

Serotonergic endings also have been seen directly on motoneurons, and these excitatory contacts probably originate in the raphe obscurus. Large injections of horse radish peroxidase (HRP) into the lumbar spinal cord in *M. fascicularis* label cells in NRO, NRM, and the nucleus gigantocellularis (21). A few cells also have been seen in the medial and lateral division of the NRD in squirrel monkeys and a baboon (60).

The descending pathways into the spinal cord are not yet clearly elucidated. Nobin and Bjorklund (63) described a single ventral descending tract in the human fetal brain. Felten and Sladek (40) report a dorsal descending tract from B_2 and a ventral descending tract from B_1 and B_3. However, we have observed no dorsal route but a medioventral and a lateroventral descending pathway. It appears that the fibers of B_2 (NRO) project to the motoneurons of the ventral horn using the descending MLF as a guide. Thus, it appears that the fibers in the medioventral descending tract moved into this inferior position at the level of the decussation of the pyramidal tract along with the fibers comprising the MLF. This projection to the motoneurons of the ventral horn would be consistent with the other projections from NRO to the motoneurons of the brainstem nuclei of nerves X and XII (40). We have termed this ventromedial descending tract the raphe obscurus spinal tract (ROST). The cells of B_3 complex (NRM, NPGL, and LRN) descend in the same position but in the opposite direction from the ascending sensory fibers in tractus spinal olivaris and the tractus spinal thalamicus. In the cervical levels of the spinal cord, the 5-HT–IR fibers appear to extend dorsally to innervate the substantia gelatinosa (Fig. 34, see p. 394). We have termed this lateroventral descending tract the raphe magnus spinal tract (RMST).

Ultrastructure in spinal cord

The existence of 5-HT–IR cell bodies, axons, and dendrites was reported in lamina X of the spinal cord in *M fascicularis* (56). The cytoplasm of the 5-HT–IR neurons contained considerable rough endoplasmic reticulum, neurofilaments, and a well-formed Golgi apparatus. The authors also reported "in one case a labeled myelinated axon was found approximately 40 μm from a labeled neuron" (p. 365). Also in one case, a small glial cell, presumably an oligodendrocyte, was found in close apposition to a labeled cell. The 5-HT–IR processes were seen near large central blood vessels and the central canal. This same pattern was reported in the brainstem of monkeys by Chan-Palay (27). Thus, as proposed for the brainstem, serotonin fibers in the spinal cord may have a role in vascular tone.

Recent immunocytochemical work also has been performed in the ventral horn of *M fascicularis* (66). These workers reported a large number of synaptic contacts on the soma and dendrites of motoneurons. The contacts were largely asymmetric on both of these sites. This work demonstrates that serotonergic fibers have direct access to outgoing motor activity. It should also be mentioned that direct 5-HT–IR fibers have been seen in the substantia gelatinosa of the rat (69), indicating a direct access of serotonergic fibers to incoming sensory activity.

Projections to Cerebellum

The serotonin projection to the cerebellum was radioautographically studied in the brains of *Macaca mulatta* following intraventricular infusion of [³H]5-HT (26). The areas of observation were limited to the periventricular zones where penetration by the labeled molecule was optimum. Labeled unmyelinated fibers were seen in the periventricular region of the fourth ventricle en route to the cerebellum. In the paraflocculus and flocculus the labeled fibers were predominately in the granular layers, although single fibers were seen to run the length of the folia. Both mossy fibers and fine beaded axons were labeled in the granular layer. Labeled mossy fibers were rare in the vermal and paravermal cortex. The number of [³H]5-HT–labeled fibers were greater in the molecular layer in these cerebellar regions. It was estimated that 1% of the mossy fibers and 0.1% of the fibers in the molecular layer were labeled in the parafloccular and floccular cortex, whereas in the vermal cortex, at least five times as many fibers were seen in the molecular layer.

All of the cerebellar and vestibular nuclei were labeled. The dentate and interpositus nuclei also received 5-HT fibers from the superior cerebellar peduncle. Labeled axon terminals were seen in synaptic relationships with cell bodies in the dentate nucleus. The origin of these fibers is believed to be from five raphe nuclei: the NRD, NSC, NRM, NRPo, and NRO. Ultrastructural studies identified six morphological classes of labeled axonal terminations (for details, see ref. 26).

Ascending Projections to Forebrain

Pathways and terminals

The serotonergic fibers projecting to the forebrain originate mainly in the rostral nuclei. Two main ascending bundles have been described in the primate brain (63,71,72). In the human fetus, "smooth, yellow-fluorescent fibers, apparently forming ascending axon bundles, were observed in two locations. First, in the central grey near the ependyma of the fourth ventricle and the aqueduct: and second, in a position between the medial raphe cells and the lateral cell system (AIP). This latter bundle could be traced rostrally through the descussation of the superior cerebellar peduncle" (63, p. 16).

In juvenile macaques, two ascending bundles were also seen. A dorsal bundle was seen just ventral to the MLF, originating at the level of locus ceruleus and received fibers from the NRD and the nucleus annularis (NCS dorsalis). These fibers appear to turn ventrally at the level of the red nucleus and enter the area tegmentalis ventralis mesencephali. A second bundle of ventrally flowing serotonergic fibers was seen just lateral to the NCS, originating at approximately the level of nucleus nervi trochlearis and receiving fibers from midline NRD and NCS.

These fibers appear to turn rostrally just dorsal to nucleus interpedunularis and enter the area tegmentalis ventralis mesencephali (72). In the common marmoset, only the latter serotonergic fiber bundle was seen (71).

In our own preparations, dense staining was present in the two areas described by Schofield and Everitt (72). In addition, we also saw fibers near the cerebral aqueduct in the hypothalamus and projecting lateroventrally from the NRD. Thus, all of the 5-HT fiber bundles observed in the rat (Fig. 35, see p. 395) appear to be present in the primate brainstem. In addition, it appears that the main ascending bundle through the hypothalamus may not be the medial forebrain bundle (MFB) as it is in the rat and commonly assumed to be in the primate. Examination of the caudal hypothalamic area (Fig. 36) shows two main ascending bundles previously described in the rat [the MFB and the dorsal raphe cortical tract (DRCT)]. However, in the primate, the latter tract, which ascends to the cerebral cortex via the internal capsule, appears to be larger than the MFB. The DRCT appears to have undergone a significant increase in absolute size when compared to the homologous pathway in the rat. This may represent the increase in the projection from the NRD to the primate cerebral cortex.

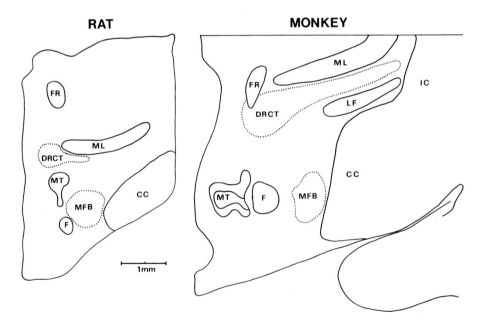

FIG. 36. Schematic drawing of coronal sections at the level of the posterior hypothalamus in the rat and monkey brain. The two main ascending pathways are the medial forebrain bundle (MFB) and the dorsal raphe cortical tract (DRCT) (outlined with dashed lines). The relative size and position of the MFB is similar in these two species. However, the DRCT is much larger in the monkey than in the rat brain, although it does occupy a similar relative position in both species. CC, crus cerebri; F, fornix; FR, fasciculus retroflexus, IC, internal capsule; ML, medial lemniscus; MT, mammillothalamic tract; LF, lenticular fasciculus. (Modified from Azmitia and Gannon, ref. 10, Fig. 1.)

Ultrastructure of ascending pathways

The main ascending projections in the monkey brain are the MFB and the DRCT (10). The comparison of these two pathways in hypothalamic coronal sections in rat and monkey is shown in Fig. 36. Ultrastructural analysis showed that the 5-HT immunoreactivity was seen predominately in unmyelinated fibers in the MFB (Fig. 37). These fibers were usually in apposition to unlabeled myelinated fibers. In addition, a significant percentage of the 5-HT-IR axons were found to be myelinated (25%, 223 of 956 profiles) (Fig. 38).

The unmyelinated fibers varied in their diameter between 0.2 and 1.25 μm, whereas the myelinated 5-HT–IR axons were generally larger, having diameters between 1.0 and 2.1 μm. The specific intraneuronal labeling was detected within the tubular profiles of the smooth endoplasmic reticulum seen in cross section (compare *a* and *b* with *c* in Fig. 37). The large number of 5-HT–IR myelinated fibers in the ascending pathways would allow serotonergic transmission to reach distal cortical regions rapidly in the primate brain. We have recently observed 5-HT–IR myelinated fibers in the cingulum bundle of *M. fascicularis (unpublished observation).* This observation of myelinated fibers argues against serotonin having an exclusively diffuse, slow-acting function, with transmitter being released throughout its axon. Although such a vegetative role may explain part of the function of serotonin in the brain, a precise and specialized role may have evolved in the primate brain.

Subcortical Distribution

Biochemistry

Humans

The majority of studies of the serotonergic system in the primate forebrain use biochemical measures of 5-HT or 5-hydroxyindoleacetic acid (5-HIAA). Table 1 presents a summary of reported values for 5-HT levels in human subcortical areas expressed as nanomoles of serotonin per gram of wet tissue weight. The highest levels are seen in the raphe nuclei of the midbrain and medulla, the substantia nigra, caudate, putamen, hypothalamus, anterior perforated substance, and the accumbens nuclei, whereas the lowest values are seen in the cerebellum, spinal cord, and ventral pons. However, there are discrepancies between laboratories both in absolute levels (see Hypothalamus and Thalamus in Table 1) and in the rank order of brain structures (see Basal Ganglion).

The distribution of 5-HIAA in human subcortical areas in shown in Table 2 and gives comparable results to the finding with 5-HT levels, except that the differences between brain regions are greater. It is interesting that the rank order in subcortical brain areas is not the same for 5-HT and 5-HIAA. Note that the globus pallidus ranks below the caudate and putamen in 5-HT concentration but above these two regions in 5-HIAA concentration. Likewise, the NRD has more 5-HT but less 5-

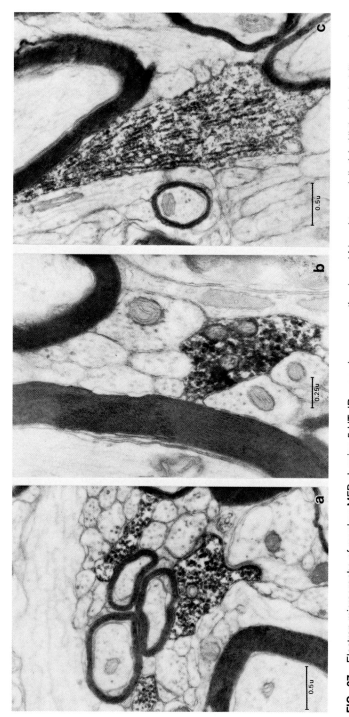

FIG. 37. Electron micrographs of monkey MFB showing 5-HT–IR axons in cross section (**a** and **b**) and tangentially (**c**). All the labeled fibers shown are unmyelinated. The reaction product associated with the serotonin immunoreactivity is located in the tubular profiles of the smooth endoplasmic reticulum (**c**).

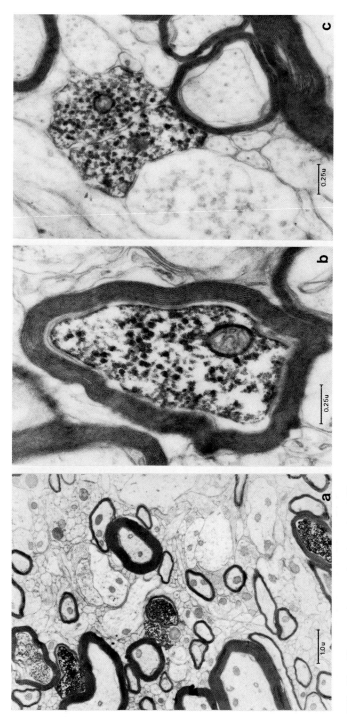

FIG. 38. Electron micrographs of monkey MFB showing 5-HT–IR axons in cross section: **a:** Low-power micrograph of a single unmyelinated axon and three myelinated axons; **b:** high-power electron micrograph showing a myelinated axon. Neurotubules appear to be only lightly stained. Specific staining is seen in the tubular profiles of smooth endoplasmic reticulum, the outer mitochondrial membranes, and in patches along the inner side of the axolemma. In **c**, a pair of labeled unmyelinated axons is shown in close apposition to an unreactive myelinated axon. IR densities in the stained axons are apposed both to myelinated and unmyelinated unreactive axons. The two IR fibers shown are separated by a glial process. (Modified from Azmitia and Gannon, ref. 10, Fig. 3.)

TABLE 1. *5-HT distribution in human subcortical area (nmol/g)*

Region	Ref. 31	Ref. 17	Ref. 18	Ref. 38	Ref. 58	Ref. 30	Ref. 19	Ref. 59	Refs. 52, 53	Ref. 78	Ref. 54	Ref. 82	Ref. 25	Ref. 80
Forebrain														
Anterior perforated substance	5.24													
Accumbens nucleus								0.42	3.66					1.7
Basal Ganglion														
Caudate	2.35	1.76	1.44		1.71		0.70	3.47	1.52	2.5		0.7	0.51	0.75
Inferior head				4.26										
Superior head				3.41		2.3								
Rostral tail				4.30										
Caudal tail				4.68										
Putamen	3.05	1.71	1.23	4.52	1.98	2.8	.91		1.42		1.42	.96		0.53
Globus pallidus	1.35	1.23	0.43			2.2			1.95					
Medial														1.44
Lateral														1.01
Fornix	1.93													
Hypothalamus														
Anterior	4.33	1.55	1.7		2.67			0.61	1.98			0.86	0.57	
Mediodorsal						2.1								
Medioventral						1.3								
Laterodorsal						2.2								
Lateroventral						1.9								
Mammillary body	2.09		1.5						1.34					
Posterior														
Mediodorsal						2.0								
Medioventral						1.2								
Laterodorsal						2.7								
Lateroventral						1.8								
Olfactory bulb			0.55											
Red nucleus					5.24	4.2	3.23	3.0	3.23					

Septum	7.59	2.94	0.16									
Substantia nigra				5.45	5.3		10.7	3.12				1.9
Subthalamus				3.21								
Thalamus												
Central (medial)	1.55	1.39	1.28		2.7	0.75	4.65	1.82	2.35		0.7	
Lateral			1.18		2.3							
Midbrain												
Tegmentum					3.1	2.03	12.9				2.46	
Quadrigemina												
Superior	4.33				2.9							
Inferior	2.51				2.3							
Raphe												
Centralis superior				12.0								
Centralis inferior				7.06								
Dorsalis				11.9				2.54				
Pons												
Tegmentum	3.74		0.94		4.4	0.25	0.27	0.27				
Ventral					0.5							
Raphe pontis				7.06								
Locus ceruleus										1.4		
Medulla	1.55		2.5			0.84		1.66	1.07			
Area postrema	3.05			5.72								
Raphe obscurus				3.26								
Raphe pallidus												
Spinal cord	0.75				0.7							
Cerebellum	0.16			0.7	0.7	0.7	0.52					
Vermis								1.02				
Dentate nucleus							0.80	1.23				

TABLE 2. *5-HIAA distribution in human subcortical area (nmol/g)*

Region	Ref. 58	Ref. 19	Refs. 51–53	Ref. 59	Ref. 78	Ref. 54	Ref. 82	Ref. 25	Ref. 32	Ref. 80
Forebrain										
Accumbens N.			9.0	3.0						7.8
Basal Ganglia										
Caudate	3.1	2.8	2.3	4.1	4.4		3.2	1.4		2.9
Putamen	5.3	5.1	2.7				5.5			4.6
Globus Pallidus										
Medial			4.5			5.4			7.0	7.7
Lateral										6.0
Hypothalamus	4.29		3.6	11.1			6.5	2.1	8.4	
Olfactory bulb				3.9						
Red nucleus			7.0							
Substantia nigra	23.3		9.0	23.1					19.4	9.5
Subthalamus	15.9									
Thalamus	10.4	5.4	3.7	8.6	5.5					
Midbrain		18	5.3	30						
Raphe										
Centralis superior	63.1									
Centralis inferior	22.9									
Dorsalis	35.9									
Pons										
Raphe pontis	39.1	4.5		26.8						
Locus ceruleus									30.2	
Ventral		7.0								
Medulla										
Raphe obscurus	14.6				5.5					
Raphe pallidus	11.6				6.5					
Cerebellum				0.6	0.97				0.55	
Vermis					0.87					

HIAA than the NCS. These differences probably reflect a greater turnover shown by the ratio of 5-HIAA to 5-HT.

Monkeys

The distribution of the 5-HT system has been measured biochemically in subhuman primates (Table 3). Table 3 shows (in nanomoles of serotonin per gram wet weight) the levels of 5-HT (columns 1–6), 5-HIAA (columns 7–10), [^{3}H]5-HT high affinity uptake (column 11), and the serotonin synthesis rate, calculated by *in vivo* 5-hydroxytryptophan (5-HTP) accumulation (columns 12 and 13) and *in vitro* tryptophan hydroxylase activity (column 14).

The distribution of 5-HT in subhuman primates is high in midbrain, substantia nigra, and hypothalamus and low in cerebellum and the basal ganglia. The levels of 5-HIAA are high in substantia nigra, thalamus, and putamen and low in caudate and accumbens. Although there appears to be some discrepancy in the rank order within the basal ganglia, most investigators reported high levels of both 5-HT and 5-HIAA in the globus pallidus. The variation noted in human studies between laboratories is also apparent in the studies on monkey brain. Note especially the values for putamen and thalamus.

The values for the [^{3}H]5-HT reuptake are shown in column 11 of Table 3 and in Fig. 39. The raphe area, medial thalamus, hypothalamus, and diagonal band are high, whereas the lateral thalamus and lateral geniculate are low in the accumulation of [^{3}H]5-HT into synaptosomal preparations. Figure 39 shows that the uptake in globus pallidus is higher than in the caudate–putamen. Also, there are differences between the various regions of the caudate, with the head being highest (Fig. 40). The reuptake measure reflects the amount of surface area in a synaptosomal preparation capable of accumulating [^{3}H]5-HT. The comparison of uptake in different regions at a single low concentration of [^{3}H]5-HT is valid only if the affinity of the uptake process is similar in these various regions. Figure 41 shows that this is indeed the case. The various brain regions concentrate different amounts of [^{3}H]5-HT, but they all have similar affinity constants (the intercept on the X axis).

The final measure in Table 3 is the measure of the serotonin synthesis rate. In the laboratory of Goldman-Rakic (22,46), this was done by *in vivo* blockade of degradation. Highest synthetic rates were seen in caudate and putamen, with slightly lower levels in brainstem, thalamus, and hypothalamus. However, if tryptophan hydroxylase activity is measured *in vitro*, the distribution in the monkey brain is very different (compare column 14 with columns 12 and 13 in Table 3). The highest levels are seen in the midbrain raphe area (87 nmol/g/hr) and then in the preoptic hypothalamic area (16 nmol/g/hr) and in the substantia nigra (14 nmol/g/hr). The lowest rates are seen in the caudate and putamen (2.4 and 2.0 nmol/g/hr, respectively). The amount of tryptophan hydroxylase activity is markedly higher in the globus pallidus (7 nmol/g/hr).

The subcortical distribution studies in humans and monkeys show the same relative distribution seen in lower vertebrates (rat, cat), but the values vary greatly among laboratories. As can be seen from Tables 1 to 3, the 5-HT and 5-HIAA

TABLE 3. 5-HT, 5-HIAA, and 5-HT reuptake (RU) and synthesis in monkey subcortical area (nmol/g)

Region	5-HT						5-HIAA				RU	Synthesis (hr)		
	1 (68)[a,b]	2 (79)[b]	3 (22)[b]	4 (73)[b]	5 (46)[b]	6 (72)[c]	7 (22)[b]	8 (14)[d]	9 (73)[b]	10 (32)[d]	11	12 (22)[b]	13 (46)[b]	14[f]
Forebrain														
Accumbens				2.1					2.6		0.3			
Basal ganglion														
Caudate	1.9	1.6	0.7	2.0	0.9	1.5	2.1	3.2	1.7		0.4	0.8	0.74	2.4
Putamen	1.7		0.5	2.2		2.9	2.8	10.4	2.9		0.3	1.3		2.0
Globus pallidus		1.2		3.0					5.5	4.6	0.4			7
Diagonal band											0.5			
Habenula											0.3			
Hypothalamus	4.1	3.2	2.0		2.1		5.2				0.5	.64	0.6	
Anterior Area						3.8								
Lateral														
Anterior						3.7								
Medial						4.1								
Posterior						4.5								
Ventral						4.2								
Arcuate/median eminence						1.1								
Dorsomedial						6.3								
Mammilary body						4.9								
Mediodorsal						4.2								
Preoptic														
Medial						3.7								
Lateral						4.7								

{16

Suprachiasm				3.0		0.6		
Ventral								
Anterior				1.5				
Medial				5.8				
Olfactory cortex					6.3			
Septum	1.3		3.7	3.6	4.5	0.4		11
Substantia nigra	0.8		5.9		11.9			14
Thalamus	3.0	2.8	3.0	8.4		0.14	0.53	
Lateral						0.54	0.5	
Medial						0.08		2.2
Lateral geniculate								
Brainstem	4.1				6.3			
Midbrain	1.5	1.9		2.4		0.65	0.66	
Dorsal raphe						0.4	0.61	87
Interpeduncular	5.0							
Quadrigeminal	1.7							
Pons	2.6	1.7						
Medulla				0.4				
Cerebellum								
Archi	0.3							
Neo	0.2							

[a]Numbers in parentheses are reference numbers.
[b]Macaca mulatta.
[c]M. mulatta, M. irus, Erythrocebus patas.
[d]Cercopithicus aethiops.
[e]Macaca fascicularis (this chapter).
[f]C. Clewans and E. C. Azmitia, unpublished observations; M. fascicularis.

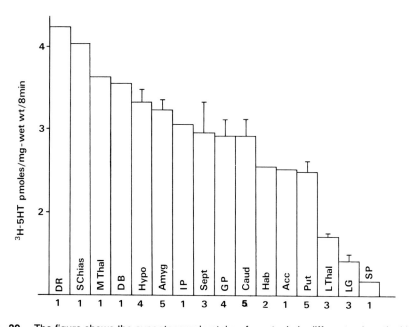

FIG. 39. The figure shows the synaptosomal uptake of serotonin in different subcortical brain regions of *M fascicularis*. *Abscissa*, number of animals sampled for each brain region (see List of Abbreviations Used in Illustrations). *Ordinate*, amount of specific uptake of serotonin (nonspecific was subtracted from total uptake) after incubating synaptosomal fractions in 5×10^{-8} M [^{3}H]5-HT for 8 min at 37°C. The bars at the top of each column are the standard deviations of the mean.

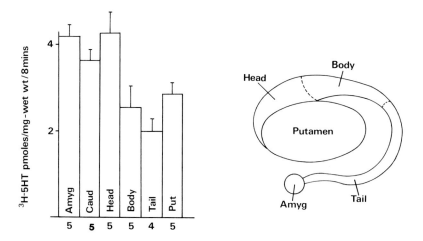

FIG. 40. Bar graph, as described in Fig. 39, shows the amount of synaptosomal uptake of serotonin in different parts of the caudate **(right)** as well as the putamen and amygdala. Note that the highest uptake in the caudate nucleus occurs in the head region. The tail is lowest although it is near the amygdala, which has very high levels of serotonin reuptake.

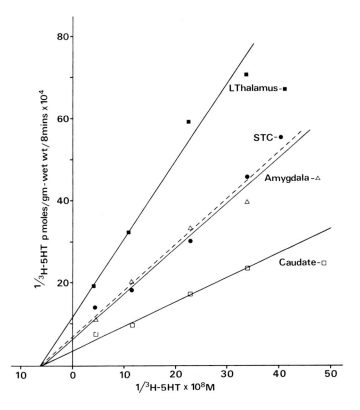

FIG. 41. Graphic analysis of the reciprocals of the [³H]5-HT molarity and the specific uptake into synaptosomes from caudate, amygdala, superior temporal cortex (STC), and the lateral thalamus of *M fascicularis*. Linear regression analysis give approximately a Km = 1.5 × 10⁻⁷ M for all brain regions, although the V_{max} values (Y-intercept) were different.

levels are comparable in humans and monkeys. The globus pallidus appears to have the greatest 5-HT turnover in the basal ganglion, probably due to high tryptophan hydroxylase levels. Marked variations are seen in nuclei of the hypothalamus, thalamus, and brainstem.

Light Microscopy

Radioautography

Serotonergic fibers were localized by tagging the high-affinity reuptake sites in brain slices from *M fascicularis*. The slices were incubated *in vitro* with [³H]5-HT at a concentration of 5 × 10⁻⁸ M for 12 min before fixation and processing for radioautography. A high density of the uptake sites is seen in the amygdala (Fig. 42a and b) and a low density is seen in the lateral geniculate body. In both subcortical areas, silver grain aggregates (SGA) are seen near neuronal soma. A

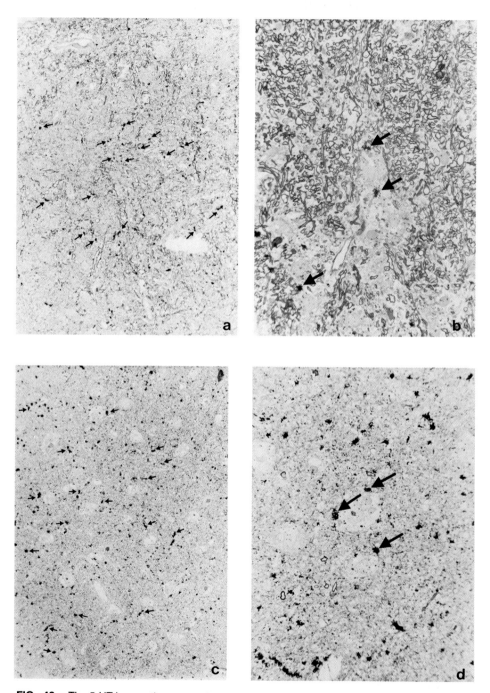

FIG. 42. The 5-HT innervation pattern in the lateral geniculate body **(a,b)** and amygdala **(c,d)** of *M fascicularis*. Photomicrographs of radioautographic-processed monkey brain 1 μm slices, using bright-field illumination. The [³H]5-HT concentrating fibers are seen as silver grain aggregates; their density is greater in the amygdala than in the lateral geniculate body. In both brain areas, the silver grain aggregates are seen in association with neuronal soma (*arrows* in high-power photomicrographs **b** and **d**). For ultrastructure of the amygdala, see Fig. 50**a**.

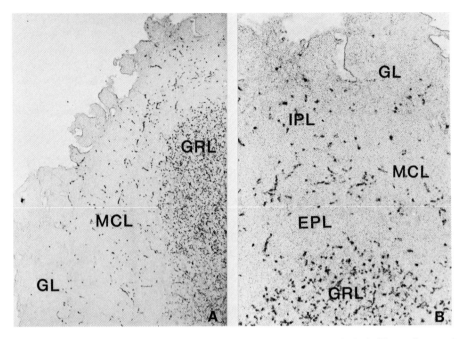

FIG. 43. The 5-HT innervation pattern in the olfactory bulb of *M fascicularis.* Photomicrographs of radioautographic-processed 10-μm slices, using bright-field illumination. The [³H]5-HT concentrating fibers are seen as silver grain aggregates, the density of which is highest in the granular layer and lowest in the glomerular layer. (See List of Abbreviations in Illustrations).

laminated labeling pattern is seen in the olfactory bulb (Fig. 43). Few SGA are visible in the glomerular region, whereas a large number of SGA are found in the granular region.

Studies of the primate brainstem have shown an extensive plexus of serotonergic axons forming a supra- and subependymal system in the walls of the ventricles, in the arachnoid sheath around major cerebral blood vessels, and in the pia over the spinal cord (27). These fibers were labeled by exogenously administered [³H]5-HT. Using the same method, the paratrigeminal nucleus was observed to receive a dense plexus of serotonergic fibers (29). A recent report relied on fluorescence histochemistry to demonstrate that NRO extended toward the hypoglossal nucleus and the dorsal motor nucleus of X (40).

The median eminence of monkeys was studied radioautographically in slices incubated *in vitro* with [³H]5-HT (24). Labeled fibers were seen in all layers but were most pronounced in the external zones. These fibers extended from the ependymal cells of the third ventricle to the external basement membrane.

Immunocytochemistry

Several studies have used immunocytochemical methods to study 5-HT fibers in the monkey. 5-HT–IR axons were seen in both regions of the substantia nigra of

M fascicularis, although mainly in the pars reticularis (47). In the neostriatum of the same species, 5-HT–IR fibers were particularly abundant in the ventromedial region of the caudate bordering the nucleus accumbens where the plexus was more dense (65). The number of fibers in the caudate was reduced in more dorsal and lateral areas. The fibers were uniformly distributed in the putamen. Fibers were fine and had irregularly spaced fusiform varicosities.

A comparative study in monkey, cat, and rat of the olfactory bulb was performed with a 5-HT antibody. Serotonergic fibers were seen in all layers except for the olfactory nerve layer in *Macaca fuscata* (77). The fibers were observed to form a chain of large varicosities in the periglomerular region. The 5-HT distribution was predominately in the internal plexiform layer. In some portions, a dense plexus of 5-HT fibers extended to the external plexiform layer. 5-HT–IR fibers were also numerous in the inner portions of the granular cell layer. A number of "stem fibers," thick axons with spindle-type varicosities, were arranged here. Finally, and in contrast to both rat and cat, the distribution of 5-HT–IR fibers was scant in the glomerular layer. In this area, only a few of the glomeruli (no more than 5%) possessed 5-HT–IR axons.

Ultrastructure of Subcortical Axons and Terminals

The first report of serotonergic axons in the primate subcortical regions was in the median eminence after *in vitro* incubation with [³H]5-HT (24). A large number of axonal varicosities were labeled, but they accounted for less than 1% of the total number of axonal profiles seen. These labeled axons had a range of 0.3 to 1.0 μm in diameter and contained both small clear vesicles and large dense-core vesicles. No synaptic contacts were seen, although close appositions to tanycytes were reported.

The [³H]5-HT–labeled axons in the supra- and subependymal system of the ventricles were also nonsynaptic (27). These axonal boutons contained large (70-nm), variable, dense synaptic vesicles and small (35-nm) vesicles. The supraependymal axons in the ventricles of the monkey brain did not form classical synaptic contacts, but specialized attachments were seen on the underlying ependymal cells.

However, other studies of serotonergic fibers in the primate subcortical regions have clearly shown classical synaptic contacts. The paratrigeminal nucleus of the rhesus monkey contains many axons that concentrate exogenously administered [³H]5-HT (27). Both unmyelinated and large myelinated (1–4 μm) axons were described. Seven types of morphologically distinct terminals were seen, four of which were synaptic. These terminals formed numerous axosomatic, axospinous, axodendritic, and possibly axoaxonal contacts with paratrigeminal neurons.

More recently, ultrastructural analysis of 5-HT–IR axons has been performed in the monkey striatum (65). The fibers were quite thin (0.1–0.5 μm) and unmyelinated. The 5-HT–IR was described as adhering "to membrane structures such as microtubules and outer mitochondrial surfaces. Most of the time, however, it appeared as round electron-dense particles, 15–35 nm in diameter filling the varicosities" (65, p. 284). Many profiles were seen to form axospinous synapses with strong asymmetric membrane specializations.

These examples of nonsynaptic and synaptic contacts from the primate subcortical regions serve to emphasize the heterogeneity of serotonergic axons. This characteristic is consistent with the observation in the rat that a single serotonergic neuron can innervate many different terminal regions (35). Thus, the types of endings that these expansive neurons make probably are determined by factors existing within the terminal fields themselves.

Cortical Distribution

Biochemistry

Humans

The serotonin distribution in the human cerebral cortex is not uniform (Table 4). The highest amounts of 5-HT are found in limbic structures such as the cingulate lobe, temporal lobe, and amygdaloid areas. High levels also are seen in the sensory cortex, such as in the visual calcarine cortex and the somatosensory area in the postcentral gyrus of the parietal lobe. Note that the motor precentral gyrus has half of the amount of 5-HT as seen in the sensory postcentral gyrus. The lowest levels are found in the frontal, parietal, and occipital lobes.

There are significant differences within a major cortical lobe. For instance, while most of the cortex in the occipital lobe has low levels, the calcarine cortex has very high levels. Likewise, the hippocampal gyrus of the temporal lobe was found to have 2.5 times the amount of serotonin as the hippocampus itself.

The distribution of 5-HIAA levels in human cortex is generally similar to that of 5-HT except that the differences between regions are less (Table 5). Note that the hippocampal gyrus is only slightly higher than the hippocampus. Furthermore, the marked differences within the major cortical subdivisions may explain why one group of investigators noted that 5-HIAA levels were twice as high in the temporal lobe than in frontal lobe (32), whereas another group found the exact opposite (78).

Monkeys

The monkey cortical serotonin system has been studied by measuring 5-HT, 5-HIAA, high-affinity uptake of [^{3}H]5-HT and the synthesis rate (Table 6). The 5-HT levels are similar in concentration and distribution to those found in human brain. There are fewer differences between regions, however. The highest levels are seen in amygdala, occipital cortex, hippocampus, and the superior and the inferior gyri of the temporal lobe. The lowest levels are seen in precentral (motor) cortex, prefrontal cortex, and postparietal cortex. Levels of 5-HIAA show the same pattern, with lowest levels seen in the superior and orbital gyri of the frontal lobe.

The distribution of 5-HT reuptake showed a greater interregional variation (Fig. 44). Highest levels are seen in amygdala, the rectus gyrus of the frontal lobe, and the inferior and superior gyri of the temporal lobe. The lowest levels are seen in the occipital lobe and the precentral (motor) cortex of the frontal lobe. Again, the

TABLE 4. 5-HT distribution in human cortex (nmol/g)

Region	Ref. 31	Ref. 17	Ref. 18	Ref. 58	Ref. 30	Ref. 19	Ref. 59	Ref. 51	Ref. 78	Ref. 54	Ref. 82	Ref. 25
Cingulate	0.214					0.16	1.32				0.107	0.320
Subcallosal gyrus	1.66											
Rostral												
Caudal												
Frontal												
Pole	0.107		0.214		0.6			0.294	4.07		0.053	
Convexity	0.075				0.5		0.487					
Orbital gyrus					0.5[a]		0.139					
Precentral gyrus (motor)		0.214					0.449					
Gray	0.251											
Occipital												
Pole	0.075		0.320		0.4		1.0		2.03			
Calcarine					0.6		0.556					
Parietal							0.936		1.23			
Postcentral gyrus (sensory)					0.65[a]		0.519		1.12	0.390		
Temporal												
Pole	0.182											
Hippocampal gyrus	0.882				1.1		1.04				1.07	
Hippocampus	0.471		0.588[b]	0.588				1.42		1.16	0.267	0.695
Rostral					0.9							
Caudal					0.9			1.07				
Dentate gyrus												
Uncus	1.18											
Amygdala	1.71			1.98	2.2		3.26	1.42				
Periamygdaloid cortex					1.4							

[a]Combined gray and white area.
[b]Includes olfactory bulb.

TABLE 5. *5-HIAA distribution in human cortex (nmol/g)*

Region	Ref. 54	Ref. 19	Ref. 59	Refs. 52, 53	Ref. 78	Ref. 54	Ref. 82	Ref. 25	Ref. 32
Cingulate			1.51				1.55	.61	
Frontal		0.71		0.59	2.76		0.72		0.87
Convexity			0.33						
Orbital gyrus			1.99						
Precentral gyrus (motor)			1.26						
Occipital					2.14				
Calcarine			1.75						
Parietal			0.59		1.28				
Postcentral (sensory)			1.63						
Temporal			0.6		1.33	1.18			1.62
Hippocampal gyrus			3.21						
Hippocampus	1.48	1.63		2.45		2.16	1.29	1.1	1.6
Dentate gyrus				1.47					
Amygdala	4.34		3.45	3.88					

differences within the major cortical lobes are very pronounced. The rectus gyrus of the frontal lobe has four times more uptake of [^{3}H]5-HT than the precentral motor cortex of the same lobe. In the occipital lobe, the calcarine region has double the uptake of the surrounding cortex. Finally, the variation within the hippocampal complex is striking. The entorhinal cortex and the dentate gyrus are high in uptake, whereas the subiculum and the cornu Ammonis (CA) are low (Fig. 45). Values obtained in a single baboon for subcortical and cortical structures are included for comparison with the results from *M fascicularis* (Fig. 46).

The synthesis rate of 5-HT in the monkey cortex (Table 6) is highest in the temporal lobe (hippocampus, inferior and superior temporal gyri) and in the sensory cortex (occipital cortex and postcentral cortex). Low levels of 5-HT synthesis are found in the frontal lobe [orbital, precentral (motor), premotor, and superior gyri].

These results emphasize the heterogeneous distribution of serotonergic fibers in the primate brain. Highest levels are associated with limbic centers (temporal lobe, amygdaloid nuclei and cingulate gyrus) and with sensory centers (visual-calcarine, auditory-superior temporal gyrus, somatosensory-postcentral cortex, olfaction-amygdaloid nuclei, and entorhinal cortex). The lowest levels are seen in the frontal lobe (with the exception of the rectus gyrus). The distribution is quite varied even within the subregions of the hippocampal complex. As a general rule, it may be proposed that serotonin levels are highest in those regions of cortex having more granule cells, since these cells are associated with sensory receiving areas and are most abundant in the dentate gyrus of the hippocampal complex.

Light Microscopy of Cerebral Cortex

Little is known of the serotonin distribution in the cerebral cortex of the rat (for review, see ref. 37). Chan-Palay (28) reported highest density of 5-HT fibers after intraventricular administration of [^{3}H]5-HT in the cingulate cortex, whereas other parts contain only low densities. Beaudet and Descarries (15), using radioautog-

TABLE 6. *5-HT, 5-HIAA, and 5-HT reuptake and synthesis in monkey cortex (nmol/g)*

Region	5-HT					5-HIAA				5-HT reuptake	Synthesis (hr)		
	1 (68)[a,b]	2 (79)[b]	3 (22)	4 (73)[b]	5 (46)[b]	6 (22)[b]	7 (14)[c]	8 (73)[b]	9 (32)	10	11 (22)[b]	12 (46)[b]	13[e]
Cingulate													
Anterior		0.5					2.1			0.15			3
Posterior										0.18			2.3
Frontal													
Orbital			0.6			0.8		3.7		0.2	0.21		1.1
Pole													
Precental (motor)			0.5		0.6	1.1				0.15	0.20		1.0
Prefrontal					0.7					0.10			
Premotor			0.45		0.6	1.0					0.21		
Rectus										0.41			
Superior (dorsolateral)			0.4			0.7				0.17	0.21		1.7
Occipital			0.6		0.9	1.3				0.10	0.37		1.1
Calcarine (visual)							0.9			0.22			1.3
Parietal													
Postcentral (sensory)			0.7		0.6	1.1				0.18	0.35		
Postparietal			0.4		0.8	1.2					0.34		1.5
Temporal													
Entorhinal												0.35	
Hippocampus	1.6f	0.75f	0.5		0.6	1.6				0.36	0.4		1.4
Cornu Ammonis										0.2			1.3
Dentate gyrus										0.1			1.3
Subiculum										0.3			2.0
										0.17			1.1
Amygdala	1.6f	0.75f	1.4	0.5		3.0	4.8			0.45	1.1		1.7
Inferior													
Anterior			0.8		1.1	1.7				0.37	0.35		
Posterior			0.4		0.7	1.3					0.30		
Pole	1.2												
Superior (Auditory)			0.8		1.1	1.8				0.34	0.46		1.1

[a] Numbers in parentheses are reference numbers.
[b] *M. mulatta.*
[c] *C. aethiops.*
[d] *M. fascicularis (this chapter).*
[e] C. Clewans and E. C Azmitia, unpublished observations; *M. fascicularis.*
[f] Combined for assay.

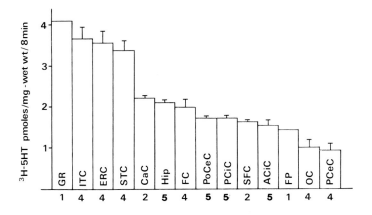

FIG. 44. Synaptosomal specific uptake of serotonin in different cortical brain regions of *M fascicularis. Abscissa,* number of animals sampled for each brain region (see List of Abbreviations Used in Illustrations). *Ordinate,* the amount of specific uptake of serotonin after incubating synaptosomal fractions in 5×10^{-8} M [^{3}H]5-HT for 8 min at 37°C. The bars at the top of each column are the standard deviations of the mean.

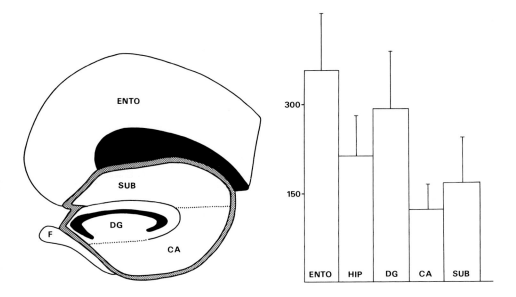

FIG. 45. Bar graph, as described in Fig. 44, shows the amount of synaptosomal uptake of serotonin (pmol/g wet wt.) in different parts of the hippocampal formation and entorhinal cortex **(left).** Note that the highest uptake in the monkey hippocampal formation occurs in the dentate gyrus (DG). The cornu Ammonis (CA) and the subiculum (SUB) have lower levels although they are continuous with the entorhinal cortex (ENTO), which has the highest levels.

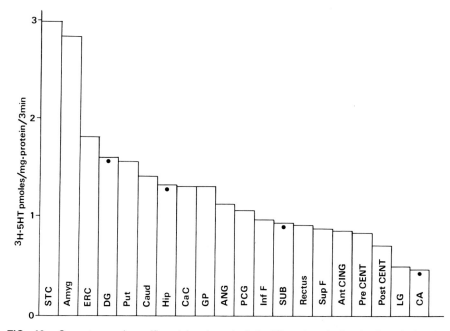

FIG. 46. Synaptosomal specific uptake of serotonin in different cortical and subcortical regions of a baboon; (●) regions within hippocampus. The specific brain region sampled is marked in each column (see List of Abbreviations Used in Illustrations); *ordinate*, as described in Fig. 44.

raphy with [³H]5-HT reported that the intralaminar density increased progressively from layer V to layer I.

The anatomy of 5-HT fibers in the cerebral cortex of primates was first studied by Nelson et al. (62). These workers used radioautography after subdural injections of [³H]5-HT and fluorescence histochemistry after incubation with 6-HT for light-microscopic analysis of postarcuate cortex (polysensory) in the squirrel monkey. They concluded that "no laminar distribution was observed" and "labeled fibers ran in all directions and the varicosities were not confined to any particular area of cortex" (p. 125).

Our results showed a clear laminar pattern in several layers of cerebral cortex. Slices were prepared from entorhinal, superior temporal, precentral, postcentral, frontal, and calcarine cortex. Radioautography was performed after *in vitro* incubation with 5×10^{-8} M [³H]5-HT for 20 min. In all regions examined, a clear lamination was observed with the highest densities in layers I and IV (Fig. 47). The density in layer IV was unexpected and suggests a preferential innervation of granule cells by 5-HT fibers (11).

Further studies were performed in slices from the hippocampal formation. The results showed that the granule cells of the dentate gyrus were very heavily innervated (Fig. 48), whereas the innervation of the CA was much weaker (Fig. 49). It is interesting that the pattern seen in the monkey dentate gyrus is similar to that observed in the rat, while the density in monkey CA is much less (Figs. 48 and

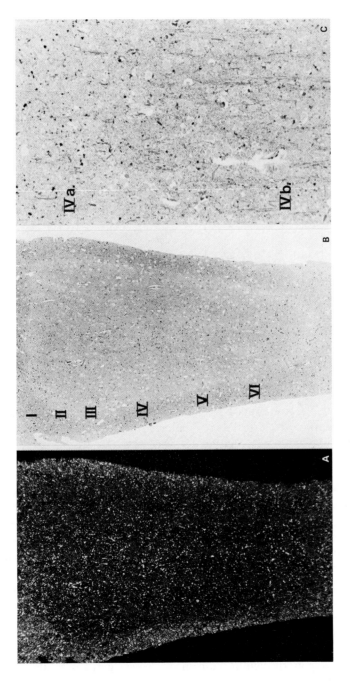

FIG. 47. The 5-HT innervation pattern in the cerebral cortex of *M fascicularis*. Dark- **(A)** and bright-field **(B)** illumination photomicrographs of radioautographic processed 1-μm coronal slice from entorhinal cortex. The [³H]5-HT concentrating fibers are seen as silver grain aggregates, the density of which is highest in layers I and IV. **(C):** Bright-field illumination high-power photomicrographs of radioautographic-processed 1-μm coronal slice from calcarine cortex. The silver grain aggregates are most abundant in layer IVa.

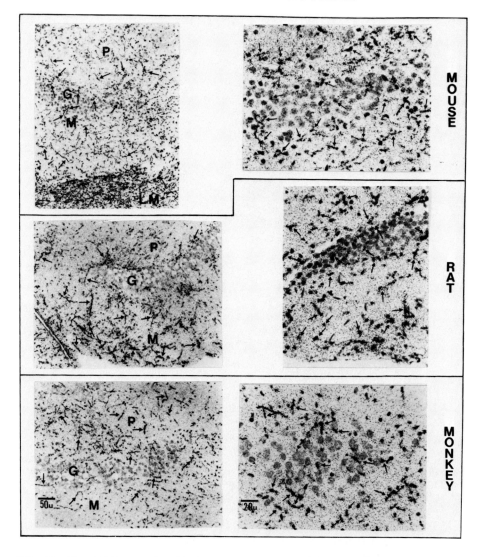

FIG. 48. The 5-HT innervation density in the dentate gyrus (M, molecular layer; G, granular layer; P, polymorphic layer) of mouse, rat, and monkey *(M fascicularis)*. Bright-field illumination photomicrographs of radioautographic-processed 5-μm coronal section. The [³H]5-HT concentrating fibers seen as silver grain aggregates in all layers, and no species difference in density of innervation is apparent. (From Azmitia, ref. 4, Plate 3, with permission.)

49). This difference between rat and monkey may represent an increased specialization in the primate brain.

An innervation of layer IV also has been reported using the immunohistochemical technique. Morrison et al. (61) found in the squirrel monkey primary visual cortex a very dense serotonergic projection in layer IV. These workers conclude that the

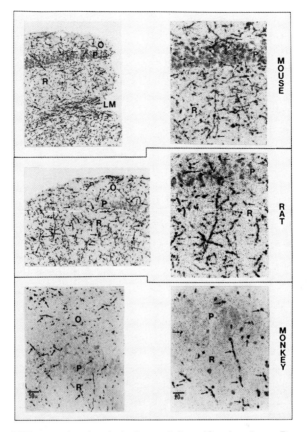

FIG. 49. The 5-HT innervation density in Ammon's horn (O, oriens layer; P, pyramidal layer; R, radiatum layer; LM, lacunosum-moleculare layer) of mouse, rat, and monkey *(M fascicularis).* See Fig. 48 for particulars. The silver grain aggregates are seen in all layers but are most dense in LM. Note that the monkey Ammon's horn has fewer silver grain aggregates than rat or mouse; those seen were often in close apposition to pyramidal soma and dendrites. From Azmitia, ref. 4, Plate 2, with permission.)

5-HT projection is in a position to modulate neuronal activity at the initial stage of signal processing in cortex. Layer IV cells are closely linked to the thalamic input" (p. 2405). Our finding that 5-HT fibers heavily innervate layer IV in a number of cortical areas, that the innervation of dentate gyrus remains constant from rat to monkey, and that 5-HT reuptake is highest in those region of cortex having a significant layer IV (e.g., sensory cortex) indicate a special relationship between serotonergic fibers and granule cells.

Ultrastructure of Terminals in Cerebral Cortex

Electron-microscopic radioautography was performed on slices of amygdala and cerebral cortex incubated *in vitro* with 5×10^{-8} M [³H]5-HT. Axonal profiles contained small clear vesicles with occasional large dense-core vesicles. In certain cases, these endings could be seen to arise from "en passant" fibers as is seen in the amygdala (Fig. 50a). A large number of asymmetrical synapses also were seen in layer IV of the cerebral cortex (Fig. 50b and c). The endings were mainly on dendritic processes. Sometimes the same dendrite received a [^{3}H]5-HT–labeled synapse and an unlabeled synapse side by side (Fig. 50b). These findings suggest that the serotonergic projection to layer IV of the cerebral cortex forms classical type-2 synaptic patterns. This result and the previously mentioned observation that serotonergic fibers are myelinated, support our hypothesis of a precise, specialized, and rapid action of serotonin in modulating cerebral cortical activity.

CONCLUSIONS

The serotonergic system in the primate brain appears to have remained remarkably stable throughout evolution (summarized in Fig. 51). The main cellular nuclei located in the brainstem first described in the rat are still present in the monkey and human brain. It has been concluded that "the pattern of organization of the three recognized aminergic systems of the brain have been preserved with remarkable consistency in the evolution of primates" (49, p. 413).

This evolutionary stability also is applicable to the main descending and ascending projections. The three descending projection nuclei (NRO, NRPa, and NRM) are still believed to innervate the substantia gelatinosa of the dorsal horn and the motor neurons of the ventral horn of the spinal cord. The ascending nuclei (NCS, NRD, and NPSL) use multiple ascending tracts to innervate most of the subcortical and cortical areas of the forebrain with a distribution pattern highly consistent with that reported in the rat. Although there has been considerable controversy, some of the minor and unusual groups seen in the rat were present in our monkey material. The B$_4$ group has not been described in any primate brain previously, yet a number of neurons were seen as part of the NRV. Furthermore, the small serotonin cells noted in the area postrema by Dahlstrom and Fuxe (33) were also seen in the pretreated primate brain.

Finally, the termination patterns seen in the spinal cord, cerebellum, median eminence, paratrigeminal nucleus, olfactory bulb, hippocampus, and cortex are largely similar to those described in subprimates. The serotonergic fibers enter the various target structures through similar pathways and appear to innervate the appropriate neurons. For instance, the labeling patterns seen in the dentate gyrus of monkey are almost indistinguishable from that seen in the rodent (4). The numerous types of morphologically distinct serotonergic terminals seen in the cerebellum and paratrigeminal nuclei were identified in both rat and monkey (27,29).

Thus, the similarities between the primate and subprimate serotonergic systems are apparent in nuclear organization, major efferent pathways, target structures, and ultrastructural relationships. Thus, it would appear that anatomical and physiological studies performed in subprimates would have direct bearing on our ap-

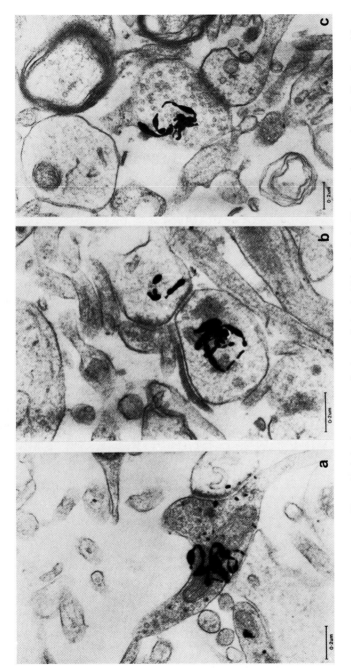

FIG. 50. Ultrastructure of 5-HT terminals in three areas of telencephalon in *M fascicularis*. Electron micrographs of radioautographic-processed brain slices after *in vitro* incubation with 5×10^{-8} M [³H]5-HT. **a:** Labeled fiber making en passant synapse on dendrite in the amygdaloid area. Small clear and dense-core vesicles are visible. Synapse has an asymmetrical density. **b:** Labeled fiber with weak asymmetrical density making a synapse on dendrite in layer IV of entorhinal cortex. The dendrite receives a second, unlabeled axon and forms a strong asymmetrical density with it. **c:** Labeled fiber making an axodendritic asymmetrical synapse in layer IV of postcentral cortex. No dense-core vesicles seen in axon.

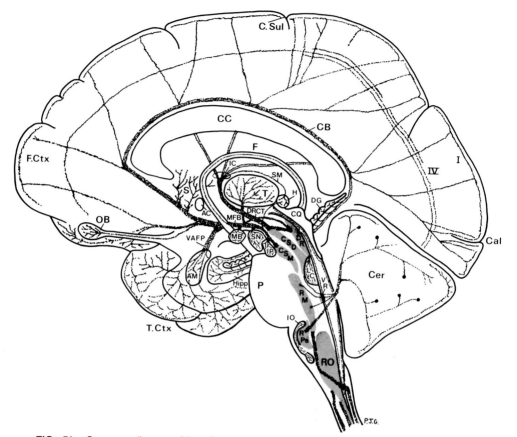

FIG. 51. Summary diagram of the primate serotonergic system. *Shading*, main nuclei; *(---)*, fiber pathways. (See List of Abbreviations Used in Illustrations.)

preciation of the primate serotonergic neurons. However, and not surprisingly, this concept of an evolutionary stable system does not appear justified when all the comparative evidence is closely scrutinized.

The nuclear organization in the primate brain does differ from that of rodents in several important aspects. First, in the rat brain, the majority of the serotonergic nuclear groups are indeed raphe nuclei; that is, the cells lie on the midline seam and extend laterally from this line. In the primate, few cells lie on the midline, and most have at best a paramedian organization. "It appears the serotonin system undergoes a "lateralization" as the phylogenetic scale is traversed towards primates" (75, p. 362). Second, the NCS is more extensive in the monkey. The inclusion of the dorsalis portion of this nucleus as proposed by Olszewski and Baxter (64) would make this the major ascending group rather than the NRD as proposed for the rat. Third, the serotonergic cells from NRO extend far more caudally in the primate brain to reach the cervical levels of the spinal cord. The location of these cells in lamina X and IX may indicate a more important relationship between serotonergic cells and motoneurons in the primate brain. Finally, the hypothalamic serotonin-concentrating cells described by several groups in the rat (15,33,41) were not seen in the primate hypothalamus.

Important differences also have been noted in the projection pathways. The descending fibers to the ventral-horn motoneurons in the rat originate from NRM and NRPa but appear to originate only from NRM in the primate (21). The ascending fibers to the forebrain in the rat use mainly the MFB (2), but in the monkey, the DRCT may be quantitatively larger (10). Finally, the fibers in the primate brain have been noted by several workers to be myelinated (8–10,27,56). Although myelinated serotonin fibers have been noted in rodents (69), we have found the occurrence in the rat (0.7%) to be much lower than in the monkey (25%) (10).

The termination pattern in certain areas also is different between primates and subprimates. We have reported that the innervation density of the CA region of the primate is markedly less than in the rat and mouse, although the innervation of the dentate gyrus is similar (4). The pattern of 5-HT–IR fibers in the olfactory bulb of the monkey also is different from that of the rat or cat (77). Takeuchi et al. (77) reported an almost total absence of serotonergic fibers innervating the glomeruli in the monkey, in sharp contrast to subprimates. Biochemical studies have revealed marked variations in the cortical distribution of the serotonin system (Tables 4–6), whereas studies in the rodent indicated a more uniform distribution (37). In the study by Schofield and Everitt (72), the amount of serotonin in the suprachiasmatic nuclei and the median eminence of rhesus monkeys was found to be low compared to other hypothalamic nuclei. This is in sharp contrast to the findings in the rat (and our results, Fig. 39), where those nuclei contain very high levels of serotonin (70). Schofield and Everitt (72) state that "these differences may reflect variations in the control of neuroendocrine events between these two species" (p. 369).

In summary, it can be stated that although the primate and subprimate serotonergic systems have many similarities, there are important differences in cellular organization, projecting pathways, and innervation patterns. The studies on the rodent serotonergic system led to the conclusion that the axons, being fine and unmyelinated, possess a slow rate of conduction and have a scarcity of postsynaptic membrane specialization, and are thus not a part of the "hard wiring" involved in the rapid stimulus–response organization of the brain (2). This view must be modified in light of the studies performed on the primate brain. It is likely that a number of concepts regarding serotonergic functions will be retained. It remains a very expansive chemical network, a part of the reticular formation, and closely integrated with nonneuronal elements of the brain. However, it appears that this primitive system has evolved certain properties in the primate to adapt to the enlargement of the cerebral cortex and the corresponding changes in the regulation of sensory, motor, endocrine, and cognitive processes.

The links between subprimate and primate research in the functioning of brain serotonin are being established with anatomy, biochemistry, and continued progress in the physiology of the system. The cost and ethics of using primates for this research cannot be taken lightly, but it appears that much additional work is required in primates to develop the basic scientific information required for clinical experimentation.

SUMMARY

This chapter has reviewed biochemical and morphological studies of the human and monkey serotonergic system. In addition, the serotonin-producing neurons of *M fascicularis* were analyzed, using immunocytochemistry, radioautography, and measurements of synaptosomal serotonin reuptake and supernatant tryptophan hydroxylase activity. The major sections of the chapter covered cell bodies, pathways, subcortical distribution, and cortical distribution, and a gross brain dissection guide of *M fascicularis* is included.

An atlas of the 5-HT–IR cell bodies was presented in Figures 7 to 33. Rostral and caudal groups of nuclei were discussed. The rostral group consists principally of the nuclei raphe dorsalis (B_7 and B_6), centralis superior (B_8, B_5, and part of B_7), and prosupralemniscus (B_9). These groups ascend mainly in tracts lying outside the medial forebrain bundle (MFB). In *M fascicularis*, 25% of the fibers within the MFB are myelinated.

The caudal 5-HT–IR nuclei consist principally of the nuclei in a dorsal cluster (raphe obscurus, B_2) and in a ventral cluster (pallidus, B_1, and magnus, B_3). The dorsal 5-HT–IR cells in raphe obscurus are associated with the MLF, and cells extend into cervical spinal cord (lamina IX and X) with the descending MLF and the TTS. Fibers from the raphe obscurus innervate the motoneurons in both the cranial nuclei (X, XII) and the ventral horn. The ventral 5-HT–IR cells lie mainly medial to the medial leminiscal fibers. A large number of these cells extend laterally into paragigantocellularis lateralis and here extend caudally lying below the lateral reticular nuclei. Cells from this group are seen dorsally joining the internal arcuate fibers. The raphe magnus of the ventral cluster projects to the dorsal horn and is believed to mediate the serotonin-induced analgesia. The descending fibers from both of these clusters are occasionally myelinated. Also, in our tryptophan- and pargyline-pretreated monkeys, small 5 HT–IR cells were visible in the area postrema.

Human and monkey biochemical data (detailed summary in Tables 1–6) provide evidence for the presence of serotonin fibers in all cortical and subcortical regions. In subcortical regions, the midbrain, medulla, amygdala, and substantia nigra have the highest, whereas the cerebellum, spinal cord, and ventral pons have the lowest amount of serotonin and its metabolite, 5-HIAA. In the basal ganglion, the globus pallidus has the highest rate of 5-HT synthesis.

The temporal lobe receives the most serotonin of the major cortical lobes. The cortical regions with a larger granular layer have a denser serotonergic innervation, with highest levels in sensory and limbic cortices. In the hippocampal complex, the dentate gyrus has the most [^{3}H]5-HT high-affinity uptake, with levels comparable to those found in the entorhinal cortex.

Radioautography of the high-affinity uptake sites of [^{3}H]5-HT was performed in slices from *M fascicularis*. The innervation pattern is very dense in the amygdala and low in the lateral geniculate body. The distribution in the olfactory bulb is laminated, with the highest density in the granular layer and lowest in the glomerular layer. The innervation in the cortex was highest in layers IV and I. Ultrastructural studies showed synaptic profiles in cortical layer IV of *M fascicularis*.

This chapter has presented many examples of differences in the serotonergic system between primates and subprimates. The primate system has unique properties in nuclear organization (e.g., 5-HT–IR cells in spinal cord), projection pathways (e.g., major ascending pathway running dorsal to MFB), axon morphology (e.g., significant number of myelinated fibers) and termination pattern (e.g., few fibers in Ammon's horn within the hippocampus). Thus, although the basic infrastructure of an expansive CNS serotonergic system is similar in all vertebrates, the primate brain appears to have evolved special characteristics.

ACKNOWLEDGMENTS

The research for this chapter was supported by the National Science Foundation with a grant from the Behavioral Neuroscience Program 83-04704. The salary of Efrain Azmitia was partially paid by a Career Scientist Award from the Irma Hirschl Trust while the author was in the Department of Anatomy at Mount Sinai School of Medicine. The authors are thankful to Dr. Carol Clewans for her work with tryptophan hydroxylase and to Vernell Daniels for her technical assistance. A special acknowledgment is extended to Dr. Patricia Whitaker for her support and help in the preparation of the manuscript.

LIST OF ABBREVIATIONS USED IN ILLUSTRATIONS

AC	Anterior commissure	CQ	Corpus quadrigimini
ACC	Accumbens	CS	Cortical spinal tract
ACiC	Anterior cingulate cortex	CSD	Cortical spinal decussation
AH	Anterior horn	CSd	Centralis superior nucleus, pars dorsalis
AIP	Ascending indoleamine pathways	CSL	Centralis superior nucleus, pars lateralis
Amyg	Amygdaloid nuclei	CSm	Centralis superior nucleus, pars medialis
ANG	Angular gyrus	Csul	Central sulcus
B	Body	DB	Diagonal band
B$_1$–B$_9$	Serotonergic nuclei of Dahlstrom and Fuxe (33)	DG	Dentate gyrus
		DPY	Decussation of pyramidal tract
BC	Brachium conjunction	DR	Dorsal raphe nucleus; dorsal raphe (Fig. 39)
CA	Cornu Ammonis (hippocampus)	DRCT	Dorsal raphe cortical tract
CaC	Calcarine cortex	DRFT	Dorsal raphe forebrain tract
Caud	Caudate nucleus	DRL	Dorsal raphe nucleus, pars lateralis
cc	Central canal (Figs. 30,33)	DRm	Dorsal raphe nucleus, pars medialis
CC	Crus cerebri (Fig. 36) corpus callosum (Fig. 51)	Ento	Entorhinal cortex (Fig. 46)
		EPL	External plexiform layer (olfactory bulb)
CG	Central gray	ERC	Entorhinal cortex

F	Fornix	NST V	Nucleus of spinal tract of V
FC	Frontal cortex	N III	Oculomotor nuclei
FP	Frontal pole	N V	Nucleus trigeminal
FR	Fasciculus retroflexus	N VII	Nucleus facial
G	Granular layer (hippocampus)	N X	Nucleus vagus
GP	Globus pallidus	N XII	Nucleus hypoglossal
GL	Glomerular layer (olfactory bulb)	n III	Oculomotor nerve
GR	Rectus gyrus	n VI	Abducens nerve
GRL	Granular layer (olfactory bulb)	n VII	Facial nerve
Hab	Habenula nucleus	n XII	Hypoglossal nerve
Hip	Hippocampus	O	Oriens layer (hippocampus)
IAF	Internal arcuate fibers	OC	Occipital cortex; optic chiasm (Fig. 2)
IC	Internal capsule	P	Pons, pyramidal layer (hippocampus)
Inf	Inferior		(Figs. 49 and 50)
InfF	Inferior frontal cortex	PC	Posterior column
IO	Inferior olivary nuclei	PCeC	Precentral cortex
IP	Interpeduncular	PCG	Posterior cingulate gyrus
IPL	Internal plexiform layer (olfactory bulb)	PCiC	Posterior cingulate cortex
IR	Immunoreactivity	POA	Preoptic area
ITC	Inferior temporal cortex	PoCeC	Postcentral cortex
Lat	Lateral	Pro SL	Nucleus prosupralemniscus
LC	Locus ceruleus	Put	Putamen
LD	Lateral dorsal	PY	Pyramidal tract (PYR in Fig. 2)
LF	Lenticular fasciculus	R	Radiatum layer (hippocampus)
LM	Lateromedial	RER	Rough endoplasmic reticulum
LRN	Lateral reticular nucleus	RF	Reticular formation
LThal	Lateral thalamus	RM	Raphe magnus
LV	Lateroventral	RM-ST	Raphe magnus–spinal tract
M	Medial	RMT	Raphe medial tract
MB	Mammillary body	RO	Raphe obscurus
MCL	Mitral cell layer (olfactory bulb)	RO-ST	Raphe obscurus spinal tract
MD	Mediodorsal	RPa	Raphe pallidus
MFB	Medial forebrain bundle	SC, S. Chiasm	Suprachiasmatic nucleus
ML	Medial lemniscus		
MLF	Medial longitudinal fasciculus	Sept	Septum
MR	Median raphe nucleus	SG	Substantia gelatinosa
MRFT	Median raphe forebrain tract	SM	Stria medullaris
MT	Mammillothalamic tract	SN	Substantia nigra
M Thal	Medial thalamus	SP	Septum pellucidum
MV	Medioventral	STC	Superior temporal cortex
NC	Nucleus cuneatus	Sub	Subicular cortex
NCS	Nucleus centralis superior	Sup	Superior
NGR	Nucleus gracilis	T	Trapezoid body
NPGL	Nucleus paragigantocellularis lateralis	TCtx	Temporal cortex
NPP	Nucleus prepositus	TSO	Tractus spino-olivaris
NRD	Nucleus raphe dorsalis	TST	Tractus spinothalamicus
NRM	Nucleus raphe magnus	TTS	Tractus tectospinalis
NRO	Nucleus raphe obscurus	vcgl	Ventrolateral geniculate body
NRPa	Nucleus raphe pallidus	V me	Mesencephalic nucleus of trigeminal
NRPG	Nucleus reticularis paragigantocellularis	VR	Raphe ventriculus
NRPO	Nucleus reticularis pontis oralis	5HIAA	5-Hydroxyindoleacetic acid
NRPo	Nucleus raphe pontis	5HT	5-Hydroxytryptamine (serotonin)

REFERENCES

1. Andrezik JA, Chan-Palay V, Palay SL. The nucleus paragigantocellularis lateralis in the rat. *Anat Embryol (Berl)* 1981;151:355–71.
2. Azmitia EC. The serotonin-producing neurons of the midbrain median and dorsal raphe nuclei. In: Iversen LL, Iversen SD, Snyder SH, eds. Handbook of Psychopharmacology; vol. 9. New York: Plenum Press, 1978:233–314.
3. Azmitia EC. Bilateral serotonergic projections to the dorsal hippocampus of the rat: simultaneous localization of retrograde transported ^{3}H-5HT and HRP. *J Comp Neurol* 1981;203:737–43.
4. Azmitia EC. The visualization and characterization of 5-HT reuptake sites in the rodent and primate hippocampus. A preliminary report. *J Physiol (Paris)* 1981;77:175–82.
5. Azmitia EC. (1982): Recent advances in serotonin methods. *J Histochem Cytochem* 1982;30(8).
6. Azmitia EC, Brennan MJ, Quartermain D. Adult development of the hippocampal serotonin system of C57BL/6N mice; analysis of high-affinity uptake of ^{3}H-5HT. *Int J Neurochem* 1983;5:39–44.
7. Azmitia EC, Gannon PJ. Visualization and characterization of serotonergic perikarya and hippocampal terminal fibers by specific reuptake and retrograde transport of ^{3}H-5HT. *Soc Neurosci Abst* 1980;6:352.
8. Azmitia EC, Gannon PJ. Immuno-reactive myelinated 5-HT axons in the medial forebrain bundle of monkey and rat. *Soc Neurosci Abst* 1982;8:134.
9. Azmitia EC, Gannon PJ. A light and electron microscopic analysis of the selective retrograde transport of ^{3}H-5HT by serotonergic neurons. *J Histochem Cytochem* 1982;30:799–804.
10. Azmitia EC, Gannon PJ. The ultrastructural localization of serotonin immunoreactivity in myelinated and unmyelinated axons within the medial forebrain bundle of rat and monkey. *J Neurosci* 1983;3:2083–90.
11. Azmitia EC, Gannon PJ, Clewans C. The cortical localization and characterization of serotonergic fibers in the primate brain. *Soc Neurosci Abst* 1981;7:790.
12. Azmitia EC, Marovitz WF. In vitro hippocampal uptake of tritiated serotonin (^{3}H-5HT); a morphological, biochemical and pharmacological approach to specificity. *J Histochem Cytochem* 1980;28:636–44.
13. Azmitia EC, Segal M. An autoradiographic analysis of the differential ascending projections of the dorsal and median raphe nuclei in the rat. *J Comp Neurol* 1978;179:641–59.
14. Bacopoulos NG, Redmond DE, Roth RH. Serotonin and dopamine metabolites in brain regions and cerebral spinal fluid of a primate species: effects of ketamine and fluphenazine. *J Neurochem* 1979;32:1215–18.
15. Beaudet A, Descarries L. Quantitative data on serotonin nerve terminals in adult rat neocortex. *Brain Res* 1976;111:301–9.
16. Beaudet A, Descarries L. Radioautographic characterization of a serotonin-accumulating nerve cell group in the adult rat hypothalamus. *Brain Res* 1979;160:231–43.
17. Bernheimer H, Birkmayer W, Hornykiewicz O. Verteilung des 5-hydroxytryptamine (serotonin) in Gehirn des Menschen und sein Verhalten bei Patienten mit Parkinson-Syndrom. *Klin Wochenschr* 1961;39:1056.
18. Bertler A. Occurrence and localization of catecholamines in the human brain. *Acta Physiol Scand* 1961;51:97–107.
19. Beskow J, Gottfries CG, Roos BE, Winblad B. Determination of monoamine and monoamine metabolites in the human brain: post mortem studies in a group of suicides and in a control group. *Acta Psychiatr Scand* 1976;53:7–20.
20. Bowden DM, German DC, Poynter WD. An autoradiographic, semistereotaxic mapping of major projections from locus coeruleus and adjacent nuclei in *Macaca mulatta*. *Brain Res* 1978;145:257–76.
21. Bowker RM, Westlund KN, Coulter JD. Origins of serotonergic projections to the lumbar spinal cord in the monkey using a combined retrograde transport and immunocytochemical technique. *Brain Res Bull* 1982;9:271–8.
22. Brown RM, Crane AM, Goldman PS. Regional distribution of monoamines in the cerebral cortex and subcortical structures of the rhesus monkey: concentrations and in vivo synthesis rates. *Brain Res* 1979;168:133–50.
23. Cajal SR. Histologie du systeme nerveux de l'homme et des vertebres; vol. 1. Paris: A. Maloine, 1909:913.

24. Calas A, Alonso G, Arnauld E, Vincent JD. Demonstration of indolaminergic fibers in the median eminence of the duck, rat and monkey. *Nature* 1974;250:241–3.
25. Carlsson A, Adolfsson R, Aquilonius SM, Gottfries CG, Oreland L, Svennerholm L, Winblad B. Biogenic amines in human brain in normal aging, senile dementia, and chronic alcoholism. In: Goldstein M et al., eds. Ergot compounds and brain function: neuroendocrine and neuropsychiatric aspects. New York: Raven Press, 1980:295–304.
26. Chan-Palay V. Fine structure of labelled axons in the cerebellar cortex and nuclei of rodents and primates after intraventricular infusions with tritiated serotonin. *Anat Embryol* 1975;148:235–65.
27. Chan-Palay V. Serotonin axons in the supra- and subependymal plexuses and in the leptomeninges: their roles in local alterations of cerebrospinal fluid and vasomotor activity. *Brain Res* 1976;102:103–30.
28. Chan-Palay V. Morphological correlates for transmitter synthesis, transport, release, uptake and catabolism: a study of serotonin neurons in the nucleus paragigantocellularis lateralis. In: Amino acids as chemical transmitter, NATO Advanced Study Symposium. New York: Plenum Press, 1978:1–30.
29. Chan-Palay V. The paratrigeminal nucleus. II. Identification and interrelations of catecholamine axons, indoleamine axons, and substance P immunoreactive cells in the neuropil. *J Neurocytol* 1978;7:419–42.
30. Cochran E, Robins E, Grote S. Regional serotonin levels in brain: a comparison of depressive suicides and alcoholic suicides with controls. *Biol Psychol* 1976;11:283–94.
31. Costa E, Aprison MH. Studies on the 5-hydroxytryptamine (serotonin) content in human brain. *J Nerv Ment Dis* 1958;126:289–93.
32. Cross AJ, Joseph MH. The concurrent estimation of the major monoamine metabolites in human and non-human primate brain by HPLC with fluorescence and electrochemical detection. *Life Sci* 1981;28:499–505.
33. Dahlstrom A, Fuxe K. Evidence for the existence of monoamine-containing neurons in the central nervous system. I. Demonstration of monoamines in the cell bodies of brainstem neurons. *Acta Physiol Scand* 1964;232(Suppl. 62):1–55.
34. de Lanerolle NC, Kapadia S, La Motte C. Serotonin and the ultrastructural organization of the raphe nuclei in the monkey: an immunohistochemical study. *Soc Neurosci Abst* 1981;7:791.
35. De Olmos J, Heimer L. Double and triple labeling of neurons with fluorescent substances: the study of collateral pathways in the ascending raphe system. *Neurosci Lett* 1980;19:7–12.
36. Descarries L, Watkins KC, Garcia S, Beaudet A. The serotonin neurons in nucleus raphe dorsalis of adult rat: a light and electron microscope radioautographic study. *J Comp Neurol* 1982;207:239–54.
37. Emson PC, Lindvall O. Distribution of putative neurotransmitters in the neocortex. *Neuroscience* 1979;4:1–30.
38. Fahn S, Libsch LR, Cutler RW. Monoamines in the human neostriatum: topographic distribution in normals and in Parkinson's disease and their role in akinesia, rigidity, chorea and tremor. *J Neurol Sci* 1971;14:427–55.
39. Felten DL, Laties AM, Carpenter MB. Monoamine-containing cell bodies in the squirrel monkey brain. *Am J Anat* 1974;139:153–66.
40. Felton DL, Sladek JR. Monoamine distribution in primate brain. V. Monoaminergic nuclei: anatomy, pathways and local organization. *Brain Res Bull* 1983;10:171–284.
41. Frankfurt M, Azmitia EC. The effect of intracerebral injections of 5,7-dihydroxytryptamine and 6-hydroxydopamine on the serotonin immunoreactive cell bodies and fibers in the adult rat hypothalamus. *Brain Res* 1983;261:91–9.
42. Garner DL, Sladek JR. Monoamine distribution in primitive brain. 1. Catecholamine-containing perikarya in the brain stem of *Macaca speciosa. J Comp Neurol* 1975;159:289–304.
43. German DC, Bowden DM. Locus ceruleus in rhesus monkey *(Macaca mulatta)*: a combined histochemical fluorescence, nissl and silver study. *J Comp Neurol* 1975;161:19–30.
44. Giesler GJ, Gerhart KD, Yezierski RP, Wilcox TK, Willis WD. Postsynaptic inhibition of primate spinothalamic neurons by stimulation in nucleus raphe magnus. *Brain Res* 1981;204:184–8.
45. Gilmore DP, Wilson CA. Indoleamine and catecholamine concentrations in the mid-term human fetal brain. *Brain Res Bull* 1983;10:395–8.
46. Goldman-Rakic PS, Brown RM. Regional changes of monoamines in cerebral cortex and subcortical structures of aging rhesus monkeys. *Neuroscience* 1981;6:177–87.

47. Holstein G, Pasik T, Pasik P. Light and electron microscopic identification of immunocytochemically labeled serotonergic axons in the substantia nigra of monkeys. *Soc Neurosci Abst* 1983;9:661.
48. Hubbard JE, Di Carlo V. Fluorescence histochemistry of monoamine-containing cell bodies in the brain stem of the squirrel monkey *(Saimiri sciureus)*. *J Comp Neurol* 1974;153:385–98.
49. Jacobowitz DM, MacLean PD. A brainstem atlas of catecholaminergic neurons and serotonergic perikarya in a pygmy primate *(Cebuella pygmaea)*. *J Comp Neurol* 1978;177:397–416.
50. Jacobs B, Gannon PJ, Azmitia EC. Atlas of serotonergic cell bodies in the cat brainstem: an immunocytochemical study. *Brain Res Bull* 1984;13:1–31.
51. Jellinger K, Riederer P. (1978): Brain monoamines in metabolic coma and stroke. *Adv Neurol* 1978;20:535–46.
52. Jellinger K, Riederer P, Kleinberger G, Wuketich St, Kothbaruer P. Brain monoamines in human hepatic encephalopathy. *Acta Neuropathol (Berl)* 1978;43:63–8.
53. Jellinger K, Riederer P, Kothbauer P. Brain monoamines in human cerebral infarcts. *Acta Neuropathol (Berl)* 1978;41:173–6.
54. Joseph MH, Baker HF, Crow TJ, Riley GJ, Risby D. Brain tryptophan metabolism in schizophrenia: a post mortem study of metabolites of the serotonin and kynurenine pathways in schizophrenic and control subjects. *Psychopharmacology* 1979;62:279–85.
55. Kapadia SE, de Lanerolle NC, LaMotte CC. An immunohistochemical and electron microscopic study of serotonin neuronal organization in the dorsal raphe of the monkey. *Soc Neurosci Abst* 1983;9:82.
56. LaMotte CC, Johns DR, De Lanerolle NC. Immunohistochemical evidence of indoleamine neurons in monkey spinal cord. *J Comp Neurol* 1982;206:359–70.
57. Lidov HGW, Molliver ME. Immunohistochemical study of the development of serotonergic neurons in the rat CNS. *Brain Res Bull* 1982;9:559–604.
58. Lloyd KG, Farley IJ, Deck JHN, Hornykiewicz O. Serotonin and 5-hydroxyindoleacetic acid in discrete areas of the brainstem of suicide victims and control patients. *Adv Biochem Psychopharmacol* 1974;11:387–97.
59. Mackay AVP, Yates CM, Wright A, Hamilton P, Davies P. Regional distribution of monoamines and their metabolites in the human brain. *J Neurochem* 1978;30:841–8.
60. Mantyh PW, Peschanski M. Spinal projections from the periaqueductual grey and dorsal raphe in rat, cat and monkey. *Neuroscience* 1982;11:2769–76.
61. Morrison JH, Foote SL, Molliver ME, Bloom FE, Lidov GW. Noradrenergic and serotonergic fibers innervate complementary layers in monkey visual cortex: an immunohistochemical study. *Proc Natl Acad Sci USA* 1982;79:2401–5.
62. Nelson CN, Hoffer BJ, Chu N-S, Bloom FE. Cytochemical and pharmacological studies on polysensory neurons in the primate frontal cortex. *Brain Res* 1973;62:115–33.
63. Nobin A, Bjorklund A. Topography of the monoamine neuron systems in the human brain as revealed in fetuses. *Acta Physiol Scand* 1973;388(Suppl):1–40.
64. Olszewski J, Baxter D. *Cytoarchitecture of the human brain stem* Philadelphia: JB Lippincott, 1954.
65. Pasik T, Pasik P. Serotonergic afferents in the monkey neostriatum. *Acta Biol Acad Sci Hung* 1982;33:277–88.
66. Pecci-Saavadra J, Pasik T, Pasik P. Immunocytochemistry of serotonergic neurons in the central nervous system of monkeys. In: Caputto R, Ajmone-Marsan C, eds. Neurotransmission, learning and memory. New York: Raven Press, 1983:81–96. (IBRO monographs series; vol. 10.)
67. Porrino LJ, Goldman-Rakic PS. Brainstem innervation of prefrontal and anterior cingulate cortex in the rhesus monkey revealed by retrograde transport of HRP. *J Comp Neurol* 1982;205:63–76.
68. Pschiedt GR, Himwich HR. Reserpine, monoamine oxidase inhibitors, and distribution of biogenic amines in monkey brain. *Biochem Pharmacol* 1963;12:65–71.
69. Ruda MA, Gobel S. Ultrastructural characterization of axonal endings in the substantia gelatinosa which take up ^{3}H-serotonin. *Brain Res* 1980;184:57–83.
70. Saavedra JM, Palkovits M, Brownstein MH, Axelrod J. Serotonin distribution in the nuclei of the rat hypothalamus and preoptic region. *Brain Res* 1974;77:157–65.
71. Schofield SPM, Dixon AF. Distribution of catecholamine and indoleamine neurons in the brain of the common marmoset *(Callithrix jacchus)*. *J Anat* 1982;134:315–38.
72. Schofield SPM, Everitt BJ. The organization of indoleamine neurons in the brain of the rhesus monkey *(Macaca mulatta)*. *J Comp Neurol* 1981;197:369–83.

73. Shannak KS, Hornykiewcz O. Brain monoamines in the rhesus monkey during long-term neuro-leptic administration. *Adv Biochem Psychopharmacol* 1980;24:315–23.
74. Sladek JR, Tabakoff B, Garver D. Certain biochemical correlates of intense serotonin histoflu-orescence in the brain stem of the neonatal monkey. *Histochemistry* 1974;75:461–71.
75. Sladek JR, Walker P. Serotonin-containing neuronal perikarya in the primate locus coeruleus and subcoeruleus. *Brain Res* 1977;134:359–66.
76. Taber E, Brodal A, Walberg F. The raphe nuclei of the brain stem of the cat. I. Normal topography and cytoarchitecture and general discussion. *J Comp Neurol* 1960;114:161–87.
77. Takeuchi Y, Kimura H, Sano Y. Immunohistochemical demonstration of serotonin nerve fibers in the olfactory bulb of the rat, cat and monkey. *Histochemistry* 1982;75:461–71.
78. Van Woert MH, Hwang EC. Biochemistry and pharmacology of myoclonus. *Clin Neuropharmacol* 1978;3:167–84.
79. Wada JA, McGeer E. Central aromatic amines and behavior. *Arch Neurol* 1966;14:129–42.
80. Walsh FX, Bird ED, Stevens TJ. Monoamine transmitters and their metabolites in the basal ganglia of Huntington's disease and control postmortem brain. In: Friedhoff AJ, Chase TN eds. Gilles de la Tourette syndrome. New York: Raven Press, 1982:165–9. (Advances in neurology; vol. 35).
81. Wiklund L, Leger L, Persson M. Monoamine cell distribution in the cat brainstem: a fluorescence histochemical study with quantification of indoleaminergic and locus coeruleus cell groups. *J Comp Neurol* 1981;203:613–47.
82. Winblad B, Bucht G, Gottries CG, Roos B-E. Monoamines and monoamine metabolites in brains from demented schizophrenics. *Acta Psychiatr Scand* 1979;60:17–28.
83. Zhou FC, Azmitia EC. Effects of 5,7-DHT on HRP retrograde transport from hippocampus to midbrain raphe nuclei. *Brain Res Bull* 1983;10:445–51.

Advances in Neurology, Vol. 43: Myoclonus,
edited by S. Fahn et al. Raven Press,
New York © 1986.

Biochemical Pharmacology of the Serotonin System

Ray W. Fuller

Lilly Research Laboratories, Eli Lilly and Company, Indianapolis, Indiana 46285

Concomitant with the elucidation of mechanisms through which serotonin neurons synthesize, store, release, and metabolize their neurotransmitters has been the development of drugs that act with some selectivity at various steps of these processes. This chapter focuses on the types of agents that are known to affect serotonin neurons, some ways in which their effects can be demonstrated in experimental animals and potentially in humans, and the possible utility of different classes of agents in the treatment of diseases, including myoclonus. At present, very few marketed drugs are known to owe their therapeutic efficacy to alteration of serotonergic function, and until recently, relatively few drugs that are highly selective in influencing serotonergic systems had been identified. The present attempt to survey various types of drugs that act on serotonergic neurons is intended to provide information mainly on drugs now available for use in humans or that may be suitable for human studies in the future.

AGENTS THAT INCREASE TOTAL SEROTONIN CONCENTRATION IN THE BRAIN

Two enzymes are involved in the synthesis of serotonin from the amino acid tryptophan (Fig. 1). The first enzyme, tryptophan 5-hydroxylase, catalyzes the hydroxylation of tryptophan to form 5-hydroxytryptophan. The second enzyme,

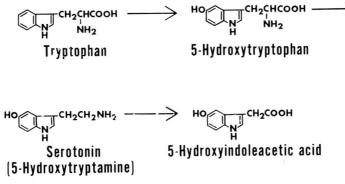

Tryptophan

5-Hydroxytryptophan

Serotonin
(5-Hydroxytryptamine)

5-Hydroxyindoleacetic acid

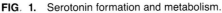

FIG. 1. Serotonin formation and metabolism.

aromatic L-amino acid decarboxylase, catalyzes the decarboxylation of 5-hydroxytryptophan to form serotonin. This latter enzyme is nonspecific and is distributed widely in many cells, where it can catalyze the decarboxylation of other amino acids, such as L-dihydroxyphenylalanine, as well. Brain concentrations of tryptophan and particularly of 5-hydroxytryptophan are not saturating with respect to the above-mentioned enzymes that metabolize them, so increasing brain concentrations of these amino acids increases the rate of formation of serotonin and total concentration of serotonin in brain. The uptake of tryptophan into the brain is related to the ratio of its serum concentration to the concentrations of other large neutral amino acids that compete with tryptophan for uptake into the brain (16). Tryptophan concentration in the brain can be increased by administration of exogenous tryptophan or by certain other manipulations that increase this ratio. An example of the latter is feeding a carbohydrate meal, which leads to insulin secretion, resulting in stimulation of amino acid uptake into various tissues and overall lowering of the serum concentration of the large neutral amino acids relative to tryptophan concentration, hence to increased tryptophan uptake into brain.

Tryptophan is a rather inefficient precursor to serotonin in the sense that 5-hydroxylation is a quantitatively minor metabolic pathway for tryptophan. The advantage to using tryptophan instead of 5-hydroxytryptophan is that tryptophan can be converted to serotonin only in those cells that normally form serotonin, i.e., those that contain tryptophan 5-hydroxylase.

5-Hydroxytryptophan concentrations in the brain normally are very low, its rate of decarboxylation to serotonin being approximately equal to its rate of formation. A large percentage of exogenously administered 5-hydroxytryptophan is converted to serotonin. But this conversion can occur in any cell containing the aromatic L-amino acid decarboxylase and is not limited to serotonin-forming cells. Thus, although 5-hydroxytryptophan is a more efficient precursor of serotonin than is tryptophan in terms of percentage of the precursor that is converted to serotonin, its disadvantage is that serotonin formation at sites other than serotonergic neurons can lead to pharmacological effects other than the desired ones, such as release of catecholamines through displacement from storage granules by serotonin.

The major pathway by which serotonin is degraded metabolically is through the action of monoamine oxidase (MAO). MAO is recognized to exist in two forms, type A and type B, and serotonin is preferentially oxidized by type-A MAO. MAO inhibitors that inhibit type-A MAO, regardless of whether they are selective for type-A MAO, can increase serotonin concentrations in the brain. However, selective inhibitors of type-A MAO, such as those shown in Fig. 2, may have the advantage of not influencing other amines that are destroyed by type-B MAO. These inhibitors do increase serotonin concentration in the brain. Recently, serotonin neurons have been shown to contain type-B MAO (46), and there has been previous evidence that type-B MAO may be able to oxidize serotonin *in vivo* when type-A MAO is inhibited (32).

Clorgyline (41) and LY51641 (19) are potent, highly selective, irreversible inhibitors of type-A MAO. The iodo analog of LY51641 has recently been described

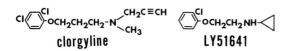

clorgyline LY51641

FIG. 2. Inhibitors of type-A MAO.

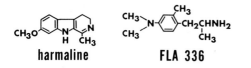

harmaline FLA 336

as another highly selective inhibitor that presumably could be used to introduce a radioiodine atom into type-A MAO (20). Harmaline and FLA 336 are reversible inhibitors of MAO. Harmaline is relatively short-acting and is highly selective for type-A MAO (21). FLA 336 is of particular interest for influencing serotonin neurons because not only is it a reversible inhibitor selective for type-A MAO but there is also evidence that FLA 336 is accumulated in serotonergic neurons by virtue of its affinity for the membrane uptake pump for serotonin, so it apparently inhibits type-A MAO present in serotonin neurons with some selectivity over type-A MAO present in other cells (3).

DRUGS THAT INCREASE SYNAPTIC CONCENTRATIONS OF SEROTONIN

Serotonin precursors and MAO inhibitors elevate total brain concentrations of serotonin; presumably most of the serotonin present at any instant is contained within neurons in storage granules, with only a small percentage being in the synaptic cleft, where its action on receptor sites causes physiological changes. When serotonin precursors and MAO inhibitors elevate serotonin, the increased intraneuronal stores of serotonin apparently lead to increased concentrations of serotonin in the synaptic cleft as well. Serotonin-releasing drugs can increase concentrations of serotonin in the synaptic cleft without altering total brain concentrations of serotonin; release of serotonin from storage granules permits its movement into the synaptic cleft, so that concentrations of serotonin at the receptor sites are increased. The major physiological means of removing serotonin from the synaptic cleft appears to be through a specific carrier mechanism located on the serotonin nerve terminal itself, this carrier mechanism transporting serotonin from the synaptic cleft back into the neuron that released it. Once inside the neuron, the serotonin is no longer able to act on synaptic membrane receptors. Inhibitors of this carrier mechanism, or uptake pump, prolong the stay of released serotonin in the synaptic cleft. Thus, both serotonin releasers and serotonin uptake inhibitors can increase concentrations of serotonin in the synaptic cleft, where the serotonin can act on receptors, without increasing total brain concentrations of serotonin.

Although amine-releasing drugs such as reserpine and tetrabenazine can release serotonin, they do not affect serotonin specifically but instead also release other amines, such as catecholamines. Two drugs that release serotonin with some specificity and that have been fairly widely used for this purpose are fenfluramine and *p*-chloroamphetamine (Fig. 3). Fenfluramine is used therapeutically as an appetite-suppressant drug, and its mechanism of reduction of food intake is believed to involve enhanced serotonergic function through serotonin release (74,75). Fenfluramine is metabolized by *N*-dealkylation to norfenfluramine, the primary amine lacking the *N*-ethyl substituent. Norfenfluramine acts similarly to fenfluramine in releasing serotonin and may account for some of the *in vivo* actions of fenfluramine. Norfenfluramine closely resembles *p*-chloroamphetamine in structure and in pharmacological action (23). *p*-Chloroamphetamine is not used clinically, though in the past it has been used experimentally as an antidepressant drug (68).

Many of the tricyclic antidepressant drugs can inhibit uptake of serotonin as well as uptake of the catecholamines, norepinephrine, epinephrine, and in some cases, dopamine. Within the past 10 years several compounds that selectively inhibit the uptake of serotonin but not catecholamines have been described. Examples of the most selective of these are in Fig. 4. Some of these drugs have now been shown to have antidepressant effects clinically. They potentiate effects of 5-hydroxytryptophan in animals (18) and in humans (69). The concern about 5-hydroxytryptophan having nonspecific effects on neurons other than serotonin neurons can be alleviated by combining low doses of 5-hydroxytryptophan with an uptake inhibitor; effects of 5-hydroxytryptophan on serotonergic neurons are potentiated so that doses of 5-hydroxytryptophan too low to have nonspecific actions on other neurons can be used.

Since the initial report of selective inhibition of serotonin uptake *in vitro* and *in vivo* by fluoxetine (73), several other selective inhibitors of serotonin uptake have been described, including zimelidine (59), fluvoxamine (8), paroxetine (5), citalopram (39), alaproclate (49) and indalpine (33). Clomipramine is a selective inhibitor of serotonin uptake suitable for *in vitro* studies, but clomipramine is metabolized *in vivo* to a compound that preferentially inhibits norepinephrine uptake, so is not useful for selectively inhibiting serotonin uptake *in vivo* (26).

DIRECT-ACTING SEROTONIN AGONISTS

Serotonin itself does not cross the blood–brain barrier and cannot be given systemically to stimulate brain serotonin receptors. In experimental animals, serotonin can be introduced directly into the brain, e.g., by intraventricular injection, direct injection into brain regions, or by microiontophoresis. Drugs that mimic the action of serotonin on the receptor (Fig. 5) represent the next most direct way of activating serotonin receptors. Several indoles related closely in structure to serotonin can activate serotonin receptors. *N,N*-Dimethyl-5-methoxytryptamine stimulates serotonin receptors, penetrates the blood–brain barrier, and is partially

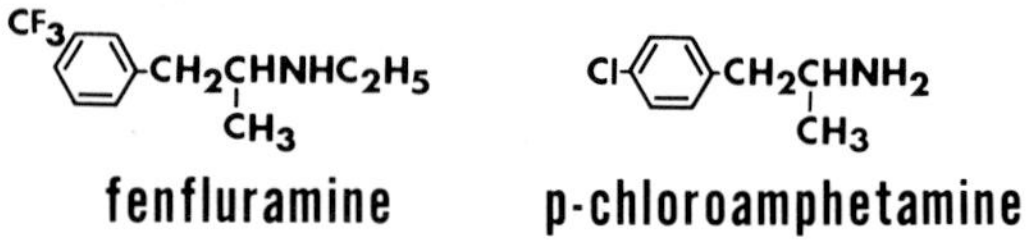

FIG. 3. Serotonin-releasing drugs.

fenfluramine   p-chloroamphetamine

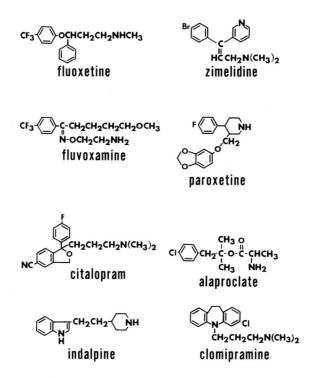

FIG. 4. Selective inhibitors of serotonin uptake.

protected from enzymatic degradation, so it can activate brain serotonin receptors when given systemically (66). Other indole-containing compounds that are serotonin agonists include RU24969 (15) and indorenate (TR3369) (36,60). Several non-indoles also are serotonin agonists. Four of these contain a piperazine ring: quipazine (37,55); MK-212 (9); *m*-chlorophenylpiperazine (61), and *m*-trifluoromethylphenylpiperazine (25). *m*-Trifluoromethylphenylpiperazine (24) and *m*-chlorophenylpiperazine (61) are potent agonists at central serotonin receptors but may be antagonists rather than agonists at peripheral serotonin receptors in the gut (70) and the vasculature (10). In the guinea pig, a species in which 5-hydroxytryptophan induces myoclonus, the piperazines quipazine, MK-212, and *m*-trifluoromethylphenylpiperazine were found not to mimic the ability of *N,N*-dimethyl-5-methoxytryptamine to cause myoclonus (50). 8-Hydroxy-*N,N*-dipropyl-2-aminotetralin (8-OH-DPAT) is a compound recently described to be a centrally acting serotonin agonist based on biochemical and behavioral measurements in rats (2,35).

SEROTONIN-DEPLETING DRUGS

The most widely used serotonin synthesis inhibitor is *p*-chlorophenylalanine (43), which causes irreversible inhibition of tryptophan hydroxylase *in vivo* through a mechanism not completely understood (29). After a single dose of *p*-chlorophen-

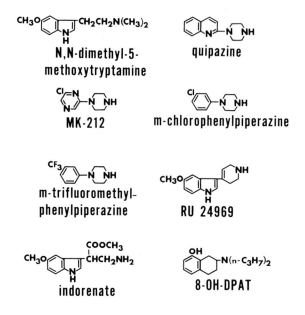

FIG. 5. Direct-acting serotonin agonists.

ylalanine, brain serotonin concentration falls to a minimum within 24 hr and remains depleted for several days. *p*-Chlorophenylalanine has been a useful pharmacological tool for animal studies and has been used in humans (13). High doses of this amino acid are required, however, and it can have other actions, such as effects on catecholamine neurons (64).

Permanent destruction of serotonin nerve terminals can be brought about by the local injection of 5,6- or 5,7-dihydroxytryptamine (4). These serotonin congeners apparently are transported into and concentrated in serotonin neurons, where they lead to neurotoxic effects probably mediated by oxidation reaction products. Although these agents are capable of influencing catecholamine neurons, they can be administered along with uptake inhibitors that prevent their uptake by catecholamine neurons to produce selective lesioning of serotonin neurons.

Fenfluramine and *p*-chloroamphetamine, whose initial effects are to elevate serotonin concentrations in the synaptic cleft due to release of intraneuronally stored serotonin, both result in long-lasting depletion of serotonin stores (23). Although these compounds may initially have some effects on catecholamine neurons, their long-term effects appear to be very specific for serotonin, and they have been useful pharmacological tools, along with 5,6- and 5,7-dihydroxytryptamine, for investigating functional consequences of serotonin depletion (40).

SEROTONIN RECEPTOR ANTAGONISTS

Among compounds known to block certain serotonin-mediated responses, some of the most useful are shown in Fig. 6. In most experimental systems, metergoline

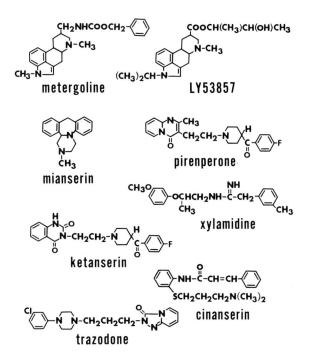

FIG. 6. Serotonin-receptor antagonists.

(28) is the most potent of the serotonin antagonists. Several others, including cinanserin (27), mianserin (53), trazodone (52), and LY53857 (22) have been described in the literature and studied in various *in vitro* and *in vivo* systems. Trazodone is an interesting serotonin antagonist because it is converted by metabolic cleavage into *m*-chlorophenylpiperazine, a serotonin agonist, which contributes to pharmacologic effects seen after trazodone in animals (7) and possibly in humans (6). Xylamidine is noteworthy because it is a potent antagonist of peripheral serotonin receptors but does not cross the blood–brain barrier well and so does not affect central serotonin receptors until very high doses are used (54). Xylamidine can therefore be useful in determining if a particular serotonergic effect is central or peripheral. After Peroutka and Snyder (56) classified central serotonin receptors by radioligand-binding studies into 5-HT$_1$ (labeled by serotonin) and 5-HT$_2$ (labeled by spiperone) types, most serotonin antagonists have been observed to have preferential affinity for 5-HT$_2$ receptors (48). Ketanserin (46) and pirenperone (11) are recently described compounds with particularly high selectivity for 5-HT$_2$ receptors distinct from 5-HT$_1$ receptors (48). However, ketanserin is also a potent blocker of α-adrenergic receptors, and evidence has been presented that certain of its cardiovascular effects are mediated by α-receptor blockade (17,42,57).

Efforts are now underway to elucidate which physiologic functions of serotonin are mediated by 5-HT$_1$ receptors and which are mediated by 5-HT$_2$ receptors through the use of selective agonists and antagonists (48). The development of antagonists that act selectively on 5-HT$_1$ receptors and of agonists that act selectively on 5-HT$_2$ receptors would help these efforts greatly, since no such agents are currently available.

FUNCTIONAL EFFECTS OF DRUGS ACTING ON SEROTONIN NEURONS

The use of direct and indirect serotonin agonists, serotonin depletors, and serotonin antagonists in experimental animals has helped to clarify physiological roles of serotonin neurons in neuroendocrine regulation (18,63,72), central control of blood pressure (45), thermoregulation (12), appetite control (62), antinociception (38), motor function (30), and various types of behavior (31,65). Possible use of direct or indirect serotonin agonists in the treatment of diseases such as depression (67), obesity (76), alcoholism (58), and chronic pain (14) has been considered; in some cases these have become realities, e.g., the use of fenfluramine as an appetite-suppressant drug and the use of zimelidine as an antidepressant drug. Serotonin precursors alone or with uptake inhibitors are useful in treating myoclonus (51,69), but I am not aware that direct-acting serotonin agonists have been evaluated. Serotonin antagonists have been suggested to be of use in treating Cushing's disease (44), migraine (34), hypertension (71), and depression (1). Some drugs that are serotonin antagonists have been beneficial in these conditions, but it is as yet unproved that their effects were due to serotonin receptor antagonism.

SUMMARY

Although relatively few drugs that specifically influence serotonin neurons have been used in humans, a wide variety of drugs has been used to modify serotonergic function in experimental animals. Several classes of agents increase serotonergic function. These include serotonin precursors (L-5-hydroxytryptophan and L-tryptophan) and monoamine oxidase inhibitors, which elevate serotonin stores; uptake inhibitors and releasers, which increase the concentration of serotonin in the synaptic cleft; and direct serotonin agonists, which mimic the action of serotonin on synaptic receptors. In addition, several kinds of drugs decrease serotonergic function, including serotonin depletors and agents that destroy serotonin neurons, as well as direct serotonin-receptor antagonists. The array of drugs now available improves the opportunities for clarifying the physiological roles of serotonin and gives promise of several therapeutic applications, including treatment of myoclonus.

REFERENCES

1. Aprison MH, Takahashi R, Tachiki K. Hypersensitive serotonergic receptors involved in clinical depression—a theory. In: Haber B, Aprison MH, eds. Neuropharmacology and behavior. New York: Plenum Press, 1978:23–53.
2. Arvidsson L-E, Hacksell U, Nilsson JLG, Hjorth S, Carlsson A, Lindberg P, Sanchez D, Wikstrom H. 8-Hydroxy-2-(di-n-propylamino)-tetralin, a new centrally acting 5-hydroxytryptamine receptor agonist. *J Med Chem* 1981;24:921–3.

3. Ask A-L, Fagervall I, Ross SB. Evidence for a selective inhibition by FLA 336(+) of the monoamine oxidase in serotonergic neurones in the rat brain. *Acta Pharmacol Toxicol (Copenh)* 1982;51:395–6.

4. Baumgarten HG, Klemm HP, Lachenmayer L, Bjorklund A, Lovenberg W, Schlossberger HG. Mode and mechanism of action of neurotoxic indoleamines: a review and a progress report. *Ann NY Acad Sci* 1978;305:3–24.

5. Buus Lassen J, Lund J, Sondergaard I. Central and peripheral 5-HT uptake in rats treated chronically with femoxetine, paroxetine, and chlorimipramine. *Psychopharmacology* 1980;68:229–33.

6. Caccia S, Fong MH, Garattini S, Zanini MG. Plasma concentrations of trazodone and 1-(3-chlorophenyl)piperazine in man after a single oral dose of trazodone. *J Pharm Pharmacol* 1982;34:605–6.

7. Cervo L, Ballabio M, Caccia S, Samanin R. Blockade of trazodone of naloxone-precipitated jumping in morphine-dependent rats: correlation with brain levels of *m*-chlorophenylpiperazine. *J Pharm Pharmacol* 1981;33:813–4.

8. Claasen V, Davies JE, Hertting G, Placheta P. Fluvoxamine, a specific 5-hydroxytryptamine uptake inhibitor. *Br J Pharmacol* 1977;60:505–16.

9. Clineschmidt BV. MK-212: a serotonin-like agonist in the CNS. *Gen Pharmacol* 1979;109:287–90.

10. Cohen ML, Fuller RW. Antagonism of vascular serotonin receptors by *m*-chlorophenylpiperazine and *m*-trifluoromethylphenylpiperazine. *Life Sci* 1983;32:711–8.

11. Colpaert FC, Niemegeers CJE, Janssen PAJ. A drug discrimination analysis of lysergic acid diethylamide (LSD): in vivo agonist and antagonist effects of purported 5-hydroxytryptamine antagonists and of pirenperone, a LSD-antagonist. *J Pharmacol Exp Ther* 1982;221:206–14.

12. Cox B, Lee TF. 5-Hydroxytryptamine-induced hypothermia in rats as an in vivo model for the quantitative study of 5-hydroxytryptamine receptors. *J Pharmacol Methods* 1981;5:43–51.

13. Cremata VY, Koe BK. Clinical and biochemical effects of fenclonine: a serotonin depletor. *Dis Nerv Syst* 1968;29:147–52.

14. De Benedittis G, Di Giulio AM, Massei R, Villani R, Panerae AE. Effects of 5-hydroxytryptophan on central and deafferentation chronic pain: a preliminary clinical trial. *Adv Pain Res Ther* 1983;5:295–304.

15. Euvrard C, Boissier JR. Biochemical assessment of the central 5-HT agonist activity of RU 24969 (a piperidinyl indole). *Eur J Pharmacol* 1980;63:65–72.

16. Fernstrom JD. Dietary precursors and brain neurotransmitter formation. *Annu Rev Med* 1981;32:413–25.

17. Fozard JR. Mechanism of the hypotensive effects of ketanserin. *J Cardiovasc Pharmacol* 1982;4:829–38.

18. Fuller RW. Serotonergic stimulation of pituitary-adrenocortical function in rats. *Neuroendocrinology* 1981;32:118–27.

19. Fuller RW, Hemrick-Luecke SK. Elevation of epinephrine concentration in rat brain by LY51641, a selective inhibitor of type A monoamine oxidase. *Res Commun Chem Pathol Pharmacol* 1981;32:207–221.

20. Fuller RW, Hemrick-Luecke SK, Molloy BB. *N*-[2-(*o*-iodophenoxy)ethyl]-cyclopropylamine hydrochloride (LY121768), a potent and selective irreversible inhibitor of type A monoamine oxidase. *Biochem Pharmacol* 1983;32:1243–9.

21. Fuller RW, Hemrick-Luecke SK, Perry KW. Influence of harmaline on the ability of pargyline to alter catecholamine metabolism in rats. *Biochem Pharmacol* 1981;30:1295–8.

22. Fuller RW, Snoddy HD. The effects of metergoline and other serotonin receptor antagonists on serum corticosterone in rats. *Endocrinology* 1979;105:923–8.

23. Fuller RW, Snoddy HD, Hemrick SK. Effects of fenfluramine and norfenfluramine on brain serotonin metabolism in rats. *Proc Soc Exp Biol Med* 1978;157:202–5.

24. Fuller RW, Snoddy HD, Mason NR, Hemrick-Luecke SK, Clemens JA. Substituted piperazines as central serotonin agonists: comparative specificity of the postsynaptic actions of quipazine and *m*-trifluoromethylphenylpiperazine. *J Pharmacol Exp Ther* 1981;218:636–41.

25. Fuller RW, Snoddy HD, Mason NR, Molloy BB. Effect of 1-(*m*-trifluoromethylphenyl)piperazine on ^{3}H-serotonin binding to membranes from rat brain in vitro and on serotonin turnover in rat brain in vivo. *Eur J Pharmacol* 1978;52:11–6.

26. Fuller RW, Snoddy HD, Perry KW, Bymaster FP, Wong DT. Importance of duration of drug

action in the antagonism of *p*-chloroamphetamine depletion of brain serotonin—comparison of fluoxetine and chlorimipramine. *Biochem Pharmacol* 1978;27:193–8.

27. Furgiuele AR, High JP, Horowitz ZP. Some central effects of SQ 10,643 [2'3-(dimethylamino-propylthio)cinnamanilide hydrochloride], a potent serotonin antagonist. *Arch Int Pharmacodyn Ther* 1965;155:225–35.

28. Fuxe K, Ogren S-O, Agnati LF, Jonsson G. Further evidence that methergoline is a central 5-hydroxytryptamine receptor blocking agent. *Neurosci Lett* 1978;9:195–200.

29. Gal EM, Whitacre DH. Mechanism of irreversible inactivation of phenylalanine-4- and tryptophan-5-hydroxylases by 4-^{36}Cl,2-^{14}C *p*-chlorophenylalanine: a revision. *Neurochem Res* 1982;7:13–26.

30. Gerson SC, Baldessarini RJ. Motor effects of serotonin in the central nervous system. *Life Sci* 1980;27:1435–51.

31. Green AR, Hall JE, Rees AR. A behavioural and a biochemical study in rats of 5-hydroxytryptamine receptor agonists and antagonists, with observations on structure-activity requirements for the agonists. *Br J Pharmacol* 1981;73:703–19.

32. Green AR, Youdim MBH. Effects of monoamine oxidase inhibition by clorgyline, deprenil or tranylcypromine on 5-hydroxytryptamine concentrations in rat brain and hyperactivity following subsequent tryptophan administration. *Br J Pharmacol* 1975;55:415–22.

33. Gueremy C, Audiau F, Champseix A, Uzan A, Le Fur G, Rataud J. 3-(4-Piperidinylalkyl)indoles, selective inhibitors of neuronal 5-hydroxytryptamine uptake. *J Med Chem* 1980;23:1306–10.

34. Hardebo JE, Edvinsson L, Owman C, Svendgaard N-A. Potentiation and antagonism of serotonin effects on intracranial and extracranial vessels. Possible implications in migraine. *Neurology* 1978;28:64–70.

35. Hjorth S, Carlsson A, Lindberg P, Sanchez D, Wikstrom H, Arvidsson L-E, Hacksell U, Nilsson JLG. 8-Hydroxy-2-(di-*n*-propylamino)-tetralin, 8-OH-DPAT, a potent and selective simplified ergot congener with central 5HT-receptor stimulating activity. *J Neural Transm* 1982;55:169–88.

36. Hong E. A serotonergic antihypertensive agent. In: Singer TP, Ondarza RN, eds. Molecular basis of drug action. New York: Elsevier North Holland, 1981:247–52.

37. Hong E, Sancilio LF, Vargas R, Pardo EG. Similarities between the pharmacological actions of quipazine and serotonin. *Eur J Pharmacol* 1969;6:274–80.

38. Hynes MD, Fuller RW. The effect of fluoxetine on morphine analgesia, respiratory depression, and lethality. *Drug Devel Res* 1982;2:33–42.

39. Hyttel J. Effect of a specific 5-HT uptake inhibitor, citalopram (Lu 10-171), on ^{3}H-5-HT uptake in rat brain synaptosomes in vitro. *Psychopharmacology* 1978;60:13–8.

40. Jacoby JH, Lytle LD, eds. Serotonin neurotoxins. *Ann NY Acad Sci* 1978;305:1–702.

41. Johnston JP. Some observations upon a new inhibitor of monoamine oxidase in brain tissue. *Biochem Pharmacol* 1968;17:1285–97.

42. Kalkman HO, Timmermans PBMWM, Van Zweiten PA. Characterization of the antihypertensive properties of ketanserin (R41468) in rats. *J Pharmacol Exp Ther* 1982;222:227–31.

43. Koe BK, Weissman A. *p*-Chlorophenylalanine: a specific depletor of brain serotonin. *J Pharmacol Exp Ther* 1966;154:499–516.

44. Krieger DT. Cyproheptadine: drug therapy for Cushing's disease. In: Muller EE, ed. Neuroactive drugs in endocrinology. Amsterdam: Elsevier North Holland, 1980:361–70.

45. Kuhn DM, Wolf WA, Lovenberg WA. Review of the role of the central serotonergic neuronal system in blood pressure regulation. *Hypertension* 1980;2:243–55.

46. Levitt P, Pintar JE, Breakefield XO. Immunocytochemical demonstration of monoamine oxidase B in brain astrocytes and serotonergic neurons. *Proc Natl Acad Sci USA* 1982;79:6385–89.

47. Leysen JE, Awouters F, Kennis L, Laduron PM, Vandenberk J, Janssen PAJ. Receptor binding profile of R 41 468, a novel antagonist at 5-HT$_2$ receptors. *Life Sci* 1981;28:1015–22.

48. Leysen JE, Tollenaere JP. Biochemical models for serotonin receptors. *Ann Repts Med Chem* 1982;17:1–10.

49. Lindberg UH, Thorberg S-O, Bengtsson S, Renyi AL, Ross SB, Ogren S-O. Inhibitors of neuronal monoamine uptake. 2. Selective inhibition of 5-hydroxytryptamine uptake by α-amino acid esters of phenethyl alcohols. *J Med Chem* 1978;21:448–56.

50. Luscombe G, Jenner P, Marsden CD. Pharmacological analysis of the myoclonus induced by 5-hydroxytryptophan in the guinea pig suggests the presence of multiple 5-hydroxytryptamine receptors in the brain. *Neuropharmacology* 1981;20:819–31.

51. Magnussen I, Mondrup K, Engbaek F, Lademann A, De Fine Olivarius B. Treatment of myoclonic syndromes with paroxetine alone or combined with 5-HTP. *Acta Neurol Scand* 1982;66:276–82.

52. Maj J, Palider W, Rawlow A. Trazodone, a central serotonin antagonist and agonist. *J Neural Transm* 1979;44:237–48.
53. Maj J, Sowinska H, Baran L, Gancarczyk L, Rawlow A. The central antiserotonergic action of mianserin. *Psychopharmacology* 1978;59:79–84.
54. Mawson C, Whittington H. Evaluation of the peripheral and central antagonistic activities against 5-hydroxytryptamine of some new agents. *Br J Pharmacol* 1970;39:223P.
55. Neuman RS, White SR. Serotonin-like actions of quipazine and CPP on spinal motoneurones. *Eur J Pharmacol* 1982;81:49–56.
56. Peroutka SJ, Snyder SH. Multiple serotonin receptors: differential binding of [³H]5-hydroxytryptamine, [³H]lysergic acid diethylamide and [³H]spiroperidol. *Mol Pharmacol* 1979;16:687–99.
57. Persson B, Hedner T, Henning M. Cardiovascular effects in the rat of ketanserin, a novel 5-hydroxytryptamine receptor blocking agent. *J Pharm Pharmacol* 1982;34:442–5.
58. Rockman GE, Amit Z, Brown ZW, Bourque C, Ogren S-O. An investigation of the mechanisms of action of 5-hydroxytryptamine in the suppression of ethanol intake. *Neuropharmacology* 1982;21:341–7.
59. Ross SB, Renyi AL. Inhibition of the neuronal uptake of 5-hydroxytryptamine and noradrenaline in rat brain by (Z)- and (E)-3-(4-bromophenyl)-N,N-dimethyl-3-(3-pyridyl) allylamines and their secondary analogues. *Neuropharmacology* 1977;16:57–63.
60. Safdy ME, Kurchacova E, Schut RN, Vidrio H, Hong E. Tryptophan analogues. 1. Synthesis and antihypertensive activity of positional isomers. *J Med Chem* 1982;25:723–30.
61. Samanin R, Mennini T, Ferraris A, Bendotti C, Borsini F, Garattini S. *m*-Chlorophenylpiperazine: a central serotonin agonist causing powerful anorexia in rats. *Naunyn-Schmiedebergs Arch Pharmacol* 1979;308:159–63.
62. Samanin R, Mennini T, Garattini S. Evidence that it is possible to cause anorexia by increasing release and/or directly stimulating postsynaptic serotonin receptors in the brain. *Prog Neuropsychopharmacol* 1980;4:363–9.
63. Smythe GA, Bradshaw JE, Cai WY, Symons RG. Hypothalamic serotoninergic stimulation of thyrotropin secretion and related brain-hormone and drug interactions in the rat. *Endocrinology* 1982;111:1181–91.
64. Tagliamonte A, Tagliamonte P, Corsini GU, Mereu GP, Gessa GL. Decreased conversion of tyrosine to catecholamines in the brain of rats treated with *p*-chlorophenylalanine. *J Pharm Pharmacol* 1973;25:101–3.
65. Valzelli L. Serotonergic inhibitory control of experimental aggression. *Pharmacol Res Commun* 1982;14:1–13.
66. Vandermaelen CP, Aghajanian GK. Intracellular studies on the effects of systemic administration of serotonin agonists on rat facial motoneurons. *Eur J Pharmacol* 1982;78:233–6.
67. Van Praag HM. Management of depression with serotonin precursors. *Biol Psychiatry* 1981;16:291–310.
68. Van Praag HM, Korf J. 4-Chloroamphetamines. Chance and trend in the development of new antidepressants. *J Clin Pharmacol* 1973;13:3–14.
69. Van Woert MH, Magnussen I, Rosenbaum D, Chung E. Fluoxetine in the treatment of intention myoclonus. *Clin Neuropharmacol* 1983;6:49–54.
70. Warrick MW, Dinwiddie WG, Lin T-M, Fuller RW, Antidiarrheal effects of quipazine and 1-(*m*-trifluoromethylphenyl)piperazine in mice. *J Pharm Pharmacol* 1981;33:675–6.
71. Wenting GJ, Man in 't Veld AF, Woittiez AF, Boomsma F, Schalekamp MADH. Treatment of hypertension with ketanserin, a new selective 5-HT₂ receptor antagonist. *Br Med J* 1982;284:537–9.
72. Willoughby JO, Menadue M, Jervois P. Function of serotonin in physiologic secretion of growth hormone and prolactin: action of 5,7-dihydroxytryptamine, fenfluramine and *p*-chlorophenylalanine. *Brain Res* 1982;249:291–9.
73. Wong DT, Bymaster FP, Horng JS, Molloy BB. A new selective inhibitor for uptake of serotonin into synaptosomes of rat brain: 3-(*p*-trifluoromethylphenoxy)-N-methyl-3-phenylpropylamine. *J Pharmacol Exp Ther* 1975;193:804–11.
74. Wurtman JJ, Wurtman RJ. Fenfluramine and other serotoninergic drugs depress food intake and carbohydrate consumption while sparing protein consumption. *Curr Med Res Opin* 1979;6(Suppl 1):28–33.
75. Wurtman JJ, Wurtman RJ. Suppression of carbohydrate consumption as snacks and at mealtime

by DL-fenfluramine or tryptophan. In: Garattini S, Samanin R, eds. Anorectic agents: mechanisms of action and tolerance. New York: Raven Press, 1981:169–182.

76. Wurtman JJ, Wurtman RJ, Growdon JH, Henry P, Lipscomb A, Zeisel SH. Carbohydrate craving in obese people: suppression by treatments affecting serotoninergic transmission. *Int J Eating Disorders* 1981;1:2–15.

Advances in Neurology, Vol. 43: Myoclonus,
edited by S. Fahn et al. Raven Press,
New York © 1986.

Motor Activity and the Brain Serotonin System

Barry L. Jacobs

*Program in Neuroscience, Department of Psychology, Princeton University,
Princeton, New Jersey 08544*

A number of different types of myoclonus have been described, with widely differing etiologies and underlying pathologies. One of the major forms of this disorder is posthypoxic action myoclonus. As discussed in detail by other authors in this volume, alterations in brain serotonin neurotransmission have been importantly implicated in this form of myoclonus. The best evidence indicates that decreased functional activity in serotonin-mediated synapses within the central nervous system (CNS) plays an important role in posthypoxic action myoclonus. This is based on the findings that serotonin precursors (5-hydroxytryptophan and L-tryptophan, in conjunction with monoamine oxidase inhibition) have been found to be clinically effective in the treatment of this disorder and that patients afflicted with this disorder often show evidence of lowered CNS serotonin metabolism (as reflected in decreased cerebrospinal fluid levels of serotonin's major metabolite, 5-hydroxyindoleacetic acid) (8). Van Woert and Rosenbaum (34) emphasize the specificity of 5-hydroxytryptophan's ameliorative effect on posthypoxic action myoclonus by reviewing evidence that this drug is not effective in the treatment of other types of myoclonus or various other types of neurological disorders.

In spite of this positive general evidence linking serotonin to posthypoxic action myoclonus, there is no definitive information regarding either the nature of the deficit or the site(s) within the CNS where the presumed dysfunction of serotonin might be localized. This lack of information is largely attributable to the complex, almost ubiquitous, distribution of serotonin axon terminal release sites within the human CNS, coupled with the general inaccessibility of the human nervous system and the lack of a reliable animal model for posthypoxic action myoclonus. In combination, these facts have made it difficult to pinpoint either the nature or locus of the dysfunction in serotonin neurotransmission thought to be operative in the CNS of those suffering from posthypoxic action myoclonus.

In the first two sections of this chapter, I shall describe animal research conducted in my laboratory that explores two aspects of the relationship between serotonin neurotransmission and CNS motor systems. A major goal of these studies was simply to provide more basic information regarding the organization and interaction between motor systems and serotonin neurons. In a third section, I shall describe a *possible* animal model for posthypoxic action myoclonus in humans.

RAT MOTOR SYNDROME STUDIES

Virtually all the serotonin-containing neurons in the mammalian brain are found on or near the midline of the brainstem, from the medulla to the mesencephalon. Most of these cells are clustered together in groups that roughly correspond to the raphe nuclei. There is abundant evidence from anatomical studies that serotonergic neurons send moderate to dense projections to a number of areas of the CNS known to be directly involved in motor control, e.g., corpus striatum, globus pallidus, red nucleus, substantia nigra, inferior olivary complex, various cranial nerve nuclei, and the ventral horn of the spinal cord (9,28).

Clear evidence that central serotonin is involved in the control or modulation of motoric processes comes from a series of simple experiments. When rats are administered any of a large set of compounds that either increase the levels of CNS serotonin, cause it to be released from its presynaptic storage sites, or directly mimic serotonin's postsynaptic effect, a dramatic motor syndrome is produced. It consists most conspicuously of hyperactivity, head shakes or "wet dog" shakes, hyperreactivity, tremor, rigidity, hindlimb abduction, Straub tail, lateral head weaving, and reciprocal forepaw treading. This syndrome is of special importance in that it represents, with the exception of the hyperactivity component (5,6), one of the few "pure" behavorial indices of central serotonergic activity (15,27).

A number of investigators in the 1950s noted that 5-hydroxytryptophan, alone or in combination with a monoamine oxidase inhibitor, produced this syndrome or a subset of its component signs. However, it was not until 1963 that aspects of this response complex were used as an analytic tool for studying the activity of serotonin-mediated synapses. In that year, Corne and his co-workers (4) suggested that the frequency of occurrence of the head-shake response in mice could be used as an index of the functional activity in serotonergic synapses. A few years later, Anden and his co-workers (2) suggested that various spinal reflexes in rat, but especially the facilitation of the hindlimb extension reflex, could be used to assess serotonergic activity in the CNS. Interest in this area was rekindled by Grahame-Smith in 1971 (10), when he proposed that the hyperactivity component (and in some instances hyperthermia) could be used as a quantifiable reflection of serotonergic activity in the CNS.

Although Corne et al., Anden et al., and Grahame-Smith had the foresight to utilize behavorial measures to index synaptic transmitter activity, the particular dependent measures chosen, i.e., head shakes, hindlimb extension reflex, and hyperactivity, lack the specificity necessary to endow such a model with the general validity required for examining the functional activity in serotonin-mediated synapses. Responses such as head shaking, increased hindlimb extension, and hyperactivity can be elicited by compounds other than those acting primarily via the serotonin system. On the other hand, tremor, rigidity, lateral head weaving, etc., represent a constellation of neurological signs whose simultaneous display is of such low probability that their occurrence can be taken as indicative of activity in a particular system, in this case, serotonin. Therefore, taking these important pioneering studies of Corne et al., Anden et al., and Grahame-Smith one step further, I proposed (13,14) that the elicitation of this response complex could be taken as unambiguous evidence for increased activity in serotonergic synapses. More specifically, I proposed that if at least four of the following six component signs were observed, the syndrome was scored as present: resting tremor (especially of the head and forelimbs), rigidity or hypertonicity (assessed both by grasping the rat around the torso and by passively extending and flexing the hindlimbs), reciprocal forepaw treading (rhythmic dorsoventral movements of the forelimbs), hindlimb abduction (a dramatic splaying out of the hindlimbs), Straub tail, and lateral head weaving (slow side-to-side head movements). This syndrome is significant for two reasons. Taken at face value, it directly tells us the types of motor responses in which CNS serotonin is involved. It is also a heuristic device, since the presence or absence of the syndrome can be used to measure, for example, the ED_{50} for a particular drug, or a significant change in the ED_{50} produced by a drug or some other manipulation.

The conclusion that this syndrome does specifically reflect central serotonergic activity is based on the following types of evidence: production or potentiation of the syndrome by serotonin precursors, releasers, agonists, and reuptake inhibitors; blockade of the syndrome by serotonin-specific antagonists or serotonin-synthesis inhibitors; and demonstration of denervation supersensitivity specific to serotonergic stimulation following destruction of serotonin nerve terminals (15,27).

This line of research has relevance beyond the laboratory rat, since a similar pattern of neurological signs is seen in a large number of animal species, including mice, hamsters, rabbits, cats, dogs, and pigeons (15). The phenomenological similarity of the syndrome across a variety of species may be reflective of a common functional role subserved by this system. Thus, across some measure of phylogenetic diversity, one of the common roles of the CNS serotonin system may be to modulate the sensorimotor systems whose activation, in the extreme, is manifested as increased extensor tone, reciprocal rhythmic forelimb movements, etc.

Of some relevance to the present discussion focusing on neurological disorders are experiments in which we have used this syndrome to provide the first behavorial evidence for the functional interaction between dopamine and serotonin (14). If L-DOPA, the immediate precursor of dopamine, is administered to rats pretreated with a monoamine oxidase inhibitor (MAOI), one observes a syndrome with all of the neurological signs described above. On the basis of the motoric similarity of these two syndromes, we hypothesized that the L-DOPA syndrome was mediated by serotonin, most likely through its displacement from presynaptic storage sites. Evidence in support of this comes from a study in which the MAOI plus L-DOPA treatment was administered to animals pretreated with a serotonin-synthesis inhibitor. In this case, the syndrome was either totally blocked or substantially attenuated; however, when the MAOI was combined with the serotonin precursor L-tryptophan, it produced a syndrome that was not affected by catecholamine synthesis inhibition but was, as expected, blocked by serotonin-synthesis inhibition. Studies from Curzon's laboratory (3,7) have indicated that not only does dopamine modulate many of the signs of the syndrome, but it appears to do so differentially. Pharmacologically induced increases in central dopaminergic activity will augment some aspects of the syndrome while inhibiting others (3,7).

We also conducted a series of studies that demonstrated that the syndrome was mediated, almost exclusively, by the action of serotonin in the brainstem and spinal cord (18). Little, if any, of the extensive forebrain innervation by serotonergic neurons appears to be importantly involved in the production of this constellation of neurological signs. If serotonin does play a role in posthypoxic myoclonus, these studies may help point the way toward elucidating the anatomical locus of its dysfunction. Since the syndrome is composed of a variety of neurological signs and simple stereotyped behaviors, we reasoned, by analogy with what is known about the dopamine system, that the neostriatum might be critically involved. Accordingly, we began by aspirating the entire neostriatum in rats. Unexpectedly, the complete drug-induced syndrome was observed in this preparation. We then began a series of experiments in which the neuraxis was to be transected in successively more caudal cuts until we abolished the syndrome. Again, somewhat unexpectedly, a cut at the caudal mesencephalic level still left the syndrome essentially intact. Complete cerebellectomy also had no distinctive effect on the syndrome.

These data indicating an important role of serotonin in brainstem and spinal mechanisms for motor control are consistent with recent neurophysiological data. In studies employing extracellular single-unit analyses, serotonin has been shown to facilitate directly the activity of motoneurons in both brainstem (25) and spinal cord (36). Thus, central serotonin may play an important role in a variety of motor disorders, e.g., tremor, rigidity, and athetosis. Such effects may be mediated primarily by means of a direct effect of serotonin on brainstem and spinal cord motoneurons.

In the intervening years since the serotonin syndrome was first described, a number of studies have indicated that the preceding description is somewhat of an oversimplification. First, not all serotonin-agonist drugs elicit these effects. Indole nucleus structure compounds elicit the syndrome, whereas piperazine-derivative compounds are not very effective (23). Second, different presumed serotonin-antagonist drugs block different aspects of the syndrome (11). Third, the relative effectiveness of various serotonin antagonists to block the syndrome depends on which agonist was employed in eliciting it (11). In light of recent neuropharmacological evidence indicating that at least two or three different serotonin receptors exist in the mammalian CNS, the most parsimonious interpretation of these data is that actions at various sertonergic receptors may be involved in mediating the various component signs of the syndrome.

Our most recent studies utilizing this syndrome are of general relevance to clinical neurology and perhaps directly relevant to myoclonus. We employed the well-known finding that destruction of serotonergic axon terminals by means of an intracerebroventricular injection of a neurotoxin (5,7-dihydroxytryptamine) results in the development of denervation supersensitivity (31). When rats pretreated in this way are tested several weeks later, they show a dramatic shift to the left in the dose-response curve for the ability of serotonin agonists or precursors to elicit the syndrome. In collaboration with Dr. Efrain Azmitia, we examined whether this supersensitivity could be reversed or "normalized" by means of transplantation of fetal rat brain serotonergic neurons into the brains of adult serotonin-denervated animals. If this treatment proved effective, it could potentially be employed clinically to reverse serotonergic dysfunction such as that seen in posthypoxic myoclonus. When fetal rat brain serotonergic neurons (15 or 16 days of gestation) are transplanted into an adult rat brain, they remain viable for at least several weeks or months. This is evidenced by their visualization with the light microscope, after the brain tissue has been processed for serotonin immunohistochemistry. In spite of this viability we have been unable, to date, to reverse the effects of serotonergic denervation with transplantation of fetal rat brain tissue into either the medulla or the thalamus of the adult rat brain. Thus, the increased sensitivity of the denervated animal to display the serotonergic syndrome or to respond with head shakes to 5-hydroxytryptophan is undiminished following transplantation of serotonergic neurons. Whether this means that the transplanted tissue, although viable, is not functional or that the transplanted tissue has not been placed in the appropriate site remains to determined. Since it is not clear precisely where the head-shake response or the various components of the syndrome are mediated, and since it is known that the processes from transplanted tissue do not migrate over a great distance, it is possible that the appropriate reinnervation simply has not occurred. On the other hand, we also have preliminary evidence in support of the nonfunctional nature of the transplanted tissue. Utilizing glass micropipettes, Dr. James Heym, in my laboratory, had very little success in finding slow and rhythmic firing cells (apparently universal characteristics of serotonergic neurons) in transplanted serotonergic neurons studied in chloral hydrate–anesthetized adult rats. I hasten to add that if this is true, it is contrary to what has been reported for transplanted dopaminergic neurons (37).

This concludes our discussion of the motoric effects of increasing CNS serotonergic activity. Other authors in this volume will discuss the direct elicitation of myoclonic responses in the guinea pig by means of 5-hydroxytryptophan. However, it should be noted that the relevance to human posthypoxic action myoclonus, of either the rat serotonin syndrome or 5-hydroxytryptophan–induced myoclonus in the guinea pig, is questionable. Recall that the human disorder is *ameliorated* by serotonin precursors, whereas reciprocally, the animal responses are *elicited* by precursor administration. However, such studies may still provide important insights into the general interaction between serotonin and motor function.

CAT SINGLE-UNIT STUDIES

Another basic research method for examining the relationship between the brain serotonergic system and motoric activity involves recording the extracellular single-unit discharge of serotonergic neurons. In my laboratory, we have been conducting such studies in awake, freely moving cats for the past 7 years. To date, we have studied serotonergic neurons in four of the major groupings of these cells in the cat brain: nucleus raphe dorsalis, nucleus centralis superior, nucleus raphe magnus, and nucleus raphe pallidus (17). One of our major findings is that the activity of serotonergic neurons in nucleus raphe dorsalis, the major source of forebrain serotonin, appears to be regulated by activity in central motor pathways or some variable tightly coupled to motor activity, e.g., sympathetic tone. We have not yet had the opportunity to examine the relationship of the other groups of serotonergic neurons to central motor activity. The following is an overview of our results in this area.

McGinty and Harper (26) were the first to report that the activity of brain serotonergic neurons changed from a slow and regular discharge pattern during waking to become virtually silent during REM sleep. Several years later, we confirmed and extended these results in my laboratory (32). We reported that across the complete sleep–wake–arousal cycle the activity of serotonergic neurons was strongly correlated with level of behavorial arousal or tonic motor activity. During these studies we were most impressed by the nearly complete suppression of serotonergic neuronal discharge during rapid-eye-movement (REM) sleep. Since REM sleep is a complex process, it was not clear whether this dramatic change in serotonergic unit activity was related to the REM sleep state per se or whether it was a correlate of one of the many physiological variables that comprise this state. Because our previous work indicated that the activity of these neurons was positively correlated with tonic motor activity, we hypothesized that the decreased unit activity during REM sleep might be related to the profound antigravity muscle atony that characterizes this state. To examine this issue experimentally, it would be necessary to separate the atonia from the REM sleep state. We have done this in two ways: by producing REM sleep without atony and, reciprocally, by producing atonia outside of REM sleep.

When bilateral lesions are placed in the pontine tegmentum of cats, the animals display REM sleep without atony (12,22). Following an extended period of slow-wave sleep, a cat with this lesion typically elevates its head and begins isolated movements of the limbs. The cat may right itself and move forward or backward and may even engage in complex behavorial acts, such as walking or attack. During this period, the eyes are open, the pupils fissurated, and the nictitating membranes relaxed. Furthermore, pontogeniculate-occipital (PGO) waves, hippocampal theta rhythm, and increased brain temperature are present, as during REM sleep in normal cats. By all criteria, these animals appear to be in REM sleep, except that they display overt behavior, presumably because the mechanism normally responsible for producing atony has been disrupted.

In normal cats, the activity of serotonergic neurons typically declines by greater than 90% in the transition from quiet waking (approximately 3 spikes/sec) to REM sleep (approximately 0.1 spikes/sec) (32). In cats displaying REM sleep without atony, this decrease in unit activity is much smaller (33). This is especially true in those animals showing the greatest degree of overt behavior and locomotion during

REM sleep. In those animals, the decrease in the transition from quiet waking to REM sleep was only 40% (from 1.5 to 0.9 spikes/sec). In fact, some of the cells studied in this latter group displayed a discharge level during REM sleep that approximated that seen during quiet waking, something never seen in normal cats. This experiment supported our hypothesis that the activity of brain serotonergic neurons is positively related to level of muscle tonus or tonic motor activity.

Another way to examine this issue is to study atony in the absence of REM sleep. If small amounts of the cholinomimetic agent carbachol are injected into the pontine tegmentum of cats, a profound atony is produced (1). Important from our perspective is the fact that these animals often manifest unambiguous periods of waking during this atony, as reflected by the animal's ability to track a visual stimulus or to respond to a looming object. In confirmation of our hypothesis, in these periods of carbachol-induced atony during waking, serotonergic unit activity was almost totally suppressed (29).

To examine whether this correlation was with central or peripheral aspects of motor activity, we administered the paralytic agent succinylcholine in a dose sufficient to block respiration completely (the cats were intubated and artificially respired) (29). In this case, the peripherally induced paralysis or atony was unaccompanied by a change in serotonergic unit activity. We tentatively concluded that the activity of these neurons is related to some aspect of the central motor system rather than the peripheral motor system. These results also make it seem unlikely that movement-generated afferent feedback exerts a major controlling influence on serotonergic neurons.

The final series of experiments in support of this hypothesis employed muscle relaxants known to act either centrally or peripherally. When a central muscle relaxant, mephenesin, was given, the activity of serotonergic neurons sharply declined in association with the occurrence of atonia. However, when dantrolene, a peripherally acting muscle relaxant, was administered, there was no alteration of unit activity associated with the atony (29).

Incidental observations from a number of studies in my laboratory are also consistent with this hypothesized relationship between serotonergic unit discharge and activity in central motor systems. Decreased unit activity occurs in conjunction with various instances of overt behavioral suppression or relaxation (17). For example, we have seen dramatic decreases in serotonergic unit activity when a cat is lifted by the scruff of the neck (as with many animals, the cat goes limp during this procedure); during defecation; and during the production of the sensorimotor rhythm (a 12–16-Hz cortical EEG rhythm associated with behavorial inhibition or response suppression).

These data indicate that the discharge of serotonergic neurons in nucleus raphe dorsalis is strongly associated with activity in central motor systems. The relationships described in the preceding sections probably involve active inhibition, rather than disfacilitation, since the depressant effect on serotonergic unit activity seen during REM sleep can be blocked, at least partially, by a pontine lesion. It may, in fact, be this area of the brain that exerts this inhibitory influence on these serotonergic neurons in the situations described in this section. We realize that a good deal more information is needed before we can conclude with any precision that this relationship is between raphe unit discharge and motor systems, rather than some concomitant of manipulating motor activity, such as alteration in sympathetic nervous system outflow. At present, we consider this a working hypothesis, but it is one that accounts for a large number of the changes that are seen in the unit activity of these serotonergic neurons. Whether such a relationship also holds for serotonergic neurons in other raphe nuclei will be determined in future experiments.

These data, in conjunction with data presented in the preceding section, indicate that serotonin neurons are involved in central motor control in at least two fundamentally different ways. First, the activity of serotonin neurons directly controls or modulates the activity of brainstem and spinal motoneurons. On the other hand, in an almost reciprocal fashion, the activity of serotonergic neurons appears to be under the control of central motor centers. It is still unclear how these two processes are interrelated.

Although these results may not have immediate relevance to the etiology, diagnosis, or treatment of posthypoxic action myoclonus, they are pertinent in a general way. They provide a description of how and, to some extent, where increased central serotonergic activity is manifested behaviorally. They also delineate the conditions under which serotonergic neurons become active or quiescent. These latter changes may be important in understanding and interpreting changes in serotonin metabolism observed in clinical studies.

AN ANIMAL MODEL FOR POSTHYPOXIC ACTION MYOCLONUS

In this final section, I shall describe some aspects of pharmacologically elicited cat behaviors that are suggestive of myoclonic jerks. This is done while recognizing full well the inherent limitations of modeling human neurological disorders with acute, drug-induced changes in animal behavior. Nonetheless, these findings are presented here in the hope that they may provide at least some additional understanding of posthypoxic action myoclonus.

In the course of studying the behavioral effects of LSD in the cat, we observed that this drug elicited a number of unusual behaviors that were rarely seen in normal, untreated animals (20,21). One of these, the limb flick response, may be relevant to myoclonus since its gross topography is characteristic of myoclonic jerk. Some animals given an LSD dose of 50 µg/kg, i.p., would emit as many as 100 of these responses in the first postdrug hour. The group mean at this dose was typically about 50 limb flicks per hour. The response is similar or identical to that seen in the normal cat whose paw comes into contact with a foreign substance (e.g., dirt or water). Typically, the paw is lifted and rapidly snapped or flicked outward from the body. It is a discrete, phasic, relatively simple, and somewhat stereotyped motor response that appears to be involuntary. As with myoclonic jerks, the limb flick response is often repetitive, with two or three occurring in rapid succession. Also like myoclonus, they are more prevalent in the forelimbs than the hindlimbs. However, unlike myoclonic jerks, we have not seen any evidence to indicate that the limb flick response can be brought on or enhanced by stimulation in various sensory modalities.

Of special importance for a model of posthypoxic action myoclonus is the fact that the limb flick response can be elicited by a number of different manipulations that decrease functional activity in central serotonergic synapses. For example, this response can be produced by the major hallucinogenic drugs [LSD, psilocin, 2,5-dimethoxy-4-methylamphetamine (DOM), and mescaline] (19,21), all of which decrease, at least to some extent, the discharge rate of serotonergic neurons. The limb flick response also can be elicited by pharmacological agents that decrease serotonergic neurotransmission by other means: synthesis inhibition, receptor blockade, or serotonin nerve terminal destruction (16). This is not, however, a necessary condition for evoking this response. Recent studies in my laboratory and in those of other investigators have shown that quipazine, lisuride, apomorphine, and pilocarpine also can elicit the limb flick response (24,30,35). Despite some question regarding which brain neurochemical system is primary to this response, one thing is clear: the limb flick response in the cat is heavily dependent on decreased serotonergic neurotransmission and increased dopaminergic neurotransmission. This fact, combined with the overt myoclonic-jerk-like nature of the response, makes it of potential use in studying the etiology and treatment of posthypoxic action myoclonus. Finally, and of special interest for the study of myoclonus, is our recent finding that quipazine-induced limb flicks can be blocked by pretreatment with 5-hydroxytryptophan (30).

CONCLUSION

This chapter has provided a brief overview of our research on the relationship of the CNS serotonin system to central motor systems. These findings may be relevant to posthypoxic action myoclonus at two different levels. The limb flick response may be directly useful as an analog of myoclonic jerks. On the other hand, our research on the complex serotonergic motor syndrome in rats and our studies of motor-relatedness of serotonergic unit activity in freely moving cats have a more general and basic relevance to myoclonus and to other forms of neuro- and psychopathology.

Three different aspects of the relationship between the brain serotonergic system and motor activity have been reviewed: the behavioral/neurological effect of pharmacologically increasing brain serotonin levels in rats; studies of the influence of autonomic and/or motoric manipulations on single-unit activity of brain serotonergic neurons in awake, freely moving cats; and description of a *possible* animal model for posthypoxic action myoclonus.

ACKNOWLEDGMENT

The author's work described in this chapter was supported by a grant from the USPHS-National Institute of Mental Health (MH 23433).

REFERENCES

1. Amatruda TT, Black DA, McKenna TM, McCarley RW, Hobson JA. Sleep cycle control and cholinergic mechanisms: differential effects of carbachol injections at pontine brain stem sites. *Brain Res* 1975;98:501–15.
2. Anden NE, Corrodi H, Fuxe K, Hokfelt T. Evidence for a central 5-hydroxytryptamine receptor stimulation by lysergic acid diethylamide. *Br J Pharmacol* 1968;34:1–7.
3. Andrews CD, Fernando JCR, Curzon G. Differential involvement of dopamine containing tracts in 5-hydroxytryptamine-dependent behaviours caused by amphetamine in large doses. *Neuropharmacology* 1982;21:63–8.
4. Corne SJ, Pickering RW, Warner BT. A method for assessing the effects of drugs on the central actions of 5-hydroxytryptamine. *Br J Pharmacol* 1963;20:106–20.
5. Crow TJ, Deakin JFW. Role of tryptaminergic mechanisms in the elements of the behavioural syndrome evoked by tryptophan and a monoamine oxidase inhibitor. *Br J Pharmacol* 1977;59:461P.
6. Deakin JFW, Dashwood MR. The differential neurochemical bases of the behaviours elicited by serotonergic agents and by the combination of a monoamine oxidase inhibitor and L-DOPA. *Neuropharmacology* 1981;20:123–30.
7. Dickenson SL, Curzon G. Roles of dopamine and 5-hydroxytryptamine in stereotyped and non-stereotyped behaviour. *Neuropharmacology* 1983;22:805–812.
8. Fahn S. Posthypoxic action myoclonus: review of the literature and report of two new cases with response to valproate and estrogen. In: Fahn S, Davis JN, Rowland LP, eds. *Advances in neurology vol. 26.* New York: Raven Press, 1979:49–84.
9. Fuxe K. Evidence for the existence of monoamine neurons in the central nervous system. IV. Distribution of monoamine terminals in the central nervous system. *Acta Physiol Scand* 1965;64 (Suppl. 247):41–85.
10. Grahame-Smith DG. Studies in vivo on the relationship between brain tryptophan, brain 5-HT synthesis and hyperactivity in rats treated with a monoamine oxidase inhibitor and L-tryptophan. *J Neurochem* 1971;18:1053–66.
11. Green AR. Pharmacological studies on serotonin-mediated behaviour. *J Physiol (Paris)* 1981;77:437–47.
12. Henley K, Morrison AR. A re-evaluation of the effects of the pontine tegmentum and locus coeruleus on phenomena of paradoxical sleep in the cat. *Acta Neurobiol Exp (Warsz)* 1974;34:215–32.
13. Jacobs BL. Effect of two dopamine receptor blockers on a serotonin-mediated behavioral syndrome in rats. *Eur J Pharmacol* 1974;27:363–6.
14. Jacobs BL. Evidence for the functional interaction of two central neurotransmitters. *Psychopharmacology* 1974;39:81–6.
15. Jacobs BL. An animal behavior model for studying central serotonergic synapses. *Life Sci* 1976;19:777–86.
16. Jacobs BL. Mechanism of action of hallucinogenic drugs: focus upon postsynaptic serotonergic receptors. In: Grahame-Smith DG, ed. *Psychopharmacology 1.* Amsterdam: Excerpta Medica, 1983:344–76.
17. Jacobs BL, Heym J, Steinfels GF. Physiological and behavioral analysis of raphe unit activity. In: Iversen LL, Iversen SD, Snyder SH, eds. *Handbook of Psychopharmacology; vol.18.* New York: Pergamon Press 1984:343–395.
18. Jacobs BL, Klemfuss H. Brain stem and spinal cord mediation of a serotonergic behavioral syndrome. *Brain Res* 1975;100:450–7.
19. Jacobs BL, Trulson ME, Stark AD, Cristoph GR. Comparative effects of hallucinogenic drugs on behavior of the cat. *Commun Psychopharmacol* 1977;1:243–54.
20. Jacobs BL, Trulson ME, Stern WC. An animal behavior model for studying the actions of LSD and related hallucinogens. *Science* 1976;194:741–3.
21. Jacobs BL, Trulson ME, Stern WC. Behavioral effects of LSD in the cat: proposal of an animal behavior model for studying the actions of hallucinogenic drugs. *Brain Res* 1977;132:301–14.
22. Jouvet M, Delorme F. Locus coeruleus et sommeil paradoxal. *CR Soc Biol* 1965;159:895–9.
23. Luscombe G, Jenner P, Marsden CD. Pharmacological analysis of the myoclonus induced by 5-hydroxytryptophan in the guinea pig suggests the presence of multiple 5-hydroxytryptamine receptors in the brain. *Neuropharmacology* 1981;20:819–31.
24. Marini JL, Jacobs BL, Sheard MH, Trulson ME. Activity of a non-hallucinogenic ergoline

derivative, lisuride, in an animal behavior model for hallucinogens. *Psychopharmacology* 1981;73:328–31.

25. McCall RB, Aghajanian GK. Serotonergic facilitation of facial motoneuron excitation. *Brain Res* 1979; 169:11–27.

26. McGinty DJ, Harper RM. Dorsal raphe neurons: depression of firing during sleep in cats. *Brain Res* 1976;101:569–75.

27. Sloviter RS, Drust EG, Connor JD. Specificity of a rat behavioral model for serotonin receptor activation. *J Pharmacol Exp Ther* 1978;206:339–47.

28. Steinbusch HWM. Distribution of serotonin-immunoreactivity in the central nervous system of the rat—cell bodies and terminals. *Neuroscience* 1981;6:557–618.

29. Steinfels GF, Heym J, Strecker RE, Jacobs BL. Raphe unit activity in freely moving cats is altered by manipulations of central but not peripheral motor systems. *Brain Res* 1983;279:77–84.

30. Trulson ME, Brandstetter JW, Crisp T, Jacobs BL. Behavioral effects of quipazine in the cat. *Eur J Pharmacol* 1982;78:295–305.

31. Trulson ME, Eubanks EE, Jacobs BL. Behavioral evidence for supersensitivity following destruction of central serotonergic nerve terminals by 5,7-dihydroxytryptamine. *J Pharmacol Exp Ther* 1976;198:23–32.

32. Trulson ME, Jacobs BL. Raphe unit activity in freely moving cats: Correlation with level of behavioral arousal. *Brain Res* 1979;163:135–50.

33. Trulson ME, Jacobs BL, Morrison AR. (1981): Raphe unit activity during REM sleep in normal cats and in pontine lesioned cats displaying REM sleep without atonia. *Brain Res* 1981;226:75–91.

34. Van Woert MH, Rosenbaum D. L-5-hydroxytryptophan therapy in myoclonus. In: Fahn S, Davis JN, Rowland LP, eds. *Advances in Neurology; vol. 26.* New York: Raven Press, 1979:107–15.

35. White FJ, Holohean AM, Appel JB. Lack of specificity of an animal behavior model for hallucinogenic drug reaction. *Pharmacol Biochem Behav* 1981;14:339–43.

36. White SR, Neuman RS. Facilitation of spinal motoneurone excitability by 5-hydroxytryptamine and noradrenaline. *Brain Res* 1980;188:119–27.

37. Wuerthele SM, Freed WJ, Olson L, Morihisa J, Spoor L, Wyatt RJ, Hoffer BJ. Effect of dopamine agonists and antagonists on the electrical activity of substantia nigra neurons transplanted into the lateral ventricle of the rat. *Exp Brain Res* 1981;44:1–10.

Advances in Neurology, Vol. 43: Myoclonus,
edited by S. Fahn et al. Raven Press,
New York © 1986.

Reengineering the Brain Serotonin System: Localized Application of Specific Neurotoxins and Fetal Serotonergic Neurons into the Adult CNS

Efrain C. Azmitia

Department of Biology, New York University, New York, New York 10003

There are a number of experimental procedures for changing whole-brain levels of serotonin. These techniques have proved very useful in defining the role of serotonin in a large number of biobehavioral phenomena, which include aggression, sleep, pain sensitivity, motor reflex, memory, punishment, sexual activity, locomotor activity, hormone secretion, and food intake. The anatomy of the CNS serotonin system (Azmitia and Gannon, *this volume*) argues against these neurons being directly involved in the organization of such diverse functions. The few thousand cells that comprise the 5-hydroxytryptamine (5-HT) system can give rise to axons with millions of varicosities, thousands of branches, and a number of target brain areas. However, one should not consider these neurons as comprising a diffuse or a homogeneous system. There is good evidence from anatomical studies that each group of serotonergic cells innervates a set of specific interacting target areas. Thus, the neurons of the median raphe nucleus innervate the septum, cingulate cortex, and hippocampus; the neurons of the dorsal raphe nucleus innervate the substantia nigra, caudate, and accumbens; the neurons of the raphe pallidus innervate the inferior olivary nuclei and the cerebellum; the neurons of the raphe obscurus innervate the motoneurons of the cranial nuclei and of the spinal cord. [For more detail, see Azmitia (1) and Deakin (19).]

Whole-brain reduction of serotonin is not a suitable method to analyze this complex and varied chemical network. Direct injection or iontophoretic application of serotonin to specific areas of the brain has provided useful information on the acute effects of 5-HT. In this chapter, experimental methods will be presented for altering serotonergic innervations of localized brain regions in a paradigm suited for studying the chronic effects of serotonin deafferentation or hyperinnervation.

USE OF CHEMICAL NEUROTOXINS: SPECIFIC AND LOCAL DESTRUCTION

The selective destruction of serotonergic fibers by a chemical neurotoxic drug was first shown by Baumgarten and his colleagues in 1971 (10a). These workers demonstrated that intraventricular injection of 25 to 75 μg of 5,6-dihydroxytryptamine (5,6-DHT) resulted in a significant fall of whole-brain serotonin levels in the rat. The use of 5,7-dihydroxytryptamine (5,7-DHT) is now considered superior to 5,6-DHT since it has a higher *in vivo* neurotoxic potency (10). The injection of 5,7-DHT must be used in conjunction with uptake blockers that protect catecholaminergic neurons. Desipramine and nomifensine have been proposed to offer optimum protection of norepinephrine (NE) and dopamine (DA) uptake mechanism.

The injection of 5,7-DHT directly into the brain provides a powerful tool to manipulate the serotonergic system. Bjorklund et al. (12) first showed that a midline injection of 4 μg of 5,7-DHT (in a 4-μl vehicle) into ventromedian midbrain tegmentum surrounding the interpeduncular nucleus produced a substantial reduction of 5-HT content (-85%) and ^{3}H-5HT uptake (-90 to -94%) in the forebrain of rats. Similar injections of the neurotoxins into midbrain were subsequently made to study specific serotonin functions (27,32). Fuxe et al. (22) used intracerebral injections to compare ascending and descending serotonergic fibers. Both biochemical and functional studies were performed on these animals. The next step toward a more localized depletion was microinjections unilaterally into medial forebrain bundle (8,25,29). This procedure caused substantial loss of the ipsilateral forebrain serotonergic fibers. This model is useful for pharmacological (29), anatomical (8), and biochemical (25) studies performed in conjunction with an asymmetrical turning model of serotonin function.

However, all of these earlier studies produced depletion of serotonergic fibers in a number of different target areas. It was therefore impossible to ascribe a single function to a depletion of serotonin in a localized area of the brain. The important question remained; do individual 5-HT terminal fields have unique functions in the control of behavior? It had already been shown that serotonergic nuclei subserved different functions, since lesions of the median raphe nucleus produced increased locomotor activity, whereas lesions of the dorsal raphe nucleus produced changes in pain-elicited aggression (28,30). Compatible results were described by Geyer et al. (24) and Srebro and Lorens (40).

However, both the median and dorsal raphe nuclei have multiple connections in the rat (8) and the cat (15). Do all the neurons within a single nucleus subserve the same function despite projecting to different areas of the brain? This would suggest that the serotonergic system has a diffuse and homogeneous role in brain activity. If, in contrast, serotonergic fibers do subserve unique functions in different neuroanatomical locations, then the system should be viewed as having precise but heterogeneous roles in brain activity.

The approach to this problem required that intracerebral injections be made in selected branches of the serotonergic fiber network so that localized areas of the brain could be depleted of their serotonergic afferents while the vast majority of the system remained intact. This chapter will describe our method of intracerebral injection of 5,7-DHT into various forebrain target sites and the type of information we have found with our procedure.

USE OF BRAIN TRANSPLANTATION: THE PROMISES
AND THE PROBLEMS

One of the major developments of neural science research in the last two decades has been the discovery of the tremendous plasticity of the brain. The organ subserving the mind was once considered a complex collection of hard-wired circuits that slowly ceased working with age. Recent work has refuted this static concept, and the brain is now regarded as existing in a highly dynamic state, with connections being made and broken throughout life. The most extreme example of this plasticity is brain transplantation.

Brain transplantation studies generally consist either of grafting pieces of fetal brain tissue onto the surface of the brain and into the fluid-filled ventricle (17,41) or of microinjections of fetal cells (13). This latter procedure is more useful when the fetal cells are implanted deep into the substance of a mature brain. When the donor fetal neurons and the host adult neurons are combined, both immediately begin growing new processes (sprouting). The sprouts from the fetal neurons extend for long distances throughout the adult nervous tissue and seek out specific regions to form terminal branches. It seems as if the process of brain development is reenacted, but now the interacting cells are of completely different ages. The brains of old mice (which already show clear signs of neuronal deterioration) (3) are quite capable of attracting and supporting the sprouts from the donor fetal neurons (7). Recent evidence indicates that fetal sprouts may actually reverse some age-related behavioral deficits (23).

This ability to change the functioning of the adult brain by transplantation of fetal neurons explains the excitement concerning this new technique. It has already been established that abnormalities can be produced when specific chemical systems are destroyed. It is now firmly established that replacement of the destroyed systems by transplanting fetal cells of the same chemical system leads to a reinstatement of the normal behavior (20,36). In our experiments, the ability of hormones to induce female sexual activity can be greatly enhanced by selective and localized destruction of serotonergic fibers (33) in the hypothalamus. This facilitation is completely reversed when fetal serotonergic neurons are microinjected into the same hypothalamic area (34). The transplantation of fetal cortex (a different neuronal system from the one destroyed) does not restore normal sexual behavior.

Brain transplantation is still in its early stages, and many problems are not yet solved. For example, we have observed that a dense glial scar forms around the transplant when the fetal cells are injected into the adult brain (9). These glial cells are a natural defense against any form of brain injury, and one of their functions is to digest foreign substances. Although many sprouts from the fetal neurons escape through this barrier to enter the adult brain, it appears that a complete integration between fetal and adult neurons is inhibited. How can this scar be prevented without harming the fetal neurons?

A second problem we have encountered is the lack of a readily available and consistent source of fetal neurons. Ideally, we desire a suspension of well-characterized cells at a known concentration and in a form that can be stored indefinitely. Thus, a frozen, homogeneous preparation of a neuronal system of known chemical transmitter content is required (such preparations of glial cells are already available). This chapter will describe our transplant procedure and briefly describe some of our results in dealing with both the promise and problems arising from introducing fetal serotonergic cells into the adult brain.

MATERIALS AND METHODS

Animals

Adult rodents are used for most of our studies. The rats are Sprague-Dawley, weighing just over 200 g. In aging studies, we have used mice (C57BL) because it is more economical than purchasing aged rats. Care should be taken to maintain a normal light/dark cycle and to study animals at the same times of the day. It should also be emphasized that yearly rhythms may play crucial roles in hormone and transmitter synthesis.

Micropipettes

The most crucial factor for obtaining reliable results is to have a reproducible means of injecting small volumes (less than 1 μl). We have developed a simple and inexpensive microsyringe (Fig. 1). A glass micropipette is pulled, using the tip of a disposable Pasteur pipette. These should be pulled by hand after even heating over a small flame. The micropipettes we use have a shank of at least 2 cm. The tip diameter is between 50 and 90 μm for neurotoxin injections, between 150 and 200 μm for dissociated cells, and between 250 and 400 μm for tissue suspensions. The tip is attached to a 19-gauge needle using 5-min epoxy cement. Care should be taken to have the cement move along the base of the pipette and the needle up to the tip of the needle. The pipette and needle should be relatively straight, although this is not crucial, since the movement of the tip of the pipette is governed by the stereotaxic arm. After the glass pipette is secured to the needle, the assembly should be stored in 70% alcohol until needed.

A plunger from a 10-μl Hamilton syringe (or similar-diameter wire) is attached to a micrometer (available from a good hardware store for about \$20). The micrometer is secured to the vertical arm of a stereotaxic frame. The micropipette assembly is filled with a sterile light oil. (The best pipettes are those that have no air pockets, especially between the glass pipette and the syringe needle. The plunger is then coated with a heavy grease and slowly inserted into the needle. The needle is attached to the bottom of a Kopf syringe arm. The turning of the micrometer will now displace 100 nl of oil for every 1 mm of vertical travel of the plunger.

The micropipette is filled under visual inspection with the aid of a dissecting microscope. A small air bubble is drawn up to mark the top of the solution. The exact amount of solution to be injected is drawn up into the micropipette by slowly turning the micrometer and observing that the air bubble moves up smoothly. The

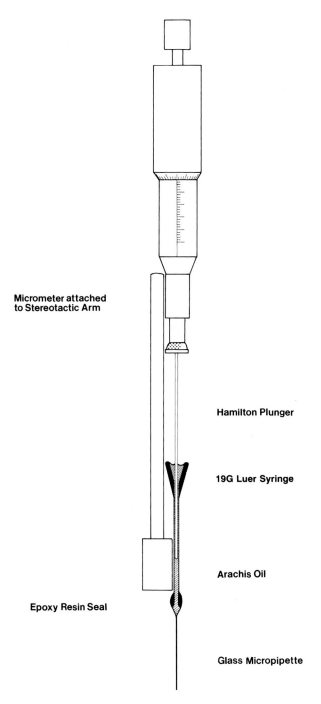

FIG. 1. Diagram of micropipette system.

remaining solution is kept at 5°C in the dark. The solution is ejected into the brain at a slow rate (5–50 nl/min) under visual inspection to ensure smooth and complete delivery into the injection site. The pipette can be raised 0.5 mm if more than 500 nl is to be injected. At the conclusion of the pressure injection, the tip should be left in the brain for several minutes to allow the solution to diffuse and not flow back up the pipette track as it is slowly removed from the brain.

Stereotaxic Microsurgery

The delivery of small amounts of solution into deep structures within the brain requires that accurate coordinates be established in all three planes (vertical, horizontal, and lateral). Coordinates obtained from a stereotaxic atlas or from published studies should serve only as a general guide. There are several reasons why this is true. First, the reference points on the rodent skull are usually the suture lines lambda and bregma. A landmark of earbar zero obtained from the stereotaxic apparatus also can be measured and used to locate internal brain structures. These landmarks are not constant to internal brain tissue from strain to strain, within strains, and even within an individual during adult development. In our studies, many trial injections with dyes are made in order to establish a reliable relationship between a location within the brain and one (or more) of the external landmarks. We have found that in certain cases the distance between lambda and bregma may be useful to locate accurately a precise point in the brain (43,44). Therefore, all three external coordinates (bregma, lambda, and earbar zero) should be utilized during trial injections to increase the accuracy of establishing a reliable indicator of soft brain tissue sites.

Pre- and Postinjection Care

In order to minimize infection, several precautions are taken with our rats. The rats are first completely anesthetized with a long-lasting drug (e.g., chloropent). The dorsal surface of the head is shaved and swabbed with alcohol. A long incision of the skull skin is made ($\approx$2 cm) so the lambda and bregma landmarks are easily visible after gently cleaning the skull. Using a 2-mm drill bit, a circular hole ($\approx$3 mm in diameter) is made in the skull up to, but not damaging, the dura. With the aide of a dissecting scope, a pin is inserted through the dura at the site where the micropipette will pass. Extreme care should be taken to avoid damage to the surface blood vessels. This is the reason a large enough surface of skull dura is exposed by drilling. Nothing is gained, and serious bleeding is risked, by drilling a small hole ($\approx$1 mm) through skull, dura, and cerebral surface.

The skin flaps are sutured tightly after the surgery is completed. The exposed surface is swabbed with an iodine solution, and a topical antibiotic is then sprayed over the incision. Rats are returned to a clean cage and kept warm (do not overheat) until recovery.

Preparation and Injection of Neurotoxin Solution

We usually purchase 5,7-DHT from Sigma Chemical Corp., St. Louis, and store it desiccated, in the dark, and at $-20°C$. The vial is brought to room temperature in a desiccated jar and approximately 2 mg weighed into a 1-ml conical-shaped tube. The amount of free-base neurotoxin is determined by multiplying the percent purity (provided by Sigma) and then dividing by 1.87 (to compensate for the weight of the salt–creatinine sulfate). The 5,7-DHT is then dissolved in ice-cold sterile Ringer's solution (or any balanced salt preparation) containing 0.2 mg/ml ascorbic acid (other reducing protecting agent can be substituted) to achieve a final concentration of 10 $\mu g/\mu l$ (2–12.5 $\mu gm/\mu l$ ranges have been used). The solution is stored in the dark and at $0°$ to $5°C$.

When the animal is ready to receive an injection, the micropipette is filled immediately before use. This is done not only to insure that the proper amount is injected but also to protect the 5,7-DHT from decomposition from the heat and light present during surgery. The pipette is lowered to the precise point; 50 nl is injected immediately, and this amount is subsequently injected every minute. If the fluid appears blocked (the upper meniscus does not move), the pipette can be raised 0.2 mm and another 50-nl turn made. This sequence can be repeated if the pipette remains blocked. However, after a maximum of three attempts, it is best to remove the syringe and clean the tip, because if too much pressure is built up, the eventual ejection of several hundred nanoliters can produce nonspecific damage to the tissue. Usually, smooth ejections are achieved if the tip size is greater than 50 μm and no external bleeding occurred. After all the solution has been injected, the syringe is then left in place for an additional 2 min before being slowly removed.

Preparation and Injection of Fetal Brain Tissue

We normally inject minced-tissue or dissociated-cell suspensions. The rat fetuses are removed between 14 and 17 days of gestation by a sterile cesarian procedure. The brains are removed to sterile balanced salt solution (e.g., Hank's or Ringer's), and a midbrain raphe strip is dissected using sterile procedures. The midbrain strip lies in the region between the mescencephalic and pontine flexures and extends vertically from just under the cerebral aqueduct to the ventral floor of the midbrain. Carefully remove the underlying pia. These strips (2 mm long, 1 mm wide, and 1 mm high) are placed in ice-cold balanced salt solution containing 1% glucose. If dissociated cells are desired, the strips are placed in 5 ml of Versene 1:5,000 [a sterile ethylenediamine-tetraacetic acid (EDTA) solution obtained from Gibco, Grand Island, New York] and gently repipetted through a Pasteur pipette in which the tip was flamed. When most of the tissue is no longer visible, the solution is allowed to settle, and the cloudy supernatant is removed and centrifuged at 500 to 800 G for 5 min. The pellet is resuspended in a balanced salt solution and recentrifuged. The final pellet is resuspended in glucose solution to give a volume of approximately 2 μl per raphe strip.

When the animal is ready to receive a suspension transplant, a single raphe strip is placed on a clean surface and minced into 6 to 10 pieces. The resultant slurry is then drawn up into the micropipette. Care should be taken to collect all of the tissue without introducing air bubbles. *Do not let tissue dry out.* Immediately after filling the microsyringe, lower it into the brain and begin to eject. The total volume is usually between 1.3 and 2.0 µl. This is ejected at a rate of 100 nl/min. In our work, the pipette tip is lowered 0.2 mm below our vertical coordinate, and the pipette is slowly raised 0.2 mm before the first tissue ejection. The pipette is raised 0.2 mm every five turns of the micrometer. After complete injection, the pipette is left 2 min.

RESULTS

The results to be summarized in this chapter deal almost exclusively with the serotonergic innervation of the dorsal hippocampus. This projection has been previously summarized by us in detail (1,2,8).

Briefly, there are three main projection routes to the dorsal hippocampus. The two routes from the median raphe nucleus are a supracallosal one, which travels above the corpus callosum with the cingulum bundle (CB), and an infracallosal one, traveling below the corpus callosum with the fornix–fimbria system. The third projection originates in the dorsal raphe nucleus and innervates the ventral hippocampus, using a ventrolateral route through the amygdala and entorhinal cortex.

Localized 5-HT Deafferentation

The intracerebral method of injecting 5,7-DHT can be selective and very effective. Two microinjections of 5,7-DHT (5 µg) were made in a desipramine-pretreated rat; one into the fornix–fimbria and one into each of the CB pathways. The amount of ^{3}H-5HT taken up into the dorsal hippocampal slices was essentially completely eliminated within 6 days (6). This was confirmed by showing that the percentage of total radioactivity in the slices remaining after 5,7-DHT injections (31%) was similar to the nonspecific uptake estimated by incubating with excess of unlabeled 5-HT (27%) or fluoxetine (37%) (Table 1). Furthermore, partial elimination of the fibers to the hippocampus can be produced by injections either into the CB or the fornix–fimbria. These single injections produce a hippocampal decrease of 30 to 60% in high-affinity uptake (4,43) and in tryptophan hydroxylase activity (16).

In contrast to these biochemical studies indicating a marked removal of hippocampal serotonergic fibers, pharmacological studies after fornix–fimbria and CB injections of 5,7-DHT failed to show any change in the receptor binding of serotonin, spiroperidol, or ketanserin in dorsal hippocampus (37). These results are in agreement with earlier studies finding no change in serotonin cortical binding after 5,7-DHT (42).

The specific removal of serotonergic fibers by 5,7-DHT has been verified by several anatomical procedures. Injections of 5,7-DHT into the CB blocked the

TABLE 1. *[³H]5-HT (5 × 10⁻⁸ M) uptake in hippocampal slices*[a]

Treatment	No. of determinations	Conc. (M)	Averages + SD (pmol/g)	Percentage[b]
Normal	12	—	245 ± 59	100
5-HT	9	1×10^{-5}	67 ± 18	27
5,7-DHT	3	*In vivo*	77 ± 9	31
Fluoxetine	3	1×10^{-4}	91 ± 7	37
	3	1×10^{-6}	111 ± 17	45
	4	1×10^{-7}	140 ± 29	57
Tryptophan	3	1×10^{-5}	233 ± 27	95
Norepinephrine	4	2×10^{-3}	90 ± 13	37
	4	1×10^{-4}	161 ± 20	66
	4	1×10^{-5}	195 ± 40	80
	3	1×10^{-6}	213 ± 33	87
Desipramine (DMI)	4	2×10^{-4}	84 ± 7	34
	4	1×10^{-5}	177 ± 19	72
	3	1×10^{-6}	222 ± 6	91
	3	1×10^{-7}	186 ± 51	76
5-HT and DMI	5	1×10^{-5}	46 ± 27	19
Cold	7	—	13 ± 5	5
Cold + 5-HT	3	1×10^{-5}	3.4 ± 0.3	1

[a]The drugs and chemicals are added before [³H]5-HT, incubation for 15 min in oxygenated Ringer's solution with pargyline, ascorbic acid, and dextrose at 37°C. (From ref. 6.)
[b]Based on 100% control uptake.

anterograde transport of radioactive proteins into the dorsal hippocampus 24 hr after injections of [³H]proline into the median raphe nucleus (4). This neurotoxin can also immediately block the retrograde transport of horseradish peroxidase from the dorsal hippocampus to the median raphe nucleus but does not block transport in noradrenergic fiber from the locus ceruleus (46). The 5-HT immunoreactive (IR) fibers in part of the hippocampus and in all of the CB can be eliminated by prior microinjections of 5,7-DHT into the CB (47). Finally, high-affinity ³H-5HT uptake sites can be visualized by fixation and radioautography. These sites correspond to axonal varicosities and terminals (Azmitia and Gannon, *this volume*). The prior injection of 5,7-DHT virtually removes all of these high-affinity uptake sites, which are seen as aggregates of silver grains (6).

The 5,7-DHT deafferentation of hippocampal serotonergic input also leads to electrophysiological changes. The stimulation of the medial septal nucleus can produce theta rhythms in the hippocampus between 6 and 10 Hz in the rat; normally the threshold current is minimum at 7.7 Hz. However, removal of serotonergic fibers produces a minimum threshold current at 6.9 Hz (35). In another protocol, the stimulation of the perforant pathway (pp) elicits a characteristic evoked action potential (EAP) in the granule cell layer of the dentate gyrus. The EAP was recorded in rats depleted of hippocampal serotonin by prior injection of *p*-chloroamphetamine (PCA) or 5,7-DHT as well as in untreated animals during two behavioral states, slow-wave sleep (SWS) and still-alert behavior (SAL). In untreated rats, the amplitude of the EAP response was significantly greater during SWS than SAL. In contrast, in animals injected with PCA or 5,7-DHT, there was no difference in the amplitude of the EAP during SWS and SAL (40a). It is concluded that 5-HT innervation of the dentate gyrus may be involved in the behavioral modulation of the EAP response. These two results demonstrate that removal of 5-HT causes electrical changes within the hippocampus.

The intracerebral injections also can be used to change the behavior of animals. Our initial observation demonstrated that microinjections of 5,7-DHT into the fornix–fimbria produced a dose-dependent decrease only in the hippocampal high-affinity ^{3}H-5HT uptake (43). These animals also showed a dose-dependent increase in nocturnal locomotor activity that was significantly negatively correlated to the uptake of serotonin in individual rats (r, -0.89; p, 0.001). We were able subsequently to establish that a single unilateral injection in the CB could produce an asymmetrical orientation response after injections of 5-HTP (4). Other sites outside of the hippocampus have been injected with 5,7-DHT by us to produce changes in turning (medial forebrain bundle) (8), circadian rhythm of corticosterone (suprachiasmatic nucleus) (44), and sexual lordosis in response to estrogen (ventromedial nucleus of hypothalamus) (34). Thus, localized 5-HT deafferentation can lead to behavioral changes, even if only part of the total serotonergic innervation is removed (43).

The removal of serotonergic fibers can lead to reorganization of the remaining chemical systems. Our own work has been directed at studying homotypic collateral sprouting: the expansion of undamaged serotonergic cells into areas of the brain vacated by destroyed serotonergic fibers. Our plasticity model consists of selective lesioning with 5,7-DHT of the serotonergic fibers traveling in the cingulum bundle. The reorganization of the serotonergic system within the hippocampus can thus be studied over time using a variety of methods, including retrograde (48) and anterograde (4) transport, measurement of tryptophan hydroxylase (16), 5-HT–IR axons (47), and behavior (4). The use of neurotoxins to study homotypic and heterotypic plastic changes is an area of study that deserves much more attention.

Raphe Transplantation

The introduction of fetal serotonergic cells into discrete areas results in serotonin cell hyperinnervation. The first report of transplantation of fetal serotonergic neurons was by Bjorklund et al. (14). This group reported that placing a piece of fetal raphe tissue in a cortical cavity resulted in an abnormal innervation of the hippocampus by the serotonergic fibers. Extensive studies with this grafting procedure led to the conclusions "that good survival rate is obtained only when the graft is in contact with the richly vascularized choroidal fissure or its extended vascular bed" (46, p. 6) and that "neural transplants seem to grow better in the brains of neonatal animals than in those of the adult animals" (17, p. 152).

Microinjection of minced or dissociated tissue is a better means of transplanting fetal neuronal cells into the brain parenchyma because stereotaxic placement in deep areas is possible without severe damage to the adult brain. Excellent survival and proper innervation of host target sites has been obtained with this microinjection approach (7). Trypsin-dissociated fetal cells survive and will function after transplantation (13,23,38). However, mechanical dissociation procedures provide a better yield of healthy serotonergic neurons *(unpublished observation)*, and this preparation is compatible with brain transplantation procedures (9). Routinely, 1 to 2 μl of mechanically dissociated or minced fetal neurons are microinjected directly into the dorsal hippocampus. Injecting fetal (E 14-17) cells into a normal hippocampus results in a hyperinnervation of appropriate target sites (7). Thus, even if the endogenous serotonergic fiber system is intact, the adult homeostatic balance between target tissue and afferent neurons can be altered by increasing the latter. Conversely, the transplantation of a serotonergic target tissue, such as the hippocampus, will result in ingrowth (expansion) of the adult serotonergic fibers into the donor fetal hippocampus (7). In summary, brain transplantation of fetal tissue provides an effective means of resetting the normal chemical balance in discrete brain regions.

The adult brain is, of course, not static but constantly changing. In the mouse, the serotonergic innervation to the hippocampus increases for many months after birth and then begins to decrease after about 20 months (3). This interaction between age and serotonergic density answers important questions about neuronal aging. Neonates are better hosts than adult animals (17), probably because the host brain is immature and plastic [e.g., see Lewis and Cotman (31) and Harvey and Lund (26)]. However, can fetal neurons survive in an aged brain? The answer is yes (7,23,39).

Fetal serotonergic neurons survive, mature, and appropriately innervate the hippocampus of aged mice. A resultant hyperinnervation was demonstrated by high-affinity uptake studies *(unpublished observation)*. Gage and his co-workers (23) noted that certain aged-related motor impairments were reversed by intrastriatal nigral grafts. These studies strongly indicate that chemical changes in the brain can be altered by fetal transplants, even when it appears that the endogenous neurons of the host animals are failing because of some age-related phenomenon. This application of fetal neuronal transplantation has tremendous promise.

There are problems associated with brain transplantation studies. We shall mention two. First, complete integration of fetal neurons into the adult brain is rarely accomplished. Even when the cells are dissociated prior to injection, immunocytochemical studies indicate that the donor fetal cell bodies remain largely segregated from the adult neuropil (9). One explanation for this observation is that a glial scar forms around the injected tissue, and this barrier prevents the mixing of the neuronal cell bodies, although many processes penetrate the barrier. The existence of a glial barrier was verified by staining the recipient adult host with an antibody raised against glial fibrillary acidic protein (GFA) (9). The amount of GFA within an astrocyte increases when these glial cells become reactive. This occurs after damage to the brain. Studies performed by Hakan Bjorklund and his colleagues (11) indicate that the formation of the glial scar after transplantation into neonatal rats is due to existing glial cells becoming reactive (migration and transformation), not increasing in number. Studies to control the formation of a glial scar should be of great benefit to the usefulness and applicability of brain transplantation. A second problem concerns the source of tissue for transplantation studies. Das and his co-workers (18) have demonstrated that fetal tissue can be stored frozen before transplantation. This requires the use of 10% DMSO as a cryoprotectant. The source of donor tissue remains unresolved. Homogenous cells for transplantation may be derived from enodcrine glands. This is being pioneered by transplantation of adrenal medullary cell (21). The availability of stable cells of known transmitter content will expedite the study of brain transplantation.

DISCUSSION

Our results demonstrate the feasibility of chemically changing the serotonergic innervations in discrete areas of the adult mammalian brain. These manipulations produce morphological, biochemical, and physiological changes. The main conclusion is that small local alterations in the serotonergic system have effects on the working of the brain.

These observations with chemical toxins and fetal transplants emphasize the central role played by serotonin in many regions of the CNS. As described by Azmitia and Gannon *(this volume)* the serotonergic fibers reach every area of the primate brain and can regulate neuronal interactions. Given this expansive distribution and given that local alterations can influence the physiology of the region, it is no wonder that serotonin has been directly implicated in so many disease states, including myoclonus. The question remains: where is the disturbance located?

Serotonergic fibers are probably not unique in their ability to influence local brain activity. It has been shown that selective removal of adrenergic, dopaminergic, cholinergic, and substance-P neuronal systems cause a disruption of normal brain functioning. Therefore, the brain can be considered to be in a chemical balance, and removal of one chemical system is sufficient to modify the function of the whole. This would be analogous to the fact that disruption of a single electrical contact can stop a computer. Furthermore, deletion of serotonergic fibers can result in expansion of the nonserotonergic cells, both neuronal and glial. Thus, eliminating one chemical system alters the equilibrium among the remaining systems. Changes in transmitter release, postsynaptic receptors, firing rate, glial transformation, and other events need to be considered. The appropriate treatment of disease states requires attention to all of these factors. To achieve this goal, the exact brain location of the fault must be identified and appropriate corrective measures applied locally.

ACKNOWLEDGMENT

The research work reported in this chapter was supported by a grant from the National Science Foundation, BNS 83-04704.

REFERENCES

1. Azmitia EC. The serotonin producing neurons of the midbrain median and dorsal raphe nuclei. In. Iversen SD and Snyder S, eds. The handbook of psychopharmacology; vol. 9. New York: Plenum Press, 1978:233–314.

2. Azmitia EC. Bilateral serotonergic projections to the dorsal hippocampus of the rat: simultaneous localization of retrograde transported ^{3}H-5HT and HRP. *J Comp Neurol* 1981;203:737.

3. Azmitia EC, Brennan MJ, Quartermain D. Adult development of the hippocampal serotonin system of C57BL/6N mice; analysis of high-affinity uptake of ^{3}H-5HT. *Int J Neurochem* 1983;5:39–44.

4. Azmitia EC, Buchan AM, Williams JH. Structural and functional restoration by collateral sprouting of hippocampal 5-HT axons. *Nature* 1978;274:374–7.

5. Azmitia EC, Gannon PJ. The ultrastructural localization of serotonin immunoreactivity in myelinated and unmyelinated axons within the medial forebrain bundle of rat and monkey. *J Neurosci* 1983;3:2083–90.

6. Azmitia EC, Marovitz WF. In vitro hippocampal uptake of tritiated serotonin (^{3}H-5HT); a morphological, biochemical and pharmacological approach to specificity. *J Histochem Cytochem* 1980;28:636–44.

7. Azmitia EC, Perlow MJ, Brennan MJ, Lauder JM. Fetal raphe and hippocampal transplants in adult and aged C57BL/6N mice; an immunohistochemical study. *Brain Res Bull* 1981;7:703–10.

8. Azmitia EC, Segal M. An autoradiographic analysis of the differential ascending projections of the dorsal and median raphe nuclei in the rat. *J Comp Neurol* 1978;179:641–67.

9. Azmitia EC, Whitaker PM. Formation of a glial scar following microinjection of fetal raphe neurons into the dorsal hippocampus or midbrain of the adult rat; an immunocytochemical study. *Neurosci Lett* 1983;38:145–50.

10. Baumgarten HG, Klemm HP, Sievers J, Schlossberger HG. Dihydroxytryptamine as tools to study the neurobiology of serotonin. *Brain Res Bull* 1982;9:131–50.

10a. Baumgarten HG, Björklund A, Lachenmayer L, Nobin A, Stenevi U. Long-lasting selective depletion of brain serotonin by 5,6-dihydroxytryptamine. *Acta Physiol Scand* 1971;(Suppl) 373:1–16.

11. Bjorklund H, Dahl D, Haglid K, Rosengren L, Olson L. Astrocytic development in fetal parietal cortex grafted to cerebral and cerebellar cortex of immature rats. *Dev Brain Res* 1983;9:170–81.

12. Bjorklund A, Nobin A, Stenevi U. The use of neurotoxic dihydroxytryptamines as tools for morphological studies and localized lesioning of central indoleamine neurons. *Z Zellforsch* 1973;145:479–501.

13. Bjorklund A, Schmidt RH, Stenevi U. Functional reinnervation of the neostriatum in the adult rat by use of intraparenchymal grafting of dissociated cell suspensions from the substantia nigra. *Cell Tissue Res* 1980;212:39–45.

14. Bjorklund A, Stenevi U, Svendgaard N-A. Growth of transplanted monaminergic neurons into the adult hippocampus along the perforant path *Nature* 1976;262:787–90.

15. Bobillier P, Seguin S, Petitijean F, Salvert D, Touret M, Jouvet M. The raphe nuclei of the cat brainstem: a topographical atlas of their efferent projections as revealed by autoradiography. *Brain Res* 1976;113:449–86.

16. Clewans C, Azmitia EC. Compensatory changes in tryptophan hydroxylase after induced homotypic collateral sprouting of hippocampal serotonergic fibers. *Brain Res* 1984;307:125–33.

17. Das GD, Hallas BH, Das KG. Transplantation of neural tissue in the brains of laboratory mammals: technical details and comments. *Experientia* 1979;35:143–53.

18. Das GD, Houle JD, Brasko J, Das KG. Freezing of neural tissues and their transplantation in the brain of rats: technical details and histological observations. *J Neurosci Methods* 1983;8:1–15.

19. Deakin JFW. Roles of serotonergic systems in escape, avoidance and other behaviours. In: SJ, Cooper ed. Theory in psychopharmacology. London: Academic Press, 1983;150–93.

20. Dunnett SB, Bjorklund A, Stenevi U, Iversen SD. Behavioural recovery following transplantation of substantia nigra in rats subjected to 6-OHDA lesions of the nigrostriatal pathway. I. Unilateral lesions. *Brain Res* 1981;215:147–61.

21. Freed WJ, Morihisa JM, Spoor E, Hoffer BJ, Olson L, Seiger A, Wyatt RJ. Transplanted adrenal chromaffin cells in rat brain reduce lesion-induced rotational behaviour. *Nature* 1981;292:351–2.

22. Fuxe K, Ogren S-O, Agnati LF, Jonsson G, Gustafsson J-A. 5,7-Dihydroxytryptamine as a tool

to study the functional role of central 5-hydroxytryptamine neurons *Ann NY Acad Sci* 1978;305:346–69.

23. Gage FH, Dunnett SB, Stenevi U, Bjorklund A. Aged rats: recovery of motor impairments by intrastriatal nigral grafts. *Science* 1983;221:966–9.

24. Geyer MA, Puerto A, Menkes B, Segal DS, Mandell AJ. Behavioral studies following lesions of the mesolimbic and meostriatal serotonergic pathways. *Brain Res* 1976;106:257–70.

25. Giambalvo CT, Snodgrass SR, Uretsky NJ. Effects of serotonin neurotoxins on rotational behavior in the rat. *Ann NY Acad Sci* 1978;305:524–31.

26. Harvey AR, Lund RD. Transplantatin of tectal tissue in rats. II. Distribution of host neurons which project to transplants. *J Comp Neurol* 1981;202:505–20.

27. Hole K, Fuxe K, Jonsson G. Behavioral effects of 5,7-dihydroxytryptamine lesions of ascending 5-hydroxytryptamine pathways. *Brain Res* 1976;385–99.

28. Jacobs BL, Cohen A. Differential behavioral effects of lesions of the median or dorsal raphe nuclei in rats: open field and pain elicited aggression. *J Comp Psychol* 1976;90:102–8.

29. Jacobs BL, Simon SM, Ruimy DD, Trulson ME. A quantitative rotational model for studying serotoninergic function in rats. *Brain Res* 1977;124:271–81.

30. Jacobs BL, Wise WD, Taylor KM. Differential behavioral neurochemical effects following lesions of the dorsal or median raphe nuclei in rats. *Brain Res* 1974;79:353–62.

31. Lewis ER, Cotman CC. Mechanisms of septal lamination in the developing hippocampus revealed by outgrowth of fibers from septal implants. I. Positional and temporal factors. *Brain Res* 1980;196:307–30.

32. Lorens SA, Guldberg HC, Hole K, Kohler C, Srebro B. 1976. Activity, avoidance learning and regional 5-hydroxytryptamine following intra-brainstem 5,7-dihydroxytryptamine and electrolytic midbrain raphe lesions in the rat. *Brain Res* 1976;108:97–113.

33. Luine VN, Frankfurt M, Rainbow TC, Biegon A, Azmitia EC. Intrahypothalamic 5,7-dihydroxytryptamine facilitates feminine sexual behavior and decreases ³H-imipramine binding and 5-HT uptake. *Brain Res* 1983;264:344–8.

34. Luine V, Renner KJ, Frankfurt M, Azmitia EC. Raphe transplants into the hypothalamus of 5,7-DHT treated female rats alters hormonal dependent sexual behavior. *Science* 1984;226:1436–39.

35. McNaughton N, Azmitia EC, Williams JH, Buchan A, Gray JA. Septal elicitation of hippocampal theta rhythm after de-afferentation of serotonergic fibers. *Brain Res* 1980;200:259–69.

36. Perlow MJ, Freed WJ, Hoffer BJ, Seiger A, Olson L, Wyatt RJ. Brain grafts reduce motor abnormalities produced by destruction of nigrostriatal dopamine system. *Science* 1979;204:643–7.

37. Quik M, Azmitia E. Selective destruction of the serotonergic fibers of the fornix-fimbria and cingulum bundle increases 5-HT$_1$ but not 5-HT$_2$ receptors in rat midbrain. *Eur J Pharmacol* 1983;90:377–84.

38. Schmidt RH, Bjorklund A, Stenevi U. Intracerebral grafting of dissociated CNS tissue suspension: a new approach for neuronal transplantation to deep brain sites. *Brain Res* 1981;218:347–56.

39. Sladek JR, Gash DM. The use of neural grafts as a means of restoring neuronal loss associated with aging. *Anat Rec* 1982;202:178A.

40. Srebro B, Lorens SA. Behavioral effects of selective midbrain raphe lesions in the rat. *Brain Res* 1975;89:303–25.

40a. Srebro B, Azmitia EC, Winson J. Effects of selective depletion of hippocampal 5-HT on neuronal transmission from perforant path through dentate gyrus. *Brain Res* 1982;235:142–7.

41. Stenevi U, Bjorklund A, Svendgaard NA. 1976. Transplantation of central and peripheral monoamine neurons to the adult rat brain: techniques and conditions for survival. *Brain Res* 1976;114:1–20.

42. Whitaker PM, Deakin JFW. Does (³H) serotonin label presynaptic receptors in rat frontal cortex? *Eur J Pharmacol* 1981;73:349–51.

43. Williams JH, Azmitia EC. Hippocampal serotonin reuptake and nocturnal locomotor activity after micro-injections of 5,7-DHT in the fornix-fimbria. *Brain Res* 1981;207:95–107.

44. Williams JH, Maill-Allen VM, Klinowska M, Azmitia EC. Effects of microinjections of 5,7-dihydroxytryptamine in the suprachiasmatic nuclei of the rat on serotonin reuptake and the circadian variation of corticosterone levels. *Neuroendocrinology* 1985;36:431–5.

45. Zhou FC, Azmitia EC. Induced collateral sprouting of hippocampal 5-HT fibers; a quantitational HRP study in the rat. *Soc Neurosci Abst* 1981;7:68.

46. Zhou FC, Azmitia EC. Effects of 5,7-dihydroxytryptamine on HRP retrograde transport from hippocampus to midbrain raphe nuclei in the rat. *Brain Res Bull* 1983;10:445–51.
47. Zhou FC, Azmitia EC. Induced homotypic sprouting of hippocampal 5-HT fibers: an immuno-cytochemical study of the rat. *Soc Neurosci Abst* 1983;9:985.
48. Zhou FC, Azmitia EC. Homotypic collateral sprouting of hippocampal serotonergic fibers demonstrated by retrograde transport of horseradish peroxidase in the rat. *Brain Res* 1984;308:53–62.

Advances in Neurology, Vol. 43: Myoclonus,
edited by S. Fahn et al. Raven Press,
New York © 1986.

L-5-HTP–Induced Myoclonic Jumping Behavior in Guinea Pigs: An Update

Paul Carvey, J. E. Paulseth, Christopher G. Goetz,
and Harold L. Klawans

*Department of Neurological Sciences, Rush-Presbyterian St. Lukes Medical Center,
Chicago, Illinois 60612*

In 1973, Klawans et al. (11) reported the production of myoclonus in intact guinea pigs following subcutaneous injections of 5-hydroxytryptophan (5-HTP), the immediate precursor of serotonin (5-HT). The temporal pattern of the response is outlined in Table 1. All animals given 300 mg/kg or more developed myoclonus. When fully developed, the myoclonus involved all major muscle groups and was symmetric, generalized, and rhythmic. Some animals simultaneously lifted all four feet off the floor and were propelled forward by the myoclonic jerks.

This behavior represents the only model of myoclonus in intact animals treated with a single agent. Other investigators have presented animal behaviors termed myoclonic but have always pretreated animals with a toxin or performed a neurosurgical procedure before administration of myoclonus-inducing agents (14). On the other hand, the use of this agent alone has produced more complex behaviors in species other than the guinea pig (8,16). The 5-HTP myoclonic model in guinea pigs, studied pharmacologically, anatomically, and physiologically, forms the basis of this presentation.

METHODS

We have found that myoclonus of similar frequency can be produced by 300 mg/ kg of 5-HTP, 125 mg/kg of L-5-HTP, or 35 mg/kg of L-5-HTP after pretreatment

TABLE 1. *Response to 300 mg/kg 5-HPT, s.c.*

Minutes	Response
0–10	Self-limited variable neck jerks, also induced by acidic medium alone
10–35	Piloerection, defecation, increased grooming, vasodilation of ear vessels
20–35	Irregular shocklike neck jerks (extension or lateral)
35–90	Generalized symmetric rhythmic jerking, variable limb stretching, writhing, or "wet-dog shakes"
90–120	Return to normal behavior

with carbidopa 25 mg, p.o., 2 hr and 4 hr before L-5-HTP. We currently use the latter regimen because the total volume injected is lower, thus reducing the acid load, and the mortality rate is lower. These amounts represent the threshold doses that produce myoclonus in all animals treated. The L-5-HTP is prepared as a supersaturated solution in distilled water, at a concentration of 40 mg/ml, and gradually acidified with 4 N HCl until it is in solution, usually requiring a pH between 2.5 and 3.5. The behavior is easily quantified by counting the number of jumps per minute, at 10-min intervals, throughout the duration of the behavior. We have then used the sum of these scores as the animal score. Even though all animals are given threshold doses and all do develop myoclonus, there is a large variance in animal scores. Furthermore, our scoring does not consider intensity, and when the jerks are low in amplitude it can be difficult to differentiate them from normal behavior. Such responses preclude the use of mechanical counters. We are currently trying to reduce the variance in the model by correcting for variable absorption of L-5-HTP. We have found that the behavior correlates quite well with plasma levels of 5-HTP (r, 0.75).

SEROTONERGIC PHARMACOLOGICAL STUDIES

There is considerable evidence that this behavior is mediated by central serotonergic systems, but the anatomic pathways remain unknown. The behavior correlated with whole-brain 5-HT levels (11) (see Table 2) and could be blocked by the 5-HT antagonists methergoline and cyproheptadine, whereas it was not blocked by antagonists of the cholinergic, α- and β-adrenergic, or dopaminergic systems (scopolamine, atropine, phentolamine, propranolol, haloperidol, pimozide, and chlorpromazine) (6,11,17). Furthermore, other serotonergic agents also have been shown to produce this behavior. Although the 5-HT precursor L-tryptophan did not produce myoclonic jumping behavior (MJB) when used alone in doses of 125 mg/kg, it did when combined with the monoamine oxidase inhibitors tranylcypromine (17) or pargyline (6). The 5-HT agonist 5-methoxy-N,N-dimethyltryptamine, and quipazine, a 5-HT releaser and uptake inhibitor, both produced myoclonus (6,17).

These data all suggest that MJB is predominantly due to activation of the 5-HT transmitter system. However, this does not preclude modification by other neurotransmitter systems. This will be discussed below.

TABLE 2. *Effect of 300 mg/kg of 5-HPT on whole-brain serotonin concentration*

Time (min)	N	Serotonin conc. (μg/g)	Time (min)	N	Serotonin conc. (μg/g)
0	6	0.25 ± 0.018	30	4	0.53 ± 0.051
7½	4	0.23 ± 0.013	60	4	0.75 ± 0.032
15	4	0.38 ± 0.043	60[a]	4	0.84 ± 0.043

[a]These animals also were given methysergide, 0.8 mg/kg.

PHYSIOLOGICAL STUDIES

Chadwick et al. (6) found that the myoclonus consisted of a synchronous 40-to-50-msec burst of EMG activity in forelimbs and hindlimbs, followed by a 50-to-75-msec period of electrical silence, then variable EMG activity up to 400 msec. The EMG activity was not accompanied by cortical EEG activity. Electrical stimuli to the limbs and photic and auditory stimuli did not affect the myoclonus. Cortical evoked potentials induced by auditory or electrical stimuli were not augmented by 5-HTP. These results are most compatible with a subcortical focus, perhaps in the brainstem.

ANATOMICAL STUDIES

The postulate of a brainstem-mediated mechanism underlying MJB gained further support when Chadwick et al. (6) found that MJB persisted after midcollicular decerebration but was abolished by midthoracic sectioning of the spinal cord. Thal and Wolfson (15) studied this further by means of autoradiography using [^{14}C]-desoxyglucose given 15 min after varying doses of L-5-HTP. These experiments revealed increased metabolic activity in the central thalamus, ventral anterior nucleus, and thalamic commissure, and decreased activity in the hippocampus and cerebral cortex, in animals given 150 mg/kg or more of L-5-HTP. These changes occurred with or without the actual development of myoclonus, which suggested that the observed alterations were not merely a reflection of the motor behavior. No mention was made of activity in the brainstem caudal to the red nucleus. The

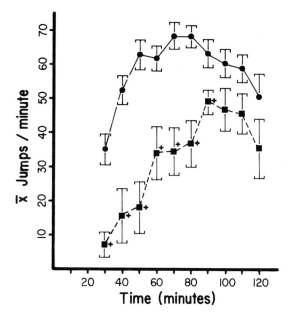

FIG. 1. The effect of apomorphine (Apo.) 0.5 mg/kg (■) on myoclonic jumping behavior induced by 100 mg/kg L-5-HTP (●). Each point represents the mean ± SEM of eight animals (+ = $p < 0.005$). N.S., normal saline.

authors suggested that serotonergic input from the dorsal raphe led to thalamic activation, either directly or indirectly via input to the cerebellum and then the thalamus. The cortical inhibition could be secondary to input from the dorsal raphe or secondary to thalamocortical input. Serotonin is inhibitory in the raphe and cerebral cortex (1) but excitatory in the facial nucleus (13) and reticular formation (3). Receptors for 5-HT are scanty in the thalamus but do exist (2). Nonetheless, it seems unlikely that the thalamus represents a final common pathway, given the results of the lesioning experiments already cited.

OTHER ACUTE PHARMACOLOGICAL STUDIES

Dopaminergic Agents

It has been shown that activity of other neurotransmitter systems can modify MJB. Acute administration of dopaminergic agents caused a significant reduction in the myoclonic response (18). The response to apomorphine is shown in Fig. 1. Similar responses were seen with the dopamine (DA) precursor, levodopa (as Sinemet® 40/400 mg/kg, p.o.), and the direct dopaminergic agonists lergotrile mesylate (50 mg/kg, s.c.), M-7(2[dimethylamino]5,6-dihydroxytetraline (2 mg/kg, s.c.) (18), and PBD (*N-n*-propyl-*N-n*-butyl-beta-(3,4-dihydroxyphenyl) ethylamine HCl (5 mg/kg, i.p.) (17), as well as DA-releaser amphetamine (7). It was also noted that stereotyped chewing behavior (SB), a manifestation of dopaminergic activity, was diminished by 5-HTP.

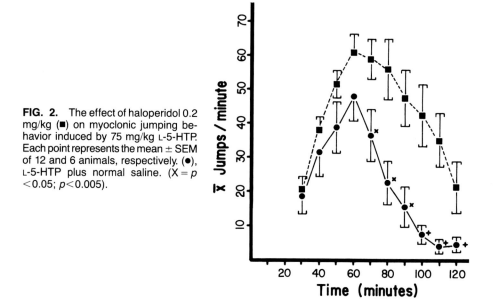

FIG. 2. The effect of haloperidol 0.2 mg/kg (■) on myoclonic jumping behavior induced by 75 mg/kg L-5-HTP. Each point represents the mean ± SEM of 12 and 6 animals, respectively. (●), L-5-HTP plus normal saline. ($X = p < 0.05$; $p < 0.005$).

Lisuride

More recently, we have also studied the effects of lisuride hydrogen maleate on this model (5). Lisuride is a direct DA agonist that also has central 5-HT activity (9). Not surprisingly, acute administration of this agent caused MJB that first appeared about 10 min after injection. This peaked at 25 min, then waned as DA-induced SB developed, and could no longer be observed approximately 40 min after injection.

MJB was produced by doses above 0.05 mg/kg, s.c., was maximal at 0.25 mg/kg, and was decreased again at 0.9 mg/kg (presumably due to the greater level of DA activity, which antagonized MJB).

Dopaminergic Antagonists

The administration of haloperidol, 1.5 mg/kg, i.p., 90 min after L-5-HTP, produced an insignificant increase in MJB (6), whereas 1 mg/kg, i.p., did not

TABLE 3. *Effect of morphine and naloxone on MJB[a]*

Group	MJB
Control	256 ± 18
Morphine (3.0 mg/kg, i.p.)	211 ± 21
Naloxone (0.9 or 1.2 mg/kg, i.p.)	295 ± 18

[a]All animals received L-5-HPT 35 mg/kg, s.c., after pretreatment with carbidopa. $N = 8$ in each group. Scores represent sum of jumps per minutes scored at 10-min intervals from 30 to 120 min ± SEM. Differences not significant ($t = 0.58$ morphine vs. controls; $t = 0.58$ naloxone vs. controls).

TABLE 4. *Effect of scopolamine and tremorine on MJB[a]*

Group	MJB
Controls	471 ± 17
Scopolamine	
0.1 mg/kg, i.p.	545 ± 23
0.25 mg/kg, i.p.	543 ± 33
0.50 mg/kg, i.p.	516 ± 7
Tremorine	
0.50 mg/kg, i.p.	209 ± 69
1.0 mg/kg, i.p.	251 ± 43
2.0 mg/kg, i.p.	22 ± 8[b]

[a]All animals received L-5-HTP 35 mg/kg, s.c., after pretreatment with carbidopa. $N = 8$ for controls, 4 for other groups. Scores as in Table 3.

[b]Significant for tremorine 2.0 vs. controls ($t = 0.584$, $p < 0.01$).

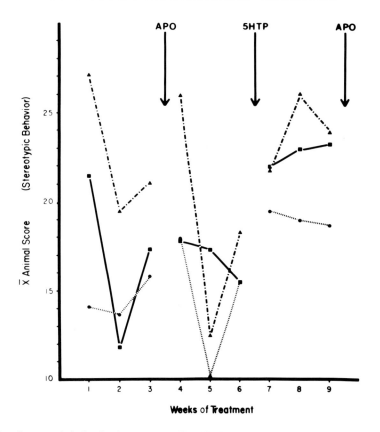

FIG. 3A. Stereotypic behavioral response to lisuride during chronic lisuride treatment: (●) 0.05, (■) 0.25, (▲) 0.50 mg/kg.

affect MJB alone but did block the decrease induced by apomorphine (17). The latter authors also found that pimozide, 2 mg/kg, i.p., had no effect on MJB. The effect of antidopaminergic agents was clarified when Weiner et al. (18) found that haloperidol, 0.2 mg/kg, s.c., given simultaneously with L-5-HTP, produced a significant augmentation of MJB (Fig. 2), whereas 1.0 mg/kg, s.c., produced an insignificant decrease in MJB. Thus, the response appears dose related, with only low doses of DA antagonists producing augmentation of MJB, i.e., the opposite effect of DA agonists. The high-dose effect of DA antagonists may be the result of nonspecific effects of these agents at high doses.

Reserpine, 2 mg/kg, s.c., 4 hr prior to 5-HTP, increased MJB (7). This can be explained as the effect of a DA depletor on MJB, or alternatively as the effect of a drug that blocks storage of 5-HT in granules, leading to the buildup of an active pool and hence an exaggerated response to a precursor load. A similar mechanism has been postulated to explain the increased SB seen when reserpine is used in conjunction with apomorphine or amphetamine.

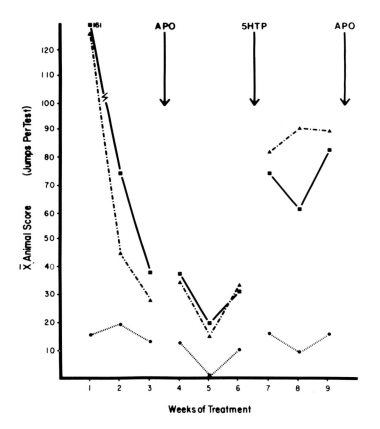

FIG. 3B. Myoclonic jumping response to lisuride: (●) 0.05, (■) 0.25, (▲) 0.50 mg/kg.

Clonazepam

Clonazepam, a drug that is useful in many types of myoclonus in humans, caused a mild increase in brain 5-HT levels after doses of 5 to 50 mg/kg, i.p., but this was less than the increase caused by threshold doses of 5-HTP, and it did not alter MJB (19). This finding suggests that its efficacy for myoclonus in humans may not be due to increased serotonergic activity. Indeed, this drug may actually decrease 5-HT release (12).

Opiates

Manipulation of the opiate system did not affect L-5-HTP–induced MJB. The response of MJB to morphine or naloxone is shown in Table 3.

Cholinergics

Manipulation of the cholinergic system did affect MJB. As noted previously, scopolamine, in doses of 0.1 to 0.5 mg/kg, i.p., had no significant effect. But the muscarinic agonist tremorine produced a dose-dependent decrease in L-5-HTP–induced MJB that did not appear to be due to excessive sedation (Table 4).

CHRONIC PHARMACOLOGIC STUDIES

The effects of chronic exposure to various agents are not always predictable from the acute effects. Furthermore, the results of chronic exposure may be more clinically relevant.

With this in mind, we recently conducted a pilot study in which the effect of oral L-5-HTP, 60 mg/kg/day, plus varying doses of carbidopa, was studied over a 3-week period. There was a trend toward increased MJB over time, but the variability exceeded that seen in the parenteral model, so that further study is needed. A chronic parenteral study is impossible, however, because of the frequent development of granulomas at injection sites due to the low pH of the HTP solution.

We have also studied the effects of chronic dopaminergic exposure. One hundred forty guinea pigs were treated with levodopa (as Sinemet 20/200 mg/kg/day, p.o.) for 12 weeks. These animals developed behavioral supersensitivity to levodopa. But after 48-hr washout periods, they were found to be subsensitive to apomorphine-induced SB (0.4 mg/kg, s.c.) and supersensitive to L-5-HTP–induced MJB (33 mg/kg, s.c., after pretreatment with carbidopa) (4). Thus, chronic administration of levodopa produces increased MJB, the opposite effect to that of acute levodopa administration. A clinical example of this DA and 5-HT interaction is the myoclonus that develops in some patients following chronic but not acute levodopa therapy. This myoclonus responds to methysergide (10). Bromocriptine, on the other hand, has produced inconsistent effects on L-5-HTP–induced MJB (5).

Chronic administration of lisuride (5) in several doses of 96 guinea pigs for 9 weeks produced a rapid tolerance to lisuride-induced MJB by 2 weeks, but by 9 weeks the behavior in the groups receiving 0.25 or 0.50 mg/kg/day had started to return to base-line values. SB also showed profound tolerance by 2 weeks, but by 7 weeks it had returned to base-line values and might well have exceeded base line had the study been longer. These responses are shown in Figs. 3A,B. The group receiving 0.50 mg/kg/day was compared to control animals at 9 weeks, in response to 0.50 mg/kg of lisuride, s.c. MJB was significantly decreased in the chronically treated animals (although Figs. 3A,B suggests this might have reversed with a longer exposure) and

TABLE 5. *Comparative profile of L-DOPA, bromocriptine, and lisuride*

Drug	Response to itself over time	Crossover to apomorphine[a]	Crossover to 5-HTP[a]
L-DOPA (200 mg/kg)	↑	↓	↑
Bromocriptine (5 mg/kg)	↔ ↓	↓ ↔ ↑	↔
Lisuride (0.50 mg/kg)	(SB) ↑ (MJB) ↑ (?)	↓	↓

[a]After a 48-to-72-hr washout.

SB was significantly increased. This treatment group also showed diminished MJB in response to L-5-HTP 35 mg/kg (after a 72-hr washout, then pretreatment with carbidopa) when compared to controls after 6 weeks, and diminished SB in response to apomorphine 0.3 mg/kg after 9 weeks of treatment and a similar washout period. The results of these chronic protocols are summarized in Table 5.

ACKNOWLEDGMENTS

This work was supported in part by grants from the United Parkinson Foundation, Chicago, and the Boothroyd Foundation, Chicago. Dr. Goetz is the recipient of the NINCDS Teacher/Investigator Award. Dr. Paulseth is the recipient of a Medical Research Council of Canada Fellowship.

REFERENCES

1. Aghajanian GK, Wang RY. Physiology and pharmacology of central serotonin neurons. In: Lipton MA, DiMascio A, Killum KF, eds. Psychopharmacology: a generation of progress. New York: Raven Press, 1978:171–83.
2. Bennett JL, Snyder SH. Serotonin binding of D-lysergic acid diethylamide (LSD) to brain membranes: relationship to serotonin receptors. *Brain Res* 1975;94:523–44.
3. Boakes RJ, Bradley PB, Briggs I, et al. Antagonism of 5-hydroxytryptamine by LSD-25 in the central nervous system: a possible neuronal basis for the actions of LSD-25. *Br J Pharmacol* 1970;40:202–18.
4. Carvey PM, Goetz CG, Klawans HL. (1983): The effect of chronic levodopa treatment on stereotypic and myoclonic jumping behavior in the guinea pig. *Neurology* 1983;33(Suppl. 2):67.
5. Carvey PM, Klawans HL. Effect of chronic lisuride treatment on stereotypical and myoclonic jumping behavior in guinea pigs. In: Calne DB, Horowski R, McDonald RJ, Wuttke W, eds. Lisuride and other dopamine agonists. New York: Raven Press, 1983:97–107.
6. Chadwick D, Hallett M, Jenner P, Marsden CD. 5-hydroxytryptophan-induced myoclonus in guinea pigs: a physiological and pharmacological investigation. *J Neurol Sci* 1978;35:157–65.
7. Goetz CG, Klawans HL. (1974): Studies on the interaction of reserpine, *d*-amphetamine, apomorphine and 5-hydroxytryptophan. *Acta Pharmacol Toxicol* 1974;34:119–30.
8. Jacobs BL. An animal behavioral model for studying central serotonergic synapses. *Life Sci* 1976;19:777–86.
9. Kehr W. Effect of lisuride and other ergot derivatives on monoaminergic mechanisms in rat brain. *Eur J Pharmacol* 1977;41:261–73.
10. Klawans HL, Goetz C, Bergen D. Levodopa-induced myoclonus. *Arch Neurol* 1975;32:331–4.
11. Klawans HL, Goetz C, Weiner WJ. 5-hydroxytryptophan-induced myoclonus in guinea pigs and the possible role of serotonin in infantile myoclonus. *Neurology* 1973;23:1234–40.
12. Lidbrink P, Corrodi H, Fuxe H, Olson L. The effects of benzodiazepines, meprobamate, and barbiturates on central monoamine neurons. In: Garrattini S, Mussini E, Randall LO, eds. The benzodiazepines, New York: Raven Press, 1973:203.
13. McCall RB, Aghajanian GK. Serotonergic facilitation of facial motor neuron excitation. *Brain Res* 1979;169:11–28.
14. Stewart RM, Growdon JH, Carcian D, Baldessarini RJ. Myoclonus after 5-hydroxytryptophan in rats with lesions of indoleamine neurons in the central nervous system. *Neurology* 1976;26:690–2.
15. Thal LJ, Wolfson LI. (1981): Functional anatomy of L-5-hydroxytryptophan-induced myoclonus in the guinea pig. *Neurology* 1981;31:955–60.
16. Vetulani J, Bednarczyk B, Reichenberg K, Rokosz A. Head twitches induced by LSD and quipazine: similarities and differences. *Neuropharmacology* 1980;19:155–8.
17. Volkman PH, Lorens SA, Kindel GH, Ginos JZ. L-5-hydroxytryptophan-induced myoclonus in guinea pigs. A model for the study of central serotonin-dopamine interactions. *Neuropharmacology* 1978;17:947–55.
18. Weiner WJ, Carvey PM, Nausieda PA, Klawans HL. Dopaminergic antagonism of L-5-hydroxytryptophan-induced myoclonic jumping behavior. *Neurology* 1979;29:1622–5.
19. Weiner WJ, Goetz CG, Nausieda PA, Klawans HL. Clonazepam and 5-hydroxytryptophan-induced myoclonic stereotypy. *Eur J Pharmacol* 1977;46:21–4.

Advances in Neurology, Vol. 43: Myoclonus,
edited by S. Fahn et al. Raven Press,
New York © 1986.

Serotonin Models of Myoclonus in the Guinea Pig and Rat

Leslie I. Wolfson, Leon J. Thal, and Lucy L. Brown

Department of Neurology, Albert Einstein College of Medicine, Bronx, New York 10461

Myoclonus has been associated with abnormalities of the serotonergic system in both humans and animal experimental models. In posthypoxic patients with intention myoclonus, the 5-hydroxyindoleacetic acid (5-HIAA) concentration in cerebrospinal fluid is often diminished (11,24). These patients often improve after treatment with the serotonin precursor L-5-hydroxytryptophan (L-5-HTP) (3,6,10,17–19,24,26). This contrasts with the response of infants with Down's syndrome treated with L-5-HTP, who may develop myoclonus after such treatment (5).

The behavioral effects of L-5-HTP treatment in animals are species specific. After rats are given L-5-HTP following reserpine and the monoamine oxidase inhibitor pargyline, they develop a serotonergic behavioral syndrome that includes resting tremor, rigidity, reciprocal forepaw treading, hindlimb abduction, and lateral head weaving, (7–9,12–15). Klawans et al. (16) produced myoclonus in young guinea pigs following subcutaneous injection of L-5-HTP, without the accompanying serotonin behavioral syndrome seen in rats. After a brief delay, the guinea pigs developed an increase in grooming behavior and then changes in peripheral autonomic activity (piloerection and increased defecation). Myoclonus initially involved the head and neck but spread to become synchronous jerks of the entire body, which could be elicited by sensory stimuli. The myoclonus could be prevented by treatment with methysergide. Subsequently, Chadwick et al. (4) demonstrated that other serotonin agonists and precursor combinations also elicited the myoclonus. Myoclonus was blocked by both centrally acting decarboxylase inhibitors or serotonin antagonists but not by catecholamine or cholinergic antagonists. The L-5-HTP–induced myoclonus was unaccompanied by any electroencephalographic (EEG) discharges. It was not abolished by a brainstem transection at the level of the superior colliculus (which produced decerebrate posturing). The myoclonus was, however, abolished beneath a thoracic spinal cord transection.

The development of the [^{14}C]deoxyglucose (DG) technique (21) for regional quantification of glucose utilization provided the opportunity to observe L-5HTP–induced changes in metabolism in specific brain regions. Our initial series of experiments used a semiquantitative version of the DG technique (25), and we are now in the midst of updating these data with quantitative determinations of local cerebral glucose utilization in myoclonic and control guinea pigs.

METHODOLOGY OF DG AUTORADIOGRAPHIC EXPERIMENTS

Four- to six-week-old male Hartley guinea pigs (average weight 250–300 mg) received an intraperitoneal injection of L-5-HTP (Calbiochem, San Diego) and then were observed behaviorally, and in some instances the EEG was recorded. After the guinea pigs developed myoclonus, they received an intravenous injection of 60 μCi of [^{14}C]2-deoxy-D-glucose (2-DG) through a femoral vein cannula that had been implanted earlier that day under halothane anesthesia. Control animals received intraperitoneal saline. Thirty minutes later the guinea pigs were sacrificed, and the brains were quickly removed and frozen. Serial 20-μm sections were cut on a cryostat for both autoradiography and histologic verification. Relative isotope accumulation was determined in regions of interest (ROI) by transmission densitometry (Photovolt Model 520 Transmission Densitometer, Photovolt, New York) fitted with a 0.25-mm aperture. Each ROI had at least four densitometric measurements, which were averaged. To allow for comparison of individual guinea pigs, a mean white matter densitometric reading was obtained from the white matter of several regions in each animal. The relative density of each structure was computed as the ratio of gray to white matter density.

BEHAVIORAL AND EEG OBSERVATIONS

With increasing doses of L-5-HTP, a progressively higher fraction of the guinea pigs demonstrated myoclonus (Fig. 1). Below 75 mg/kg, there was no myoclonus, and above 200 mg/kg, the majority of guinea pigs developed myoclonus. The dose necessary for all guinea pigs to develop myoclonus (ED_{100}) was 400 mg/kg, whereas the ED for myoclonus induction in half of the animals (ED_{50}) was 174 mg/kg (calculated by method of least squares). The addition of carbidopa (in a ratio of

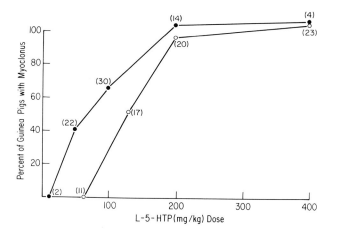

FIG. 1. L-5-HTP dose is plotted against the percentage of guinea pigs developing myoclonus. Numbers in parentheses indicate number of animals at each dose; (○) animals pretreated with only L-5-HTP; (●) animals pretreated with carbidopa and then injected with L-5-HTP.

1:4 with L-5-HTP, injected 30 min before the L-5-HTP) halved the ED_{50} and ED_{100} to 85 and 200 mg/kg, respectively.

Within 10 min after injection of the ED_{50} dose, the guinea pigs manifested neck and forelimb myoclonus that went on to generalized myoclonus at a rate of 25 to 35 jerks per minute lasting for 2 hr. At the ED_{100}, the myoclonus occurred within a few minute at a rate of 60 jerks per minute.

At a dose of 50 mg/kg, the guinea pig EEG was normal (12–16 Hz low-voltage fast), but at 150 and 400 mg/kg, there was slowing of the EEG to 2 to 4 Hz high-amplitude activity. The slowing disappeared 3 hr after administration of the L-5-HTP. The myoclonus was demonstrated on electromyographic (EMG) recording as polyphasic motor unit activity in both agonist and antagonist muscles. No clear-cut EEG discharges were noted during the myoclonus, although movement artifact may have obscured any paroxysmal EEG discharges present during the jerk.

AUTORADIOGRAPHIC OBSERVATIONS

In the myoclonic guinea pigs, the most striking changes in regional metabolism seen on visual inspection of the autoradiograms occurred in the thalamus (Fig. 2a and b). The densitometric readings from the ventrolateral nucleus and centromedian nucleus indicated that metabolism in these structures was higher than controls. Metabolism in other thalamic nuclei (e.g., dorsal lateral and ventroanterior) did not change significantly from controls. In both the centromedian and ventrolateral nuclei, the metabolic increases correlated with increasing L-5-HTP dose and were present in both the myoclonic and nonmyoclonic guinea pigs at the ED_{50} (Table 1).

In addition, there was widespread decrease in cortical glucose uptake (Fig. 2). This was substantiated by densitometric determinations, which showed diminished glucose uptake in the frontal and sensorimotor cortex of myoclonic guinea pigs at both the ED_{100} and ED_{50} but not in nonmyoclonic guinea pigs at the ED_{50} (Table 1). Preliminary analysis of our quantitative DG autoradiograms suggest that the cortical glucose utilization was diminished by as much as 50%.

The molecular layer of the hippocampus is usually clearly discernible on the normal guinea pig autoradiograms (Fig. 2a and b). This structure is no longer visible in the myoclonic guinea pigs. The third nerve nucleus and cerebellar nodulus appeared on the autoradiograms to have increased glucose uptake, although we were unable to substantiate this with our densitometric indices (Table 1) because of high interanimal variability.

MYOCLONUS INDUCED BY MICROINJECTION INTO THE DORSAL RAPHE REGION

Twenty young guinea pigs (250 g) were stereotaxically implanted with chronic indwelling cannulae directed at the dorsal raphe region. Ten days later they were injected with 60 to 200 μg per 0.5 to 2 μl of serotonin hydrochloride in saline. Eight of the animals developed pure myoclonus (15–60 jerks/min) 20 to 90 min

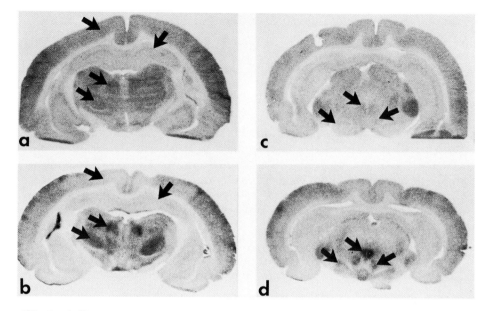

FIG. 2. [¹⁴C]deoxyglucose autoradiograms of coronal sections from a normal guinea pig **(a,c)** and an L-5-HPT–treated (400 mg/kg) myoclonic guinea pig **(b,d).** **a:** Coronal section through the thalamus of a normal guinea pig. *Arrows* are for comparison with **b.** **b:** Section through the thalamus of an L-5-HTP–treated myoclonic guinea pig. **Bottom arrow:** The ventral lateral thalamus shows increased glucose uptake compared to **a.** **Middle arrow:** The dorsomedial nucleus parafascicular nucleus region also shows increased glucose utilization. **Top arrow:** This cortical region shows decreased glucose utilization. **Right arrow:** The molecular layer of the hippocampus is now absent. **c:** A section through the midbrain of a normal guinea pig. *Arrows* are for comparison with **d.** **d:** Section through the mesencephalon of an L-5-HTP–treated myoclonic guinea pig. **Left arrow:** The lateral portion of the substantia nigra demonstrates increased glucose uptake. **Center arrow:** The third-nerve nucleus shows markedly increased glucose uptake. **Right arrow:** The red nucleus has increased glucose uptake.

following the injection. Four animals that were injected with the highest dose (200 μg/2 μl) developed seizures and died.

The myoclonus was preceded by increased preening activity, consisting of bursts of scratching the face with a hindpaw. Also, small twitches were present in individual limbs or the face. The animals were sensitive to touch but not to sound. The animals that never developed myoclonus showed a variety of movements: alternate forepaw movements, occasional jerks (one every 5 min) of a limb or the head, extension of the neck, rotation, head bobs, excessive preening, and scratching of the face area with a hindpaw. Histologic verification showed the cannulae were just dorsal and lateral to the dorsal raphe region in the myoclonic animals. In animals that did not show myoclonus, the cannulae were in the aqueduct or dorsal central gray. Previous studies with microinjection in other regions indicate the likelihood of high concentration of serotonin at the cannula tip, with some dorsal spread along the cannula track.

TABLE 1. *Changes in glucose utilization with various doses of L-5-HTP[a]*

	Animal groups				
L-5-HTP (mg/kg)	0	50	150	150	400
Myoclonus	−	−	−	+	+
No. of animals	5	4	3	7	5
Structure					
Frontal cortex	1.59 ± 0.075	1.55 ± 0.052	1.55 ± 0.047	1.40 ± 0.037[b]	1.37 ± 0.049[b]
Sensorimotor cortex	1.60 ± 0.054	1.58 ± 0.052	1.67 ± 0.140	1.48 ± 0.053	1.36 ± 0.039[c]
Striatum	1.54 ± 0.058	1.54 ± 0.045	1.54 ± 0.107	1.36 ± 0.053	1.50 ± 0.104
Hippocampus	1.23 ± 0.076	1.27 ± 0.045	1.41 ± 0.182	1.18 ± 0.053	1.20 ± 0.045
Centromedian nucleus	1.40 ± 0.044	1.62 ± 0.073	1.79 ± 0.077	1.85 ± 0.065[d]	2.14 ± 0.294[b]
Ventrothalamic nucleus	1.48 ± 0.037	1.55 ± 0.064	1.74 ± 0.025	1.80 ± 0.071[c]	1.92 ± 0.159[b]
Ventroanterior thalamic nucleus	1.52 ± 0.097	1.56 ± 0.048	1.70 ± 0.112	1.77 ± 0.071	1.82 ± 0.120
Dorsolateral thalamic nucleus	1.48 ± 0.119	1.48 ± 0.059	1.48 ± 0.143	1.30 ± 0.033	1.36 ± 0.067
Third-nerve nucleus	1.59 ± 0.097	1.73 ± 0.045	1.72 ± 0.128	1.73 ± 0.053	1.79 ± 0.145
Red nucleus	1.47 ± 0.127	1.53 ± 0.073	1.55 ± 0.145	1.50 ± 0.064	1.57 ± 0.136
Cerebellar nodulus	1.59 ± 0.110	1.66 ± 0.080	1.56 ± 0.015	1.74 ± 0.077	1.79 ± 0.108
Cerebellar cortex	1.14 ± 0.073	1.31 ± 0.081	1.25 ± 0.012	1.28 ± 0.063	1.16 ± 0.040
Substantia nigra reticulata	1.12 ± 0.049	1.33 ± 0.053	1.25 ± 0.070	1.14 ± 0.063	1.22 ± 0.042

[a] Each value represents the gray matter: mean white matter ratios (± SE) obtained from transmission densitometry as detailed in Methodology of DG Autoradiographic Experiments. Statistical significance for each group was calculated by comparing the isotope density of the experimental group to the control group using a two-tailed Student's *t* test. (Data from Thal et al., ref. 25.)

[b] $p < 0.05$.

[c] $p < 0.01$.

[d] $p < 0.001$.

RAT MYOCLONUS MODELS

We attempted to produce myoclonus in rats by manipulation of the serotonergic system, as had been shown previously (7). Adult male Sprague-Dawley rats were injected with doses of L-5-HTP ranging from 50 to 400 mg/kg. No animal developed spontaneous myoclonus, although mild tremulousness developed at the highest doses. Rats were subsequently treated with reserpine (2 mg/kg, i.p) to deplete serotonin and catecholamines. Twenty-four hours later, they were injected with the monoamine oxidase inhibitor pargyline (75 mg/kg, i.p). Two hours after that, they were given doses of L-5-HTP ranging from 3 to 200 mg/kg. All animals receiving 6 mg/kg of L-5-HTP or higher developed symptoms that consisted of tremor, then head and neck myoclonus, and piloerection followed by reciprocal forepaw movements. The animals then developed rapid low-amplitude myoclonus at a rate of 120 per min. The manifestations of the serotonin behaviorial syndrome persisted throughout the period of myoclonus and lasted for 2 hr. Doses of 12 mg/kg resulted in death within 2 hr, whereas doses lower than 6 mg/kg did not reliably induce the syndrome. Omission of pargyline pretreatment failed to induce myoclonus.

A second group of rats was pretreated with desmethylimipramine (DMI) 25 mg/kg, i.p, to protect catecholamine neurons. One hour later, under light halothane anesthesia, 200 μg of the serotonergic neurotoxin 5,7-dihydroxytryptamine (5,7-DHT) in 25 μl artificial cerebrospinal fluid was injected intracisternally. Pentobarbital at a dose of 15 mg/kg was subsequently injected subcutaneously to prevent seizures.

Following the injection of neurotoxin, all animals appeared to be normal. Three days later, each rat was injected with 65 mg/kg of L-5-HTP. Within 5 min, all animals developed generalized tremulousness and then intermittent twitching of the head, neck, and forepaws. Following this, an exaggerated startle response developed, and then piloerection and intermittent myoclonus occurred. This was followed by generalized myoclonus. Local twitching, as well as the other behavioral manifestations described, accompanied the myoclonus at all times. Thirty-five to 90 min postinjection, six of six injected animals expired.

We also tried to induce myoclonus in rats by making them hypoxic, because such a syndrome would closely mimic postanoxic action myoclonus. Ten-day-old and 30-day-old male rats were used. Animals were placed in a chamber in which the atmosphere was rapidly replaced with nitrogen gas. Both 10-day-old and adult animals stopped breathing within 3 to 10 min. Twenty percent of the 10-day-old rats and 80% of the adult rats died. Twenty percent of each of the surviving groups developed a few brief myoclonic jerks followed by full recovery. No animal developed permanent myoclonus. Similar data were obtained in the mouse and guinea pig.

DISCUSSION

A number of animal models of myoclonus were investigated. Since posthypoxic myoclonus in humans is often secondary to an acute hypoxic insult, this model was studied. Although transient myoclonus followed hypoxia in some animals, permanent myoclonus did not ensue. Others have reported similar findings in the adult rat (20), suggesting that the mouse, rat, and guinea pig may be more resistant to hypoxia than are humans.

Administration of L-5-HTP to guinea pigs results in stereotyped dose-dependent myoclonus. By contrast, administration of L-5-HTP to rats failed to induce myoclonus, suggesting that the site(s) responsible for the induction of myoclonus in the guinea pig is considerably more sensitive to the administration of serotonin precursors than in the rat. Rats, however, do develop myoclonus if receptor sensitivity is increased by amine depletion or destruction of serotonin neurons with a selective neurotoxin. This syndrome has been described by others (7–9,12–15) and represents a serotonin behavioral syndrome. However, the behavioral output in the rat following the induction of myoclonus is considerably more complex than that seen in the guinea pig, suggesting that the pathways activated during the rat serotonin behavioral syndrome may differ from those activated in myoclonic guinea pigs. The guinea pig myoclonus model has several drawbacks, including species specificity, paradoxical induction by L-5-HTP, and rhythmicity at rest rather than isolated action myoclonus. Nevertheless, we conclude that the guinea pig L-5-HTP model of myoclonus is preferable to the rat model for anatomical analysis since it is a purer myoclonus model, highly dose dependent, and readily reproducible.

The myoclonus induced by injection directly into the dorsal pons also was pure myoclonus similar to systemic L-5-HTP–induced myoclonus, except that it was not sound sensitive. These data, and previous studies by others who demonstrated that collicular transections do not abolish myoclonus (4), strongly suggest that the origin may be in lower brainstem structures.

Prominent changes in glucose uptake occurred in the thalamus, cortex, and hippocampus. Each of these changes may have been caused by a direct effect on serotonin receptors or by indirect effects via afferent stimulation. The decreased glucose uptake observed in cortex is very likely due to a direct effect on serotonin receptors because there is a wide distribution of serotonin in the cortex (2,22) and serotonin has been shown to inhibit cortical activity. The complex glucose utilization changes in the thalamus do not correlate closely to the distribution of serotonin (22) and thus probably represent indirect effects.

The role of the observed cortical and thalamic changes in myoclonus is an open question. Myoclonus can still be induced after a collicular transection, indicating that cortex is not necessary for myoclonus. However, a decrease in cortical metabolism occurred only in the myoclonic guinea pigs, suggesting that a relationship may exist between cortical inhibition and myoclonus.

The descending serotonin projection from the ventral raphe to the spinal cord may be an important system in myoclonus. Our efforts to induce myoclonus by local raphe injections may have been successful because we affected the serotonergic cell bodies or serotonin-sensitive cells projecting to the spinal cord. A dual effect by the systemically injected L-5-HTP may produce inhibition within the cortex with diminished cortical control of brainstem structures, as well as serotonergic activation of brainstem projections to the spinal cord.

We have not observed prominent changes in glucose uptake in the raphe region. We are currently investigating the possibility that small changes in glucose utilization in this structure may account for substantial changes in the serotonergic functional status we have observed behaviorally. In future studies, serotonin microinjection into the brainstem in conjunction with DG autoradiography may allow us to identify the structures involved in the guinea pig myoclonus model.

SUMMARY

Myoclonus could not be induced in rats with either L-5-HTP alone or hypoxia. Following amine depletion or destruction of the serotonin neurons with 5,7-DHT, myoclonus appeared as part of a complex serotonergic behavioral syndrome induced by serotonin agonists. On the other hand, in the guinea pig, L-5-HTP induces a pure myoclonic syndrome in a dose-dependent fashion. Myoclonus also was induced by injection of serotonin into the dorsal pons of the guinea pig. This is additional evidence confirming the importance of the brainstem structures in the L-5-HTP guinea pig model of myoclonus.

Deoxyglucose (DG) autoradiography in guinea pigs following systemic L-5-HTP administration demonstrated increased glucose metabolism within thalamic and third nerve nuclei, with decreased metabolism in the cortex, and the molecular layer of the hippocampus. Since serotonin is an inhibitory transmitter, we hypothesize that the decreases observed in cortex may be the result of direct serotonergic inhibition, whereas the increases observed in the thalamus probably represent indirect effects via polysynaptic pathways.

REFERENCES

1. Aghajanian GK, Wang RY. Physiology and pharmacology of central serotonin neurons. In: Lipton MA, DiMascio A, Killum KF, eds. Psychopharmacology: a generation of progress. New York: Raven Press, 1978:171–83.
2. Bennett JP, Snyder SH. Serotonin binding of D-lysergic and diethylamide (LSD) to brain membranes: relationship to serotonin receptors. *Brain Res* 1975;94:523–44.
3. Chadwick D, Hallett M, Harris R, et al. Clinical, biochemical, and physiological features distinguishing myoclonus responsive to 5-hydroxytryptophan, tryptophan with a monoamine oxidase inhibitor and clonazepam. *Brain* 1977;100:455–87.
4. Chadwick D, Hallett M, Jenner P, et al. 5-Hydroxytryptophan induced myoclonus in guinea pigs. *J Neurol Sci* 1978;35:157–65.
5. Coleman M. Infantile spasms associated with 5-hydroxytryptophan administration in patients with Down's syndrome. *Neurology* 1971;21:911–9.
6. DeLean J, Richardson JC, Hornykiewicz O. Beneficial effects of serotonin precursors in postanoxic action myoclonus. *Neurology* 1976;26:863–8.
7. Gerson SC, Baldessarini RJ. Motor effects of serotonin in the central nervous system. *Life Sci* 1980;27:1435–51.
8. Grahame-Smith DG. Inhibitory effect of chlorpromazine on the syndrome of hyperactivity produced by L-tryptophan or N-methoxy-N,N-dimethyltryptamine in rats treated with monoamine oxidase inhibitor. *Br J Pharmacol* 1971;43:856–64.
9. Grahame-Smith DG. Studies in vivo on the relationship between brain tryptophan, brain 5HT

synthesis and hyperactivity in rats treated with a monoamine oxidase inhibitor and L-tryptophan. *J Neurochem* 1971;18:1053–66.

10. Growdon JH, Young RR, Shahani BT. L-5-hydroxytryptophan in treatment of several different syndromes in which myoclonus is prominent. *Neurology* 1976;26:1135–40.
11. Guilleminault C, Thorp BR, Cousen D. HVA and 5-HIAA CSF measurements and 5-HTP trials in some patients with involuntary movements. *J Neurol Sci* 1973;18:435–41.
12. Jacobs BL. Effect of two dopamine receptor blockers on a serotonin mediated syndrome in rats. *Eur J Pharmacol* 1974;27:363–6.
13. Jacobs BL. Evidence for the functional interaction of two central neurotransmitters. *Psychopharmacology (Berlin)* 1974;39:81–6.
14. Jacobs BL. An animal behavioral model for studying central serotinergic synapses. *Life Sci* 1976;19:777–86.
15. Jacobs BL, Klemfuss H. Brainstem and spinal cord mediation of a serotinergic behavioral syndrome. *Brain Res* 1975;100:450–7.
16. Klawans HL Jr, Goetz C, Weiner WJ. 5-Hydroxytryptophan-induced myoclonus in guinea pigs and the possible role of serotonin in infantile myoclonus. *Neurology* 1973;23:1234–40.
17. Lhermitte F, Marteau R, Degos CF. Analyse pharmacologique d'un nouveau cas de myoclonies d'intention et d'action post-anoxiques. *Rev Neurol (Paris)* 1972;126:107–14.
18. Lhermitte F, Peterfalvi M, Marteau R, et al. Analyse pharmachologique d'un cas de myoclonies d'intention et d'action post-anoxiques. *Rev Neurol (Paris)* 1971;124:21–31.
19. Magnussen I, Dupont E, Engbaek F. Post-hypoxic intention myoclonus treated with 5-hydroxytryptophan and an extracerebral decarboxylase inhibitor. *Acta Neurol Scand* 1978;57:289–94.
20. Sharma JN, Snider SR, Fahn S, Hiesiger E. Anoxic myoclonus in the rat. *Adv Neurol* 1979;26:181–9.
21. Sokoloff L, Reivich M, Kennedy C, DesRossiers MH, Patlak CS, Pettigrew KD, Sakurada O, Shinohara M. The [^{14}C]deoxyglucose method for the measurement of local cerebral glucose utilization: theory, procedure and normal values in the conscious and anesthetized albino rat. *J Neurochem* 1977;28:897–916.
22. Steinbusch HMW. Distribution of serotonin-immunoreactivity in the central nervous system of the rat—cell bodies and terminals. *Neuroscience* 1981;6:557–618.
23. Stewart RH, Growdon JH, Cancean D, Baldessarini RJ. 5-Hydroxytryptophan induced myoclonus: increased sensitivity to serotonin after intracranial 5,7 dihydroxytryptamine in the adult rat. *Neuropharmacology* 1976;15:449–55.
24. Thal L, Sharpless NS, Wolfson L, et al. Treatment of myoclonus with L-5-hydroxytryptophan and carbidopa: clinical, electrophysiological and biochemical observations. *Ann Neurol* 1980;7:570–6.
25. Thal LJ, Wolfson LI. Functional anatomy of L-5-hydroxytryptophan induced myoclonus in the guinea pig. *Neurology* 1981;31:955–60.
26. Van Woert MH, Rosenbaum D, Howieson J, et al. Long term therapy of myoclonus and other neurologic disorders with L-5-HTP and carbidopa. *N Engl J Med* 1977;296:70–5.

Advances in Neurology, Vol. 43: Myoclonus,
edited by S. Fahn et al. Raven Press,
New York © 1986.

5-HT–Mediated Myoclonus in the Guinea Pig as a Model of Brainstem 5-HT and Tryptamine Receptor Action

G. Luscombe, P. Jenner, and C. D. Marsden

*University Department of Neurology, Institute of Psychiatry and King's College Hospital
Medical School, London SE5, United Kingdom*

Postanoxic and some other forms of human myoclonus may be due to a functional deficit of brain 5-hydroxytryptamine (5-HT) action. Drugs increasing brain 5-HT, such as L-5-hydroxytryptophan (5-HTP), or L-tryptophan plus a monoamine oxidase (MAO) inhibitor, suppress the myoclonus.

In contrast, in the guinea pig, the converse appears to occur. Klawans and his colleagues (17,18) made the original observation that administration of 5-HTP to guinea pigs produced "brief, shocklike repetitive movements that appeared to be myoclonic in nature" (17,18). Our own studies have confirmed and extended this finding (3,20–23).

The frequency and intensity of 5-HTP–induced myoclonic jerking is dose dependent and correlates with elevation of whole-brain 5-HT concentrations (17). Other drug treatments increasing brain 5-HT content or acting as 5-HT agonists also cause myoclonus. Myoclonus is evoked by L-tryptophan plus an MAO inhibitor and by 5-methoxy-N,N-dimethyltryptamine (3,17,20,37).

The 5-HTP myoclonus model did not, however, fulfill the criteria for a model of human reticular reflex myoclonus as we had hoped. Although evoked from the brainstem, 5-HTP myoclonus is not stimulus sensitive, is characterized by prolonged bursts of EMG activity in active muscles, and is not inhibited by administration of clonazepam (3,39). However, 5-HTP–induced myoclonus appears to be a relatively specific model of 5-HT function in the guinea pig. The syndrome is antagonized by 5-HT receptor blockers but not by drugs blocking dopamine or norepinephrine receptors (3,17). In addition, myoclonus in guinea pigs is a pure behavioral model not complicated by the appearance of more complex behaviors (such as forepaw treading, head weaving, or "wet-dog shakes"), which often are evoked by the administration of 5-HT precursors and 5-HT agonists to other rodent species (14,16). Thus, 5-HTP–induced myoclonus in the guinea pig provides a readily observed behavioral model for specifically studying brainstem 5-HT function.

In a series of recent studies we have utilized this model to investigate indoleamine mechanisms in the guinea pig brainstem. We have been particularly concerned to discover (a) how the different classes of brain 5-HT receptors (30,31) are involved in the production of myoclonus, and (b) whether we could find any evidence for the involvement of the pharmacologically distinct tryptamine receptors thought to be present in the brain (5,6,32). Although the model itself may not be of direct relevance to human myoclonic disorders, it may be useful for study of the organization of 5-HT systems in the brainstem.

BEHAVIORAL STUDIES

The extent of myoclonus occurring in the guinea pig was assessed using a 0 to 4 observer rating system reflecting both the frequency and intensity of jerking: 0, no jerking; 1, very occasional jerking; 2, head jerking (frequency >very occasional); 3, whole-body jerking (frequency >very occasional, <continuous); 3.5, almost continuous whole-body jerking; 4, continuous rhythmic whole-body jerking.

Comparison of the Ability of 5-HT Precursors and Indole-Containing and Piperazine-Containing 5-HT Agonists to Induce Myoclonus

Currently available 5-HT agonists can be divided into those that structurally resemble 5-HT itself, namely, the indole-containing compounds such as 5-methoxy-N,N-dimethyltryptamine, and a group of piperazine-containing agonists such as quipazine or MK 212. A striking observation from previous studies (3,37) was that the piperazine-containing compounds rarely induced myoclonus, compared with the indole-containing group. We investigated, therefore, the ability of a range of 5-HT agonists of both classes to induce myoclonus in the guinea pig (20,21).

Administration of 5-HTP (5–120 mg/kg, s.c.) to guinea pigs pretreated with the peripheral decarboxylase inhibitor carbidopa (25 mg/kg, i.p., 1 hr previously), or of 5-HTP (20–200 mg/kg, s.c.) alone, induced dose-dependent myoclonus (Table 1). L-Tryptophan (25–200 mg/kg, i.p.) also evoked dose-related myoclonic jerking but only following inhibition of MAO by pargyline (75 mg/kg, i.p., 1 hr previously). However, 5-HT (1–36 mg/kg, i.p.) did not induce myoclonus, confirming the central origin of this behavior.

Tryptamine (6–160 mg/kg, i.p.) evoked dose-dependent myoclonus in pargyline-pretreated (75 mg/kg, i.p. 1 hr previously) animals. A range of other indole-containing 5-HT agonists (Table 1) similarly induced dose-dependent myoclonus in guinea pigs.

In marked contrast, 5-HT agonists containing a piperazine moiety (Table 2) evoked only occasional myoclonus at toxic doses, which often caused seizures sometimes resulting in death. Myoclonus was observed very rarely following administration of these piperazine-containing agonists in doses that are effective in producing other behavioral and biochemical changes indicative of 5-HT agonist action (4,11,12,33). So the doses of the piperazine-containing 5-HT agonists used were adequate to stimulate 5-HT receptors. The compounds certainly penetrated into the brain and exerted central actions. Quipazine, MK 212, or 1-(m-trifluoro-methylphenyl)piperazine (all at 20 mg/kg, i.p.) potentiated the occasional jerking

TABLE 1. *The ability of 5-HT precursors and indole-containing 5-HT agonists to induce myoclonic jerking in guinea pigs*

Name	Doses tested (mg/kg)	Threshold myoclonic dose (mg/kg)	Maximum myoclonus score ± SEM	Dose (mg/kg)	Mean duration[a] of myoclonus (min)
L-Tryptophan (plus pargyline 75 mg/kg i.p.)	25–200, i.p.	25	2.9 ± 0.3	150	360
L-5-HTP	5–200, s.c.	20	3.8 ± 0.2	200	215
L-5-HTP (plus carbidopa 25 mg/kg i.p.)	1–120, s.c.	5	3.9 ± 0.1	75	360
5-HT	1–36, i.p.	36	0		
Tryptamine (plus pargyline 75 mg/kg i.p.)	1–160, i.p.	6	3.6 ± 0.2	80	95
N,N-dimethyltryptamine	1–160, i.p.	20	3.4 ± 0.2	160	110
5-methoxy-N,N-dimethyltryptamine	0.1–20, i.p.	2.5	3.8 ± 0.2	20	30
Bufotenine	10–160, i.p.	80	1.9 ± 0.6	160	25
Psilocin	2.5–160, i.p.	10	3.0 ± 0.0	160	85
Psilocybin	1–80, i.p.	10	2.5 ± 0.5	80	50
RU 24969[b]	1–120, i.p.	40	3.0 ± 0.0	80	270
d-LSD[b]	0.1–8.0, i.p.	0.25	3.9 ± 0.1	8.0	60

[a]The mean duration of myoclonus was that observed for the dose of each compound causing the maximum myoclonus score shown.
[b]d-LSD, d-lysergic acid diethylamide tartrate; RU 24969, 5-methoxy-3(1,2,3,6-tetrahydro-4-pyridinyl)-1H-indole, succinate.

TABLE 2. *The ability of piperazine-containing 5-HT agonists to induce myoclonic jerking in guinea pigs*

Name	Doses tested mg/kg, i.p.	Threshold myoclonic dose (mg/kg)	Maximum myoclonus[a] score ± SEM	Dose (mg/kg)	Mean duration[b] of myoclonus (min)	Threshold seizure dose (mg/kg)
Quipazine	1–200	30	2.3 ± 0.5	160	10	80
MK 212[c]	1–80	40	2.0 ± 0.0	80	1	20
2-(1'-piperazinyl)-quinoxaline	1–40	5	0.6 ± 0.3	10	10	20
1-(m-trifluoromethyl-phenyl)piperazine	1–160	40	2.0 ± 1.0	120	55	80
m-Chlorophenylpiperazine	1–160	80	1.7 ± 0.5	160	5	160
p-Chlorophenylpiperazine	1–160	—	0		—	160
Phenylpiperazine	1–160	—	0		—	40

[a]Such myoclonus was seen intermittently and only occasionally during the time period stated.
[b]The mean duration of myoclonus was that observed for the dose of each compound causing the maximum myoclonus score shown.
[c]MK 212, 6-chloro-2-(1-piperazinyl)pyrazine.

induced in guinea pigs by a threshold dose of 5-HTP (20 mg/kg, s.c., plus carbidopa 25 mg/kg, i.p. 1 hr previously) (20).

The marked difference in ability of the two structurally distinct groups of 5-HT agonists to evoke myoclonus may reflect the differing capacity of these drugs to interact with those 5-HT receptors in guinea pig brainstem responsible for the induction of myoclonus. Different populations of 5-HT receptors are thought to exist in the brain (30,31). We recently have investigated the ability of the same range of 5-HT agonists to interact with brainstem 5-HT receptors in the guinea pig, using ligand-binding techniques.

Evidence for the Involvement of 5-HT-1 Receptors in the Induction of Myoclonus

There has been much recent interest in the possible existence of multiple 5-HT receptors in brain. Ligand-binding studies have shown the presence of two receptor populations in rat brain, one labeled selectively by [³H]5-HT (5-HT-1) and the other by [³H]spiperone (5-HT-2), each with different regional distribution and with different agonist and antagonist affinities (19,28–31). No information was available on which receptors were present in the guinea pig brainstem or which population might be involved in 5-HT–dependent myoclonus. So we examined the interaction of [³H]spiperone and [³H]5-HT with guinea pig brainstem homogenates and the ability of 5-HT agonists to displace these ligands.

Specific [³H]5-HT (0.5–64 nM, as defined using 10^{-5} M 5-HT) (2,27) binding to guinea pig brainstem preparations involved both a high-affinity (B_{max} 1.97 ± 0.01 pmol/g wet weight of tissue; K_D 3.70 ± 1.02 nM) and low affinity site (B_{max} 9.23 ± 2.18 pmol/g wet weight of tissue; K_D 29.1 ± 4.0 nM). Specific binding of [³H]spiperone (0.125–4.0 nM, as defined using 10^{-5} M 5-HT or d-LSD) was very low and could not be accurately or reproducibly measured.

The specific binding of [³H]5-HT (4 nM) to guinea pig brainstem preparations was potently displaced by indole-containing 5-HT agonists (range of IC_{50}, 3.4–519 nM) but was only weakly displaced by piperazine-containing 5-HT agonists (range of IC_{50}, 408–42,551 nM) (Table 3).

The results of these experiments suggest that the 5-HT receptor present in the guinea pig brainstem has the characteristics of a 5-HT-1 site and that it is 5-HT agonist action at this site that induces myoclonus. Clearly, there is not a direct linear relationship between induction of myoclonus and activity of indole-containing agonists at 5-HT-1 sites. Such in vitro actions do not reflect the in vivo pharmacokinetic differences between these agents.

Differential Action of 5-HT Antagonists and 5-HT Reuptake Blockers on 5-HTP–Induced Myoclonus

If the concept that 5-HT–dependent myoclonus in the guinea pig brainstem is mediated via one receptor subpopulation, then drugs acting as 5-HT receptor antagonists or as 5-HT reuptake blockers may show different actions on 5-HTP–induced myoclonus (20).

TABLE 3. *Displacement of specific [³H]5-HT binding from guinea pig brainstem preparations by 5-HT agonists*[a]

Indole-containing 5-HT agonists	IC_{50}[a] (nM ± SEM)	Piperazine-containing 5-HT agonists	IC_{50}[a] (nM ± SEM)
d-LSD	3.4 ± 1.7	1-(m-trifluoromethyl phenyl) piperazine	407.6 ± 124.0
Bufotenine	22.5 ± 12.0	m-Chlorophenylpiperazine	3261 ± 2738
RU 24969	30.2 ± 6.0	Quipazine	7241 ± 2714
5-Methoxy-N,N-dimethyltryptamine	158.1 ± 23.6	Phenylpiperazine	7476 ± 2725
Psilocin	240.8 ± 80.9	p-Chlorophenylpiperazine	8729 ± 4303
Dimethyltryptamine	280.0 ± 105.0	MK 212	17260 ± 9714
Psilocybin	519.3 ± 82.0	2-(1'-piperazinyl) quinoxaline	42551 ± 21742

[a]IC_{50}, concentration of drug required to inhibit 50% of the specific binding of [³H]5-HT (4 nM); d-LSD, d-lysergic acid diethylamide tartrate; RU 24969, 5-methoxy-3(1,2,3,6-tetrahydro-4-pyridinyl)-1H-indole, succinate; MK 212, 6-chloro-2-(1-piperazinyl)pyrazine.

5-HTP was selected at a dose (75 mg/kg, s.c., plus carbidopa 25 mg/kg, i.p., 1 hr previously) generally producing continuous whole-body jerking 90 min after 5-HTP administration (average score, 3.8 ± 0.1). A number of indoleamine receptor antagonists were injected in a dose range of 1.0 to 20 mg/kg, i.p., either 60 min prior to or at the time of 5-HTP administration. We found that methergoline, cyproheptadine, mianserin, methysergide, and cinanserin differed markedly in their ability to inhibit 5-HTP–induced myoclonus (Table 4). Methergoline and cyproheptadine were potent antagonists of 5-HTP–evoked myoclonus, mianserin was only moderately active, and methysergide and cinanserin were weak inhibitors of jerking.

For experiments employing 5-HT reuptake blockers, 5-HTP was chosen at a threshold dose (20 mg/kg plus carbidopa 25 mg/kg 1 hr previously) that rarely induces myoclonus. A number of 5-HT reuptake blockers were tested for their efficacy in potentiating myoclonus, by injecting in a dose range of 1.0 to 20 mg/kg, i.p., 10 min prior to 5-HTP administration. 5-HTP-induced myoclonus was potently enhanced by chlorimipramine, paroxetine, and Org 6582 ((±)-8, chloro-11-antiamino-benzo-(b)-bicyclo-3,3,1-nona-3,6-a(10a)-diene HCl) but was only weakly potentiated by femoxetine, fluoxetine and desmethylimipramine. Femoxetine and fluoxetine, however, are potent and selective 5-HT reuptake blockers (26,38).

The results of these experiments suggest that either inhibitors of 5-HT uptake and 5-HT receptor antagonists vary in their ability to alter 5-HT function in different brain areas or the drugs show differing selectivity for the various 5-HT receptor populations and their associated neurons.

Evidence that Myoclonus Induced by Tryptamine May Be Produced Through a Different Indoleamine Receptor Population from That Mediating 5-HTP–Induced Myoclonus

In addition to the evidence suggesting that different subpopulations of 5-HT receptors may exist in the brain, there is also a considerable literature that proposes

TABLE 4. *Comparison of the ability of indoleamine receptor antagonists to inhibit 5-HT-dependent and tryptamine-induced behaviors in rodents*

Antagonist	Dose (mg/kg)	Reduction of myoclonus score induced in guinea pigs %		ED_{50} values (mg/kg) in rats as inhibitors	
		5-HTP[a]	Tryptamine[b]	5-HTP–induced head twitch[c]	Tryptamine-induced forepaw clonus[d]
Methergoline	5	65	68	0.47	0.14
Cyproheptadine	10	92	36	0.12	5.0[f]
Mianserin	10	48	55	—	1.5[e]
Methysergide	10	15	55	2.5[f]	2.3
Cinanserin	10	12	18	1.5	40

[a]5-HTP–induced myoclonus in guinea pigs. Indoleamine receptor antagonists were intraperitoneally administered immediately prior to 5-HTP (75 mg/kg, s.c.) plus carbidopa (25 mg/kg, i.p. 60 min previously). This combination generally produced continuous, rhythmic myoclonus, and the table shows the % reduction of the myoclonus score by the antagonist, assessed 90 min after 5-HTP treatment (20; *unpublished data*).

[b]Tryptamine-induced myoclonus in guinea pigs. Indoleamine receptor antagonists were intraperitoneally administered either before or after tryptamine (40 mg/kg, i.p., plus pargyline (75 mg/kg, i.p., 60 min previously). This combination usually induced myoclonus, and the table shows the % reduction of the myoclonus score by the antagonist, assessed 30 min after tryptamine administration (22).

[c]5-HTP–induced head twitch in rats. Indoleamine receptor antagonists were intraperitoneally administered 30 min prior to 5-HTP (270 mg/kg, i.p.), a dose evoking head twitches in all rats. The number of animals exhibiting at least one head twitch was determined 60 min after 5-HTP administration. The dose of antagonist needed to prevent the response in 50% of the rats (ED_{50}) was estimated by regression analysis (5).

[d]Tryptamine-induced forepaw clonus in rat. 5-HTP antagonists were administered intraperitoneally 60 min prior to tryptamine (40 mg/kg, i.v.), a dose consistently evoking clonus of the forepaws. Using 5 sec or more of uninterrupted clonus as the end point, the antagonists were evaluated for their ability to inhibit forepaw clonus. The antagonist dose required to prevent the response in 50% of the rats (ED_{50}) was estimated by regression analysis (5).

[e]Tryptamine-induced forepaw clonus in rats. Mianserin was intraperitoneally administered 30 min prior to tryptamine (15 mg/kg, i.v.). A rat was considered protected when no behavior was observed to last for more than 5 sec. Under these conditions the ED_{50} for cyproheptadine was 5 mg/kg, i.p. (36).

[f]Dose-response curve unsuitable for estimation of 95% confidence interval, since greater than 60% antagonism was not observed even at doses as high as four times the quoted ED_{50} value (5).

distinct tryptamine and 5-HT receptors (5,6,32). In an attempt to distinguish between actions at these latter sites, we have investigated the ability of 5-HT antagonists and 5-HT reuptake blockers to influence tryptamine-induced myoclonus, and compared their effects with those observed using 5-HTP to induce myoclonus (22).

Tryptamine was chosen at a dose (40 mg/kg, plus pargyline 75 mg/kg 1 hr previously) consistently producing myoclonus. This myoclonus, although less consistent, closely resembled that induced by 5-HTP (plus carbidopa), suggesting the involvement of a final common mechanism. The pattern of inhibition of tryptamine-induced myoclonus by the range of indoleamine receptor antagonists, however, was different from that for inhibition of 5-HTP–evoked myoclonus (Table 4). Methergoline, mianserin, and methysergide antagonized tryptamine-induced myoclonus, whereas cyproheptadine and cinanserin only weakly inhibited jerking (Table 4).

Reuptake blockers were administered 10 min prior to either (a) tryptamine (40 mg/kg) plus pargyline (75 mg/kg 1 hr previously) to investigate their ability to antagonize myoclonus, or (b) tryptamine (10 mg/kg) plus pargyline (75 mg/kg 1 hr previously) to examine their capacity to potentiate the jerking occasionally induced by this small dose of tryptamine. The myoclonus evoked by either tryptamine 40 mg/kg or 10 mg/kg administration to pargyline-pretreated guinea pigs was not altered by any of the reuptake blockers.

The differential inhibition by indoleamine receptor antagonists of myoclonus induced by tryptamine and by 5-HTP suggests that pharmacologically distinct postsynaptic tryptamine and 5-HT receptors are involved in the production of myoclonus. This is confirmed by the experiment using 5-HT reuptake blockers.

The results from these experiments suggest that release of 5-HT by tryptamine does not contribute to the myoclonus induced in guinea pigs by tryptamine in pargyline-pretreated animals. However, as described above, at least some 5-HT reuptake blockers potentiate the myoclonus induced by 5-HTP. So it might be expected that tryptamine myoclonus would have been affected by some of these compounds. In the present experiments, animals were pretreated with an MAO inhibitor not used in the 5-HTP studies, which may have so increased synaptic 5-HT concentration that a reuptake blocker would have no further effect.

Presynaptic 5-HT Function Is Required for Tryptamine to Induce Myoclonus

Even though tryptamine and 5-HT (derived from 5-HTP) may induce myoclonus through distinct postsynaptic receptors, and tryptamine-induced myoclonus is not affected by 5-HT reuptake blockers, these data do not negate the possibility that tryptamine's action requires intact 5-HT neuronal function. We have looked at this possibility by both decreasing and increasing the amount of 5-HT available in presynaptic 5-HT terminals.

Depletion of presynaptic neuronal stores of 5-HT, using para-chlorophenylalanine (PCPA) (150 mg/kg administered 48, 24, and 2 hr prior to tryptamine), completely abolished the jerking induced by tryptamine (40 mg/kg) in pargyline-pretreated (75 mg/kg 1 hr previously) animals (22). This dosage regimen of PCPA decreased 5-HT levels in the frontal cortex by 40%.

Preloading of presynaptic neuronal stores of 5-HT by the administration of L-tryptophan (15 mg/kg) 1 hr following administration of pargyline (75 mg/kg) and 1 hr prior to the administration of tryptamine (6 mg/kg) potentiated the behavioral effects of this threshold dose of tryptamine (22).

These data suggest that, although tryptamine receptors may be separate from 5-HT receptors, an action of tryptamine to induce myoclonus is dependent on intact presynaptic 5-HT function.

Summary of Behavioral Studies

The behavioral studies of indoleamine-induced myoclonus in the guinea pig have led us to propose the following (Table 5):

1. A 5-HT receptor subpopulation may be responsible for indoleamine-induced myoclonus. The major evidence supporting this conclusion is as follows: (a) myoclonus may be induced in guinea pigs by 5-HT precursors and by indole-containing 5-HT agonists but not by piperazine-containing 5-HT agonists; (b) only 5-HT-1 receptors are present in guinea pig brainstem preparations; (c) indole-containing 5-HT agonists potently displace [^{3}H]5-HT from these brainstem 5-HT-1 receptors, but piperazine-containing 5-HT agonists do not; (d) different 5-HT antagonists show differing abilities to inhibit 5-HTP–induced myoclonus; (e) different 5-HT reuptake blockers show differing abilities to potentiate 5-HTP–induced myoclonus.

2. Tryptamine acts on receptors different from those activated by 5-HT to induce myoclonus, but tryptamine's effect is dependent on intact 5-HT presynaptic function. The major evidence supporting this conclusion is as follows: (a) 5-HT antagonists differentially block myoclonus induced by 5-HTP and tryptamine; (b) 5-HT

TABLE 5. *Summary of the ability of 5-HT precursors or 5-HT agonists to induce myoclonus, 5-HT reuptake blockers to potentiate 5-HTP–induced myoclonus and indoleamine antagonists to inhibit either 5-HTP- or tryptamine-induced myoclonus in the guinea pig*

5-HT precursors or agonists	
Did produce myoclonus	Did not produce myoclonus
Tryptophan (plus pargyline)	Tryptophan alone
5-HTP (with or without carbidopa)	Tryptamine alone
Tryptamine (plus pargyline)	Piperazine-containing 5-HT agonists;
Indole-containing 5-HT agonists;	e.g., quipazine, MK 212
e.g., d-LSD, dimethyltryptamine	

5-HT reuptake blockers	
Strongly potentiated myoclonus	Little or no potentiation of myoclonus
Chlorimipramine	Femoxetine
Paroxetine	Fluoxetine
Org 6582	Desmethylimipramine

Indoleamine antagonists	
Potently antagonized	Weak or no effect
5-HTP myoclonus	on 5-HTP myoclonus
Methergoline	Mianserin
Cyproheptadine	Methysergide
Potently antagonized	Cinanserin
tryptamine myoclonus	Weak or no effect on
Methergoline	tryptamine myoclonus
Methysergide	Cyproheptadine
Mianserin	Cinanserin

From Luscombe et al. (20–22).

reuptake blockers differentially potentiate 5-HTP–induced myoclonus but do not potentiate or antagonize tryptamine-evoked jerking; (c) The inhibition by PCPA, and enhancement by L-tryptophan pretreatment of tryptamine-induced myoclonus suggest a dependence on intact presynaptic function.

BIOCHEMICAL STUDIES

Our behavioral investigations suggested a role for both 5-HT and tryptamine receptor activation in the production of brainstem myoclonus in the guinea pig. However, we could not distinguish between the relative importance of 5-HT and tryptamine in the induction of myoclonus using these behavioral techniques. We have therefore carried out biochemical investigations to ascertain the relationship between altered 5-HT concentration in the brain and the induction of myoclonus following administration of 5-HTP, L-tryptophan, or tryptamine, and the changes in brain tryptamine content induced by each of these treatments (23).

We measured the regional tryptophan, 5-HT, and 5-hydroxyindoleacetic acid (5-HIAA) levels, and the whole-brain tryptamine content, following administration of 5-HT precursors or tryptamine. The following brain areas were analyzed: frontal cortex, tuberculum olfactorium and nucleus accumbens (mesolimbic area), striatum, hippocampus, hypothalamus, midbrain, pons, and cerebellum. Animals were sacrificed at the time of maximal drug-induced myoclonus, that is, 30 min following tryptamine administration, 60 min following 5-HTP administration, 90 min following L-tryptophan administration, 120 min following carbidopa administration, and 90 min or 120 min following administration of pargyline. Regional tryptophan content was determined by a modification (9) of the fluorimetric technique of Denckla and Dewey (8), and regional 5-HT and 5-HIAA levels were assayed by the fluorimetric technique of Curzon and Green (7). Whole-brain tryptamine content also was measured fluorimetrically (23). The results of the studies are summarized in Table 6.

Alterations in Brain Tryptophan, 5-HT and 5-HIAA Levels Following Administration of Indoleamine Precursors or Tryptamine

L-Tryptophan

L-Tryptophan (50–500 mg/kg) did not evoke myoclonus in guinea pigs despite producing a dose-related elevation of tryptophan, 5-HT, and 5-HIAA concentrations in all brain regions (23). Administration of L-tryptophan (50–200 mg/kg) to pargyline-pretreated (75 mg/kg 30 min previously) guinea pigs induced dose-dependent myoclonus. L-Tryptophan 100 to 200 mg/kg plus pargyline (75 mg/kg) caused a dose-related increase in both tryptophan and 5-HIAA levels in all brain regions, compared to the effect of pargyline (75 mg/kg) treatment alone. Cerebral 5-HT concentrations, however, were equally elevated following administration of either 100 or 200 mg/kg L-tryptophan to pargyline-pretreated animals, despite the increase in intensity of myoclonus produced by doubling the L-tryptophan dose.

TABLE 6. *Effect of indoleamines (L-tryptophan, 5-HTP, and tryptamine), pargyline, and carbidopa on whole-brain tryptamine content, pontine 5-HT levels, and guinea pig behavior*

Treatment	Whole-brain tryptamine (ng/g) (mean ± SEM)	Myoclonus score[a] (mean ± SEM)	Pontine 5-HT(ng/g) (mean ± SEM)
Saline	29 ± 6	0 ± 0	835 ± 79
L-Tryptophan (200 mg/kg)	279 ± 14[b]	0 ± 0	1955 ± 248[b]
Pargyline (75 mg/kg; 2 hr previously)	72 ± 4[b]	0 ± 0	1709 ± 278[b]
Pargyline (75 mg/kg) plus L-tryptophan (200 mg/kg)	175 ± 29[c]	2.8 ± 0.5	2909 ± 136[c]
5-HTP (200 mg/kg)	9 ± 4[b]	3.1 ± 0.4	4367 ± 594[b]
Carbidopa (25 mg/kg)	47 ± 8	0 ± 0	447 ± 40[b]
Carbidopa (25 mg/kg) plus 5-HTP (80 mg/kg)	21 ± 3[d]	3.5 ± 0.2	2764 ± 196[d]
Tryptamine (40 mg/kg)	ND[e]	0 ± 0	683 ± 31
Pargyline (75 mg/kg;1.5 hr, previously)	ND	0 ± 0	805 ± 61
Pargyline (75 mg/kg) plus tryptamine (10 mg/kg)	354 ± 35[c]	0 ± 0	ND
Pargyline (75 mg/kg) plus tryptamine (40 mg/kg)	2798 ± 345[c]	2.8 ± 0.5	1210 ± 132[c]

[a]Myoclonus score. This value represents the mean value of all myoclonus scores recorded prior to measurement of either cerebral 5-HT levels or brain tryptamine content, since a similar behavioral response was observed in each instance (total N = 8 guinea pigs).
[b]$p < 0.05$ vs. saline.
[c]$p < 0.05$ vs. appropriate pargyline pretreatment.
[d]$p < 0.05$ vs. carbidopa.
[e]ND, not determined. n = 4 guinea pigs for all biochemical determinations. Animals killed at times indicated in "Methods." Biochemical data analyzed by 2-tailed Student's t test. From Luscombe et al. (23), with permission.

This lack of association between cerebral 5-HT content and the intensity of myoclonus suggests that other active substances are at least partly responsible for the induction of myoclonus by L-tryptophan plus pargyline.

L-5-HTP

5-HTP (50–200 mg/kg) administration evoked dose-dependent myoclonus in naive guinea pigs and caused a dose-related elevation of 5-HT and 5-HIAA levels in all brain regions. Similar behavioral and biochemical data were reported following administration of 5-HTP (20–80 mg/kg) to carbidopa-pretreated (25 mg/kg 1 hr previously) animals (23).

Tryptamine

Tryptamine (40 mg/kg) administration to naive guinea pigs did not induce myoclonus or alter cerebral 5-HT levels (23). Administration of tryptamine (40 mg/kg) to pargyline-pretreated (75 mg/kg 1 hr previously) guinea pigs evoked myoclonus, although 5-HT levels were elevated notably (by 50%) only in the pons and cerebellum, compared to the effect of pargyline (75 mg/kg) alone.

Alterations in Whole-Brain Tryptamine Content Following Administration of Indoleamine Precursors or Tryptamine

Pargyline (75 mg/kg) or L-tryptophan (200 mg/kg) administration to naive guinea pigs elevated the tryptamine content of whole brain, but myoclonus was not evoked (23). Myoclonus induced by administration of L-tryptophan (200 mg/kg) to pargyline-pretreated (75 mg/kg 30 min previously) guinea pigs, however, was accompanied by an increase in whole-brain tryptamine content, although this was less than that produced by L-tryptophan or pargyline alone.

Administration of 5-HTP (200 mg/kg) to naive guinea pigs, or of 5-HTP (80 mg/kg) to carbidopa-pretreated (25 mg/kg 1 hr previously) animals, induced marked myoclonus but reduced whole-brain tryptamine levels compared to the respective effects of saline and carbidopa (25 mg/kg) alone.

Tryptamine (10 or 40 mg/kg) administration to pargyline-pretreated (75 mg/kg 1 hr previously) guinea pigs caused a dose-related increase in whole brain tryptamine content compared to the effect of pargyline (75 mg/kg) alone, but jerking was seen only following the larger dose of tryptamine.

Summary of Biochemical Studies

Administration of 5-HTP to naive or carbidopa-pretreated guinea pigs, or of either L-tryptophan or tryptamine to pargyline-pretreated animals, induced a similar behavioral response but different biochemical changes.

Administration of 5-HTP to naive or carbidopa-pretreated guinea pigs markedly elevated brain 5-HT levels but reduced or did not alter cerebral tryptamine content. Administration of L-tryptophan (200 mg/kg) to pargyline-pretreated animals increased cerebral concentrations of both 5-HT and tryptamine. Tryptamine administration to guinea pigs pretreated with pargyline caused only a small increase in brain 5-HT levels but markedly elevated cerebral tryptamine content. Thus, 5-HT appears to be the indoleamine responsible for 5-HTP–induced myoclonus, but tryptamine predominates in tryptamine-induced myoclonus. Both 5-HT and tryptamine may contribute to myoclonus evoked by L-tryptophan in pargyline-treated animals.

DISCUSSION

These investigations of myoclonus in the guinea pig show that although this is a relatively pure model of indoleamine action, the organization of indoleamine systems in the brainstem is complex. However, the model provides a ready means of investigating those brainstem neuronal systems that might be of importance in some human myoclonic disorders.

The findings we have described have led us to two main conclusions. First, that myoclonus is initiated through a brainstem 5-HT receptor subpopulation and, second, that tryptamine receptors, distinct from the 5-HT sites, also may be involved.

The evidence for involvement of a 5-HT receptor subpopulation grew mainly from the division between the actions of different agonist drugs. The ability of indole-containing 5-HT agonists both to evoke dose-dependent myoclonus in guinea pigs and to potently displace [³H]5-HT from its specific binding sites in guinea pig brainstem contrasted markedly with the negligible ability of piperazine-containing 5-HT agonists either to induce myoclonus or to displace specific [³H]5-HT binding (Table 3). The relationship between induction of myoclonus and *in vivo* with *in vitro* receptor action strongly suggests that the brainstem receptor protein responsible for the induction of myoclonus may possess a distinct physical conformation rendering it accessible to 5-HT agonists with an indole nucleus but not to those with a piperazine group. Obviously, there is no exact correlation between these parameters, but this is not surprising since pharmacokinetic factors will be critically important *in vivo*.

How does the 5-HT receptor in the brainstem, at which indoleamines act to cause myoclonus, relate to previously reported postsynaptic 5-HT receptor populations? Based on ligand-binding experiments, 5-HT receptors have been divided into 5-HT-1 and 5-HT-2 receptors which possess different regional distributions (19,29,31,34). 5-HT-1 receptors are selectively labeled *in vitro* by [³H]5-HT and are not linked to adenylate cyclase. [³H]5-HT binding is preferentially displaced by 5-HT agonists. 5-HT-2 receptors, which also appear not to be linked to a 5-HT–sensitive adenylate cyclase, are specifically labeled *in vitro* by [³H]spiperone, which is preferentially displaced by 5-HT antagonists (19,30,31). Since guinea pig brainstem preparations possess specific binding sites for [³H]5-HT but do not reliably demonstrate specific [³H]spiperone binding, it appears that the brainstem 5-HT receptor involved in the production of myoclonus is a 5-HT-1–type receptor.

At present, most functional effects of 5-HT receptor occupation have been associated with the 5-HT-2 receptor. Inhibition of 5-HTP–induced head twitching in mice and of tryptamine-induced forepaw clonus in rats by indoleamine receptor antagonists correlates with their ability to displace specific [³H]spiperone binding to 5-HT-2 receptors in rat frontal cortex preparations (19,30). This contrasts with the ability of 5-HT agonists in the present studies to induce myoclonus that correlates with 5-HT-1 activity. However, previous studies have concerned themselves with the actions of 5-HT antagonists rather than agonists, and it may be that different sites are involved for agonists and antagonists. An alternative explanation for this discrepancy is that the head twitching and clonus behaviors previously used for correlation studies are brainstem-mediated responses, but the ligand-binding studies performed in these investigations used forebrain tissue. It would seem more appropriate to correlate biochemical data from the same area that generates the behavioral change. In our investigations, [³H]5-HT binding to brainstem homogenates was compared to myoclonus generated from this same area (3).

The existence of pharmacologically distinct tryptamine receptors in the brain has been postulated by others from the differential inhibition of tryptamine-induced and 5-HT–dependent behaviors by indoleamine receptor antagonists (5,6,32) (Table 4). Evidence for the presence of tryptamine receptors in the guinea pig brainstem is provided by the present data, showing that indoleamine receptor antagonists differentially inhibit the myoclonus induced in guinea pigs by 5-HTP or tryptamine (Table 4). However, the behavioral response of guinea pigs to tryptamine or 5-HTP was similar, indicating a final common mechanism. Previously, distinct 5-HT and tryptamine receptors have been postulated to exist only if the amines produced contrasting behavioral changes in the same animal (6,24). The similar behavioral response of guinea pigs to 5-HTP and tryptamine administration, however, was accompanied by different biochemical changes (Table 6). These indicated that 5-HT is the indoleamine responsible for 5-HTP–evoked jerking, whereas tryptamine predominates in tryptamine-evoked myoclonus. Both 5-HT and tryptamine may be implicated in myoclonus provoked by L-tryptophan, since this amino acid is a precursor for both amines.

Different receptor systems may only partly explain how tryptamine induces myoclonus. Our data indicate that 5-HT neuronal pathways may be involved in the action of tryptamine. Thus, depletion of 5-HT stores by PCPA pretreatment abolished both the myoclonus induced in guinea pigs and the hyperactivity evoked in rats, by administration of tryptamine to animals pretreated with an MAO inhibitor (10,22,25). This suggests that myoclonus induced via tryptaminergic systems is critically dependent on intact presynaptic 5-HT function. Indeed, preloading of 5-HT terminals using L-tryptophan potentiated the myoclonus evoked by a threshold dose of tryptamine in pargyline-pretreated guinea pigs (22). Such an effect could represent a direct action of tryptamine on 5-HT neurons since there is evidence that tryptamine may both cause release of 5-HT (1,13) and inhibit 5-HT reuptake (1,13,15,35). The lack of effect of 5-HT reuptake blockers on tryptamine-plus-pargyline–induced myoclonus in guinea pigs suggests, however, that release of 5-HT induced by a direct action of tryptamine is not a contributing factor to the behavioral response (22).

In conclusion, the original observation of Klawans and his colleagues (17,18) that 5-HTP induces myoclonus in guinea pigs has resulted in the discovery of indoleamine systems in the brainstem mediating myoclonic activity. Our studies have revealed that a discrete indoleamine population is responsible for this myoclonus.

SUMMARY

Indoleamine-induced myoclonus in guinea pigs is a specific model of brainstem 5-HT function that can be used to characterize the indoleamine systems initiating myoclonus.

5-HT precursors and indole-containing 5-HT agonists induce myoclonus in guinea pigs, but piperazine-containing compounds do not. This selectivity of action correlates with the ability of 5-HT agonists to act at 5-HT-1 receptors. Further evidence for the involvement of a brainstem 5-HT receptor subpopulation in the initiation of myoclonus is shown by the differential ability of 5-HT antagonists to inhibit 5-HTP–induced myoclonus and of 5-HT reuptake blockers to potentiate threshold myoclonus.

Distinct tryptamine receptors also may be involved in producing myoclonus, since indoleamine antagonists show differing potencies in inhibiting 5-HTP- and tryptamine-induced myoclonus. Tryptamine-induced myoclonus is, however, dependent on intact presynaptic 5-HT function.

Biochemical studies indicate that 5-HT is primarily responsible for 5-HTP–evoked myoclonus, whereas tryptamine predominates in tryptamine-induced myoclonus. Both 5-HT and tryptamine may contribute to myoclonus produced by L-tryptophan.

Indoleamine-induced myoclonus in guinea pigs may be valuable in studying the organization of brainstem indoleamine systems that may be involved in some forms of human myoclonus.

ACKNOWLEDGMENTS

This study was supported by the Research Funds of the Bethlem Royal and Maudsley Hospitals and King's College Hospital. G. L. was an SRC CASE award student who worked in conjunction with Organon Laboratories Ltd.

REFERENCES

1. Baker GB, Hiob LE, Martin IL, Mitchell PR, Dewhurst WG. Interactions of tryptamine analogs with 5-hydroxytryptamine and dopamine in rat striatum *in vitro*. *Proc West Pharmacol Soc* 1980;23:167–70.
2. Bennett JP Jr, Snyder SH. Serotonin and lysergic acid diethylamide binding to rat brain membranes: relationship to postsynaptic serotonin receptors. *Mol Pharmacol* 1976;12:373–89.
3. Chadwick D, Hallett M, Jenner P, Marsden CD. 5-Hydroxytryptophan-induced myoclonus in guinea pigs. *J Neurol Sci* 1978;35:157–65.
4. Clineschmidt BV. MK-212; a serotonin like agonist in the CNS. *Gen Pharmacol* 1979;10:287–90.
5. Clineschmidt BV, Lotti VJ. Indoleamine antagonists: relative potencies as inhibitors of tryptamine and 5-hydroxytryptophan-evoked responses. *Br J Pharmacol* 1974;50:311–3.
6. Cox B, Lee TF, Martin D. Different hypothalamic receptors mediate 5-hydroxytryptamine- and tryptamine-induced core temperature changes in the rat. *Br J Pharmacol* 1981;72:477–82.
7. Curzon G, Green AR. Rapid method for the determination of 5-hydroxytryptamine and 5-hydroxyindoleacetic acid in small regions of the brain. *Br J Pharmacol* 1970;39:653–5.
8. Denckla WS, Dewey HK. The determination of tryptophan in plasma, liver and urine. *J Lab Clin Med* 1967;69:160–9.
9. Eccleston EG. A method for the estimation of free and total acid soluble plasma tryptophan using an ultrafiltration technique. *Clin Chim Acta* 1973;48:269–72.
10. Foldes A, Costa E. Relationship of brain monoamine and locomotor activity in rats. *Biochem Pharmacol* 1975;24:1617–21.
11. Fuller RW, Snoddy HD, Mason NR, Molloy BB. Effect of 1-(*m*-trifluoromethylphenyl)-piperazine on ^{3}H-serotonin binding to membranes from rat brain *in vitro* and on serotonin turnover in rat brain *in vivo*. *Eur J Pharmacol* 1978;52:11–6.
12. Fuller RW, Snoddy HD, Mason NR, Owen JE. Disposition and pharmacological effects of *m*-chlorophenylpiperazine in rats. *Neuropharmacology* 1981;20:155–62.
13. Fuxe K, Ungerstedt U. Histochemical studies on the effect of (+)-amphetamine, drugs of the imipramine group and tryptamine on central catecholamine and 5-hydroxytryptamine neurones after intraventricular injection of catecholamines and 5-hydroxytryptamine. *Eur J Pharmacol* 1968;4:135–44.
14. Grahame-Smith DG. Studies *in vivo* on the relationship between brain tryptophan, brain 5HT synthesis and hyperactivity in rats treated with a monoamine oxidase inhibitor and L-tryptophan. *J Neurochem* 1971;18:1053–66.

15. Horn AA. Structure activity relations for the inhibition of 5HT uptake into rat hypothalamic homogenates by serotonin and tryptamine analogues. *J Neurochem* 1973;21:883–8.

16. Jacobs BL. An animal behaviour model for studying central serotonergic synapses. *Life Sci* 1976;19:777–86.

17. Klawans HL, Goetz C, Weiner WJ. 5-Hydroxytryptophan-induced myoclonus in guinea pigs and the possible role of serotonin in infantile myoclonus. *Neurology* 1973;23:1234–40.

18. Klawans HL, Goetz C, Westheimer R, Weiner WJ. 5-Hydroxytryptophan induced behavior in intact guinea pigs. *Res Commun Chem Pathol Pharmacol* 1973;5:555–9.

19. Leysen JE. Serotonergic receptors in brain tissue: properties and identification of various ³H-ligand binding sites *in vitro*. *J Physiol (Paris)* 1981;77:351–62.

20. Luscombe G, Jenner P, Marsden CD. Pharmacological analysis of the myoclonus induced by 5-hydroxytryptophan in the guinea pig suggests the presence of multiple 5-hydroxy tryptamine receptors in the brain. *Neuropharmacology* 1981;20:819–31.

21. Luscombe G, Jenner P, Marsden CD. Myoclonus in guinea pigs is induced by indole-containing but not piperazine-containing 5HT agonists. *Life Sci* 1982;30:1487–94.

22. Luscombe G, Jenner P, Marsden CD. Tryptamine-induced myoclonus in guinea pigs pretreated with a monoamine oxidase inhibitor indicates pre- and post-synaptic actions of tryptamine upon central indoleamine systems. *Neuropharmacology* 1982;21:1257–65.

23. Luscombe G, Jenner P, Marsden CD. Alterations in brain 5HT and tryptamine content during indoleamine-induced myoclonus in guinea pigs. *Biochem Pharmacol* 1983;32:1857–64.

24. Marley E, Nistico G. Tryptamines and some other substances affecting waking and sleep in fowls. *Br J Pharmacol* 1975;53:193–205.

25. Marsden CA, Curzon G. The contribution of tryptamine to the behavioural effects of L-tryptophan in tranylcypromine-treated rats. *Psychopharmacology* 1978;57:71–6.

26. Mireylees SE, Goodlet I, Sugrue MF. Effects of Org 6582 on monoamine uptake *in vitro*. *Biochem Pharmacol* 1978;27:1023–7.

27. Nelson DL, Herbet A, Bourgoin S, Glowinski J, Hamon M. Characteristics of central 5HT receptors and their adaptive changes following intracerebral 5,7-dihydroxytryptamine administration in the rat. *Mol Pharmacol* 1978;14:983–95.

28. Nelson DL, Herbet A, Enjalbert A, Bockaert J, Hamon M. Serotonin-sensitive adenylate cyclase and ³H-serotonin binding sites in the CNS of the rat. I. Kinetic parameters and pharmacological properties. *Biochem Pharmacol* 1980;29:2445–53.

29. Pedigo NW, Yamamura HI, Nelson DL. Discrimination of multiple ³H-5-hydroxytryptamine binding sites by the neuroleptic spiperone in rat brain. *J Neurochem* 1981;36:220–6.

30. Peroutka SJ, Lebovitz RM, Snyder SH. Two distinct central serotonin receptors with different physiological functions. *Science* 1981;212:827–9.

31. Peroutka SJ, Snyder SH. Multiple serotonin receptors: differential binding of ³H-5-hydroxytryptamine, ³H-lysergic acid diethylamide and ³H-spiroperidol. *Mol Pharmacol* 1979;16:687–99.

32. Quock RM, Weick BG. Tryptamine-induced drug effects insensitive to serotonergic antagonists: evidence of specific tryptaminergic receptor stimulation? *J Pharm Pharmacol* 1978;30:280–3.

33. Rokosz-Pelc A, Antkiewicz-Michaluk L, Vetulani J. 5-Hydroxytryptamine-like properties of m:chlorophenylpiperazine: comparison with quipazine. *J Pharm Pharmacol* 1980;32:220–2.

34. Seeman P, Westman K, Coscina D, Warsh JJ. Serotonin receptors in hippocampus and frontal cortex. *Eur J Pharmacol* 1980;66:179–91.

35. Tuomisto L, Tuomisto J. Inhibition of monoamine uptake in synaptosomes by tetrahydroharmane and tetrahydroisoquinoline compounds. *Naunyn-Schmiedebergs Arch Pharmacol* 1973;279:371–80.

36. Vargaftig BB, Coigent JL, de Cos CJ, Grysen H, Bonta IL. Mianserin hydrochloride. Peripheral and central effects in relation to antagonism against 5-hydroxytryptamine and tryptamine. *Eur J Pharmacol* 1971;16:339–46.

37. Volkman PH, Lorens SA, Kindel GH, Ginos JZ. L-5-Hydroxytryptophan-induced myoclonus in guinea pigs; a model for the study of central serotonin-dopamine interactions. *Neuropharmacology* 1978;17:947–55.

38. Waldmeier PC, Baumann PA, Maitre L. CGP 6085A, a new, specific, inhibitor of serotonin uptake: neurochemical characterization and comparison with other serotonin uptake blockers. *J Pharm Exp Ther* 1979;211:42–9.

39. Weiner WJ, Goetz C, Nausieda PA, Klawans HL. Clonazepam and 5-hydroxytryptophan-induced myoclonic stereotypy. *Eur J Pharmacol* 1977;46:21–4.

Advances in Neurology, Vol. 43: Myoclonus,
edited by S. Fahn et al. Raven Press,
New York © 1986.

A New Animal Model for Action Myoclonus

*Esther Shohami, **Shmuel Evron, *Marta Weinstock,
†Dov Soffer, and ‡Amiram Carmon

*Department of Pharmacology, The Hebrew University, Hadassah Medical School;
**Department of Anesthesia, Hadassah University Hospital; †Department of Pathology,
Hadassah University Hospital; and ‡Brain and Behavior Research Unit, Hadassah
University Hospital, Jerusalem, Israel 91120*

Action myoclonus is a syndrome characterized by a sudden contraction or a series of contractions of a single muscle or of a group of muscles. This syndrome can be activated by the intention to move or by visual or acoustic stimuli.

One of the predominant causes for the human syndrome is cerebral hypoxia. It was first reported by Lance and Adams (6) to persist in patients who recovered from hypoxic coma, and they therefore named it "Post hypoxic action myoclonus".

Several attempts have been made to establish an animal model of this neurological disorder. Klawans et al. induced myoclonus in guinea pigs by the injection of 5-HTP (5) or levodopa (4), whereas Chadwick et al. (1,2) used either 5-HTP or chloralose in this species. Muscimol (7) and chloro-organic coupounds (11) were shown to cause myoclonic activity in mice. Sharma et al. (8) attempted to induce myoclonus in the rat by anoxia but succeeded only in obtaining a few isolated jerks of short duration in the early anoxic phase and again during transformation from an atmosphere of nitrogen to room air. All of the animal models hitherto reported failed to show a behavior consistent with the arrhythmic stimulus-sensitive and movement-initiated jerks that typify action myoclonus.

While investigating the analgesic efficacy of epidural morphine in rats, we occasionally observed a phenomenon that resembled action myoclonus and that lasted for about 1 hr (9). Tang and Schoenfeld (10) noted that intrathecal injection of morphine-induced myoclonus to human myoclonus, which was confirmed by S. Fahn *(personal communication)*, led us to conduct a thorough, methodological study of this behavior. This was of particular relevance in view of a recent clinical survey of postanoxic myoclonus (3), from which it can be implied that the majority of the subjects had received opiates.

study of this behavior. This was of particular relevance in view of a recent clinical survey of postanoxic myoclonus (3), from which it can be implied that the majority of the subjects had received opiates.

METHODS

Male Sabra rats (Hebrew University, Jerusalem) weighing 180–200 g were used in this study.

Surgical Procedure

Implantation of Intrathecal Catheters

Rats were chronically implanted with polyethylene (PE-10) catheters under sodium pentobarbital anesthesia (35 mg/kg). A midline incision of 2 cm was made in the skin above the lumbar vertebrae, the skin was pulled aside, and the attachments of the muscles to the spinal processes were cut and retracted. A tiny part of the dura was exposed, and the catheter was inserted into the subdural space and advanced about 8 to 9 cm to the upper thoracic–lower cervical level in one group of rats, and 2 cm to the lumbar region in another. The catheter was attached to the exposed laminae with acrylic bone cement, and the muscles and skin were sutured. The free end of the catheter was bent and passed subcutaneously to the neck area; 2 to 3 cm of it was left protruding from the skin to allow for drug administration. The catheter was washed with 0.03 ml saline and plugged with a drop of cement. In three rats from each group, we have verified the location of the catheters by injection of 0.03 ml of indigo. Approximately 5% of the rats developed paralysis of the lower limbs and were discarded from the study. The experiments were carried out one to three days after surgery.

Preparation of Spinal Rats

The spinal column was exposed at the lower thoracic level of 8 rats followed by laminectomy. Then, the spinal cord was transected and the canal blocked with bone wax to prevent diffusion of injected material. The intrathecal catheter was then implanted in the lumbar region.

Drugs

Drugs for intrathecal administration were dissolved in normal saline so that the dose required was in 20 or 40 µl. Control groups were injected with an identical volume of the vehicle. Morphine hydrochloride (U.S. Vitamins Laboratories Division, New York) at a dose of 0.4 mg was used throughout the study to produce the myoclonic activity. Methadone (Eli Lilly, Indianapolis), 0.2 and 0.4 mg, was administered to a group of 20 rats, and pethidine (Janssen Pharmaceutical Research Laboratories Beerse, Belgium), 0.2 to 0.5 mg, to eight rats. Etorphine (Reckett & Sons, United Kingdom) 12.5 µg and 25 µg was given to six rats.

Naloxone (Endo Laboratories, Garden City, New York) was injected either into the catheter (0.04 mg) or intraperitoneally (0.4 mg) at the peak of the myoclonic activity.

Measurement of Myoclonic Activity

Some of the animals were placed on an animal movement monitor (a platform with strain gauge produced by Columbus Instruments, Columbus, Ohio). During the experiments, the output of the strain gauge was fed through amplifiers into a paper-chart recorder. This produced a permanent record of the animals' movements, which enabled us to make more accurate measurements of their timing and amplitude.

Measurement of Blood Gases and Effect of Hypoxia

In another eight rats, an additional catheter, PE-50, was inserted under anesthesia into the carotid artery. On the following day, when the animals were fully awake, arterial blood samples (0.2 ml) were taken before and at various time points after the injection of morphine or saline. The samples were analyzed for blood gases (Pa_{CO_2} and Pa_{O_2}) on a gas analyzer (IL 313 Instrumentation Laboratory, Lexington).

In order to evaluate whether hypoxia would facilitate myoclonic activity, a group of eight rats was prepared with 2 cannulae as described above and injected with 0.2 mg morphine. This dose was found to produce myoclonic activity of a weaker intensity and of shorter duration than that induced by 0.4 mg morphine. Five minutes after morphine administration, the rats were exposed to atmospheric nitrogen for 1 to 2 min, and blood samples were taken to determine the level of hypoxia.

Neuropathological Examination

At the peak of the myoclonic activity, five rats were processed for pathological examination, together with two control rats. Another two rats were examined 1 week later. The animals for histopathologic evaluation were killed by perfusing the cardiovascular system with 10% buffered formaldehyde solution. Brains were removed, immersed in the same fixative for 10 days and processed for paraffin embedding. Five sections were examined from each brain, from different levels including neocortex, hippocampus, thalamus, hypothalamus midbrain, pons medulla and cerebellum. Sections were examined by one examiner (D.S.) without prior knowledge of the group of rats to which the brains belonged.

RESULTS

Behavior

After morphine administration, a stereotypic sequence of disrupted behavior started. It was observed in 80% of the animals irrespective of the length of the intrathecal catheter. This sequence can be divided into the following, overlapping, stages:

1. Piloerection, and dragging of the lower limbs that started immediately. This stage lasted for 10 to 20 min. Some animals also exhibited transitory erection of the tail.
2. About 5 min after injection, the animals started to scratch themselves, mainly at the level of the tip of the catheter. These movements were sometimes violent; the upper limbs were entangled around the torso for many seconds in an attempt to scratch the lower neck. Such "seizures" lasted 10 to 20 sec

each time and could occur once or twice a minute. Usually, this phenomenon lasted from 3 to 15 min.

3. Before the violent scratching was terminated, myoclonic jerks were noticed. These appeared at irregular intervals and were clearly augmented by two factors, initiation of a movement and external stimulation. When precipitated by movement, the jerks usually involved the limbs, but sometimes the neck and head only. Jerking was invariably initiated by an acoustic stimulus such as hand clapping. Such stimuli often aroused violent generalized jerks that in some cases made the animal jump an inch or two in the air. Stimulus-sensitive movements could be elicited only if enough time (5–10 sec) was allowed between the stimulus and the previous jerk.

The myoclonic manifestations were visually observed, and notice was taken of the time of onset, variations, duration, and frequency as well as sensitivity to external stimuli.

The frequency of the jerks increased from their onset and reached a maximum of 10 to 15 bursts of jerks per minute at 10 to 15 min after onset. Then the rats became progressively less active, and after 40 to 50 min, jerking ceased. The stimulus sensitivity, however, lasted longer, up to 1.5 hr.

Figure 1 shows a record of the spontaneous jerks and response to an acoustic stimulus (hand clap, marked by an arrow) of the same rat before (Fig. 1A) and after (Fig. 1B) morphine injection. No spontaneous jerks were recorded in the control period before injection. Only after morphine administration did the animals exhibit the abrupt spontaneous myoclonic activity.

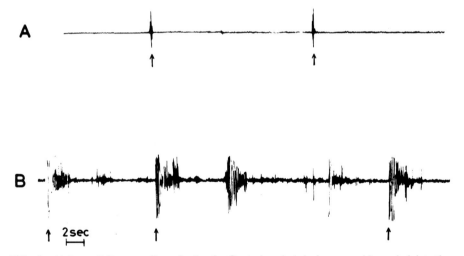

FIG. 1. Motor activity recording of rat. **A:** Control period, before morphine administration. **B:** 10 min after 0.4 mg morphine injection into the intrathecal space. *Arrow*, acoustic stimulus (hand clap).

Most rats (80%) survived the myoclonic episode and seemed to return to normal activity. One day after the experiment, myoclonus could be induced again in those rats by the same dose of morphine.

The rats with spinal transection were tested with morphine 1 day after surgery to determine which neuronal pathways were involved in the genesis and expression of this syndrome. All spinal-transected rats had paralysis of the lower limbs but were otherwise normal. Administration of morphine intrathecally below the level of transection did not result in any myoclonic activity.

Administration of Other Drugs

Three other analgesic drugs were employed in the study, to test whether this effect of morphine can be induced by other opiate agonists. One day after myoclonus had been induced by morphine in eight rats, they were given either 0.2 mg ($N = 4$) or 0.4 mg ($N = 4$) of methadone. Another group of 12 rats was given methadone only, without prior morphine treatment. Methadone failed to induce myoclonic activity in any of these rats. Pethidine, given to eight rats, resulted in an instantaneous hindlimb paralysis that lasted for 20 to 30 min but did not produce the myoclonic syndrome. These rats suffered from respiratory depression, and three died as a consequence. The rats that received etorphine became catatonic within seconds of injection. This catatonia lasted for 2 hr, after which time the rats returned to normal activity.

In order to determine whether morphine produced the myoclonus by activation of specific opiate receptors, the opiate antagonist naloxone was injected in a number of rats at the peak of the myoclonic activity. Naloxone injected either intraperitoneally or intrathecally caused an obvious, yet temporary reduction in both the amplitude and frequency of the jerks.

Blood Gases

In view of the clinical association between myoclonus and hypoxia, it was of interest to determine whether the myoclonic activity induced by intrathecal morphine was associated with respiratory depression. Arterial blood gases were monitored in six of the eight rats that developed myoclonus. The results of the blood gas levels are summarized in Table 1. It can be seen that intrathecal injections of morphine did not cause any significant respiratory depression. Although the myoclonic attacks did not appear to be correlated with hypoxia, we nevertheless decided to check whether there is an additive effect of morphine and hypoxia on the myoclonus in another group of rats. Eight rats were exposed to nitrogen and their level of Pa_{O_2} was reduced to 20 to 35 mm Hg. Five of the rats developed myoclonus, which was of the same intensity and duration as that developed by nonhypoxic rats injected with the same dose of morphine. When the myoclonic activity ceased, these rats were exposed to nitrogen for another 2 min. No change

TABLE 1. *Blood gas values at various times after injection of morphine into the intrathecal space*

Time after injection (min)	Pa$_{O_2}$ (mm Hg ± SE)	Pa$_{CO_2}$ (mm Hg ± SE)
0	98.8 ± 7.3	20.3 ± 2.0
5	108 ± 9	19.8 ± 2.3
10	100 ± 10	17.8 ± 3.9
20	88 ± 6	23 ± 4
30	105 ± 11	26.5 ± 1.5
60	95 ± 6	25.6 ± 2.3

in their motor activity was noticed. The other three rats did not develop myoclonus even after 2 min of hypoxia.

Dye injection experiments in the rats with long catheters verified that the catheters had been placed in the intrathecal space and that their tips were about 1.0 to 1.5 cm caudal to the medulla oblongata. We noticed that the dye stayed close to the point of application to the spinal cord, did not diffuse toward the cisterna magna, and had no access to the entire neuraxis. In the rats with the short catheters, the dye did not diffuse more than a few millimeters from the point of application.

Neuropathology

The myoclonic rats displayed marked hypoxic–ischemic cell change in certain neuronal groups. This change was characterized by shrinkage of neuronal cell bodies, which stained uniformly eosinophilic. The nucleus appeared shrunken, angulated, and pyknotic, and the nucleolus was invisible. Changes were most pronounced in the Purkinje cell layer of the cerebellum, in which it was estimated that 70 to 80% of the neurons were affected. In Sommer's sector of the hippocampus, 30 to 90% of the pyramidal neurons were injured, and in the bulbar reticular formation, approximately 20 to 50% of the neurons were involved. Scattered hypoxic neurons were observed in other brain regions, mainly in the cerebral cortex. There was no apparent neuronal loss nor significant glial reaction. Brains of control animals usually displayed mild changes of hypoxic–ischemic type in occasional neurons in various brain regions. The brains of two rats were examined 1 week after morphine administration and myoclonic episode. The same regions that seemed to be affected at the peak of the myoclonic activity displayed hypoxic–ischemic cell changes of similar intensity.

DISCUSSION

The myoclonus induced by intrathecal morphine was irregular, unpredictable, stimulus-sensitive, and initiated by movement. As such, it resembled closely the human syndrome of myoclonus and may therefore serve as a novel animal model for the study of this neurological disturbance. Since the myoclonus induced by morphine was antagonized by naloxone, one may conclude that it is mediated by specific opiate receptors. The experiments with methadone, pethidine, and etorphine were performed to determine whether the myoclonic syndrome induced by intrathecal morphine also occurs with other opiate analgesic drugs. The present results demonstrate that methadone, which is as potent an analgesic drug as morphine, does not produce myoclonic activity. No conclusive results could be obtained regarding the action of pethidine or etorphine, since the rats developed paralysis or catatonia when given these drugs. These conditions could have prevented the appearance of myoclonic activity. It is therefore suggested that morphine induces the myoclonic syndrome by a mechanism that is not common to all other opiate analgesics.

It is likely that the syndrome resulted from an action of morphine on the spinal cord, since it occurred when the drug was injected at either the lumbar or thoracocervical level. The experiments with the spinally transected rats were designed to demonstrate whether the effect of morphine was local, at the spinal cord level, and could be expressed even though all neuronal pathways that connect the site of application to higher brain regions had been severed. The results of these experiments demonstrate that an intact spinal cord is required for the myoclonus syndrome to occur as a result of intrathecal morphine administration.

Most of the clinical reports of myoclonus have been associated with a hypoxic episode during surgery, often in conjunction with the use of opiate analgesic drugs. In the present model, we could find no evidence that hypoxia resulting from morphine-induced respiratory depression occurred before or during the myoclonic episode. We were also unable to demonstrate any facilitation of the phenomenon by hypoxia. It is therefore possible that the phenomenon in humans and that described in the present study result from the same final neurological changes which are initiated differently. Hypoxia however did occur in various brain regions, as described above (Results). These changes were irreversible, as was seen from the pathological examination performed 1 week following the myoclonic episode. These preliminary results suggest that the brain damage is a result of the myoclonic activity, which, although transient in its neurologic manifestation, causes permanent cell damage in the brain.

The results presented here demonstrate that the myoclonic activity induced by intrathecal morphine does not result from respiratory depression. However, as a result of these prolonged myoclonic seizures, hypoxic changes occur in the brain.

It should be stressed that at present the relationship between this animal model and the clinical syndrome are only phenomenological. The mechanism by which intrathecal morphine induces myoclonus is not yet understood. It is hoped that a study of the effect of morphine on neurotransmitters in the spinal cord will clarify the mode of action.

SUMMARY

Morphine was injected into a catheter implanted chronically into the intrathecal space of rats. Three to eight minutes after drug administration, 80% of the rats developed arrhythmic stimulus-sensitive jerks that lasted up to 1 hr. The morphine-induced myoclonic activity was markedly reduced by naloxone. Methadone, pethidine, and etorphine failed to produce the syndrome. In spinally transected rats, morphine injected below the level of transection did not produce the syndrome. No significant changes in Pa_{CO_2} and Pa_{O_2} were produced by morphine before and throughout the period of myoclonic activity. Neither did induced hypoxia augment the effect of morphine. However, irreversible hypoxic–ischemic cell changes were noticed in some brain regions. The phenomenon described here resembles the human syndrome of action myoclonus and may serve as an animal model for studying the mechanism of that neurological disorder.

ACKNOWLEDGMENT

We wish to thank Miss H. Avissar for her skillful technical assistance. This work was partially supported by a grant from the joint fund of the Hebrew University and Hadassah Medical Organization, Jerusalem, and by the Seiden Family and the Myoclonus Foundation.

REFERENCES

1. Chadwick D, Hallett M, Jenner P, Marsden CD. 5-Hydroxytryptophan–induced myoclonus in guinea pigs. *J Neurol Sci* 1978;35:157–65.
2. Chadwick D, Hallett M, Jenner P, Marsden CD. Observation on chloralose-induced myoclonus in guinea pigs. *Br J Pharmacol* 1980;69:535–40.
3. Fahn S. Posthypoxic action myoclonus: review of the literature and report of two new cases with response to valproate and estrogen. In: Fahn S, Davis JN, Rowland LP, eds. Advances in Neurology; vol. 26. New York: Raven Press, 1979:49–84.
4. Klawans HL, Goetz C, Bergen D. Levodopa induced myoclonus. *Arch Neurol* 1975;32:331–4.
5. Klawans HL, Goetz BA, Weiner WJ. 5-Hydroxytryptophan–induced myoclonus in guinea pigs and the possible role of serotonin in infantile myoclonus. *Neurology* 1973;23:1234–40.
6. Lance JW, Adams RD. The syndrome of intention or action myoclonus as a sequel to hypoxic encephalopathy. *Brain* 1963;86:111–36.
7. Menon MK, Vivonia CA. Muscimol induced myoclonic jerks in mice. *Neuropharmacology* 1981;20:441–4.
8. Sharma JN, Snider SR, Fahn S, Hiesiger E. Anoxic myoclonus in the rat. In: Fahn S, Davis JN, Rowland LP, eds. Advances in Neurology; vol. 26. New York: Raven Press, 1979:181–9.
9. Shohami E, Evron S. Intrathecal morphine induces myoclonic seizures in the rat. *Acta Pharmacol Toxicol* 1985;56:50–4.
10. Tang AH, Schoenfeld MJ. Comparison of subcutaneous and spinal subarachnoid injections of morphine and naloxone on analgesic tests in the rat. *Eur J Pharmacol* 1978;52:215–23.
11. Van Woert MH, Chung Hwang E. Animal models of myoclonus. In: Fahn S, Davis JN, Rowland LP, eds. Advances in Neurology; vol. 26. New York: Raven Press, 1979:173–80.

Advances in Neurology, Vol. 43: Myoclonus,
edited by S. Fahn et al. Raven Press,
New York © 1986.

Urea-Induced Stimulus-Sensitive Myoclonus in the Rat

S. Muscatt, J. Rothwell, J. Obeso, N. Leigh, P. Jenner,
and C. D. Marsden

*University Department of Neurology, Institute of Psychiatry and King's College Hospital
Medical School, London SE5, United Kingdom*

Stimulus-sensitive myoclonus occurs in a variety of neurological and metabolic disorders in man, notably postanoxic action myoclonus and uremia. The physiology of stimulus-sensitive myoclonus is complex, but at least in some patients the myoclonic jerks appear to originate in the brainstem rather than in the cerebral cortex. This has been termed reticular reflex myoclonus (3). This form of stimulus-sensitive myoclonus may involve a deficit in brain 5-hydroxytryptamine (5-HT) function and may be responsive to the administration of clonazepam or 5-hydroxy-tryptophan (2).

A variety of abnormal movements occur in patients with renal failure, including muscle fasciculation, asterixis, and myoclonus (4,7). Chadwick and French (1) have provided a recent detailed description of uremic-induced myoclonus. Such myoclonus usually was absent at rest but was provoked by voluntary movement. Myoclonus was also provoked by a variety of sensory stimuli, which often caused widespread proximal and distal muscle jerks. In these respects, it closely resembled the reticular reflex myoclonus sometimes observed after recovery from cerebral anoxia. A further similarity was the marked ability of clonazepam to suppress myoclonus in uremic patients. Based on their observations. Chadwick and French (1) proposed that uremic myoclonus arose in the lower brainstem reticular formation, as in the case in some patients with postanoxic action myoclonus.

At the present time no animal model of postanoxic action myoclonus exists. Since it seems probable that both uremia and anoxia may cause myoclonus mediated by similar mechanisms, the ability of urea infusions in animals to induce myoclonus may be of relevance to the mechanisms responsible for both forms of myoclonus in man. The object of the present work has been to evaluate this model by reference to the work of Zuckerman and Glaser (8) in the cat and to our own studies in the rat.

UREA-INDUCED MYOCLONUS IN THE CAT

Previous studies had shown that increasing the plasma concentration of urea in animals induces a syndrome strikingly reminiscent of the excitatory neuromuscular events seen in clinical uremia (5,6). However, it was the careful investigations of Zuckerman and Glaser (8) that determined the mechanism underlying these paroxysmal events and the brain structures that were involved.

Behavioral Effects of Urea Infusion in the Cat

In an initial series of studies, conscious cats with 19 implanted electrodes in the brain were infused with urea (33% solution in 10% invert sugar) at a rate of 0.07 to 0.09 ml/min/kg body weight, into either the internal jugular vein or the peripheral end of the internal carotid artery. The behavior of the animals and their cardiac, muscular, and brain activity were monitored.

During the first 80 min of urea infusion, no behavioral changes were observed. After 80 to 120 min, all animals developed typical motor manifestations. Small asynchronous fascicular twitches appeared at different levels, initially in the facial musculature. The twitches increased in magnitude, became synchronous, and merged into clear-cut localized myoclonic jerks that induced some limb displacement. During this period, loud noises and proprioceptive stimuli induced generalized jerks and startle reactions. During the following 15- to 20-min period, a continuous increase in incidence and amplitude of these phenomena occurred. This was followed by more generalized myoclonic jerking, occurring either spontaneously or induced by voluntary movements of the animal or by sensory stimuli. After a further 10- to 15-min interval, these jerks were followed by generalized clonic convulsions lasting 5- to 10-sec. During the next 30- to 60-min period, the myoclonic jerks occurred continuously. Finally, generalized tonic-clonic convulsions took place, and the animals died in status epilepticus.

Zuckerman and Glaser (8) found that if the urea infusion was stopped as soon as the myoclonic changes became apparent, then a milder syndrome developed, without tonic-clonic seizures, and gradually subsided over the following 1 to 3 hr. When the urea infusion was stopped later, but before the onset of generalized seizures, and a hypotonic saline infusion was substituted, recovery also usually occurred.

The Electrophysiology of Urea-Induced Myoclonus in the Cat

A detailed electrophysiological study showed that supramesencephalic structures were not involved in the production of the myoclonus, although they were active during the stage of generalized tonic-clonic seizures. Myoclonus was associated with paroxysmal activity in the brainstem, particularly from the reticular formation. This began after the first 60 to 70 min of urea infusion, before myoclonic jerks were observed visually or were apparent in EMG recordings. Irregular spikes and sharp waves occurred intermittently. These changes were more evident in the bulbar reticular formation, especially at the level of the nucleus gigantocellularis and nucleus reticularis caudalis. During the final period, when generalized tonic–clonic seizures developed, the location of the epileptic activity shifted toward neocortical and paleocortical structures. Microelectrodes implanted into the reticular formation of the lower brainstem during urea infusion showed that each EEG spike, associated with a spontaneous or a stimulus-evoked myoclonic jerk, represented a large depolarization wave lasting 30 to 160 msec, with a high frequency burst of 700- to 900-per-second spikes superimposed on its rising phase.

Effect of Brainstem and Cord Transection and of Tubocurarine on Urea-Induced Myoclonus in the Cat

In a second series of experiments, animals that had recovered from a first urea infusion received transections to the brainstem at different levels. Some of these animals received tubocurarine before or during a subsequent urea infusion.

The basic pattern of the urea-induced myoclonic seizures was not changed in animals with a supracollicular, intercollicular or subcollicular brainstem section. The behavioral and electrical events occurred in the same sequence as described above but with a slight delay in their appearance. In contrast, after sectioning the upper cervical cord, or treatment with tubocurarine to induce complete neuromuscular block, the EEG and behavioral manifestations of urea-induced myoclonic seizures were markedly decreased. Both maneuvers depressed the paroxysmal activity in the reticular formation during urea infusion.

These results suggested that the reticular formation's paroxysmal activity during urea infusion was generated locally without involvement of supramesencephalic structures. Since cervical cord section and curarization reduced, but did not completely abolish, the paroxysmal activity in the reticular formation, such activity appeared to be dependent to a large extent on sensory input.

The experiments of Zuckerman and Glaser (8) established that urea infusions in the cat could reproduce myoclonus similar to that seen in man. However, because of costs, it was not possible to carry out a pharmacological analysis of the phenomena in the cat. We therefore turned our attention to the possibility that urea infusions in the rat might provide a viable and cheaper model of human reticular reflex myoclonus.

UREA-INDUCED MYOCLONUS IN THE RAT

Based on the findings of Zuckerman and Glaser in the cat, we embarked on a series of studies designed to evaluate whether urea would induce a similar myoclonus in the rat that could be used for pharmacological experiments.

Behavioral Effect of Urea Infusion in the Rat

In initial experiments, female Wistar rats (230 g) were anesthetized with chloral hydrate (300 mg/kg, i.p.) and the right external jugular vein was cannulated with fine Portex tubing. The cannulae were filled with sterile 0.9% sodium chloride and secured to the skin of the neck. The rats then were allowed to recover for at least 24 hr. After this period, rats received an intravenous infusion of urea (22 to 65% solution in distilled water) via a constant infusion pump at a rate of 0.045

ml/min (≡0.015 g/min). Behavioral observations were made throughout the period of infusion.

To characterize the behavioral syndrome induced by urea infusion, we initially utilized a 33% concentration as employed by Zuckerman and Glaser. During the first 30 min of urea infusion, no gross abnormality in the rats was observed. Between 30 to 50 min following the start of infusion, animals appeared ataxic with loss of balance and coordination and a swaying of the head and trunk. Some 10 to 20 min later, bursts of rapid shaking movements became apparent, accompanied by an increase in the degree of incoordination. These movements may represent the production of tremor or bursts of fine myoclonic activity. No distinction could be made between these possibilities on gross behavioral observation. Approximately 1 hr after the infusion was initiated, the shaking movements became stimulus sensitive. Sudden noise, touch, or movement would stimulate shaking. Within approximately another 20 min, clear-cut stimulus-sensitive myoclonus became apparent, initially affecting the limbs but later becoming more generalized. The duration of myoclonus following each stimulus increased, and the threshold of stimulation decreased, until long bursts of apparently spontaneous myoclonic activity occurred. Continued infusion then led to tonic–clonic convulsions ending in death.

Using this description of myoclonic activity obtained during infusion of a 33% urea solution, a scoring system for behavioral change was devised as shown in Table 1. The average times of onset of the various stages of the behavioral syndrome seen during the urea infusion are shown in Table 2. This behavioral scoring system was used to assess the progression of the syndrome in subsequent experiments.

Varying the concentration of the urea solution infused between 22 and 60.5% showed the time of onset of the components of the behavioral syndrome to be concentration-related. As shown in Figure 1A, the onset of stimulus-sensitive myoclonus occurred after approximately 4 hr infusion at 22% urea, but the time of onset fell rapidly with increasing concentrations of urea. Only approximately

TABLE 1. *Behavioral syndrome induced by the intravenous infusion of a 33% solution of urea in the rat*

Score	Behavior
1	Ataxia
2	Loss of coordination accompanied by swaying of head and trunk
3	Shaking movements with increasing incoordination of movement
4	Stimulus-sensitive shaking movements
5	Onset of stimulus-sensitive myoclonus initially affecting limbs but becoming generalized
6	Long bursts of myoclonic activity with maintained extension of limbs
7	Generalized tonic-clonic seizures
8	Death

TABLE 2. *Time of onset of components of
the behavioral syndrome induced
by the intravenous infusion of a
33% solution of urea in the rat*

Score	Time of onset[a] (min)
1 + 2	40.5 ± 2.4
3	55.4 ± 2.6
4	66.7 ± 3.3
5	86.6 ± 2.9
6	96.8 ± 2.9
7	99.3 ± 4.1
8	112.0 ± 2.5

[a]Means ± 1 SEM; $N = 12$.

1.5-hr infusion was required to obtain myoclonus with the 33% concentration. A 60.5% concentration caused myoclonus after some 40 min of infusion. Calculation of the total amount of urea infused (Fig. 1B) showed that with urea concentrations of between 22 and 33%, the time to onset was inversely related to the total amount of urea infused. With concentrations of 33 to 60.5%, the total amount of urea infused in the time to onset of myoclonus was almost constant, perhaps explaining the less dramatic decrease in onset time with concentrations of above 33%.

The stimulus-sensitive myoclonic component of this behavioral syndrome was of current interest, so attempts were made to prevent myoclonus developing into generalized seizure activity leading to the death of the animals. However, unlike the findings of Zuckerman and Glaser (8) in the cat, discontinuing infusion at the time of onset of stimulus-sensitive myoclonus in the rat did not reliably prevent the syndrome from progressing. When the infusion was terminated at the first signs of behavioral change, the subsequent occurrence of myoclonus was unpredictable. Attempts were also made to vary the infusion rate once myoclonus was established, but this too did not provide any consistent means of provoking myoclonus alone.

Electrophysiology of Urea-Induced Myoclonus in the Rat

In subsequent experiments animals were prepared with silver electrodes implanted over the sensorimotor cortex, the cerebellar cortex, and the brainstem at the level of nucleus reticularis gigantocellularis. Several days later, animals received an infusion of a 33% urea solution, and EEG and EMG activity following spontaneous or electrically triggered myoclonus was analyzed.

As shown in Fig. 2, spontaneous muscle jerks were preceded by a time-locked discharge in the lower brainstem and ipsilateral cerebellum, as previously shown in the cat. This is consistent with the idea of a focus present in hindbrain structures, which then spreads to the rest of the brain and to the muscles. The effect of electrical stimulation of the hindlimb, with ring electrodes around the foot, is shown in Fig. 3. In limb muscles, the stimulation provoked an initial short-latency

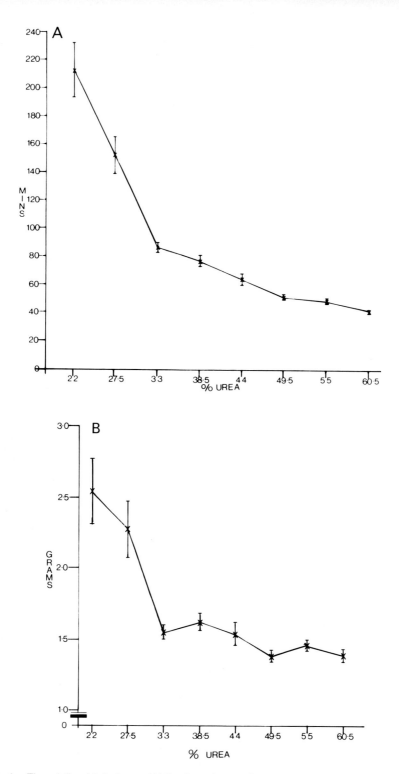

FIG. 1. The relationship between **(A)** the time of onset (in minutes after starting urea infusion) of stimulus-sensitive myoclonus to the concentration of urea solution infused, and **(B)** the total amount (in grams) of urea infused at each concentration required to induce stimulus-sensitive myoclonus.

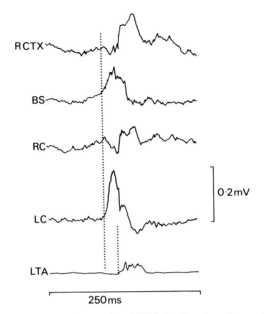

FIG. 2. Average of 16 EEG **(top 4 traces)** and EMG **(bottom trace)** recordings of spontaneous jerks in a rat during the 75 to 100 min of a continuous intravenous 33% urea infusion. Electrodes were implanted over the right parietal cortex (RCTX), brainstem (BS), and right and left cerebellum (RC, LC). All were refered to an electrode implanted in midfrontal cortex. The rectified EMG is from an electrode implanted in the left tibialis anterior muscle (LTA). The ongoing EEG was back-averaged from the take-off of the muscle action potential in tibialis anterior. No obvious cortical event preceded the muscle contractions. However, some 20 msec prior to the EMG onset *(smaller dotted line)*, there is a clear EEG event (with onset at the larger dotted line) maximal in the electrode recording over the left cerebellum. A similar potential is evident in the electrode over the brainstem, and a smaller potential, of opposite polarity, is seen in the electrode from the right cerebellum.

response followed by a longer-lasting and less synchronous polyphasic EMG contraction. In the masseter muscle, only the late response was seen. Such stimulation in normal rats usually evokes the first component of the response, which we suggest is a withdrawal reflex. It rarely produces late responses unless the stimulation intensity is extremely high. We interpret the data in Fig. 3 as showing an ascending spinal withdrawal reflex, followed by a later descending, myoclonic jerk (dotted lines). The evoked response in the ipsilateral cerebellum and brainstem precedes the late jerk in the leg by approximately the same time as that seen in spontaneously jerking animals (Fig. 2). Thus, the ascending sensory volley, produced by hindlimb stimulation, may activate the excitable focus in the hindbrain and provoke a myoclonic discharge that travels down the spinal cord to the limb muscles and up the brainstem to the fifth cranial nerve nucleus of the masseter muscle.

Effect of Clonazepam on Urea-Induced Myoclonus in the Rat

The data suggest that urea infusion in the rat produces a myoclonic syndrome that is stimulus sensitive and that resembles, electrophysiologically, reticular reflex

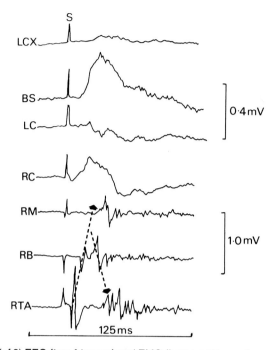

FIG. 3. Average (of 8) EEG **(top 4 traces)** and EMG **(bottom 3 traces)** responses to electrical stimulation of the right foot during the course of an intravenous 33% urea infusion in the rat. The stimulation was given via ring electrodes around the foot, at an intensity was sufficient to provoke a small visible withdrawal response in the animal prior to infusion. EEG electrodes implanted over left parietal cortex (LCX), brain stem (BS) and left and right cerebellum (LC; RC), referred to a mid-frontal cortical electrode. EMGs were recorded from bipolar wire electrodes in the right masseter (RM), biceps brachii (RB) and tibialis anterior (RTA). Following stimulation, a short-latency synchronous EMG response occurs in both limb muscles, followed by a later polyphasic contraction. In the masseter, only the latter is evident. We interpret the two components as being due to spinal withdrawal reflex produced by the ascending sensory volley in the cord, followed by a descending reflex jerk produced by sensory activation of the excitable "center" in the hind-brain. Thus, the initial spinal withdrawal occurred in tibialis anterior before biceps brachii. But the later polyphasic contraction appeared in biceps brachii before tibialis anterior *(dotted lines, arrows)*. Such foot stimulation in a normal rat produces a small early response in tibialis anterior followed by a very small and inconsistent late response in that muscle. In biceps brachii, there is a small early response but no late response in the normal animal.

myoclonus in humans. Finally, we examined whether this myoclonus was sensitive to the administration of clonazepam.

In a series of animals receiving a 44% urea infusion, clonazepam (0.4–2 mg/ kg, i.p.) was administered at the time of onset of stimulus-sensitive myoclonus (50.8 ± 1.6 min). There was a dose-related delay in the development of the myoclonic syndrome, but clonazepam did not prevent myoclonus or the development of the subsequent tonic–clonic convulsions (Fig. 4).

In electrophysiological experiments, rats received a 33% infusion of urea until the onset of myoclonus, when the EEG and EMG recordings of electrically triggered myoclonus were taken. Animals then received clonazepam (0.4 mg/kg), and the

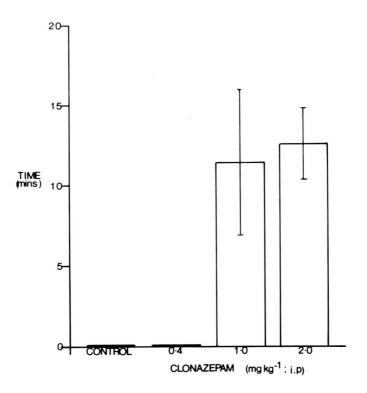

FIG. 4. The ability of clonazepam (0.4–2.0 mg/kg, i.p.) administered at the onset of stimulus-sensitive myoclonus to delay the subsequent occurrence of myoclonus in animals receiving an intravenous 44% infusion. Animals were infused with a 44% urea infusion until the occurrence of stimulus-sensitive shaking and occasional stimulus-sensitive myoclonus. Clonazepam was then administered and caused an immediate cessation of shaking and myoclonus. The urea infusion was continued and the time at which consistent stimulus-sensitive myoclonus reappeared was recorded; $N = 6$; $p < 0.05$, using a two-tailed Student's t-test.

recordings were repeated. As can be seen in Fig. 5, the responses occurring in the cerebellum and brainstem and the subsequent myoclonic jerks were markedly reduced by clonazepam treatment.

DISCUSSION

Intravenous infusion of urea in both the cat and rat appears to be a valid model of reticular reflex myoclonus occurring both in uremia and following anoxic episodes in humans. In both animal species, the infusions resulted in stimulus-sensitive myoclonus of brainstem origin, which was sensitive, to some extent, to clonazepam. However, our initial purpose in reexamining this animal model was to find a reliable and simple pharmacological means of screening drugs that might be useful in the treatment of human myoclonic disorders. Unfortunately, urea infusion in the rat did not meet these criteria. It took a considerable time to initiate myoclonus.

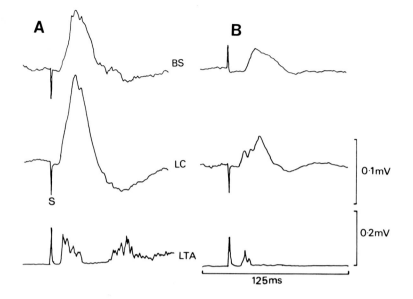

FIG. 5. Averaged EEG recordings ($N = 16$) from electrodes implanted over the brainstem (BS) and left cerebellum (LC), all referred to a midfrontal reference, and the rectified EMG from an electrode implanted in the left tibialis anterior (LTA) of reflex jerks in response to electrical stimulation (S) of the left foot. Records are *(left panels)* before and *(right panels)* 30 min following administration of clonazepam (0.4 mg/kg, i.p.) to an animal receiving an intravenous 33% urea infusion. Before administration of clonazepam, the stimulus evoked the typical double EMG jerk in LTA, which we interpret as a spinal withdrawal response followed by a later reflex jerk. After clonazepam, both phases of the muscle jerk were much reduced and resembled those seen in a normal rat. In addition, the evoked responses in brainstem and ipsilateral cerebellum were attenuated by over 50%.

When myoclonus appeared, it was unstable and progressed into seizures and death. Finally, the complexity of the syndrome made it difficult to document behavioral change with any reliable accuracy.

In conclusion, although mimicking reticular reflex myoclonus in humans, the urea infusion model in the rat (and cat) has not provided the means of assessing drug action that we would have liked. It does, however, provide a means of understanding the electrophysiological and biochemical mechanisms involved in such myoclonus.

SUMMARY

Uremia in humans can cause spontaneous and stimulus-sensitive myoclonus that responds to clonazepam. Uremic myoclonus in humans resembles the reticular reflex form of postanoxic action myoclonus.

Previous investigations have established that urea infusions in the cat can produce spontaneous and stimulus-sensitive myoclonus. This has been shown, electrophysiologically, to arise in the brainstem medullary reticular formation, and it does not require forebrain structures. Our own studies in the rat have shown that urea infusions also produce spontaneous and stimulus-sensitive myoclonus. Electrophysiologically, this resembles human reticular reflex myoclonus. It can be reduced by clonazepam.

The myoclonus produced by urea infusions in the rat progresses very rapidly into uncontrollable tonic-clonic convulsions. Although the urea model in the rat mimics some forms of human myoclonus that arise in the brainstem, it is not suitable as a routine animal model for pharmacological investigations.

ACKNOWLEDGMENTS

This study was supported by the Research Funds of the Bethlem Royal and Maudsley Hospitals and King's College Hospital and the Medical Research Council.

REFERENCES

1. Chadwick D, French AT. Uraemic myoclonus: an example of reticular reflex myoclonus? *J Neurol Neurosurg Psychiatry* 1979;42:52–5.
2. Chadwick D, Hallett M, Harris R, Jenner P, Reynolds EH, Marsden CD. Clinical, biochemical and physiological factors distinguishing myoclonus responsive to 5-hydroxytryptophan, tryptophan plus a monoamine oxidase inhibitor and clonazepam. *Brain* 1977;100:455–87.
3. Hallett M, Chadwick D, Adam J, Marsden CD. Reticular reflex myoclonus: a physiological type of human post-anoxic myoclonus. *J Neurol Neurosurg Psychiatry* 1977;40:253–64.
4. Locke S, Merrill JP, Tyler WR. Neurological complication of acute uraemia. *Arch Intern Med* 1961;108:519–30.
5. Mason MF, Resnik H, Minot AS, Rainey J, Pilcher C, Harrison TR. Mechanisms of experimental uraemia. *Arch Intern Med* 1937;60:312–36.
6. Teschan PE. On the pathogenesis of uraemia. *Am J Med* 1970;48:671–7.
7. Tyler HR. Neurological disorders in renal failure. *Am J Med* 1968;44:734–48.
8. Zuckermann EG, Glaser GH. Urea-induced myoclonic seizures. *Arch Neurol* 1972;27:14–28.

Advances in Neurology, Vol. 43: Myoclonus,
edited by S. Fahn et al. Raven Press,
New York © 1986.

Urea Myoclonus: Possible Involvement of Glycine

Eunyong Chung and Melvin H. Van Woert

*Departments of Neurology and Pharmacology, Mount Sinai School of Medicine,
New York, New York 10029*

In clinical uremia, neurological symptomatology is prominent and includes generalized myoclonus, asterixis, seizures, and obtundation (1,9,12). Infusion of urea into laboratory animals produces abnormal movements similar to those seen in uremia in humans (6,11,14). Zuckerman and Glaser (14) injected urea intravenously into cats and observed generalized stimulus-sensitive myoclonus, which correlated with spike-and-sharp-wave electrical discharges in the lower brainstem reticular formation, mostly in nucleus gigantocellularis (NRG). The mechanism by which urea produces excitation of the medullary reticular formation, and the resultant myoclonus had not been previously investigated.

We have found that unilateral local infusions of p,p'-DDT [1,1,1-trichloro-2,2-bis-(p-chlorophenyl)ethane] or strychnine into the medullary reticular formation (including NRG) of the rat also induced bilateral stimulus-sensitive myoclonus (2). DDT slows sodium-channel closure in neurons, which results in repetitive discharges after a single stimulus (7); this may be the mechanism by which DDT produces a stimulus-sensitive myoclonus. In contrast, strychnine is a glycine receptor antagonist and may increase reticular neuronal discharges by blocking inhibitory glycinergic input to this brain region. In the present study, we investigated whether urea might also block glycinergic neurotransmission in the rat medulla.

METHODS

Male Sprague-Dawley rats weighing 125 to 150 g were used. Urea 2 g/kg (33% in 10% invert sugar) was injected intraperitoneally every 15 min for 4 doses. Rats were sacrificed at the time of maximum intensity of myoclonus, which was 45 min after the last injection. After removing proteins with sodium tungstate, glycine levels were measured by the method of Sardesai and Provido (10). Urea levels were determined according to Henry (4).

In vitro competition of urea with [^{3}H]strychnine and [^{3}H]γ-aminobutyric acid (GABA) binding to membranes from rat medulla were carried out by a modification of a method of Young and Snyder (13) and Enna and Snyder (3), respectively. Frozen medulla was homogenized in 50 vol of 0.05 M TRIS HCl buffer (pH 7.7) and centrifuged at $28,000 \times g$ for 15 min. The pellet was washed once and resuspended in 100 vol of 0.05 M TRIS HCl buffer (pH 7.5). Aliquots of this homogenate were incubated with 1×10^{-9} M [³H]strychnine for 10 min or [³H]GABA for 30 min at 4°C. The reaction was terminated by centrifugation, and the pellet was surface-washed twice with ice-cold buffer. Radioactivities in the pellets were extracted with ethanol and counted by liquid scintillation spectrometry. For [³H]GABA binding, membranes were treated with 0.05% Triton X-100, and 10^{-5} M aminooxyacetic acid was included in the incubation medium. 10^{-4} M of unlabeled strychnine or GABA was used to determine nonspecific binding.

RESULTS

We observed that generalized myoclonic movements occurred in rats after administration of urea 2 g/kg, i.p., every 15 min for 4 doses. After the third dose, the animals developed tremor and myoclonus associated with movement. After the fourth dose, all animals showed spontaneous myoclonus, appeared cyanotic, and had decreased locomotion. Forty-five minutes to 1 hr after the last urea injection, myoclonus reached maximum intensity followed by tonic-clonic convulsions and death.

We measured glycine and urea levels in the medulla of these rats sacrificed during maximum myoclonic movements (Table 1). There was no change in glycine levels, and brain urea levels increased about sevenfold after urea treatment. Plasma urea was elevated 18-fold.

We next examined the effect of urea on glycine receptor binding using [³H]strychnine as a ligand; 10^{-2} and 10^{-1} M urea significantly decreased [³H]strychnine binding by 30 and 43%, respectively. Inhibition of [³H]strychnine binding by urea was reversible and could be restored by repeated washing of the membrane fractions with buffer (data not shown). On the other hand, urea had no effect on [³H]GABA receptor binding (Table 2).

DISCUSSION

Uremia produces multisystem manifestations, one of which is a stimulus-sensitive generalized myoclonus. Numerous biochemical abnormalities have been identified in uremia. In addition to the elevation of urea, increased concentration of other nitrogenous substances, such as aliphatic and aromatic amines, phenolic derivatives,

TABLE 1. *Effects of urea[a] on glycine and urea levels in rats*

	Control[b]	Urea-treated[b]
Medulla glycine (μg/mg protein)	3.03 ± .07	2.78 ± .11
Medulla urea (mg/g wet weight)	0.61 ± .05	4.12 ± .68
Plasma urea (mg/ml)	0.84 ± .04	14.88 ± 1.26

[a]2 g/kg i.p. × 4 every 15 min.
[b]Each value is the mean ± SE of six rats each.

TABLE 2. *Effect of urea (in vitro) on glycine and GABA binding in rat medulla*

	[^{3}H]-strychnine binding[a]	[^{3}H]-GABA binding[a]
Control	3.05 ± 0.19	2.35 ± 0.05
10^{-4} M urea	3.15 ± 0.14	2.51 ± 0.01
10^{-3} M urea	2.80 ± 0.11	2.35 ± 0.01
10^{-2} M urea	2.14 ± 0.12[b]	2.30 ± 0.01
10^{-1} M urea	1.73 ± 0.04[c]	2.19 ± 0.10

[a]Each value (in pmol/g wet weight) is the mean ± SE of 4 samples.
[b]$p < 0.02$.
[c]$p < 0.001$ compared to control.

indoles, amino acids, and other organic acids, have been found in uremic plasma (11). These substances in uremic plasma have been reported to inhibit glycolysis, oxidative phosphorylation, and enzymes involved in other metabolic processes. Because of this diffuse cellular dysfunction in uremia, it has been difficult to link specific chemical changes to uremic symptoms in human patients.

In experimental animals, increasing plasma urea concentration produces generalized stimulus-sensitive myoclonus similar to that observed in clinical uremia (6,11,14). In cats, intravenous infusion of urea induced generalized myoclonus, which occurred either spontaneously or associated with voluntary movements and stimuli such as loud noises and proprioceptive stimulation (14). Electrical activity, recorded from a number of different brain structures during urea infusion, revealed seizure activity, consisting of irregular spikes and sharp waves confined to the bulbar reticular formation, especially at the level of the NRG and nucleus reticularis caudalis. There was a direct correlation between plasma urea concentration and the gradual increase in intensity of epileptic activity.

In the present study, 8 g/kg of urea, in four divided intraperitoneal injections over a 45-min period, produced myoclonus in rats similar to that described in cats by Zuckerman and Glaser (14) after intravenous infusion. Since the glycine receptor antagonist strychnine produces a similar myoclonic syndrome in rats when locally infused into the medullary reticular formation (2), we examined the effect of urea on glycine receptor binding. A reversible 43% inhibition of [^{3}H]strychnine binding in the rat medulla was produced by 0.1 M urea. Urea had no effect on brain glycine levels. Since brain urea concentration was 0.068 M at the time of maximum myoclonic movements, this urea-induced decrease in medullary glycine receptor binding could be responsible for the myoclonus. Thus, urea might inhibit glycine action at the receptor site, like strychnine, or produce allosteric changes in glycine receptor by denaturing the receptor protein. High concentrations of urea have been shown to change the tertiary structure of some proteins, and to a certain extent, this effect can be reversible (5). This is compatible with the reversibility of myoclonus in uremic encephalopathy after hemodialysis. Neuropathological examinations of the brains in patients dying with uremic encephalopathy have revealed only nonspecific changes (8), further suggesting that the neurological signs are probably the result of reversible biochemical changes. GABA receptor binding was not altered by urea, indicating that interference with glycinergic neurotransmission may be a relatively specific effect.

Since the clinical manifestations of experimental urea infusion in animals is similar to the excitatory neuromuscular phenomena in uremic patients, the role of disinhibition of glycinergic neurotransmission by urea in clinical uremia deserves further investigation. Other clinical myoclonic syndromes also could be due to a loss of glycinergic inhibition of medullary reticular neurons.

ACKNOWLEDGMENTS

The authors thank M. Dvorozniak for his technical assistance. This work was supported by USPHS grants NS 17258, NS 12341, and The Gateposts Foundation, Inc.

REFERENCES

1. Chadwick D, French AT. Uremic myoclonus: an example of reticular reflex myoclonus? *J Neurol Neurosurg Psychiatry* 1979;42:52–5.
2. Chung E, Van Woert MH. DDT myoclonus: sites and mechanism of action. *Exp Neurol* 1984;85:273–82.
3. Enna SJ, Snyder SH. Properties of γ-amino-butyric acid (GABA) receptor binding in rat brain synaptic membrane fractions. *Brain Res* 1975;100:81–97.
4. Henry RJ. *Clinical chemistry: principles and techniques.* New York: Harper and Row, 1967:266–70.
5. Katz S, Denia J. Mechanisms of denaturation of bovine serum albumin by urea and urea-type agents. *Biochem Biophys Acta* 1969;188:247–54.
6. Mason MF, Resnik H, Minot AS, Rainey J, Pilcher C, Harrison TR. Mechanism of experimental uremia. *Arch Intern Med* 1937;60:312–36.
7. Narahashi T, Haas H. Interaction of DDT with the component of lobster nerve membrane conductance. *J Gen Physiol* 1968;51:177–98.
8. Olsen S. The brain in uremia. *Acta Psychiatr Scand* 1961;36:(suppl 156) 1–128.
9. Plum F, Posner JB. (Eds.) Metabolic brain diseases causing coma. In: The diagnosis of stupor and coma. 2nd ed. Philadelphia: FA Davis, 1972:141–216.
10. Sardesai VM, Provido HS. The determination of glycine in biological fluids. *Clin Chim Acta* 1970;29:67–71.
11. Teschan PE. On the pathogenesis of uremia. *Am J Med* 1970;48:671–7.
12. Tyler HR. Neurologic disorders in renal failure. *Am J Med* 1968;44:734–8.
13. Young AB, Snyder SH. Strychnine binding associated with glycine receptors of the central nervous system. *Proc Natl Acad Sci USA* 1973;70:2832–2936.
14. Zuckerman EG, Glaser GH. Urea-induced myoclonic seizures. *Arch Neurol* 1972;27:14–28.

Advances in Neurology, Vol. 43: Myoclonus,
edited by S. Fahn et al. Raven Press,
New York © 1986.

DDT Myoclonus: Site of "Myoclonus Center" in the Brain

Eunyong Chung and Melvin H. Van Woert

Departments of Neurology and Pharmacology, Mount Sinai School of Medicine, New York, New York 10029

The insecticide 1,1,1-trichloro-2,2-bis(*p*-chlorophenyl)ethane (p,p'-DDT)(200–600 mg/kg intragastrically) produces generalized, irregular, stimulus-sensitive myoclonus in mice and rats (4,16). DDT-induced myoclonus in rodents is an excellent animal model for serotonin-responsive human intention myoclonus. We previously reported that the myoclonus produced by 600 mg/kg DDT in mice is reduced by intraperitoneal injections of L-5-hydroxytryptophan (L-5-HTP) concomitantly with the serotonin uptake inhibitor chlorimipramine, other serotonin agonists, and clonazepam. In rats, myoclonus induced by 300 mg/kg DDT intragastrically was also reduced by L-5-HTP plus chlorimipramine or clonazepam (4). Various agonists and antagonists of dopamine, γ-aminobutyric acid (GABA), acetylcholine, and norepinephrine were found to have no effect on DDT myoclonus, with the exception of phenoxybenzamine, which also produced a marked amelioration of myoclonic activity (5).

We also reported that transection of the rat spinal cord at the lower thoracic level eliminated DDT-induced myoclonus below the level of transection, whereas transection through the anterior midbrain did not affect DDT myoclonus, indicating that the myoclonic activity is generated within either the brainstem or the cerebellum (4). In order to further localize the neuronal pathways involved in myoclonus, we have infused DDT directly into various brain areas.

METHODS

Male Sprague-Dawley rats weighing 270–320 g were anesthetized with methohexital (Brevital®, Lilly) 50 mg/kg, i.p. A stainless steel needle (60 μm outside diameter) attached to a Hamilton microsyringe was positioned stereotaxically in the various regions of the brain (left side) according to the atlas of Pelligrino et al. (131). One milligram of DDT in 10 μl of dimethylsulfoxide (DMSO) was infused over 67 sec using an infusion pump. The needle was left in place for 6 min before withdrawing. We have verified the position of the needle and the size of DDT diffusion by using 1% Evans blue dye in the injection solution. Equal volumes of DMSO with Evans blue were injected in the same regional areas for controls. Intensity of myoclonus was scored on a scale of 0 to + + +: 0, no myoclonus; +, mild transient myoclonus; + +, moderate transient myoclonus; + + +, severe continuous myoclonus.

RESULTS

Figure 1D is a section through a site of DDT injection that produced maximum intensity of myoclonus (+ + +). The DDT is localized in the medullary reticular formation. Similar unilateral stereotaxic injections of DDT in other parts of the medullary reticular formation (MRF) (8.0–11.0 mm posterior to bregma) also produced generalized arrhythmic, stimulus-sensitive myoclonus comparable to that observed in rats administered intragastric injections of DDT (Table 1). However, no myoclonus was observed when DDT was injected into the pontine, mesencephalic, and most caudal region of MRF (greater than 11.0 mm posterior to bregma). Myoclonus was first observed 30 min to 1 hr after infusion and increased to a maximum intensity at 3 to 4 hr, which persisted unchanged for another 2 hr. Subsequently, the myoclonus gradually decreased, and the animals returned to normal motor function by 18 to 24 hr after DDT infusion. The intensity of myoclonus increased after stimuli such as touch and air puffs. Injection of vehicle alone into the medullary reticular formation had no effect on behavior. Other areas of the brain where unilateral injections of DDT produced generalized stimulus-sensitive myoclonus are cerebellar nuclei, inferior olive, and red nucleus (Fig. 1C, Table 1). Injection of DDT into the following brain areas did not produce myoclonus or any other behavioral abnormality: caudate (Fig. 1A), substantia nigra, hippocampus, motor cortex, cerebellar cortex, amygdala, inferior colliculus, superior colliculus, hypothalamus, ventral thalamus (Fig. 1B), mediodorsal thalamus, subthalamic nucleus, midbrain reticular formation, pontine reticular formation, and most caudal MRF.

DISCUSSION

Myoclonus may be due to hyperexcitable and hyperresponsive neurons secondary to the loss of inhibitory input. Since inhibitory afferent fibers can arise from various regions of the brain, it is not unexpected that the pathological changes in patients with myoclonus have been diffuse and variable. On the other hand, a primary functional abnormality in certain neurons, such as from a metabolic defect (e.g., Lafora body myoclonus), can produce a focus of hyperexcitability resulting in paroxysmal neuronal discharges. It would appear that DDT myoclonus can be attributed to this latter mechanism, i.e., primary neuronal hyperexcitability rather than loss of inhibitory input. DDT-induced myoclonus is reversible, and neurohistological studies have not revealed significant pathological changes (5,12). Furthermore, electrophysiological experiments have demonstrated that the major action of DDT on neurons is prolongation of the negative (depolarizing) afterpotential without altering resting potential (11). This effect of DDT has been shown to be due to a delay in the normal closing of sodium channels. DDT does not open sodium channels that are closed; therefore, it does not initiate an action potential. The net effect of these electrophysiological changes is to increase the number of neuronal discharges after a single stimulus; this may be the mechanism by which DDT produces a stimulus-sensitive myoclonus.

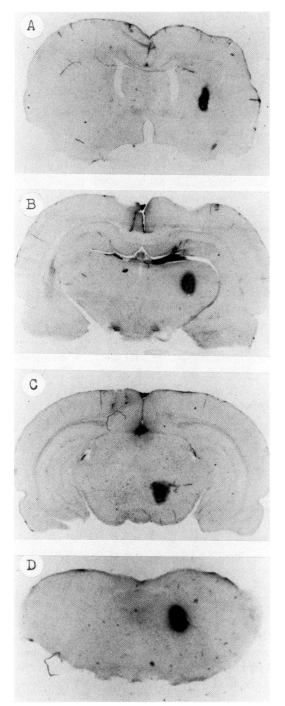

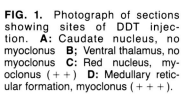

FIG. 1. Photograph of sections showing sites of DDT injection. **A:** Caudate nucleus, no myoclonus **B;** Ventral thalamus, no myoclonus **C:** Red nucleus, myoclonus (+ +) **D:** Medullary reticular formation, myoclonus (+ + +).

TABLE 1. *Regional areas of rat brain where DDT infusion produces myoclonus*

Area	Intensity of myoclonus	No. of observations
Medullary reticular formation (AP, −8.0 to −11.0)	+ + to + + +	38
Red nucleus	+ to + +	5
Inferior olive	+ to + +	6
Cerebellar nuclei	+ to + +	18

In the present study, we have localized the anatomical sites of DDT-induced neuronal hyperexcitability that is associated with myoclonic activity. The local infusion of DDT into certain brain regional areas unilaterally, i.e., medullary reticular formation, cerebellar nuclei, red nucleus, and inferior olive, produces the same generalized stimulus-sensitive myoclonus as occurs after intragastric administration of DDT. Unilateral DDT infusions produce bilateral diffuse myoclonus, presumably due to a lack of somatotopic organization in these brain regions (2). DDT produced the greatest intensity of myoclonus when injected into the medullary reticular formation. The region of the medullary reticular formation where DDT infusion produces myoclonus roughly corresponds to the "inhibitory region" of Magoun (10).

Anatomically, the "inhibitory region" of Magoun coincides with the medullary region that gives rise to reticulospinal fibers. The great majority of medullary reticulospinal neurons originate from the nucleus reticularis gigantocellularis (NRG). Cutaneous nerve stimulation activates a long spinal reflex system, the spinoreticular-spinal reflex, which depends on relay through the bulbar reticular formation with a projection by reticulospinal fibers to flexor alpha motorneurons (14). Halliday (7) has proposed that bilateral myoclonic responses to somatic stimuli could be due to an accentuation of this physiological spinoreticular-spinal reflex. DDT may enhance this spinoreticular-spinal reflex by causing repetitive firing of reticulospinal neurons in response to stimuli from spinoreticular neurons, thus producing a stimulus-sensitive type of myoclonus. Cesa-Bianchi et al. (3) reported that local injections of metallic cobalt powder into the lower brainstem (including NRG) also induced bilateral, generalized, stimulus-sensitive myoclonic muscle jerks, which occurred as early as 24 hr after cobalt implantation and disappeared within 5 to 6 days. Like DDT, cobalt may also produce myoclonus by increasing excitability of the spinoreticular-spinal loop. The work of Zuckerman and Glaser (18) provides further support for this hypothesis. They found that stimulus-sensitive myoclonus produced by intravenous infusions of urea in cats was associated with spike discharges largely confined to NRG and nucleus reticularis caudalis in the medulla.

FIG. 2. Rat cortical EEG following unilateral local injection of DDT into left NRG. Recording electrodes were placed at 2.5 mm posterior to bregma and 4.5 mm lateral to the midsagittal line bilaterally. Reference electrodes were positioned at 2.0 mm anterior to bregma and 3.0 mm lateral to midsagittal line bilaterally.

Normal rat

60 min after DDT injection (in left NRG); appearance of spikes on left side

85 min after DDT injection; bilateral spikes

100 min after DDT injection; bilateral spikes unrelated to myoclonic jerks

101 min after DDT injection; synchronous spike and wave discharge (2.5 sec⁻¹) bilaterally

120 min after DDT injection

Left cortical EEG with EMG of paraspinal muscles after light tactile stimulation of tail

The effect of oral administration of DDT in awake rats chronically implanted with electrodes has been reported (9,17). Frequencies and amplitudes of electrical activities in multiple brain areas were increased. We have recorded cortical EEG's in rats injected with DDT into the left medullary reticular formation (Fig. 2) (M. Onofri, I. Bodis-Wollner, M. Van Woert, E. Chung, *unpublished observations*). Following control EEG recording (Fig. 2, first panel), 1 mg DDT in 10 μl DMSO was infused into left NRG through a previously implanted cannula. In about 30 min, mild generalized myoclonus was first observed with no change in the EEG recording. At 60 min, spikes appeared on the left side, and by 85 min., bilateral spikes were observed. Generalized arrhythmic stimulus-sensitive myoclonus developed, and periodic runs of EEG spikes were observed. However, these EEG spikes had no temporal relationship to spontaneous or tactile stimulus-induced myoclonus. Left cerebral cortex EEG spikes preceded right EEG spikes by approximately 100 msec. One hundred twenty minutes after the DDT injection, cortical EEG returned to normal, although the myoclonus was still present. The last panel of Fig. 2 shows that myoclonic jerks per se, induced by tactile stimulation of the tail at 125 min, do not produce artifacts in the cortical EEG (M. Onofri, I. Bodis-Wollner, M. Van Woert, E. Chung, *unpublished observations*). These results are in contrast to cobalt implantation in the caudal pons and bulbar region in cats, which produces cerebral cortex discharges associated with the myoclonic jerks (3). Thus, the DDT-induced hyperexcitability of neurons in the medullary reticular formation spreads rostrally as well as caudally. Further, since transection of the brain at the anterior midbrain region does not modify DDT myoclonus (4), the electrocortical discharges are not responsible for the myoclonus.

Myoclonus is also produced when DDT is infused into cerebellar nuclei, red nucleus, and inferior olive, although the intensity in each case is less than that observed in the medullary reticular formation. There are afferent projections to the medullary reticular formation from the fastigial nucleus of the cerebellum and from the red nucleus (2). We are not aware of any direct neuronal projections from the inferior olive to the medullary reticular formation. However, the inferior olive can modulate the medullary reticular formation via a relay through the cerebellum (1). Alternatively, the close proximity of the inferior olive to the MRF makes it difficult to eliminate the possibility that DDT infusions to the inferior olive might also make contact with adjacent reticular neurons.

We believe the DDT animal model of myoclonus should be useful for understanding the neuronal pathways and neurotransmitters involved in certain types of myoclonus in humans. Myoclonus has been described in humans accidentally exposed to DDT and other organochlorine pesticides (6,8). Presumably, the neuronal pathways involved in the production of DDT myoclonus are similar in humans and rodents. Further, the DDT animal model has neurological and pharmacological similarities to serotonin-responsive myoclonus in patients (e.g., postanoxic intention myoclonus) (15). We do not exclude the likelihood that other pathways may be involved in other types of myoclonus.

ACKNOWLEDGMENTS

The authors thank M. Dvorozniak for his technical assistance. This work was supported by USPHS grants NS 17258 and NS 12341.

REFERENCES

1. Achenback KE, Goodman DC. Cerebellar projections to pons, medulla and spinal cord in the albino rat. *Brain Behav Evol* 1968;1:43–57.
2. Brodal A. *Neurological anatomy in relation to clinical medicine.* 3rd ed. Oxford: Oxford University Press, 1981:206.
3. Cesa-Bianchi MG, Mancia M, Mutani R. Experimental epilepsy induced by cobalt powder in lower brain-stem and thalamic structures. *Neurophysiology* 1967;22:525–36.
4. Chung Hwang E, Plaitakis A, Magnussen I, Van Woert MH. Relationship of inferior olive-climbing fibers to p,p'-DDT induced myoclonus in rats. *Neurosci. Lett.* 1981;24:103–8.
5. Chung Hwang E, Van Woert MH. p,p'-DDT-induced neurotoxic syndrome: experimental myoclonus. *Neurology* 1978;10:1020–25.
6. Eskenasy JJ. Status epilepticus by dichlorodiphenyltrichlorethane and hexachlorocyclohexane poisoning. *Rev Roum Neurol* 1972;6:435–42.
7. Halliday AM. The neurophysiology of myoclonic jerking—a reappraisal. In: Charlton MH, ed. *Myoclonic seizures.* Amsterdam: Excerpta Medica, 1975:1–29.
8. Hayes WJ Jr. Dieldrin poisoning in man. *Publ Health Rep.* 1957;72:1087–91.
9. Joy RM. Electrical correlates of preconvulsive doses of chlorinated hydrocarbon insecticides in the CNS. *Neuropharmacology* 1973;12:63–76.
10. Magoun HW, Rhines R. An inhibitory mechanism in the bulbar reticular formation. *J Neurophysiol* 1946;9:165–71.
11. Narahashi T, Haas H. Interaction of DDT with the components of lobster nerve membrane conductance. *J Gen Physiol* 1968;51:177–98.
12. Nelson AA, Draize JH, Woodward G, Fitzhugh OC, Smith RB, and Calvery HO. Histopathological changes following administration of DDT to several species of animals. *Publ Health Rep* 1944;59:1009–20.
13. Pelligrino LJ, Pelligrino AS, Cushman AJ. *A Stereotaxic Atlas of the Rat Brain.* New York: Plenum Press, 1979.
14. Shimamura M, Aoki M. Effects of spino-bulbo-spinal reflex volleys on flexor motoneurons of hindlimb in the cat. *Brain Res* 1969;16:333–49.
15. Van Woert MH, Chung Hwang E. Animal models of myoclonus. In: Fahn S, Davis JN, Rowland LP, eds. *Advances in neurology; vol. 26.* New York: Raven Press, 1979;173–80.
16. Van Woert MH, Chung Hwang E. Role of brain serotonin in myoclonus. In: Lloyd KG, Morselli PL, eds. *Neurotransmitters seizures and epilepsy.* New York; Raven Press, 1981:239–49.
17. Woolley DE, Barron BA. Effects of DDT on brain electrical activity in awake, unrestrained rats. *Toxicol Appl Pharmacol* 1968;12:440–54.
18. Zuckermann EG, Glaser GH. Urea-induced myoclonic seizures. *Arch Neurol* 1972;27:14–28.

Advances in Neurology, Vol. 43: Myoclonus,
edited by S. Fahn et al. Raven Press,
New York © 1986.

p,p'-DDT-Induced Myoclonus in the Rat and Its Application as an Animal Model of 5-HT-Sensitive Action Myoclonus

J. A. Pratt, J. Rothwell, P. Jenner, and C. D. Marsden

*University Department of Neurology, Institute of Psychiatry and King's College Hospital
Medical School, Denmark Hill, London SE5, United Kingdom*

Many attempts have been made to find an animal model that mimics the 5-hydroxytryptamine (5-HT)–sensitive action myoclonus of brainstem origin occurring in humans. In 1978, Chung Hwang and Van Woert (4) described the production of stimulus-sensitive myoclonus in mice and rats following administration of *p,p'*-DDT [1,1,1-trichloro-2,2-bis-(*p*-chlorophenyl)ethane]. In mice, they found that drugs that act as 5-HT agonists or that prolong the action of 5-HT in the brain, such as L-5-hydroxytryptophan (L-5-HTP), quipazine, fluoxetine, and Org 6582, decreased myoclonus induced by *p,p'*-DDT. Drugs antagonizing 5-HT receptors, such as methysergide, methergoline, and cinanserin, all increased the intensity of *p,p'*-DDT–induced myoclonus. These findings were interpreted as indicating that *p,p'*-DDT–induced myoclonus was a result of drug-induced deficiency of 5-HT in the brain. This myoclonus appeared initially to be a useful animal model of postanoxic action myoclonus.

Following the introduction of L-5-HTP for treatment of human postanoxic action myoclonus, clonazepam was found to be equally effective (2,3). So when Chung Hwang and Van Woert (4) reported the induction of myoclonus following *p,p'*-DDT administration, we examined the effects of clonazepam on this drug-induced myoclonus in rats. We were unable to demonstrate an effect of clonazepam on *p,p'*-DDT–induced myoclonus in this species, so were surprised when Chung Hwang and Van Woert (5) reported that clonazepam could block the myoclonus induced by *p,p'*-DDT in mice. These findings led us to carry out a detailed pharmacological, biochemical, and physiological investigation of the rat model in an attempt to clarify the mechanism by which *p,p'*-DDT induces myoclonus in the rat and its relationship to action myoclonus in humans. Although most of the published work of Van Woert and his colleague was on studies in the mouse, we used the rat for our investigations because of our electrophysiological expertise in analysis of the source and type of myoclonus in this species. We scarcely expected any major differences in the response of the mouse and the rat to *p,p'*-DDT.

BEHAVIORAL ASSESSMENT

Following p,p'-DDT administration (50–600 mg/kg, p.o., dissolved in corn oil) male Wistar rats (170–230 g) were placed in individual plastic boxes ($35 \times 25 \times 18$ cm) and their motor behavior observed for up to 5 hr. In all of their studies, Chung Hwang and Van Woert employed automated activity meters for assessment of drug effects on p,p'-DDT myoclonus. Such a technique measures all forms of body movement, including myoclonus, tremor, locomotion, and fits. In our studies, we employed a technique of direct observation of individual animals specifically looking for myoclonus, which we defined as spontaneous repetitive limb and body jerks. We also compared the effect of assessing myoclonus using activity meters with the rating system.

The intensity of the behavioral response was assessed by two methods:

1. Behavioral observations at 30-min intervals on a 0 to 6 scale of increasing severity of myoclonus as follows:

   0 The appearance of the animals no different from vehicle-treated controls.
   1 Hyperreactive response to external stimulus but no obvious myoclonus.
   2 Increased stimulus sensitivity accompanied by tremor but without myoclonus.
   3 Intermittent myoclonus involving head and limbs accompanied by tremor.
   4 Continuous myoclonus of head and limbs accompanied by tremor.
   5 Severe continuous myoclonus accompanied by gross tremor.
   6 Intermittent convulsions often leading to death.

2. In automated activity meters. Total activity was recorded in rats previously treated with p,p'-DDT (600 mg/kg, p.o.) by placing individual rats in double photocell activity meters (constructed in the Neurology Department by Mr. H. C. B. Bertoya). Total activity counts were recorded every 5 min for periods of up to 5 hr after p,p'-DDT administration. Animals were simultaneously rated by an observer, as described above.

The effect of drug administration on myoclonus induced by p,p'-DDT (600 mg/ kg, p.o.) was assessed by observation of the intensity of the behavioral response at 30-min intervals following p,p'-DDT administration. At least 6 rats were treated with each drug and compared to control animals pretreated with p,p'-DDT in the same dose but given vehicle rather than active drug. The procedure was modified for examination of drugs expected to potentiate myoclonus by using a subthreshold dose of p,p'-DDT (100 mg/kg, p.o.), with and without the drug under examination.

To increase brain functional 5-HT activity, animals received L-tryptophan (200 mg/kg, i.p.) 1.0 hr following p,p'-DDT administration, L-5-HTP (200 mg/kg, i.p.) 1.5 hr or 3 hr following p,p'-DDT administration, or quipazine (10 mg/kg, i.p.) 1.75 hr following p,p'-DDT administration. In addition, other animals received either nialamide (100 mg/kg, i.p.), tranylcypromine sulfate (25 mg/kg, i.p.), or pargyline hydrochloride (75 mg/kg, i.p.), all administered simultaneously with *p,p'*-DDT. 5-HT reuptake was inhibited by the administration of Org 6582 (10 mg/ kg, i.p.) 1 hr or 2.5 hr following *p,p'*-DDT. To reduce functional 5-HT activity, *p*-chlorophenylalanine methyl ester hydrochloride (PCPA) (200 mg/kg, i.p.) was administered 18 hr and 2 hr prior to *p,p'*-DDT (600 mg/kg, p.o.). Methergoline (5 mg/kg, i.p.), methysergide (5 mg/kg), or cinanserin (10 mg/kg i.p.) were administered 1 hr following *p,p'*-DDT administration (100 or 600 mg/kg, p.o.). Clonazepam (2 or 4 mg/kg, i.p.) was administered 2.5 hr following *p,p'*-DDT administration (600 mg/kg, p.o.).

BEHAVIORAL EFFECTS OF *p,p'*-DDT

Myoclonus appeared gradually after oral administration of *p,p'*-DDT (600 mg/ kg, p.o.) to rats. Initially, tremor developed, followed after 2 to 2.5 hr by intermittent jerking, which became continuous by 3 hr. Between 3 and 5 hr, myoclonus was continuously repetitive and became increasingly severe.

p,p'-DDT (3 hr prior to behavioral assessment) produced a dose-dependent increase in the number of animals exhibiting myoclonus and in the intensity of the behavioral response. At 50 mg/kg *p,p'*-DDT, the appearance of the animals did not differ from vehicle-treated controls. With 100 mg/kg, the animals showed tremor and were hyperreactive in their response to external stimuli. Increasing the dose of *p,p'*-DDT to 200 mg/kg produced intermittent myoclonus in approximately 60% of the animals, although only a small number exhibited continuous myoclonus (10%). At 400 mg/kg, *p,p'*-DDT produced continuous myoclonus in over 80% of animals, and with 600 mg/kg *p,p'*-DDT, all animals developed continuous myoclonus.

EFFECT OF CLONAZEPAM ON *p,p'*-DDT–INDUCED MYOCLONUS

Administration of clonazepam (2 and 4 mg/kg) to rats 2.5 hr following *p,p'*-DDT administration (600 mg/kg) did not inhibit myoclonus as assessed by observer rating (Fig. 1). The number of animals developing continuous myoclonus over the observation period did not differ in the clonazepam or vehicle-treated groups. Following administration of clonazepam (2 and 4 mg/kg), the animals were flaccid and immobile for a period of approximately 1 hr. Clonazepam-treated animals were jerking continuously but were ataxic, unlike vehicle-treated animals, who developed continuous myoclonus but remained upright. The activity of the animals was assessed in parallel using activity meters (Fig. 1). Two-way analysis of variance revealed no overall difference in the activity of animals between different drug treatments. Similarly, there was no interaction between treatment and time. However, analysis of the activity data using the same method as Chung Hwang and Van Woert (5) (paired *t*-test) showed that clonazepam (4 mg/kg) reduced the number of activity counts following drug treatment but that total activity remained unchanged after clonazepam (2 mg/kg) or vehicle (Table 1).

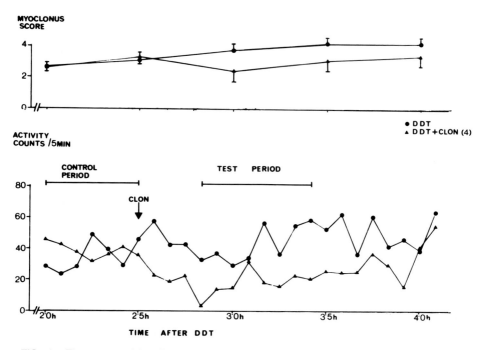

FIG. 1. Time course of the effects of clonazepam on *p,p'*-DDT–induced myoclonus in rats when administered after the onset of myoclonus. Clonazepam 4 mg/kg, i.p. (▲) was administered 2.5 hr following *p,p'*-DDT administration (600 mg/kg, p.o.); (●), animals receiving *p,p'*-DDT in combination with clonazepam vehicle. Results for six animals are expressed as the mean myoclonus score ± SEM, as assessed by observer ratings, and as the number of activity counts per-min period, as determined using activity meters.

TABLE 1. *Effect of clonazepam on motor activity assessed by activity meters in p,p'-DDT–treated rats*

Treatment	Dose (mg/kg, i.p.)	Control[a]	After drug treatment[a]	Paired t-test[a]
Clonazepam vehicle	—	33 ± 6	42 ± 6	NS
Clonazepam	2	23 ± 6	35 ± 8	NS
Clonazepam	4	38 ± 9	18 ± 8	$p < 0.05$[b]

[a]Each value (counts per 5 min) is the mean ± SEM of 7 to 10 rats.
[b]p values refer to the comparison of average activity counts for a period of 30 min prior to drug treatment (control period) with those obtained for a period of 40 min after drug treatment (test period).

EFFECT OF INCREASING BRAIN 5-HT FUNCTION ON *p,p'*-DDT– INDUCED MYOCLONUS

Administration of L-5-HTP (200 mg/kg) 1.5 hr after *p,p'*-DDT (600 mg/kg, p.o.), prior to the onset of myoclonus, delayed the appearance of myoclonus and

TABLE 2. *Influence of drugs that alter 5-HT function on myoclonus in rats induced by p,p'-DDT*

Drug[a]	Dose (mg/kg)	Time after p,p'-DDT (hr)	Change in mean myoclonus score over 3–5 hr[b]
L-5-HTP	200	1.5	Reduced
L-5-HTP	200	3.0	Reduced
L-tryptophan	200	1.0	Reduced
Org 6582	10	1.0	No change
Org 6582	10	2.5	No change
Methergoline	5	1.0	No change
PCPA	200 × 2	18 and 2 hr prev.	No change
Methergoline[c]	5	1.0	No change
Methysergide[c]	5	1.0	No change
Cinanserin[c]	10	1.0	No change

[a]Drugs in the doses shown were injected at the times stated following *p,p'*-DDT (600 mg/kg p.o.).

[b]Average myoclonus score 3–5 hr following the administration of *p,p'*-DDT in combination with each drug was compared to that in animals receiving *p,p'* DDT alone using a Mann–Whitney U test.

[c]Animals receiving a subthreshold dose of *p,p'*-DDT (100 mg/kg p.o.).

reduced its intensity over the observation period. L-5-HTP administered in another experiment 3 hr after the same dose of *p,p'*-DDT, at a time when most animals exhibited continuous myoclonus, reduced the intensity of myoclonus; this effect lasted until the end of the observation period (Table 2).

L-Tryptophan (200 mg/kg) administered 1 hr after *p,p'*-DDT (600 mg/kg, p.o.), prior to the onset of continuous, myoclonus delayed the appearance of the myoclonus and reduced the intensity of myoclonus until the end of the experiment.

Administration of the selective 5-HT reuptake blocker Org 6582 (10 mg/kg) 1 hr following *p,p'*-DDT administration or 30 min following the onset of *p,p'*-DDT–induced myoclonus did not alter the onset of myoclonus or intensity of myoclonus over the 5-hr observation period.

Quipazine (10 mg/kg) administered 1.75 hr after *p,p'*-DDT (600 mg/kg, p.o.) caused a reduction in the mean myoclonus score 2 to 2.5 hr following *p,p'*-DDT administration. However, 3 hr after *p,p'*-DDT, quipazine-treated rats showed gross tremor, forepaw treading, and prostration with splayed hindlimbs, making behavioral assessment impossible.

EFFECT OF DRUGS DECREASING 5-HT FUNCTION ON *p,p'*-DDT–INDUCED MYOCLONUS

Methergoline (5 mg/kg) had no effect on the onset or intensity of myoclonus induced by *p,p'*-DDT (600 mg/kg, p.o., 1 hr previously). Methergoline (5 mg/kg), methysergide (5 mg/kg), and cinanserin (10 mg/kg) administered 1 hr after a subthreshold dose of *p,p'*-DDT (100 mg/kg, p.o.) did not alter the numbers of animals exhibiting myoclonus over the following 4-hr period. Pretreatment with PCPA (200 mg/kg), 18 and 2 hr prior to p,p'-DDT (600 mg/kg, p.o.), which in parallel experiments produced a 65% depletion of cerebral 5-HT concentration, did not alter the severity of p,p'-DDT (600 mg/kg, p.o.)-induced myoclonus.

EFFECT OF MONOAMINE OXIDASE INHIBITORS ON p,p'-DDT–INDUCED MYOCLONUS (FIG. 2)

Pargyline (75 mg/kg) administered simultaneously with p,p'-DDT (600 mg/kg, p.o.) completely prevented the appearance of myoclonus. Animals appeared quite normal, with the exception of some tremor and sensitivity to external stimuli.

Similarly, tranylcypromine (25 mg/kg) or nialamide (100 mg/kg) administered simultaneously with p,p'-DDT (600 mg/kg, p.o.) reduced the intensity of myoclonus but, unlike pargyline, did not completely prevent it. In the tranylcypromine-treated group five of six animals developed intermittent myoclonus, but this did not develop into continuous myoclonus. Nialamide in combination with p,p'-DDT only produced continuous myoclonus in 26% of rats as compared to 73% in the corresponding p,p'-DDT–treated control animals.

CHANGES IN 5-HT PARAMETERS IN p,p'-DDT–TREATED RATS

Whole-brain 5-HT and tryptophan concentrations were unchanged at the onset of continuous myoclonus 3 hr after p,p'-DDT (50–600 mg/kg, p.o.) in comparison to control animals. Brain 5-HIAA concentrations were increased at this time interval but only after p,p'-DDT (600 mg/kg, p.o.) administration ($p = 0.05$). Continuous myoclonic jerking was established in all animals at this time following administration of p,p'-DDT (600 mg/kg, p.o.) and in over 50% of animals receiving p,p'-DDT (200 mg/kg or 400 mg/kg).

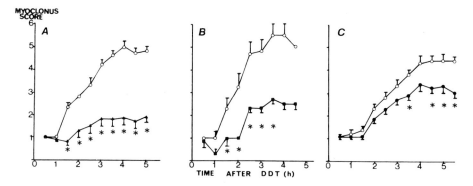

FIG. 2. Time course of the effects of monoamine oxidase inhibitors on p,p'-DDT–induced myoclonus in rats. **(A)** Pargyline 75 mg/kg, i.p. (▲), **(B)** tranylcypromine 25 mg/kg, i.p. (■), or **(C)** nialamide 100 mg/kg, i.p. (●) were administered simultaneously with p,p'-DDT (600 mg/kg, p.o.); (○), animals receiving p,p'-DDT in combination with appropriate vehicle as control. Results are expressed as the mean myoclonus score ± SEM for at least six animals. (*) $p < 0.05$ compared with p,p'-DDT + vehicle-treated control animals (Mann-Whitney U test).

After a period of prolonged myoclonus (4.5 hr after *p,p'*-DDT administration) brain 5-HIAA and tryptophan concentrations were elevated following *p,p'*-DDT administration (200–600 mg/kg, p.o.) ($p = 0.01$) although 5-HT concentrations were unchanged.

PHYSIOLOGY OF *p,p'*-DDT–INDUCED MYOCLONUS

Although a large dose (600 mg/kg, p.o.) of *p,p'*-DDT was employed for all pharmacological and biochemical experiments, it was impossible to obtain uncontaminated electrical recordings from muscle or brain in such rats. The intensity of their jerking led to considerable movement artifact in the electrical records. Accordingly, physiological recordings were undertaken with a smaller dose of *p,p'*-DDT (300 mg/kg, p.o.). Approximately 2 hr afterward, the animals chosen for investigation had developed whole-body jerking, which occurred regularly at a frequency of 1 to 1.5 Hz. Each jerk, which involved many muscles all over the body, consisted of a short asynchronous burst of EMG activity lasting about 50 msec. The relative timing of these bursts in different muscles was estimated for a number of spontaneous jerks in four rats. The sequence of muscle bursting indicated an origin in the lower brainstem activating first the neck muscles innervated by the first three cervical nerves, then subsequently spreading upward to the cranial nerves and downward to the spinal cord, innervating fore- and hindlimbs (Fig. 3A).

Ring electrode stimulation of the limbs did not evoke time-licked generalized muscle jerking, although the local nocioceptive response occurred with much smaller voltages than needed in control animals and also failed to habituate. Cortical evoked potentials were recorded on stimulating the forelimb with shocks insufficient to provoke a nocioceptive response, but there was no change in the latency (8.5– 10 msec) or amplitude (10–15 μV) recorded from central electrodes as compared to untreated animals.

Back-averaging of cortical activity using the EMG jerks recorded from neck muscles failed to reveal any cortical event occurring prior to the earliest EMG burst in the neck muscles. Onset of cortical activity was approximately simultaneous with the muscle jerks and may have been due to "pick-up" of remote muscle activity by the implanted scalp electrodes (Fig. 3B).

Thus, these electrophysiological recordings suggested that the first muscle activity occurred in areas innervated by the lower brainstem. No preceding cortical activity was found that could have caused the muscle jerking. Finally, although animals treated with *p,p'*-DDT exhibited considerable auditory sensitivity (a clap would provoke an obvious jerk), myoclonus was not sensitive to electrical limb stimulation.

DISCUSSION

Following oral administration of *p,p'*-DDT to rats, animals developed fine whole body tremor and stimulus-sensitive myoclonus confirming the initial observations of Chung Hwang and Van Woert in rats and mice (4). The myoclonus was dose dependent, and as in the studies of Chung Hwang and Van Woert (4), the onset of

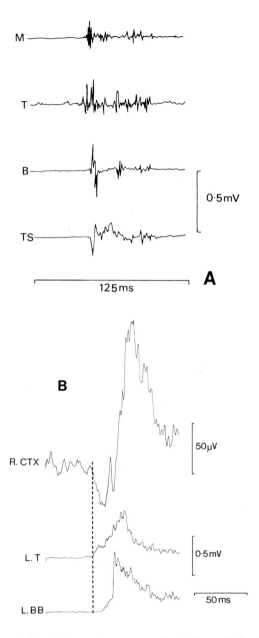

FIG. 3. A. EMG record of a single spontaneous muscle jerk in a rat following administration of *p,p'*-DDT (300 mg/kg). Hooked wire recording electrodes inserted into masseter (M), trapezius (T), biceps brachii (B), and triceps surae (TS). The jerk began with activity in trapezius, followed by activity in masseter and the limb muscles. **B.** Average EEG **(top trace)** and rectified EMG **(bottom traces)** records from 45 spontaneous, whole-body, muscle jerks. The EEG was taken from an electrode implanted over the right sensorimotor cortex, referred to a linked earlobe reference. EMGs taken from the left trapezius (L.T) and left biceps brachii (L.BB). No cortical activity precedes the first sign of EMG activity (see dotted line).

p,p'-DDT myoclonus at a dose of 600 mg/kg, p.o., occurred between 2.0 and 2.5 hr following administration. In mice, Chung Hwang and Van Woert (4) found that drugs that enhanced brain 5-HT activity reduced *p,p'*-DDT–induced myoclonus, whereas 5-HT receptor antagonists generally enhanced myoclonus. They postulated that *p,p'*-DDT–induced myoclonus may be a result of a functional deficiency of 5-HT at its receptor site.

It was the effect of clonazepam that led us to repeat much of Chung Hwang and Van Woert's original work on the myoclonus produced by *p,p'*-DDT, since this compound may be effective in the treatment of human postanoxic myoclonus (2,3).

We adopted an identical protocol to that of Chung Hwang and Van Woert (5) but used rats instead of mice. Clonazepam (2 or 4 mg/kg, i.p.) was administered 30 min after the onset of myoclonus (2.5 hr after *p,p'*-DDT administration) and myoclonus measured as activity counts in activity meters. In addition, in our studies we made parallel assessments of myoclonus by observer rating. Clonazepam (2 and 4 mg/kg, i.p.) did not inhibit or reduce the intensity of myoclonus at any time following *p,p'*-DDT administration as assessed by observer rating. Similarly, two-way analysis of variance of the activity data revealed no difference in activity between animals that had received clonazepam plus *p,p'*-DDT and those that received *p,p'*-DDT alone, nor was there any interaction between treatment and time. Chung Hwang and Van Woert (5), however, used a different method for assessing their activity data. Rather than comparing control and treated animals over the same time period they compared, by a paired Student's *t*-test, the mean activity of animals during a period prior to the administration of clonazepam with a further period following clonazepam. Using an identical method of analysis, we found, in agreement with Chung Hwang and Van Woert (5) that clonazepam in doses of 4 mg/kg, but not 2 mg/kg, reduced the number of activity counts when compared to the pre-clonazepam activity. Such a method, however, neglects any effects on activity produced by clonazepam itself. Indeed, it was observed that clonazepam (4 mg/kg) rendered animals immobile and ataxic for some time following administration, but these rats still exhibited myoclonus. Thus, in our hands, activity meter recordings gave a false impression of the effects of clonazepam. Reduced activity counts were not due to a reduction in intensity of myoclonus but, at least partially, were the result of sedation.

The present pharmacological investigation of *p,p'*-DDT–induced myoclonus in the rat has shown a more complex involvement of monoamine systems in the modulation of myoclonus than was shown by the similar experiments of Chung Hwang and Van Woert in the mouse (4).

In agreement with Chung Hwang and Van Woert's findings in mice (4), we found that L-5-HTP and L-tryptophan reduced *p,p'*-DDT (600 mg/kg, p.o.)–induced myoclonus in the rat, but in contrast, we could find no effect of Org 6582 (10 mg/kg, i.p.) when administered prior to or following the onset of *p,p'*-DDT–induced myoclonus. Likewise, Chung Hwang and Van Woert (4) reported that quipazine (10 mg/kg, i.p.) reduced *p,p'*-DDT–induced myoclonus in mice, but the same dose in our investigation produced such profound changes in behavior that it was difficult to assess any effect on myoclonic activity. Such animals exhibited gross tremor, forepaw treading, head weaving, and prostration.

The 5-HT antagonists methergoline, methysergide, and cinanserin, all at a dose of 5 mg/kg, i.p., potentiated *p,p'*-DDT–induced myoclonus in mice (4), but in our study in rats, using the same or larger doses were ineffective. For example, methergoline (5 mg/kg, i.p.) did not influence the time to onset or severity of myoclonus in rats. Similarly, depletion of 5-HT by PCPA administration was ineffective. Because *p,p'*-DDT (600 mg/kg, p.o.) produces continuous myoclonus in all animals tested, it would have been difficult to potentiate this effect, so we examined the effect of methergoline (5 mg/kg), methysergide (5 mg/kg), and cinanserin (10 mg/kg, i.p.) on a subthreshold dose of *p,p'*-DDT (100 mg/kg, p.o.). None of these compounds influenced the severity of myoclonus.

Taken overall, the data suggest that *p,p'*-DDT–induced myoclonus is probably not a result of a deficiency of cerebral 5-HT. However, increased 5-HT neuronal activity in brain can inhibit established *p,p'*-DDT–induced myoclonus, even though reduction of 5-HT function does not appear to initiate or modulate myoclonic activity.

Why the results obtained in this study differ from those of Chung Hwang and Van Woert (4,5) is unclear. One reason may be that they used mice in their studies, whereas we employed rats. This seems unlikely, however, since in their investigations of agents from a range of pharmacological classes on myoclonic activity in the mouse, they state "similar results were observed in rats but only the mice were counted with the activity meters" (4). Assuming that we employed similar doses and a similar protocol, one possible reason for the discrepancy in results may be the different assessment techniques employed; observer rating scale versus activity meters to measure the severity of myoclonus.

In agreement with the behavioral findings, biochemical results also suggest that *p,p'*-DDT–induced myoclonus is not a result of a deficiency of cerebral 5-HT. The onset of myoclonus did not appear to be associated with any change in brain 5-HT, 5-HIAA or tryptophan. The elevations of brain 5-HIAA and tryptophan concentrations observed when myoclonus had become well established would suggest that they are a consequence rather than a cause of the myoclonus. These findings are in accord with those of Chung Hwang and Van Woert (4), who observed elevations of 5-HIAA concentrations in seven regions of rat brain in animals that had experienced myoclonus for a 2-hr period following prior treatment with *p,p'*-DDT.

Altered monoamine function did seem important in the control of *p,p'*-DDT–induced myoclonus. Elevation of monoamine levels following administration of monoamine oxidase inhibitors (MAOIs) dramatically reduced *p,p'*-DDT–induced myoclonus. In the doses used, pargyline was more effective than either tranylcypromine or nialamide. The protective effect of MAOIs was much longer lasting than that of either L-5HTP or L-tryptophan. The effect of pargyline and other MAOIs on *p,p'*-DDT myoclonus has not been reported previously. Chung Hwang and Van Woert (4–6) did not examine the effect of MAOIs, and so this finding would not have influenced their concept of the genesis of *p,p'*-DDT myoclonus.

In conclusion, unlike Chung Hwang and Van Woert's (4–6) studies of *p,p'*-DDT–induced myoclonus in the mouse, we have found no consistent evidence that changes in 5-HT function are involved in the production of *p,p'*-DDT–induced myoclonus in the rat. Neither behavioral assessment following pharmacological manipulation, nor biochemical determinations of cerebral 5-HT and 5-HIAA concentrations following *p,p'*-DDT administration, suggested a role for 5-HT in the production of myoclonus. What is clear, however, is that increasing 5-HT activity can decrease the intensity of *p,p'*-DDT–induced myoclonus, although the converse does not appear to be true. Other experiments showed that MAOIs produced a greater protection against *p,p'*-DDT myoclonus than either of the 5-HT precursors, although the mechanism of this protection by MAOIs has not been established. Clonazepam, a benzodiazepine effective in the treatment of action myoclonus in man, did not influence the severity of *p,p'*-DDT–induced myoclonus in this study in the rat, although it appears to do so in the mouse (5).

The electrophysiological experiments suggest that *p,p'*-DDT–induced myoclonus in the rat may be similar to reticular myoclonus seen in humans. The order of muscle activation in spontaneous jerks indicates an origin of the discharge in the lower brainstem. This first activates neck muscles, innervated by the first three cervical nerves, and then spreads up the cranial nerve nuclei (masseter) and down the spinal cord (biceps). Absence of any cortical event preceding the earliest jerk also is consistent with this hypothesis.

At present, the mechanism by which *p,p'*-DDT produces myoclonus is unknown. The possibility of involvement with other neurotransmitter systems required further investigation. For example, reduced brain γ-aminobutyric acid (GABA) concentrations have been reported to occur following *p,p'*-DDT administration to rats (8,10). However, *p,p'*-DDT–induced myoclonus is not blocked by GABA agonists (5). Indeed, *p,p'*-DDT may have diverse effects on many neuronal systems in brain since it slows the closing of sodium channels that open during depolarization and elicits repetitive firing in various nerve fibers (1,9) and also may affect prostaglandin function (7). Clearly, *p,p'*-DDT–induced myoclonus in rats is not a simple model for examining the basis of action myoclonus or to investigate the potential screening of drugs for the treatment of postanoxic action myoclonus.

SUMMARY

p,p'-DDT–induced myoclonus in mice has been proposed as a model of stimulus-sensitive action myoclonus responsive to L-5-HTP and clonazepam treatment. However, we have been unable to confirm the ability of clonazepam to reduce myoclonus induced by *p,p'*-DDT in the rat. A detailed pharmacological, biochemical, and physiological investigation in the latter species shows *p,p'*-DDT–induced myoclonus not to resemble stimulus-sensitive action myoclonus occurring in humans.

Precursors of 5-HT (L-tryptophan and L-5-HTP) reduced the intensity of myoclonus, but the 5-HT agonists quipazine and Org 6582 did not. 5-HT antagonists (methergoline, methysergide, and cinanserin) did not potentiate myoclonus induced by p,p'-DDT. In contrast, administration of MAOIs (pargyline, nialamide, and tranylcypromine) markedly attenuated the myoclonus.

No observable changes in cerebral 5-HT biochemical parameters occurred at the onset of myoclonus, although brain tryptophan and 5-HIAA were increased following periods of prolonged myoclonus.

Electrophysiological analysis of p,p'-DDT–induced myoclonus in the rat revealed changes in EEG and EMG activity that were different from those observed in human reticular reflex myoclonus.

In conclusion, in contrast to the mouse, myoclonus induced by p,p'-DDT in the rat does not appear to be a suitable model of 5-HT–sensitive action myoclonus in man.

ACKNOWLEDGMENTS

This study was supported by the Research Funds of Bethlem Royal and Maudsley Hospitals and King's College Hospital and the Medical Research Council.

REFERENCES

1. Århem P, Frankenhaeuser B. DDT and related substances: effects on permeability properties of myelinated Xenopus nerve fibre. Potential clamp analysis. *Acta Physiol Scand* 1974;91:502–11.
2. Boudouresques J, Roger J, Khalil R, Vigouroux RA, Gossett A, Pellisier JF, Tassinari CA. A propos de 2 observations de syndrome de Lance et Adams. Effet thérapeutique du RO-05-4023. *Rev Neurol (Paris)* 1971;125:306–9.
3. Chadwick D, Harris R, Jenner P, Reynolds EH, Marsden CD. Manipulation of brain serotonin in the treatment of myoclonus. *Lancet* 1975;2:434–5.
4. Chung Hwang E, Van Woert MH. p,p'-DDT-induced neurotoxic syndrome: experimental myoclonus. *Neurology* 1978;28:1020–5.
5. Chung Hwang E, Van Woert MH. Antimyoclonic action of clonazepam: the role of serotonin. *Eur J Pharmacol* 1979;60:31–40.
6. Chung Hwang E, Van Woert MH. p,p'-DDT-induced myoclonus: serotonin and α-noradrenergic interaction. *Res Commun Chem Pathol Pharmacol* 1979;23:257–66.
7. Chung Hwang E, Van Woert MH. Role of prostaglandins in the antimyoclonic action of clonazepam. *Eur J Pharmacol* 1981;71:161–4.
8. Kar PP, Matin MA. Possible role of cerebral amino acids in acute neurotoxic effects of DDT in mice. *Eur J Pharmacol* 1974;25:36–9.
9. Lund AE, Narahashi T. Interaction of DDT with sodium channels in squid giant axon membranes. *Neuroscience* 1981;6:2253–8.
10. Matin MA, Jaffery FN, Siddiqui RA. (1981) A possible neurochemical basis of the central stimulatory effects of p,p'-DDT. *J Neurochem* 1981;36:1000–5.

Advances in Neurology, Vol. 43: Myoclonus,
edited by S. Fahn et al. Raven Press,
New York © 1986.

Animal Models of Myoclonus Using 1,2-Dihydroxybenzene (Catechol) and Chloralose

A. Angel

Department of Physiology, The University, Sheffield S10 2TN, United Kingdom

The use of catechol (1,2-dihydroxybenzene) as a model system for studying myoclonus came as a result of a series of correlative observations between the effects of this chemical in animals and certain myoclonic states in man. Halliday (42) had suggested, from clinical evidence, that myoclonus in man may be of three main types: (a) associated with an abnormal cortical discharge; (b) with disruption of "extrapyramidal" function; and (c) produced by segmental spinal or brainstem lesions.

It was with the first type of myoclonus that catechol showed some interesting correlations. First, Dawson (34,35) and Halliday (41) had shown that in patients with myoclonus presumed to be of cortical origin, the initial parts of the cortical response to sensory stimulation were abnormally large and, second, that there appeared to be a correlation with the incidence of jerks and the amplitude of the early negative wave of the cortical response (41). Similar observations were made after the administration of catechol to animals.

For similar reasons, chloralose has also been used as a model for myoclonic activity. Hanriot and Richet (45) originally demonstrated that this chemical also produced a stimulus-sensitive state wherein any abrupt sensory stimulus produced a muscle jerk, which was shown later (1) to be accompanied by a recognizable motor cortical potential and a discharge of impulses down the pyramidal tract.

Bearing in mind that myoclonus in humans is usually a chronic state and that most model systems are by their very nature acute, these two models are now examined.

CATECHOL

General Properties

Catechol is a simple hydroxyphenol that appears to be uncommon as a plant constituent, although plant polyphenols contain catechol and its isomers resorcinol and hydroxyquinone (46). Catechol itself has been reported in only a few plants: the broomlike *Ephedra*; the grapefruit, *Citrus paradisi*; and the scales of the onion, *Alium cepa*. Catechol is a derivative of the tannin pyrocatechuic acid or catechu that used to be extracted from the climbing shrub *Uncaria gambier* and from the heartwood of the leguminous plant *Acacia catechu*. Its name is derived from the Greek *katecho*, "I restrain" (the catechins were once a group of mythical substances that were supposed to prevent any excessive action by the four classical cardinal humors: blood, phlegm, choler, and melancholy).

Catechol is a relatively toxic substance; its LD_{50}, after subcutaneous administration, is 225 mg/kg in the rat and mouse (24). Much of the early work on catechol was concerned with the activity of sympathomimetic amines that contain the catechol nucleus. Bacq (19,20) first showed that catechol, in common with several other polyhydroxyphenols, possessed no sympathomimetic activity but could potentiate the actions of endogenous and exogenous epinephrine and norepinephrine. Subsequently, this was shown to be due to a competitive action for the enzyme catechol-ortho-methyltransferase (COMT) (21). The most potent effect of catechol is its action as a convulsant, first described by Brieger in 1879 (28), giving a spectrum of muscular activity that depends on the dose administered, ranging from tremor to muscular jerks after auditory or tactile stimuli, and at high doses, spontaneous convulsions that can show a typical "Jacksonian march" (10). Occasionally, tonic extensor spasm is seen. The abnormal muscular movements are invariably accompanied by an increase in respiratory rate (4) but there appears to be no consistent effect on either the pulse rate or blood pressure (68).

Spontaneous Convulsions

Chemistry

In addition to catechol, several other derivatives of phenol also can produce convulsive activity (56,57). In order to delineate more precisely the structure activity relations of hydroxybenzenes, the convulsive dose 50 (CD_{50}) has been determined in anesthetized mice. Male albino mice (Sheffield strain) in the weight range of 20 to 25 g were used and anesthetized with ethyl carbamate (urethane 2.0 g/kg). The anesthetized animals were placed in the supine position in a quiet environment and the ambient temperature maintained at 22°C. All chemicals were dissolved in 0.9% saline and were administered intraperitoneally. The doses that induced spontaneous convulsions in 50% of the animals (CD_{50}) were determined by the method of Weil (71) with groups of six mice. The results from those hydroxybenzenes and monosubstituted phenols that were active are shown in Table 1. The only monosubstituted benzene that was found to be active was phenol; aniline, fluorobenzene, chlorobenzene, toluene, nitrobenzene, benzoic acid, benzaldehyde, benzyl alcohol, thiophenol, and methoxybenzene were all, in sublethal doses, without effect. As can be seen from Table 1, catechol was the most potent chemical. The convulsant activity of phenol was found to be increased by *o*-, *m*-, or *p*-chloro substitution, was unchanged by methyl substitution, and was decreased by amino substitution. Since catechol (*o*-hydroxyphenol) was the most potent hydroxyl-substituted phenol, other *o*-substituted phenols were analyzed for convulsant activity. Salicylic acid, salicylaldehyde, *o*-nitrophenol, and guaicol (*o*-methoxyphenol) were all inactive; *o*-fluorophenol, however, was convulsant.

TABLE 1. *Activity of hydroxybenzenes and monosubstituted phenols in producing convulsions in urethane-anesthetized mice[a]*

| Compound | Structure | | | | | CD_{50} (mM/kg) | Relative potency |
	1	2	3	4	5		
Phenol	OH	—	—	—	—	1.04	0.37
Catechol	OH	OH	—	—	—	0.38	1.0
Resorcinol	OH	—	OH	—	—	0.92	0.41
Quinol	OH	—	—	OH	—	0.90	0.42
Pyrogallol	OH	OH	OH	—	—	5.71	0.07
Phloroglucinol	OH	—	OH	—	OH	>16	<0.02
o-Chlorophenol	OH	Cl	—	—	—	0.77	0.49
m-Chlorophenol	OH	—	Cl	—	—	0.86	0.44
p-Chlorophenol	OH	—	—	Cl	—	0.90	0.42
o-Cresol	OH	CH_3	—	—	—	1.08	0.35
m-Cresol	OH	—	CH_3	—	—	0.94	0.40
p-Cresol	OH	—	—	CH_3	—	1.02	0.37
o-Aminophenol	OH	NH_2	—	—	—	3.42	0.11
m-Aminophenol	OH	—	NH_2	—	—	2.28	0.17
p-Aminophenol	OH	—	—	NH_2	—	2.53	0.15
o-Fluorophenol	OH	F	—	—	—	0.73	0.52

[a]For further details, see Angel et al., ref. 14.

It was hoped that the structure-activity relationships of the *o*-substituted phenols might show some indication of the mechanism of action of the phenol radical. However, no simple explanation can be essayed from these data. Scaling the phenols according to acidity or electron-accepting capability shows no correlation with convulsant potency. One possible mechanism of action is that the phenolic radical may form hydrogen bonds with the amide groups of proteins in the nerve cell membrane that could alter permeability and result in hyperexcitability. A restriction must be added to the size, or electron-attracting power, of the group next to the phenol to correlate with the decrease in potency of the substituted phenols. One must suppose that the hypothetical receptor site is large enough to accept a hydroxyl group and that the bond must be formed by the hydroxyl group and not its neighbor. Thus, catechol with two such hydroxyl groups in close apposition can readily form such bonds.

In order to be able to describe the quantitative effects of catechol injection, unanesthetized mice were placed in an ordinary animal cage suspended on a continuous length of silicon rubber tubing filled with mercury to form a strain gauge and passed back and forth between two supporting bars. The anesthetized animals were placed in a plastic beaker suspended by a rigid wire from a beam with two semiconductor strain gauges bonded to it. The strain gauges were used in a Wheatstone bridge circuit, the output from which was rectified and integrated, thus giving a measure of the deformation of the gauge and hence the movement of the animal. The time course of the convulsant activity produced by equal doses of catechol (Fig. 1) is different in the two preparations. In the unanesthetized mouse, the convulsant activity (catechol 0.55 mM/kg) usually lasts for 3 to 5 min (mean, 4.68 ± 0.44 SEM; N, 40) and is followed by a prolonged period of postictal depression. In the anesthetized animal, the convulsion lasts for 10 to 20 min (mean, 13.93 ± 0.92 SEM; N, 20). It is of interest to note that catechol convulsions cannot be totally inhibited with anesthetic. Anesthetics always proved fatal before the catechol convulsion was blocked. Comparison of the effects of equipotent doses of

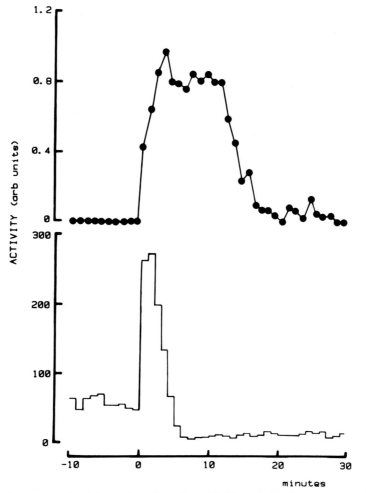

FIG. 1. Time course of activity produced by catechol (0.55 mM/kg) in the unanesthetized **(bottom)** and anesthetized mouse (urethane 2 g/kg) **(top)**. Each graph is the mean effect of catechol in 12 individual animals. (Modified from Angel and Rogers, ref. 14.)

catechol, phenol, quinol, and resorcinol shows that the time course of the effects of each chemical are not the same. The time to reach the peak effect was 2 min for catechol and phenol, 8 min for quinol, and approximately 12 min for resorcinol. The decay of the effect of these four chemicals was found to be of a simple exponential nature, which allowed a comparison of their half-lives: 3 min for catechol, 20 min for resorcinol and quinol, and 30 min for phenol (14). The simple exponential decay for catechol would suggest a single mechanism for its destruction, which is probably via COMT. Evidence for this is given by the effect of pretreatment with pyrogallol, which increases the effect of a subsequent injection of catechol and also increases its half-life to 10.5 min. That the mechanism of action of catechol is probably not due to any adrenergic effect is shown by the fact that pyrogallol is not convulsant until doses are given that render the animal obviously anoxic and that pyrogallol is a more potent competitive inhibitor of COMT. Furthermore, the most potent COMT competitive inhibitor, alpha-methyl-tropolone, does not show any convulsant activity.

As well as possessing COMT-inhibiting properties, catechol has been shown to inhibit glycolysis in brain cells (49) and thereby reduce the cerebral supply of adenosine triphosphate (ATP). Thus, the action of catechol could be simply to give what are in effect anoxic convulsions. However, the measurement of cerebral ATP levels after catechol and pyrogallol (13) showed that this was not so. Figure 2 shows the effect of intraperitoneal injections of 60 mg/kg of both catechol (0.55 mM/kg) and pyrogallol (0.48 mM/kg) on the levels of these two hydroxybenzenes in the brain, the change in locomotor activity, and the change in cerebral ATP levels. It can be seen that both chemicals gave approximately the same decrease in ATP levels: catechol, 28.6% decreased (SD $\pm$ 4.8); pyrogallol, 23.7% decrease (SD $\pm$ 5.8) but that catechol produces a convulsion, whereas pyrogallol does not. Subconvulsive doses of catechol also produced a fall in brain ATP levels. Furthermore, in animals respiring a 95% O_2 and 5% CO_2 gas mixture, the change in ATP level is almost eliminated, but the duration and intensity of the catechol convulsion is unaffected. These observations suggest that the fall in brain ATP levels are a consequence of the convulsion rather than the cause and are in accord with other workers who have studied different convulsants (50,61).

Pharmacology

For the assessment of drugs on the effectiveness of catechol as a convulsant, two techniques were used. First, if the drug pretreatment required a prolonged period of time to reach its maximum effect, then the CD_{50} for catechol was determined. Care was taken in this determination to keep the environment as quiet as possible, since the CD_{50} for auditory evoked jerks is less than that for the spontaneous convulsions (0.28 mM/kg compared to 0.37 mM/kg, respectively). Second, if the drug pretreatment showed a rapid effect, then the determination was that of the ratio of the total activity in the second convulsion to that in the first. Although the variation in individual mice was enormous, it was found that the ratio of second

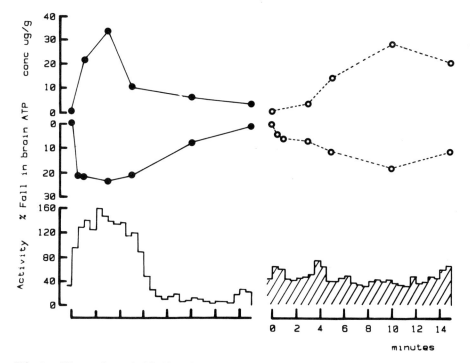

FIG. 2. Effects of catechol **(left)** and pyrogallol **(right)** injections (0.55 mm/kg, i.p.) on the concentrations of the chemical in the brain **(top)**, the % fall in the cerebral ATP levels **(middle)**, and the locomotor activity **(bottom)** in two mice. (Modified from Angel et al., ref. 13.)

to first convulsive activity was fairly constant in any one animal, provided that the time between successive doses was not less than 40 min and that the animal's rectal temperature was maintained at 37°C. All of the drugs with rapid effect were administered so that their time to peak effect coincided with the peak effect of the second catechol convulsion. The dose of catechol used was fixed at 0.73 mm/kg. The convulsive activity was defined as the total activity in the 20 min after the injection of catechol minus the total activity in the 20-min period preceding the injection. No pretreatment drugs were found to alter the activity of the anesthetized mice.

Catecholamines

Gross levels of cerebral catecholamines can be altered by reserpine (51) and the monoamine oxidase (MAO) inhibitors (73). Pretreatment with any of these drugs had no effect on the catechol convulsions (Table 2). Similarly, destruction of brain adrenergic and dopaminergic neurons with the neurotoxin 6-hydroxydopamine (69) or pretreatment with the dopamine precursor L-DOPA was also without effect. The effect of pretreating with pyrogallol is probably due to competition for COMT. Although treatment with pyrogallol does increase cerebral catecholamine levels

TABLE 2. *Effects of drugs requiring long pretreatment times on the CD_{50} to catechol*

Drug[a]	Dose (mg/kg)	CD_{50} (mM/kg)	p
Pargyline	50	0.34	—
Control		0.34	
Iproniazid	50	0.39	—
Control		0.35	
Reserpine	1	0.31	—
Control		0.34	
L-DOPA	200	0.36	—
Control		0.38	
PCPA	150	0.58	<0.05
Control		0.39	
PCPA + 5-HTP	150 + 100	0.59	<0.05
Control		0.40	
6-Hydroxydopamine	80 μg	0.40	—
Control		0.40	
Atropine	50	0.58	<0.05
Control		0.39	

[a]All drugs were administered intraperitoneally except 6-hydroxydopamine, which was given directly into the cerebral ventricles.
For further details, see Angel et al. ref. 8.

(25), the absence of effect with reserpine and MAO inhibitors, together with the observation that catechol does not elevate cerebral norepinephrine or dopamine levels (63), seems to rule out a presynaptic effect of catechol on aminergic neurons. A postsynaptic effect can be similarly dismissed. Phentolamine had no effect, and the effect of (+ −)-propranolol is matched by the (+) form of propranolol; the latter has a weaker β-blocking action but similar membrane-stabilizing effects. This would seem to imply that the effect of propranolol is due to its local anesthetic action.

That dopamine is probably not involved in the action of catechol is shown both by the absence of effect of reserpine, MAO inhibitors, and L-DOPA and by the ineffectiveness of apomorphine (a dopamine agonist) (38) and amphetamine (which releases endogenous catecholamines) (70).

5-Hydroxytryptamine

The results with drugs modulating the putative central transmitter 5-hydroxytryptamine (5-HT) were found to be inconclusive. Para-chlorophenylalanine (PCPA), which causes 85% depletion of mouse brain 5-HT with little change in catecholamine levels (62), was found to increase significantly the catechol CD_{50}, and L-tryptophan, a specific elevator of 5-HT levels (31), potentiated the convulsions. However, a combination of PCPA to deplete and 5-hydroxytryptophan (5-HTP) to restore 5-HT levels caused a similar increase in CD_{50} to that obtained with PCPA alone, and methysergide, a 5-HT receptor blocker, had no effect. Furthermore, the absence of effect of reserpine and the MAO inhibitors would also seem to preclude this amine from the genesis of convulsive activity with catechol (8). A similar conclusion, for the guinea pig, has been reached by Chadwick et al. (30), although they present no data concerning any of the 5-hydroxytryptaminergic drugs they employed, and the levels of 5-HT and 5-hydroxyindoleacetic acid (5-HIAA) they report as unchanged were determined during the declining phase of the catechol convulsions. Thus, this amine remains as possibly being involved in the genesis of catechol convulsions.

γ-Aminobutyric acid

Treatment with γ-aminobutyric acid (GABA) or the GABA-transaminase inhibitor amino-oxyacetic acid had no effect on the catechol convulsions. In addition, the benzodiazepines clonazepam and Librium® also were ineffective in altering the convulsions. These two drugs are possibly glycine or GABA agonists (32).

Acetylcholine

Drugs affecting this transmitter all showed a clear-cut effect (Tables 2 and 3). Both muscarinic and nicotonic blockers decreased the effectiveness of catechol, and anticholinesterases gave a clear increase in the catechol convulsions, these latter

TABLE 3. *Effects of drugs requiring short pretreatment times on catechol convulsions[a]*

Drug	Dose (mg/kg)	Median activity ratio	*p*
Saline	—	1.36	
Pyrogallol	100	2.30	<0.05
Phentolamine	5	1.27	ns
(+ −)-Propranolol	2	1.07	<0.05
(+)-Propranolol	5	0.98	<0.01
Sotalol	5	1.42	ns
L-Tryptophan	200	1.90	<0.01
Methysergide	2	1.39	ns
Apomorphine	20	1.18	ns
(+)-Amphetamine	5	1.55	ns
GABA	100	1.89	ns
Amino-oxyacetic acid	25	1.37	ns
Atropine	10	0.86	<0.05
Hyoscine	20	0.84	<0.001
Atropine methyl nitrate	5	1.46	ns
Mecamylamine	2	1.08	<0.01
Pempidine	5	0.94	<0.05
Hexamethonium	2	0.90	<0.05
Dihydro-β-erythroidine	0.5	0.87	<0.001
Physostigmine	0.002	3.40	<0.001
Neostigmine	0.025	2.12	<0.001
Oxotremorine	0.01	1.86	ns

[a]Modified from Angel et al. ref. 8.

without causing multiple firing of the muscles to a single motor nerve volley. Interestingly, catechol also causes a decrease in cerebral acetylcholine levels from 2.1 µg/g to 1.25 µg/g (8).

Physiology

To study this aspect of catechol convulsions, female rats in the weight range of 190 to 210 g were used, anesthetized with urethane to abolish reflex withdrawal of the hindleg to a strong pinch (1.3–1.5 g/kg). The limbs were fixed in a perspex frame and electromyographic activity recorded from triceps and biceps brachii and from gastrocnemius and tibialis anterior. All other muscles of the limbs were denervated. Preliminary determinations showed that catechol 0.07 mM/kg, i.p., produced no effect, doses between 0.14 and 0.28 mM/kg produced pronounced hyperventilation without convulsive activity, and convulsions were seen at doses between 0.32 and 0.36 mM/kg. The onset of convulsions at a dose of 0.55 mM/kg was very rapid, usually occurring between 1 and 1.5 min; they reached their maximum intensity at 4 to 5 min and disappeared within 20 to 25 min. In the same way as in the mouse, near fatal concentrations of anesthetic (urethane 3.0 g/kg) failed to abolish the catechol effect. Examination of the jerks produced in the gastrocnemius, by attaching its tendon to a strain gauge, showed that the contractions were twitchlike and occurred at frequencies up to 150 per minute. Comparison of the activity in the gastrocnemius to that in the tibialis anterior showed that (a) the contractions were occasionally exactly synchronous and (b) the extensor muscle contracted more often, the mean ratio of total extensor:flexor jerks being 1.5:1.0. The variation in total activity was considerable from animal to animal, but the ratio of total activity in each of the muscles in response to two identical doses separated by not less than 45 to 60 min was constant. For example, in 10 experiments, the ratio of the total number of jerks occurring after the second dose to that after the first dose was found to be 0.98 (±0.07 SD) and 0.99 (±0.14 SD) in the triceps brachii and gastrocnemius muscles, respectively.

The effects of various lesions of the neuraxis are shown in Table 4. For this series of experiments, the second dose of catechol was given not less than 1 hr after the lesion. One additional observation was made in unanesthetized decerebrate rats, in which it was found that convulsant doses of catechol initially intensified their rigidity. No activity was seen in response to catechol in de-efferented muscles.

From these lesion experiments, it can be seen that catechol activates a system that extends from the intercollicular level down to the spinal cord. As far as the ankle extensors are concerned, this system appears to be tonically inhibited, even in the surgically anesthetized animal, by the sensorimotor cortex and cerebellum as well as by structures rostral to the colliculi. That this system then exerts its effect on the spinal cord indirectly via the gamma motoneurons and not directly on the alpha motoneurons is shown by the observations that (a) the convulsions are severely attenuated in the deafferented animal and (b) the decerebellate, deafferented animal shows only a slight but statistically significant ($p<0.05$) increase in convulsive activity when compared to the intact deafferented animal.

TABLE 4. *Alteration produced by various lesions of the neuraxis to the second of an identical pair of doses of catechol (0.55 mm/kg)[a]*

Lesion	Dorsal roots L4–S1	Effect[b] (%) Extensor	Flexor
None	Intact	100 (7)	97 (8)
Decorticate[c]	Intact	221 (40)	69 (11)
Decerebrate	Intact	714 (169)	58 (12)
Decerebellate	Intact	217 (69)	69 (11)
Spinal	Intact	16 (11)	12 (8)
None	Cut	15 (5)	4 (2)
Decerebrate	Cut	12 (5)	18 (7)
Decerebellate	Cut	38 (10)	41 (16)
Spinal	Cut	5 (3)	5 (3)

[a]Modified from Angel and Lemon, ref. 10.
[b]The effect is expressed as the percentage of the activity to the second dose compared to that of the first (SD in parentheses) for the gastrocnemius (extensor) and tibialis anterior (flexor) muscles in the urethane-anesthetized rat.
[c]Decorticate refers to a lesion restricted to the sensorimotor cortex contralateral to the hindlimb under study.

Thus, the system activated by catechol must (a) be located within the brainstem; (b) be subjected to tonic cortical, supracollicular, and cerebellar inhibition; (c) exert reciprocal effects on extensor and flexor motoneurons (see Table 4); and (d) exert its effect via the gamma-motoneuronal system. Such a system can be readily identified with the brainstem reticulospinal areas of Magoun and his co-workers (55). Further experiments have shown that the discharge from hindlimb muscle spindle afferents, both primary and secondary, show an increase in their frequency of discharge that parallels the convulsive activity consequent on catechol administration (7); and that some muscle jerks are preceded by an increase in spindle discharge. Furthermore, this spindle activity is increased by anticholinesterases and decreased by muscarinic blocking agents (8).

The muscle responses during the spontaneous convulsions are not related to any discharge in the electrocorticogram. The effect of catechol is to give a generalized arousal reaction with no spike-and-wave deflections being seen (4,5). One peculiar feature of the change in electrocorticographic activity is that although it is changed from a pattern of high-voltage, low-frequency activity to low-voltage, high-frequency activity, oscillations of a very low frequency (approximately 0.1 Hz) and high amplitude appear during the catechol effect (5).

Subconvulsive doses of catechol were found to be without effect on blood pressure; and the small increases seen with convulsant doses were always transient, blood pressure returning to normal long before the convulsion had ceased. Sub- and convulsive doses of catechol always increased the respiratory rate, producing on average a twofold increase in respiratory minute volume and a 3½-fold increase in respiratory rate. Little variation in arterial pO_2 was seen, but as was to be expected from the marked hyperventilation, some hypocapnia was present, the arterial pCO_2 falling by 6 to 10 mm Hg. However, the convulsive activity was unchanged in animals respiring a 5% CO_2, 95% O_2 gas mixture.

Evoked Convulsions

Physiology

Stimulation of the fore- and hindlimbs via gauze strips soaked in 3 M NaCl loosely wrapped around the wrist or ankle (− ve) and a digit or toe (+ ve) was found not to elicit any detectable electromyographic responses from any muscles in the surgically anesthetized rat. In contrast, shortly after an intraperitoneal injection of catechol (0.55 mM/kg), each stimulus was accompanied by a series of three bursts of electromyographic activity restricted to the muscles of the stimulated limb (Table 5), with mean latencies of 4.3, 13.4, and 40.0 msec in the forelimb elbow extensors and flexors, and at 8.1, 19.4, and 51.4 msec in the hindlimb ankle extensor. Figure 3 shows a typical record obtained from the gastrocnemius. The mean latency and probability of occurrence of each component of the response are shown in Table 5. An identical triple response, but at longer latency (Table 5), was seen in response to mechanical stimuli applied to the tactile pads of the fore- and hindpaws. The first response was always the highest in amplitude and had the least latency scatter and the highest probability of occurrence. (The probability was

TABLE 5. *Latency and probability of occurrence of evoked muscle responses to electrical, mechanical, or auditory stimulation[a]*

Muscle[b]	First response mean msec (SD)	Second response mean msec (SD)	Third response mean msec (SD)
Triceps brachii			
Latency			
Electrical	4.3 (0.6)	13.4 (1.6)	40.0 (7.0)
Mechanical	5.5 (0.9)	15.8 (2.5)	44.8 (5.4)
Auditory	5.7 (0.7)	19.3 (3.5)	—
Probability			
Electrical	0.97 (0.04)	0.59 (0.09)	0.17 (0.10)
Gastrocnemius			
Latency			
Electrical	8.1 (0.9)	19.4 (3.7)	51.4 (7.3)
Mechanical	8.9 (1.4)	21.6 (2.5)	48.1 (3.5)
Auditory	8.4 (0.8)	21.8 (3.2)	—
Probability			
Electrical	0.91 (0.05)	0.35 (0.03)	0.14 (0.03)
Tibialis anterior			
Latency			
Electrical	8.3 (1.1)	20.0 (2.4)	—
Probability			
Electrical	0.90 (0.09)	0.57 (0.09)	—

[a]Modified from Angel and Lemon, ref. 11.
[b]Electrical and mechanical stimuli were applied to the forepaw (triceps brachii response) or hindpaw (gastrocnemius and tibialis anterior responses).

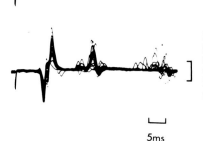

FIG. 3. Electromyographic activity recorded from the gastrocnemius to electrical stimulation of the ipsilateral ankle before **(top)** and after **(bottom)** an i.p. injection of catechol 0.55 mм/kg in a rat anesthetized with urethane (1.25 g/kg). Each record is of 20 superimposed responses.

5ms

taken as unity if the response occurred to each stimulus applied during the convulsive period.) The second and third responses were of smaller amplitude and showed a greater scatter in their latencies and a smaller probability of occurrence. The second response was easier to obtain from forelimb than hindlimb muscles, and in the hindlimb it was more frequently observed in the flexor muscle. Examination of single efferents teased from the central stump of the lateral gastrocnemius nerve showed that the pattern of activation of single units mirrored that of the integrated muscle activity. In most experiments, it was found that units with the highest recorded voltage, and therefore presumably from the larger diameter fibers, responded only to peripheral stimulation within the latency span of the first component. Those with smaller recorded amplitudes responded at times consistent with all three components, usually responding only once during the first component but repetitively during the second and third components.

In the rat, the ED_{50} for obtaining the jerks evoked by electrical stimulation of the periphery, determined by the method of Weil (71), was 0.27 mм/kg compared with 0.45 mм/kg for the spontaneous convulsions. One feature of the jerks was that they could be obtained from direct antagonists at similar latencies and with similar probabilities of occurrence. Auditory stimuli (binaural clicks) were found to evoke a double response from the muscles (Table 5), but visual stimulation in the albino rat was without effect.

After acute or chronic (8-day) section of the spinal cord (Th 13), the gastrocnemius response to electrical stimulation of the ankle consisted of the first component of the response alone. The second and third responses were never seen in the spinal animal, although all three responses were seen in the forelimb muscles of the same animals. In addition, the time course of the effect of catechol was prolonged below the level of the section, increasing to 40 to 45 min compared with 20 to 25 min in the intact animals. Further analysis showed that the first response to peripheral stimulation represented a simple disynaptic reflex.

The second component of the response is present in the decerebellate animal but absent in the decerebrate animal. This component was always preceded by a large-amplitude, early negative wave in the cortical response evoked by the peripheral stimulus. Further analysis of this component (12) showed that in the cat, rabbit, and rat it was specifically abolished in the forelimb by lesions confined to the contralateral forelimb sensorimotor cortex. Such lesions had no effect on the second component in the hindlimb. In the cat, the second component in the hindlimb muscles was specifically abolished by lesions confined to that hindlimb's sensorimotor cortex. In the rat and rabbit, on the other hand, this component vanished only after bilateral cortical lesions in the hindlimb sensorimotor cortices. These animals were subsequently shown to have bilateral primary motor and sensory cortical representations for the hindlimb. These experiments show that the integrity of the appropriate sensorimotor cortical area is essential for the production of this component of the response to peripheral stimulation. Electrical stimulation of the appropriate part of the sensorimotor cortex also can elicit a muscle response in the catechol-treated animal. Analysis of the temporal relations of the second component (Table 6) also shows that it occurs at a time consistent with its generation via a peripheral-cortical-muscle loop. The difference between the afferent plus efferent times and that of the occurrence of the second response to peripheral stimulation of -1.4 msec and -2.1 msec for the flexor carpi and tibialis anterior muscles, respectively, can be taken to represent the synaptic delay in the cortex. Further evidence that this component represents a direct corticospinal effect is given by the observation that the muscle response to cortical stimulation is equal to the sum of the latencies of the muscle response to stimulation in the medullary decussation of the pyramidal tract plus the antidromic cortical response latency to the same stimulus. This rules out a brainstem relay for the cortical response.

In accord with this postulate is the effect of catechol on the centripetal transmission of sensory information. After catechol administration, there is a net increase in the excitability of the dorsal column sensory pathway (4). Responses recorded from the primary cortical sensory receiving area and the ventrobasal thalamus show both an increase in size and a decrease in latency, together with its scatter. Responses recorded from the cuneate nucleus show either no change or a reduction in size. These changes are accompanied by a generalized arousal reaction of the electrocorticogram and changes in the discharge frequency of cells located in the thalamic reticular nucleus. Thus, the cortical responses are increased in size, indicating a greater discharge of cortical cells to an incoming volley as a result of

TABLE 6. *Analysis of the temporal relations of the second component[a]*

Muscle	Afferent	Efferent	Total	Second component	Difference
Forelimb (flexor carpi)	5.8 (0.49)	6.55 (0.45)	12.35 (0.76)	13.72 (0.35)	-1.37 (0.68)
Hindlimb (tibialis anterior)	8.97 (0.45)	7.93 (0.15)	16.9 (0.47)	19.0 (0.62)	-2.1 (0.37)

[a]Latency of the first positive wave of the cortical response (afferent), latency of the muscle response to cortical stimulation (efferent), total time (afferent plus efferent) time of occurrence of the second component of the peripherally evoked jerk, and the difference between this and the total time. Each statistic shows the mean time in msec obtained from six animals with the SD in parentheses. Modified from Angel and Lemon, ref. 11.

a disruption in the thalamic reticular control of the ventrobasal thalamus (6). A similar excitatory effect on brainstem reticular cells has been reported in the cat (72).

The third component of the response is present in the decerebrate animal and is presumed to be of brainstem origin.

Pharmacology

To assess the effects of drugs on the evoked activity after catechol, it was infused intravenously at a rate of 0.034 mM/kg/min to achieve a steady state of response. Drugs were then superimposed on this infusion as a bolus. None of the drugs tested to modify adrenergic and cholinergic transmitter action (Table 7) altered the response probability of the first component of the evoked myoclonic jerk to peripheral stimulation (9). The effects on the second component are shown in Table 7. Atropine and mecamylamine were shown to decrease the probability of occurrence of this component, and the absence of effect of atropine methyl nitrate, which poorly penetrates the central nervous system, indicates that this was a central phenomenon. Physostigmine was shown to enhance the occurrence of the second component. This cholinergic effect may be related to the action of catechol on afferent transmission and arousal. There is a large body of evidence, both histological (66,67) and pharmacological (27,52), suggesting that acetylcholine is a possible excitatory transmitter involved in reticulocortical arousal. Acetylcholine has also been put forward as a possible excitatory transmitter in the ventrobasal thalamus (60). The high ratio of muscarinic to nicotonic cholinoreceptors in brain tissue (48,58) offers an explanation of why atropine but not mecamylamine should be effective in blocking the second component of the myoclonic jerk.

TABLE 7. *Effects of various drug treatments on the frequency of occurrence of the second component of the jerk evoked by peripheral stimulation[a]*

Drug	Dose (mg/kg)	M2 (%)	p
Atropine	40	74.3 (18.9/7)	<0.01
Hyoscine	40	25.4 (12.3/4)	ns
Atropine methyl nitrate	20	−26.0 (17.4/5)	ns
Mecamylamine	2.5	21.7 (3.7/4)	<0.001
Hexamethonium	10	10.9 (9.5/5)	ns
Physostigmine	0.04	−19.5 (7.0/7)	<0.02
Neostigmine	0.03	−3.8 (23.8/5)	ns
Propranolol	5	41.4 (13.1/4)	ns
Phentolamine	10	1.8 (25.7/4)	ns

[a]The effect of catechol, as a constant intravenous infusion, was assessed by comparing the mean probability of occurrence of the response over a 20-min period pre-and post-drug treatment. Drugs decreasing the probability have positive values; those increasing it have negative values. Figures in parentheses show the SEM/and number of animals used. Modified from Angel and Dewhurst, ref. 9.

CHLORALOSE

General Properties

Chloralose is prepared by heating equal parts of anhydrous glucose and trichloroacetaldehyde (anhydrous chloral) in the presence of sulfuric acid at 100°C (47). The reaction product occurs in two forms, mainly as α-chloralose but with some β-chloralose. The exact structure of these two isomers is the subject of some controversy (22). Chloralose shows approximately the same lethal dose 200 mg/kg, after subcutaneous administration in the rat, as catechol and has an anesthetic dose of 55 mg/kg (23). Kruger and Albe-Fessard (53) reported that care in dissolving chloralose can produce anesthesia without convulsant activity. They state that if the chloralose solution is filtered at 60°C, then a mixture of α- and β-forms is not injected, implying that the convulsant activity is given by the β-chloralose.

Convulsive Activity

Physiology

Hanriot and Richet (44) were the first to demonstrate that animals anesthetized with chloralose gave a brief generalized muscle jerk to sensory stimulation: "le moindre attouchement détermine un soubresaut général . . . brusque et total." Subsequent studies showed that somatesthetic, acoustic, and visual stimuli also could evoke a generalized body jerk (2,45,59). Although Adrian and Moruzzi (1) showed that an abrupt stimulus would produce a convulsive movement associated with a motor cortical response and a discharge of impulses down the pyramidal tract, it was shown subsequently that the sensory myoclonic jerks to somatic and acoustic stimuli could still be observed in chronically decorticate animals (3), and those to visual stimuli in the absence of the primary visual cortex (33). After bilateral section of the medullary pyramids, the convulsive activity of chloralose was still seen (18). Convulsant activity is, however, abolished by high spinal transection (2). An extensive investigation of the genesis of chloralose jerks has been carried out by Ascher (16). In contradistinction to the localized jerks produced by catechol after stimulation of the limbs, that produced in animals anesthetized with chloralose shows a different generalized pattern. Figure 4 shows the efferent discharge from the seventh lumbar ventral root on the left-hand side to stimulation of all four appendages, as well as to auditory and visual stimuli, in a cat anesthetized with chloralose (80 mg/kg). Recording from muscle nerves showed that the jerks were more commonly found in those supplying flexor muscles. Although the generalized chloralose jerks could be obtained in the decorticate preparation, it was shown that the cortex exerted a facilitatory action on the jerk, which was somatotopically organized. Thus, the jerk produced by stimulating the left hindleg was decreased in amplitude after lesions to its cerebral projection area and showed a decrease in amplitude and increase in latency after dorsal column section (15). To explain this, Ascher hypothesized that the input was conveyed along two separate paths—one

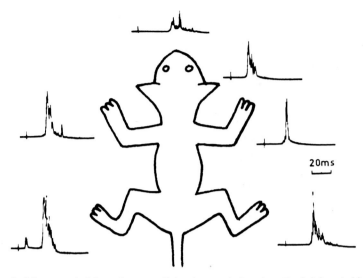

FIG. 4. Activity recorded from the seventh lumbar ventral root on the left-hand side to stimulation of the four limbs, as well as to auditory and visual stimuli. The responses have been arranged on the figurine according to the stimulus site. (Modified from Ascher, ref. 16.)

subcortical, the other via a cortical loop—and that they both converged on a subcortical efferent structure. The cortical loop appeared to be via the direct lemniscal path, and the other was conveyed in the anterolateral columns. The final efferent structure was in the bulbar reticular formation. Further evidence for this hypothesis was obtained by a study of the jerks evoked by visual stimulation (17), which showed (a) stimulation of the superior colliculus evoked generalized motor responses, (b) that the collicular visual responses were facilitated by the visual cortex, and (c) that the superior colliculus was a relay for the facilitatory influence of the visual cortex on the motor responses. Thus, they provide evidence for retinotectal and retinocortico-tectal afferent paths and a common tectoreticulospinal efferent path.

Shimamura and Yamauchi (65) further demonstrated that in the chloralose-anesthetized cat, as well as the long latency response (approximately 30 msec in the seventh lumbar ventral root) mainly to flexor muscles after stimulation anywhere on the body surface, an early segmental spinal reflex discharge was also obtained. Comparison of the effects of nerve stimulation in the decerebrate and decerebrate chloralose-anesthetized animal (65) showed that the late (generalized) jerk showed the same properties as that of the spino-bulbo-spinal reflex demonstrated by Shimamura and Livingston (64) in the decerebrate animal. The descending fastest conduction velocity for the late response was found to be 31 (± 4 SD) m/sec.

Devandan et al. (36) showed that the responses of single flexor motoneurons, to peripheral stimulation applied to the limb containing the muscle, consisted of two phases of depolarization with spike generation; the first consistent with a polysynaptic spinal reflex and the second with the spino-bulbo-spinal reflex (see Fig. 4: response to stimulation of the left hindlimb). These same authors (37) also showed that the intracellular responses from extensor motoneurons were generally hyper-polarizations temporally related to the flexor depolarizations, but they commented that the effects of peripheral stimuli on extensor motoneurons were extremely variable.

The spino-bulbo-spinal reflex has not been examined in any great detail. For example, its brainstem focus is not known with any exactitude, although examination of Fig. 4 in Shimamura and Livingston (64) would suggest that it is located within the nucleus reticularis gigantocellularis. Crude lesioning experiments indicated that the afferent path for the reflex ascends mainly on the ipsilateral side of the cord, with a smaller contralateral component, and that the efferent path descends bilaterally. Both afferent and efferent components are in or near the lateral funiculus.

Pharmacology

The two investigations into the pharmacological effects of chloralose on cerebral concentrations of 5-HT give conflicting results. In the rat, Bonnycastle et al. (26) found that a number of central depressants all gave a large increase in brain (minus cerebellum) 5-HT levels assayed biologically on Venus heart. For example, chloralose in a dose of 100 mg/kg elevated the level from 360 ($\pm$ 7.2 SEM; N, 34) pg/g to 560 ($\pm$ 36.3 SEM; N, 8) pg/g, which was statistically highly significant ($p < 0.001$). Chadwick et al. (29), on the other hand, showed that only the midbrain 5-HT levels were altered in guinea pigs given 80 mg/kg chloralose. These latter authors also state that the administration of the 5-HT precursor L-tryptophan with a monoamine oxidase inhibitor, and of L-5-HTP as well as the 5-HT receptor antagonist cyproheptadine, did not have any obvious influence on the myoclonic activity after chloralose administration. They omit, however, any quantitative evidence to substantiate this claim.

CONCLUSIONS

The major reason for the use of catechol and chloralose to produce models of sensory myoclonus was that examination, by eyeball, of the effects of these two chemicals appeared to show a state that, albeit superficially, resembled that seen in human patients.

Chloralose produces a stimulus-sensitive state seen mainly in flexor muscles, which in the stimulated limb elicits a spinal polysynaptic reflex and a generalized startle response in all other flexor muscles, possibly via a spino-bulbo-spinal mechanism. Catechol, on the other hand, produces both a stimulus-sensitive state at low doses and spontaneous convulsions, with the stimulus sensitivity retained, at higher doses. The stimulus sensitivity is seen as a series of three muscular responses in both flexor and extensor muscles but restricted to the limb stimulated.

The first is a polysynaptic spinal reflex, the second a periphero-corticospinal reflex, and the third resembles the spino-bulbo-spinal reflex.

The clinical description that some forms of myoclonus are exacerbated by either voluntary movement or sensory stimuli is characteristic of intention or action myoclonus following cerebral anoxia (54) as well as some other forms of myoclonic epilepsy (43). Two distinct forms of myoclonus are found after cerebral anoxia; reticular reflex myoclonus (39) and cortical reflex myoclonus (40).

The relevance of both of these chemicals to the human condition has been dismissed (29,30) for the following reasons:

1. Brainstem reticular reflex myoclonus, "appears to be" associated with a functional deficiency of 5-HT and "may be" treated successfully with its precursor 5-HTP or with tryptophan plus a monoamine oxidase inhibitor (29). The quotation marks have been inserted to point out that this may not be a consistent observation.

2. Chadwick et al. (29) found no change in brain 5-HT after chloralose in the guinea pig, which is in contrast with the 53% increase in the rat found by Bonnycastle et al. (26). Similarly, Chadwick et al. (30) found no change in brain 5-HT after catechol, but according to the timing of the sampling, the catechol convulsion was almost over and the animals could have been entering the period of postictal depression.

3. Chadwick et al. (29,30) state that manipulation of 5-HT levels produces no change in the catechol spontaneous or chloralose-evoked activity, with no quantitative data to support these observations. Angel et al. (8) found that their quantitative findings after manipulation of brain 5-HT levels on the catechol-induced spontaneous activity were inconclusive.

The first important point to be made here is not to dismiss an animal model unless the evidence is unequivocal—and the reverse, not to accept an animal model unless the evidence is clear. To date, nobody has investigated the midline or raphe regions of the pons and upper brainstem, which are known to be the sites of 5-HT–containing neurons, to evaluate their activity during myoclonic convulsions.

The second point to be made is that these two animal models are designed to make the intact animal myoclonic. It is not unreasonable to assume that cerebral hypoxia will have caused some damage to the nervous system. In such a circumstance, one could hypothesize that a transmitter system, which in the normal condition subserves a small role, could, in the damaged animal, assume a much more important role.

The relevance of catechol as a model comes from the observation that it increases the cortical evoked response, which is associated in terms of both amplitude and temporal relations with the second component of the evoked muscle activity. Whether or not the same mechanism of increase in cortical response seen after catechol (4,5,12) and the consequent increase in pyramidal discharge seen in the rat and the human myoclonic condition remains to be determined.

SUMMARY

A description of the physiological effects and pharmacological actions of catechol (1,2-dihydroxybenzene) and chloralose (monoglucochloralose) on muscular activity in animals has been presented. Catechol produces a stimulus-sensitive state wherein a tactile stimulus to a limb evokes a jerk in the muscles of that limb. This jerk can consist of three components: a polysynaptic spinal reflex, a periphero-corticospinal reflex, and a brainstem reflex. Chloralose also produces a stimulus-sensitive state with two components: a polysynaptic spinal reflex in the stimulated limb and a presumed spino-bulbo-spinal reflex activation of all body flexor muscles. The relevance of these agents as animal models for the mechanism of generation of human myoclonic activity has been discussed.

REFERENCES

1. Adrian ED, Moruzzi G. Impulses in the pyramidal tract. *J Physiol (Lond)* 1939;97:153–99.
2. Alvord EC, Fuortes MGF. A comparison of generalized reflex myoclonic reactions elicitable in cats under chloralose anesthesia and under strychnine. *Am J Physiol* 1954;176:253–61.
3. Alvord EC, Whitlock DG. Role of brainstem in generalized reflex myoclonic reactions in cats under chloralose anesthesia. *Fed Proc* 1954;13:1.
4. Angel A. An analysis of the effect of 1,2-dihydroxybenzene on transmission through the dorsal column sensory pathway. *Electroencephalogr Clin Neurophysiol* 1969;27:392–403.
5. Angel A. An experimental model of sensory myoclonus produced by 1,2-dihydroxybenzene in the anesthetized rat. In: Harris P, Mawdsley C. eds. Epilepsy. Edinburgh, London and New York: Churchill Livingstone, 1974:37–47.
6. Angel A. Processing of sensory information. *Prog Neurobiol* 1977;9:1–122.
7. Angel A, Clarke KA. Effect of catechol on the discharge of muscle spindle afferents from the hindlimb of the rat. *Electroencephalogr Clin Neurophysiol* 1980;49:373–81.
8. Angel A, Clarke KA, Dewhurst DG. A pharmacological study of the spontaneous convulsive activity induced by 1,2-dihydroxybenzene in the anaesthetized mouse. *Br J Pharmacol* 1977;61:433–39.
9. Angel A, Dewhurst DG. A pharmacological investigation of the electrically evoked convulsive activity induced by administration of catechol in the anaesthetized rat. *Br J Pharmacol* 1978;64:539–44.
10. Angel A, Lemon RN. The convulsive action of 1,2-dihydroxybenzene in the anaesthetized rat. *Electroencephalogr Clin Neurophysiol* 1973;34:369–78.
11. Angel A, Lemon RN. An analysis of the myoclonic jerks produced by 1,2-dihydroxybenzene in the rat. *Electroencephalogr Clin Neurophysiol* 1973;35:589–601.
12. Angel A, Lemon RN. Sensorimotor cortical representation in the rat and the role of the cortex in the production of sensory myoclonic jerks. *J Physiol (Lond)* 1975;248:465–88.
13. Angel A, Lemon RN, Rogers KJ, Banks P. The effect of polyhydroxyphenols on brain ATP in the mouse. *Exp Brain Res* 1969;7:250–7.
14. Angel A, Rogers KJ. An analysis of the convulsant activity of substituted benzenes in the mouse. *Toxicol Appl Pharmacol* 1972;21:214–29.
15. Ascher P. Rôle de la voie lemniscal dans l'élaboration de réponses motrices extrapyramidales à des stimulations somesthésiques. *J Physiol (Paris)* 1964;3:278–9.
16. Ascher P. La réaction du sursaut du chat anesthésié au chloralose [Thesis]. Paris: Faculté des Sciences de L'Université de Paris, 1965.
17. Ascher P, Gachelin G. Rôle du colliculus supérieur dans l'élaboration de réponses motrices à des stimulations visuelles. *Brain Res* 1966;3:327–42.
18. Ascher P, Jassik-Gerschenfeld D, Buser P. Participation des aires corticales sensorielles à l'élaboration de réponses motrices extrapyramidales. *Electroencephalogr Clin Neurophysiol* 1963;15:246–64.
19. Bacq ZM. Recherches sur la physiologie et la pharmacologie du système nerveux autonome. XX.

Sensibilisation à l'adrénaline et l'excitation des nerfs adréniques par les antioxygenes. *Arch Int Physiol Biochim* 1936;42:340–66.

20. Bacq ZM. Recherches sur la physiologie et la pharmacologie du système nerveux autonome. XXII. Nouvelles observations sur la sensibilisation à l'adrénaline par les antioxygènes. *Arch Int Physiol Biochim* 1936;44:15–23.

21. Bacq ZM, Gosselin L, Dresse A, Renson J. Inhibition of *o*-methyltransferase by catechol and sensitization to epinephrine. *Science* 1959;130:453–4.

22. Balis GU, Monroe RR. The pharmacology of chloralose. A review. *Psychopharmacologia* 1964;6:1–30.

23. Barnes CD, Eltherington LG. Drug dosage in laboratory animals. A handbook. Berkeley, CA: University of California Press, 1973:70.

24. Binet P. Toxicologie comparée des phénols. Rev Med Suisse Romande 1895;15:561.

25. Biscardi A, Izquierdo J. Influencia del piragalol sobre el contenido de norepinefrina en el raton. *Rev Soc Argent Biol* 1961;37:293.

26. Bonnycastle DD, Bonnycastle MF, Anderson EG. The effect of a number of central depressant drugs upon brain 5-hydroxytryptamine levels in the rat. *J Pharmacol Exp Ther* 1962;135:7–20.

27. Bradley PB, Dray A. Short-latency excitation of brain-stem neurones in the rat by acetylcholine. *Br J Pharmacol* 1972;45:372–4.

28. Brieger L. Über das physiologische Benehmen von Katechol Hydroquinone und Resorkinol und ihre Formation im tierischen Körper. *Dubois Arch Physiol* 1879;(Suppl 61).

29. Chadwick D, Hallett M, Jenner P, Marsden CD. Observations on chloralose-induced myoclonus in guinea pigs. *Br J Pharmacol* 1980;69:535–40.

30. Chadwick D, Jenner P, Marsden CD. 5-Hydroxytryptamine and myoclonus induced by 1,2-dihydroxybenzene (catechol) in the guinea pig. *Br J Pharmacol* 1979;66:358–60.

31. Chase TN, Murphy DL. Serotonin and central nervous system function. *Annu Rev Pharmacol Toxicol* 1973;13:181–97.

32. Costa A, Guidotti A, Mao CC, Suria A. New concepts on the mechanism of action of benzodiazepines. *Life Sci* 1975;17:167–86.

33. D'Argenio L, Migliorini M. Moruzzi G. Gli effetti elettroretinografici "d'illuminazione" et "di oscuramento" ritrovati in un particolare tipo di risposta motoria a stimoli luminosi. *Atti Accad Fisioc Studi Fac Med Sienna* 1943;11:134–6.

34. Dawson GD. The relation between the electroencephalogram and muscle action potentials in certain convulsive states. *J Neurol Neurosurg Psychiatry* 1946;9:5–22.

35. Dawson GD. Investigations on a patient subject to myoclonic seizures after sensory stimulation. *J Neurol Neurosurg Psychiatry* 1947;10:141–62.

36. Devandan MS, Eccles RM, Lewis DM, Stenhouse D. Responses of flexor alpha-motoneurones in cats anaesthetized with chloralose. *Exp Brain Res* 1969;8:163–76.

37. Devandan MS, Eccles RM, Lewis DM, Stenhouse D. Responses of extensor alpha-motoneurones in cats anaesthetized with chloralose. *Exp Brain Res* 1969;8:177–89.

38. Ernst AM. Mode of action of apomorphine and dexamphetamine on gnawing compulsion in rats. *Psychopharmacologia* 1967;10:316–23.

39. Hallett M, Chadwick D, Adams J, Marsden CD. Reticular reflex myoclonus: a physiological type of human post-anoxic myoclonus. *J Neurol Neurosurg Psychiatry* 1977;40:253–64.

40. Hallett M, Chadwick D, Marsden CD. Cortical reflex myoclonus. *Neurology* 1979;29:1107–25.

41. Halliday AM. Cerebral evoked potentials in familial progressive myoclonic epilepsy. *J R Coll Physicians Lond* 1967;1:123–34.

42. Halliday AM. The electrophysiological study of myoclonus in man. *Brain* 1967;90:241–84.

43. Halliday AM. The neurophysiology of myoclonic jerking—a reappraisal. *Excerpta Med Int Cong Series* 1975;307:1–29.

44. Hanriot M, Richet C. De l'action physiologique du chloralose. *C R Soc Biol (Paris)* 1893;5:1–7.

45. Hanriot C, Richet C. Effets physiologiques du chloralose. *C R Soc Biol (Paris)* 1893;5:129–33.

46. Harborne JB, Simmonds NW. The natural distribution of phenolic aglycones. In: Harbone J, ed. Biochemistry of phenolic compounds. London: Academic Press, 1964:77–127.

47. Hefter A, Über die einuirkung von ehloral auf glucose. *Chem Ber* 1889;22:1050–1.

48. Hiley CR, Burgen ASV. The distribution of muscarinic receptor sites in the nervous system of the dog. *J Neurochem* 1974;22:159–62.

49. Hochstein P, Cohen G. The inhibitory effects of quinones and dihydric phenols on glucose metabolism in sub-cellular systems of brain. *J Neurochem* 1960;5:370–8.

50. King LJ, Lowry OH, Passoneau JV, Venson V. Effects of convulsants on energy reserves in the cerebral cortex. *J Neurochem* 1967;14:599–611.
51. Kirschner N. Uptake of catecholamines by a particular fraction of the adrenal medulla. *J Biol Chem* 1962;237:2311–7.
52. Krnjevic K. Chemical transmission and cortical arousal. *Anesthesiology* 1967;28:100–5.
53. Kruger L, Albe-Fessard D. Distribution of responses to somatic afferent stimuli in the diencephalon of the cat under chloralose anaesthesia. *Exp Neurol* 1960;2:442–67.
54. Lance JW, Adams RD. The syndrome of intention or action myoclonus as a sequel to hypoxic encephalopathy. *Brain* 1963;86:111–36.
55. Magoun HW. Caudal and cephalic influences of brain stem reticular formation. *Physiol Rev* 1950;30:459–74.
56. Matsumoto J, Kiyono S, Nishi H, Koike J. Ichihashi T. The convulsive mechanism of phenol derivatives. *Med J Osaka Univ* 1963;13:313–23.
57. Matsumoto J, Nishi H. Functional mechanism of catechol in the central nervous system. I. The anatomic site of action. *Med J Osaka Univ* 1963;13:365–73.
58. McCance I, Phillis JW, Westerman RA. Acetylcholine sensitivity of thalamic neurones: its relation to synaptic transmission. *Br J Pharmacol* 1968;32:635–51.
59. Moruzzi G. Un nuovo riflesso interessante il sistema extrapyramidale. *Arch Fisiol* 1942;43:1–23.
60. Phillis JW. The pharmacology of thalamic and geniculate neurons. *Int Rev Neurobiol* 1971;14:1–48.
61. Pscheidt GR, Benitez D, Kirschner LB, Stone WE. Effects of fluoroacetate poisoning on citrate, lactate and energy-rich phosphates in the cerebrum. *Am J Physiol* 1954;176:483–7.
62. Rogers KJ. Role of brain monoamines in the interaction between pethidine and tranylcypromine. *Eur J Pharmacol* 1971;14:86–8.
63. Rogers KJ, Angel A, Buttertfield L. The penetration of catechol and pyrogallol into mouse brain and the effect on cerebral monoamine levels. *J Pharm Pharmacol* 1968;21:214–29.
64. Shimamura M, Livingston RB. Longitudinal conduction systems serving spinal and brain-stem co-ordination. *J Neurophysiol* 1963;26:258–72.
65. Shimamura M, Yamauchi T. Neural mechanisms of the chloralose jerk with special reference to its relationship with the spino-bulbo-spinal reflex. *Jpn J Physiol* 1967;17:738–45.
66. Shute CCD, Lewis PR. Cholinesterase containing systems of the brain of the rat. *Nature* 1963;199:1160–4.
67. Shute CCD, Lewis PR. The ascending, cholinergic reticular system: neocortical, olfactory and sub-cortical projections. *Brain* 1967;90:497.
68. Tainter ML. Comparative actions of sympathomimetic compounds: catechol derivatives. *J Pharmacol Exp Ther* 1930;40:43–64.
69. Thoenen H, Tranzer JP. The pharmacology of 6-hydroxydopamine. *Annu Rev Pharmacol Toxicol* 1973;13:169–80.
70. Thornberg JE, Moore KE. The relative importance of dopaminergic and noradrenergic neuronal systems for the stimulation of locomotor activity induced by amphetamine and other drugs. *Neuropharmacology* 1973;12:853–66.
71. Weil CS. Tables for convenient calculation of median-effective dose (LD50 or ED50) and instructions in their use. *Biometrics* 1952;8:249–62.
72. Yoshii N, Matsumoto J, Ogura H. Studies on the unit discharges of brainstem reticular formation in the cat. II. Effects of catechol, amphetamine, nembutal and megimide. *Med J Osaka Univ* 1960;11:19–33.
73. Zeller AE, Fouts JR. Enzymes as primary targets of drugs. *Annu Rev Pharmacol Toxicol* 1963;3:9–32.

Advances in Neurology, Vol. 43: Myoclonus,
edited by S. Fahn et al. Raven Press,
New York © 1986.

Myoclonus Induced by Intermittent Light Stimulation in the Baboon: Neurophysiological and Neuropharmacological Approaches

*R. Naquet and **B. S. Meldrum

*Laboratoire de Physiologie Nerveuse, Department of Applied Neurophysiology, C.N.R.S.
91190, Gif-sur-Yvette, France; and **Department of Neurology, Institute of Psychiatry,
London SE5 8AF, United Kingdom

In 1966, Killam et al. (21) discovered that a high percentage of *Papio papio* baboons from Casamance (Senegal) when submitted to intermittent photic stimulation (ILS) at 25 Hz presented clinical manifestation of epilepsy, the major feature being bilateral myoclonus. Killam et al. (24) classified this myoclonus in three grades: grade 1, concerning the periocular musculature; grade 2, facial and neck musculature; grade 3, generalized myoclonus involving the rest of the body. The latter can take the form of massive myoclonus, both bilateral and synchronous, of the same type as described in humans by Gastaut et al. (18). The three grades of myoclonus are accompanied by electroencephalographic (EEG) paroxysmal discharges (PDs) in the form of polyspikes, polyspikes and waves, and spikes and waves, analogous to what is found in humans in photosensitive epilepsy as first described clinically by Cobb (14) and, from the EEG point of view, by Walter et al. (87). This photosensitive epilepsy of the *P papio*, which is genetically transmitted (4,59), is still considered, in spite of some minimal differences, as a natural and unique model for the study of human photosensitive epilepsy (22,49,58,60,62,65).

In recent years, it was discovered that the same baboons, photosensitive or not, may present, without ILS, another type of myoclonus. This consists of myoclonus massively involving the muscles of the neck and trunk, especially those of the shoulder, without any facial symptoms. It is never accompanied by EEG PDs. Although it exists in some animals without any lesion or drug adjunction, it is favored by vermisectomy (5,52) or by the injection of some benzodiazepines, such as Valium® or lorazepam (11,52,78). These two types of myoclonus were recently designated "myoclonus type A" (the type induced by ILS) and "myoclonus type B" (the others) (80). This paper will be devoted to the neurophysiology and neuropharmacology of myoclonus type A.

EEG CHARACTERISTICS OF THE PD ACCOMPANYING MYOCLONUS INDUCED BY ILS

PDs induced by ILS are bilateral and synchronous. They are not generalized to the whole hemispheres, but are localized in the frontorolandic (FR) region. They may, under the continuation of ILS, radiate to some other cortical areas, but they are never truly generalized to all of the cortex; for example, they do not reach the occipital cortex. In the naturally photosensitive animal, they never originate in subcortical structures, as was demonstrated first by Fischer-Williams et al. (17) and always confirmed in later studies. But when PDs reach a certain amplitude at the cortical level, they radiate into some deep structures, such as certain nuclei of the thalamus or brainstem reticular formation. The latencies of the discharges recorded in deep structures are never shorter than the latency recorded at cortical level (Bryére et al., *in preparation*). They never radiate to the limbic structures (i.e., hippocampus and amygdala). After section of the corpus callosum, synchronization of the PDs between the two hemispheres diminishes. PDs induced by ILS may appear synchronously or asynchronously in the two FR areas (8,63). They also may appear independently in the two hemispheres. This is particularly true when the section of the corpus callosum is associated with the destruction of the FR cortex of one hemisphere. PD appears only in the nonlesioned side and clinical symptoms in the hemibody homolateral to the lesioned side.

RELATIONS BETWEEN PD AND MYOCLONUS

There exists a precise temporal relationship between the EEG spikes and the myoclonus, the latter following the PD within a few milliseconds (51). During the spikes or the spikes and waves or the polyspikes and waves induced by ILS, bursts of muscular activation are observed accompanying each spike surface element of the PD (Fig. 1). The PD slow wave is correlated to a muscular inactivation. The muscular groups involved are recruited in the following chronological order: palpebral orbicular, other facial muscles (masseter), distal musculature (biceps), prox-

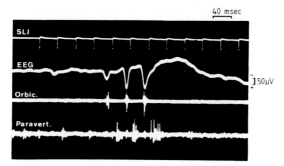

FIG. 1. EMG recording of myoclonic jerking accompanying EEG paroxysmal discharges. SLI, intermittent light stimulation at 25 Hz; EEG, frontorolandic cortical recording; Orbic., EMG recording of the palpebral orbicular; Paravert., EMG recording of the paravertebral muscle. (From Naquet et al., ref. 66, with permission.)

imal general musculature (paravertebral). The mean EMG latency from the beginning of the surface positive cortical spike of PD, for 70 tests, is respectively 4.1 msec (± 0.5) for the palpebral orbicular myoclonus, 7 msec (± 0.8) for the masseter myoclonus, 8.1 (± 1.1) for the biceps myoclonus, and 23.8 (± 1.3) for the paravertebral myoclonus (67) (Fig. 2). Furthermore, there exists a statistical relationship between the amplitude of the cortical spike and the probability that a myoclonic jerk will appear. The higher the voltage of the cortical spike, the greater is the muscular discharge, starting with an EEG spike of 100 μV amplitude. A plateau is reached for the orbicular and biceps myoclonus when this EEG spike reaches an amplitude located between 500 and 800 μV. For myoclonus of the paravertebrals, the EEG spike threshold is higher, but a plateau is never reached. It is possible also to demonstrate a close correlation between the cortical PD and the concomitant discharge recorded in the pyramidal tract at the pontobulbar level. No discharge exists at this level without PD at the cortical level. If a discharge is recorded, it is found 6.7 msec (± 0.6) after the beginning of the surface positive spike. It culminates at 11.9 msec (± 0.7) when the cortical one culminates at 6.2 msec (± 0.4) (67).

MECHANISMS RESPONSIBLE FOR THE PD AND FOR MYOCLONUS INDUCED BY ILS

The data above demonstrate that the myoclonus induced by ILS in the *P papio* has a particular topographic organization and is always preceded by PDs in the FR cortex. The reasons why myoclonus starts first in the eyelids and why ILS induces PDs in the FR cortex are still unknown. However, using different approaches and different techniques, it has been possible in the last 15 years to show the following:

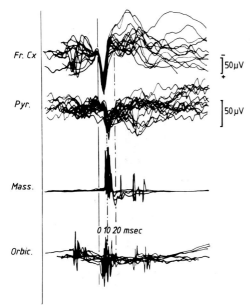

FIG. 2. Simultaneous recording of paroxysmal discharges from the frontorolandic cortex (FR. Cx), concomitant discharges from the pyramidal tract (Pyr.), and myoclonic jerking recorded at masseter (Mass.) and palpebral orbicular (Orbic.) muscle level. Zero time corresponds to the beginning of the FR spikes. (From Naquet et al., ref. 66 with permission.)

1. Electrical stimulation of the FR cortex where the PDs are predominant does not induce myoclonus of the eyelids (Menini, *personal communication*).

2. Irritative lesions of the FR cortex greatly facilitate the appearance of PDs. In contrast, destruction of this region suppresses the photosensitivity on the side of the lesion (16).

3. Destructive bilateral or unilateral lesions of the visual cortex (specific and nonspecific) block the appearance of PD in the FR region (84), but lesions of the two superior colliculi do not modify the photosensitivity (85).

4. Paralysis of the baboons by a curarizing agent diminishes considerably or suppresses completely the photosensitivity (17,61). Paralysis of the eye muscles by procaine or section or deinsertion of these muscles diminishes the photosensitivity in a transitory manner (6,61).

5. The FR cortex is a convergence zone where multiple afferents arrive, particularly visual and somatosensory (48). But although Charmasson and Catier (13) proposed a direct pathway from the occipital cortex to the frontal cortex on the basis of recording of EEG evoked potentials, a direct anatomical pathway from the occipital cortex to the FR area was not demonstrated by Riche (70,71) using horseradish peroxidase. From the occipital cortex to the FR cortex, there is no direct pathway, but connections exist between occipital cortex and parietal cortex, and between parietal cortex and FR cortex. Study of degeneration after lesions of the occipital cortex confirm these data. The lesion must be large and occupying not only area 17 but also 18 and 19 to find connections with the frontal cortex (7–9).

All of these data, which are indirect, are in favor of (a) the necessary role of the occipital cortex to generate PDs in the FR cortex (but its exact role as relay zone or control zone cannot be defined); (b) the role of multiple afferents (visual and somatosensory) reaching the FR cortex, and this afferent convergence must be considered as playing a role in changing the excitability of this cortex; (c) the special property of this cortex to produce PDs; and (d) the lack of specificity of this cortex to induce myoclonus of the eyelids by electrical stimulation, the initial symptom induced by ILS.

INTRACORTICAL RECORDINGS: UNIT AND FIELD POTENTIALS

To demonstrate the special property of the FR to generate PDs, recordings were carried out intracortically at different levels of the FR cortex (at a cellular level and with macroelectrodes) to follow the modifications of the different components of the visual evoked potential (VEP). The study of the single-unit concomitant of the PDs has been technically difficult in animals displaying myoclonic jerks. However, if these animals are paralyzed, it becomes very difficult to induce PDs. These difficulties were overcome by using allyglycine in subconvulsant dosage. This compound increases the natural photosensitivity of baboons in a stable way, for several hours, and makes it possible to induce PDs by ILS even in paralyzed animals (20,54). The similarity with the natural photosensitive animal is not perfect, allyglycine changing in some ways the excitability of the occipital cortex, where sometimes minimal PD may be induced by ILS.

It was necessary to add to this preparation a specific procedure consisting of repeating every 20 sec an ILS train lasting 10 sec, followed by a single flash generally 1 sec later and in some specific experiments at different times during the 10-sec intervals (53). Under these conditions, the VEP induced by the flash may become paroxysmal (PVEP), and its morphology is similar to that of PD (53,77,81).

During ILS, the activity of the FR cortex cells takes the form of bursts of action potentials, even before the constitution of surface PDs or PVEPs. The intrinsic frequency of these bursts increases as the PDs and the PVEPs are constituted and can attain 600 to 800 c/sec. These bursts are always correlated to the positive spikes of the surface PDs; the slow negative wave that follows them is accompanied by suppression of unit firing (51,55) (Fig. 3). Activation in bursts, PDs, and PVEPs are reversible once ILS is stopped. In other cortical areas, which do not display surface PDs, single-unit recordings do not show the bursts of activation concomitant with PD or PVEP seen in the FR cortex (51).

The precise temporal relationship that exists between the single flash that follows the train of ILS and the PVEP has established clear correlations between surface and intracortically recorded PVEPs and cellular activity. It was demonstrated that the PVEPs from the FR cortex do not correspond to the progressive enhancement of a preexisting evoked potential: In a series of trains that ended with PVEPs, the VEP evoked at the beginning of the series by a single flash is completely modified at the end. The first phenomenon to appear is a late negative wave, and the most precocious (the spike) elements of the PVEP appear only after the repetition of ILS trains, when the late wave has clearly increased in amplitude (73).

Finally, it was demonstrated that the FR VEP induced by a flash light, when it is not paroxysmal, does not originate in the same area as the PVEP. The VEPs found at different depths do not display an inversion of polarity in relation to the potential simultaneously recorded at the surface. On the other hand, the intracortical recording of a PVEP shows an inversion of its polarity in relation to the surface (73). The late part of surface potential starts to invert at a depth of 500 μm. The earliest part, i.e., the two positive spikes, inverts at 1,500 μm. This inversion zone corresponds with the layer of Betz cells.

From these results it is possible to conclude that (a) the nonparoxysmal VEPs in the FR cortex, induced by flashes, do not have their origin there and can be considered field potentials, the generator of which must be located in the neighboring cortical region or at the subcortical level; (b) the generator of the precocious spikes in the PVEP and PD is to be found at the level of the layer of giant pyramidal cells. This region receives thalamic afferents (52,66,73); when the spikes are prominent, efferent conduction may be sufficient to trigger myoclonus synchronous with the spikes; (c) the first neuronal elements to be brought into play by repetition of trains of ILS are the slow late negative waves of the VEP, waves that are generated at the superficial level of the cortex, where the afferents are probably corticocortical and/or nonspecific thalamocortical (66). The bringing into play of

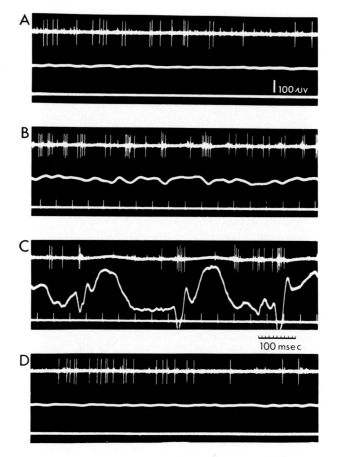

FIG. 3. Unitary recordings in the FR cortex, before **(A)**, during **(B** and **C)**, and after **(D)** the ILS. We note that under the effect of ILS, unitary activity takes the form of bursts that are synchronous with EEG spikes when these occur **(C)**, and that this burst activation is reversible and disappears when ILS is stopped. (From Naquet et al., ref. 66, with permission.)

these nonspecific afferents could be facilitated by the repetition of the trains of ILS realizing an experimental procedure of conditioning to time (56). This repetition may provoke a conditioned inhibition favoring the processes of synchronization, these being themselves the consequence of a reticular inhibition (64). On the contrary, it is known that an increase in vigilance, which corresponds to a reticular activation, provokes an inhibition of the PDs (22).

NEUROPHYSIOLOGICAL CONCLUSIONS

These results confirm that the paroxysmal EEG events induced by ILS in the *P papio* originate in the FR cortex and are responsible for the myoclonus that follows PD or PVEP. However, the hyperexcitability of this cortex is, certainly in part, regulated by the tendency to synchronization that is produced by a decrease of excitation from the reticular formation.

Some points are still under discussion.

1. How do visual afferents act and arrive in the FR cortex? Some anatomical and electrophysiological data were given, but they do not explain everything. The repetition of ILS or trains of ILS may create a state of hyperexcitability permitting a hypothetical "gate" to open and the arrival of afferents in this area that in other conditions are not effective (64).

2. What is the respective role of visual and proprioceptive afferents in determining the appearance of PD in this area? For the visual afferents, recent data (72) have shown that the problem is more complicated than expected. The proprioceptive afferents certainly play a role when the animal is not curarized, but they are not essential, as PDs may appear in FR cortex in the curarized animal, when the animal is extremely photosensitive or when the level of excitability is changed by adjunction of a subthreshold dose of a convulsant.

3. What is the role of the reticular formation in the induction of myoclonus? The myoclonus induced by ILS does not start at this level, but the state of excitability of this structure is crucial for its appearance. When the animal (not paralyzed or paralyzed without convulsant) is too much aroused, myoclonus is blocked, but it is facilitated when the animal falls asleep. It is also facilitated when the animal is awake but relaxed, with eyes closed. Possibly there exists in the *Papio papio* an abnormal way of response of the reticular formation that permits expression of the myoclonus whatever its origin. This hypothesis is reinforced by the fact that *P papio* (photosensitive or not) seems to be predisposed to show myoclonus type B in some particular conditions (5,11,78,80) and that this myoclonus is currently considered as originating at the level of the brainstem (in the reticular formation or in some related structures).

PHARMACOLOGICAL STUDIES

Studies in *P papio* have primarily utilized the acute administration of drugs, by the intravenous, intraperitoneal, or oral route. They can be classified under two headings: (a) studies of established or potential anticonvulsant drugs, and (b) studies of the possible role of different central neurotransmitters in photically induced myoclonic responses, utilizing drugs with specific actions on particular neurotransmitter mechanisms. The latter have emphasized the role of γ-aminobutyric acid (GABA)ergic and monoaminergic mechanisms in the control of myoclonic responses. By comparison, cholinergic and enkephalinergic mechanisms seem relatively unimportant (43,44,46). Preliminary data are now becoming available on the role of excitatory amino acids. We review below studies relating to anticonvulsants and to the major neurotransmitter systems. The ultimate aim of such studies is to explain the myoclonic phenomena in terms of the pathways and neuronal mechanisms acted on by the drugs. A tentative account can be given in relation to GABA (47), but definite conclusions require more basic research.

Anticonvulsant Drugs

Acute doses of anticonvulsant drugs that suppress photically induced myoclonus are shown in Table 1. Diphenylhydantoin and carbamazepine prevent tonic-clonic seizures but are relatively inactive against myoclonus. Valproate is effective, but as in other animal models of epilepsy, higher plasma concentrations are required than are necessary during chronic treatment in man.

The benzodiazepines are the most effective of all the classes of anticonvulsant drugs. The clinical usefulness of the traditional 1,4-benzodiazepines (e.g., diazepam and clonazepam) is limited by their tendency to impair complex motor performance and by the phenomenon of adaptation, or "escape" from seizure control. Interestingly, the latter phenomenon can be observed during chronic administration of clonazepam in baboons (23). These problems have prompted the testing in baboons of many novel benzodiazepines and related compounds. These have included various 1,5-benzodiazepines (33a,34,39) of which clobazam appears to offer considerable promise in clinical use. Several other classes of anxiolytic/anticonvulsant drugs act on the benzodiazepine receptor (32). Particularly interesting among these are the esters of β-carboline 3-carboxylic acid. Some of these are potent convulsants in the baboon and in low doses facilitate the induction of myoclonic responses (10,15,79). Some novel derivatives, however, are potent anticonvulsants in animal models of epilepsy. In particular ZK 91296 is as potent as diazepam when given intravenously to photosensitive baboons but has a more prolonged action and produces less alteration in EEG background rhythms (36).

TABLE 1. *Therapeutic doses and plasma levels in the photosensitive baboon* Papio papio

Drug	Acute dose (mg/kg, i.v.)	Plasma conc. (μg/ml)	Refs.
Standard agents			
Phenobarbital	15	7–17	41
Primidone	100		41
Diphenylhydantoin	50[a]	20–30	41
Carbamazepine	40[a]		41
Ethosuximide	100	80	41
Diazepam	0.5–1.0	0.5	41
Clonazepam	0.15	0.025–0.04	28
Valproate	200	200–400	27
Novel agents			
Clobazam	1–4		33
Desmethylclobazam	1–4		33
γ-Vinyl GABA	450		37
2-Amino-phosphonoheptanoic acid	200		34
ZK 91296	1.0		35
YG 19-256	1–3		39
BAU 426	1		38

[a]Incomplete therapeutic action.

GABAergic Inhibition

There is no direct evidence, biochemical or physiological, for a deficiency in GABAergic mechanisms in baboons with photically induced myoclonus. However, an abnormality in the intrinsic GABAergic system in the cortex could explain the hyperexcitability and the abnormal unit responses described above (47). Impairing the synthesis of GABA by the administration of various agents that block the activity of the enzyme glutamic acid decarboxylase enhances the myoclonic responses (30; Meldrum, *this volume*). Most attention has been paid to L-allyglycine (42,54), which readily causes animals with weak photosensitivity to give enhanced myoclonic responses to photic stimulation.

Pharmacological mechanisms for enhancing GABAergic inhibition are reviewed by Meldrum *(this volume)*. The suppression of myoclonic responses by barbiturates and benzodiazepines is at least partially due to an action on the postsynaptic GABA receptor/chloride ionophore enhancing complex GABAergic inhibition (32).

GABA Agonists

The most direct approach to enhancing GABA-mediated postsynaptic inhibition is the use of GABA agonists (i.e., compounds acting at the GABA recognition sites in the receptor complex) to reproduce the effect of GABA (25,26). Compounds that potently and selectively act at the postsynaptic receptor to open chloride channels, and whose effect is antagonized by bicuculline (GABA agonists), include muscimol and tetrahydroisooxazolopyridineol (THIP). Surprisingly, these compounds are ineffective at suppressing photically induced myoclonus in the baboon (41,67). In contrast, GABA B-agonists, which act at a bicuculline-insensitive receptor on presynaptic terminals and decrease calcium entry and neurotransmitter release, do diminish or suppress myoclonic responses (37). Progabide, which has some agonist activity at both types of GABA receptor, also decreases myoclonic responses following acute administration (12).

GABA-Transaminase Inhibitors

Aminooxyacetic acid was the first potent inhibitor of GABA transaminase shown to block photically induced myoclonus in the baboon (30). However, slightly higher doses than were needed for anticonvulsant action produced seizures, perhaps because of inhibition of glutamic acid decarboxylase activity.

Among the recently described irreversible (catalytic) inhibitors of GABA transaminase, γ-acetylenic GABA and γ-vinyl GABA produce a rather sustained suppression of the myoclonic responses (38). Among the stereoisomers of γ-vinyl GABA, only (S) γ-vinyl GABA inhibits GABA transaminase. This isomer, given at 100 to 200 mg/kg, i.v., suppresses myoclonic responses for more than 24 hr (47).

Which GABAergic Systems Control Myoclonic Responses?

Meldrum and Wilkins (47), combining psychophysical and pharmacological data, have proposed that photosensitive epilepsy in humans could arise from a diffuse cortical deficiency of the intrinsic GABAergic system. Evidently, in the baboon such a deficiency could explain the neurophysiological data described above if its major impact was in the frontorolandic regions.

Studies of the synaptic connections in the primate neocortex, using electron microscopy and degeneration techniques (74), have demonstrated the activation of the intrinsic inhibitory system (aspinous stellate neurons) by collaterals of cortical afferents and by recurrent collaterals from axons of pyramidal neurons. These inhibitory neurons provide symmetrical synapses to the soma of pyramidal neurons.

Immunocytochemical studies employing antibodies to glutamate decarboxylase have confirmed the predominance of GABAergic terminals around the soma of pyramidal neurons but also have identified prominent axoaxonic GABAergic endings surrounding the initial segments of the pyramidal neuron axon originating from particular inhibitory interneurons (75,76). As photically induced myoclonus is clearly dependent on burst firing in cortical pyramidal neurons, these GABAergic inputs to the soma and the axon initial segment represent a major defense mechanism against myoclonus. Enhancing the hyperpolarizing action of endogenous GABA at these sites is likely to be highly important in suppressing myoclonus. Endogenous GABA agonists may, however, act by desensitizing the receptors and thus facilitate myoclonus.

Excitatory Amino Acids

The role of excitatory amino acids in myoclonic phenomena, and the protective effect of antagonists that block excitation at the *N*-methyl-D-aspartate receptor, are described by Meldrum *(this volume)*. In the photosensitive baboon, the selective antagonists 2-amino-7-phosphonoheptanoic acid and 2-amino-5-phosphonovaleric acid suppress myoclonic responses for 2 to 4 hr (35) (Fig. 4). Other antagonists of excitatory amino acids that are less selective for the *N*-methyl-D-aspartate receptor,

FIG. 4. Effect of 2-amino-7-phosphono-heptanoic acid (2 APH) on photically induced myoclonus in the Senegalese baboon *Papio papio*. Responses to a standardized period of stroboscopic stimulation are graded as 0, none; 1, myoclonus of eyelids; 2, myoclonus of muscles of face and neck; 3, myoclonus of muscles of trunk and limbs; 4, myoclonus continuing beyond the period of photic stimulation. Ordinate indicates mean response (four baboons) before and after the intravenous injection of saline (control) or 2-amino-7-phosphonoheptanoic acid 1.0 mmol/kg. (Modified from Meldrum et al., ref. 35.)

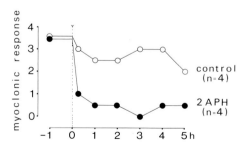

such as *cis*-2,3-piperidine dicarboxylic acid and glutamic acid diethyl ester, also have some protective action.

Monoamines

Many drugs acting on central monoaminergic transmission modify myoclonic responses, including, for example, various ergot alkaloids (33). It is often difficult to establish which monoaminergic transmitter system is principally involved in such drug effects. However, two selective actions are clearly established. These are the protective effects of dopamine agonists and of serotonergic agonists.

Dopamine Agonists

An acute protective action of apomorphine 0.5 to 1.0 mg/kg against photically induced myoclonus was initially described by Meldrum and colleagues (29). L-DOPA is not effective (31) and piribedil and bromocriptine are only weakly active. Among ergot alkaloids with dopamine agonist action, ergocornine 1 to 2 mg/kg abolishes myoclonic responses for up to 90 min (3). Among the apomorphine derivatives with dopamine agonist activity so far tested, (−)2,10,11-trihydroxy-*N*-propylnorapomorphine has the most potent and prolonged protective action (Table 2).

The site of antimyoclonic action of dopamine agonists is not definitively known. It is clearly central (i.e., within the blood–brain barrier), as the peripheral dopamine receptor antagonist domperidone does not block the protective effect of apomorphine (2).

A similar acute protective action of apomorphine against photically induced EEG signs in patients with photosensitive epilepsy has been described in humans (2,69). It is not known whether a significant proportion of patients with other forms of reflex epilepsy (including action myoclonus) respond to apomorphines.

TABLE 2. *Dopamine agonist aporphine derivatives that prevent photically induced myoclonus in* Papio papio *(1,2,3)*

Derivatives	Minimum effective dose (mg/kg, i.v.)	Duration of protection (min)
Apomorphine	0.25	15–30
Norapomorphine	>6	15–60
2,10,11-trihydroxyaporphine	5	1–4
(–)10,11-methylene-dioxy-*N*-propylnoraporphine	0.25	15–120
N-ethyl-2,10,11-trihydroxy-noraporphine	6.25	120
(–)2,10,11-trihydroxy-*N*-propylnoraporphine	0.5	15–420

Serotonergic Agonists and Antagonists

The intravenous or intraperitoneal administration of L-5-hydroxytryptophan (L-5-HTP) 15 to 30 mg/kg produces a relatively sustained suppression of myoclonic responses (33,83). This effect is associated with augmented delta rhythms on the EEG and an increase in spontaneous paroxysmal EEG activities. Similar effects on both myoclonus and background EEG activity are produced by psilocybin and by N,N-dimethyltryptamine (45). Thus, the protective action of 5-HTP can probably be attributed to an action of 5-hydroxytryptamine (5-HT) on 5-HT receptors. L-tryptophan 200 to 600 mg/kg does not prevent myoclonus but has a sustained protective effect when combined with pretreatment with tranylcypromine 10 mg/kg (31).

D-Lysergic acid diethylamide (D-LSD) also potently suppresses myoclonic responses to photic stimulation, but unlike the simpler analogs of 5-HT (psilocybin and N,N-dimethyltryptamine), it suppresses background delta activity and spontaneous spikes and waves on the EEG (82,86).

Some serotonergic antagonists, e.g., methysergide and methergoline, also decrease myoclonic responses (Table 3).

These observations can be tentatively interpreted in terms of the two functional types of 5-HT receptor described by Peroutka et al. (68). One type (5-HT$_1$ receptors) is responsible for the inhibitory effects observed with microiontophoretic application of 5-HT and binds serotonin and D-LSD with high affinity. The other type (5-HT$_2$ receptors) is responsible for excitatory effects of 5-HT and binds spiroperidol and D-LSD with high affinity. Functionally, D-LSD is an agonist at 5-HT$_1$ receptors and an antagonist at 5-HT$_2$ receptors, whereas methergoline, cyproheptadine, and methysergide are antagonists at 5-HT$_2$ receptors.

One tentative interpretation is that an antimyoclonic effect can result from agonist action at 5-HT$_1$ receptors (e.g., 5-HTP, psilocybin, and N,N-dimethyltryptamine and D-LSD) or by antagonist action at 5-HT$_2$ receptors (as with D-LSD, methysergide, methergoline, and cyproheptadine).

L-5-HTP–induced head twitches in mice have been claimed to result from an agonist action at 5-HT$_2$ receptors. Thus, the head twitches are blocked by 5-HT$_2$

TABLE 3. *Serotonergic agonists and antagonists that prevent photically induced myoclonus in* Papio papio

	Dose (mg/kg)	Duration (hr)	Refs.
L-5-hydroxytryptophan	15–30	2–4	83
L-tryptophan + tranylcypromine	100–200 10	1–6	39
D-LSD	0.025–0.05	0.5–1	86
Psilocybin	1–4	1–2	44
N,N-dimethyltryptamine	2–4	0.5–1	44
Methysergide	2–5	0.5–2	44
Methergoline	4	0.25–0.5	44

antagonists. However, they can be induced by D-LSD, which is not consistent with a 5-HT$_2$ agonist origin of the twitches.

Interpretation in terms of activity in specific 5-HT pathways is further complicated by the action of 5-HT autoreceptors, which decrease firing rate of serotonergic neurons (and respond to 5-HT, D-LSD, and *N,N*-dimethyltryptamine). In Luscombe et al.) it is proposed that myoclonus induced by 5-HTP (or D-LSD or psilocybin) in the guinea pig arises from agonist actions at 5-HT$_1$ receptors. Interestingly, this syndrome is a rather precise converse of myoclonus in the baboon, in which similar doses of the 5-HT agonists block myoclonus.

PHARMACOLOGICAL CONCLUSIONS

The pattern of pharmacological responsiveness of photically induced myoclonus in *P papio* is more closely similar to that of posthypoxic action myoclonus than is that of any other animal model of myoclonus so far described. Thus, the responses are readily suppressed by clonazepam, valproate, and L-5-HTP. It appears, therefore, to be a valuable test system for assessing novel treatments that may be of value in man. Available data suggest that dopamine agonists and excitatory amino acid antagonists merit clinical investigation.

REFERENCES

1. Anlezark GM, Blackwood DHR, Meldrum BSM, Ram VJ, Neumeyer JL. Comparative assessment of dopamine agonist aporphines as anticonvulsants in two models of reflex epilepsy. *Psychopharmacology* 1983;81:135–9.
2. Anlezark G, Marrosu F, Meldrum B. Dopamine agonists in reflex epilepsy. In: Morselli PL, Lloyd KG, Löscher W, Meldrum B, Reynolds EH, eds. *Neurotransmitters, Seizures and Epilepsy.* New York: Raven Press, 1981:
3. Anlezark G, Meldrum B. Blockade of photically induced epilepsy by "dopamine agonist" ergot alkaloids. *Psychopharmacology* 1978;57:57–62.
4. Balzamo E, Bert J, Menini Ch, Naquet R. Excessive light sensitivity in Papio papio: its variations with age, sex and geographic origin. *Epilepsia* 1975;16:269–76.
5. Brailowsky S, Menini Ch, Naquet R. Myoclonus developing after vermisectomy in photosensitive Papio papio. *Electroencephalogr Clin Neurophysiol* 1978;45:82–9.
6. Carlier E, Cherubini E, Dimov S, Naquet R. Resection des nerfs faciaux et de la musculature perioculaire chez le Papio papio photosensible. *Electroencephalogr Clin Neurophysiol* 1973;35:13–23.
7. Catier J, Charmasson G, Christolomme A. Study of ipsilateral cortico-cortical connections from the occipital lobe in the photosensitive baboon. *J Physiol (Paris)* 1973;66:93–100.
8. Catier J, Choux M, Cordeau JP, Dimov S, Riche D, Eberhard A, Naquet R. Resultats préliminaires des effets electrographiques de la section du corps calleux chez le Papio papio photosensible. *Rev Neurol (Paris)* 1970;122:521–2.
9. Catier J, Menini Ch, Charmasson G, Carlier E. Mise en evidence de projections corticales somesthesiques au niveau du lobe frontal chez le Babouin. *J Physiol (Paris)* 1971;63:121A–2A.
10. Cepeda C, Tanaka T, Besselievre R, Potier P, Naquet R, Rossier J. Proconvulsant effects in baboons of β-carboline, a putative endogenous ligand for benzodiazepine receptors. *Neurosci Lett* 1981;24:53–7.
11. Cepeda C, Valin A, Calderazzo L, Stutzmann JM, Naquet R. Myoclonies induites par certaines benzodizaèpines chez le Papio papio. Comparaison avec les myoclonies induites par la stimulation lumineuse intermittente. *Rev Electroencephalogr Neurophysiol Clin* 1982;12:32–7.
12. Cepeda C, Worms P, Lloyd KG, Naquet R. (1982). Action of progabide in the photosensitive baboon, Papio papio. *Epilepsia* 1982;23:463–70.

13. Charmasson G, Catier J. Etude electrophysiologique des connexions occipitofrontales directes au niveau du centre ovale chez Papio papio. *Electroencephalogr Clin Neurophysiol* 1975;38:161–70.
14. Cobb S. Photic driving as a cause of clinical seizure in epileptic patients. *Arch Neurol* 1947;58:70–71.
15. Croucher MJ, De Sarro GB, Jensen LH, Meldrum BS. Behavioural and convulsant actions of two methyl esters of β-carboline-3-carboxylic acid in photosensitive baboons and in DBA/2 mice. *Europ. J. Pharmacol.*, 1980, 104:55–60.
16. Dimov S, Lanoir J. (1973): Chronic epileptogenic foci in the photosensitive baboon Papio papio. *Electroencephalogr Clin Neurophysiol* 1973;34:353–67.
17. Fischer-Williams M, Poncet M, Riche D, Naquet R. Light induced epilepsy in the baboon Papio papio: cortical and depth recordings. *Electroencephalogr Clin Neurophysiol* 1968;25:557–69.
18. Gastaut H, Trevisan C, Naquet R. Diagnostic value of electroencephalographic abnormalities provoked by intermittent photic stimulation. *Electroencephalogr Clin Neurophysiol* 1958;10:194–5.
19. Haigler HJ, Aghajanian GK. (1974). Lysergic acid diethylamide and serotonin: a comparison of effects on serotoninergic neurons receiving a serotoninergic input. *J Pharmacol Exp Ther* 1974;188:688–99.
20. Horton RW, Meldrum BS. Seizures induced by allylglycine, 3 mercaptopropionic acid and 4 deoxypyridoxin in mice and photosensitive baboons, and different modes of inhibition of cerebral glutamic acid decarboxylase. *Br J Pharmacol* 1973;49:52–63.
21. Killam KF, Killam EK, Naquet R. Mise en evidence chez certains singes d'un syndrome photo-myoclonique. *CR Acad Sci (Paris)* 1966;262:1010–2.
22. Killam KF, Killam EK, Naquet R. An animal model of light sensitive epilepsy. *Electroencephalogr Clin Neurophysiol* 1967;22:497–513.
23. Killam EK, Matsuzaki M, Killam KF. Effects of chronic administration of benzodiazepines on epileptic seizures and brain electrical activity in Papio papio. In: Garattini S, Mussini E, Randall LO, eds. *The benzodiazepines.* New York: Raven Press, 1973:443–
24. Killam KF, Naquet R, Bert J. Paroxysmal response to intermittent light stimulation in a population of baboons (Papio papio). *Epilepsia* 1966;7:215–9.
25. Meldrum B. GABA-Agonists as anti-epileptic agents. In: Costa E, Di Chiara G, Gessa GL, eds. *GABA and benzodiazepine receptors.* New York: Raven Press, 1981:207–17.
26. Meldrum B. Anticonvulsant drugs and GABA-mediated inhibition. In: Sandler M, ed. *Psychopharmacology of anticonvulsant drugs.* Oxford: Oxford University Press, 1982:62–78.
27. Meldrum BS, Anlezark GM, Ashton CG, Horton RW, Sawaya MCB. Neurotransmitters and anticonvulsant drug action. In: Majkowski J, ed. *Epilepsy: post-traumatic*
28. Meldrum BS, Anlezark G, Balzano E, Horton RW, Trimble M. Photically-induced epilepsy in Papio papio as a model for drug studies. In: Meldrum BS, Marsden CD, eds. Primate models of neurological disorders. New York: Raven Press, 1975:119–28. (Advances in neurology; vol. 10).
29. Meldrum BS, Anlezark G, Trimble M. Drugs modifying dopaminergic activity and behaviour, the EEG and epilepsy in Papio papio. *Eur J Pharmacol* 1975;32:203–13.
30. Meldrum BS, Balzano E, Gadea M, Naquet R. Photic and drug-induced epilepsy in the baboon (Papio papio): The effects of isoniazid, thiosemicarbazide, pyridoxine and amino-oxyacetic acid. *Electroencephalogr Clin Neurophysiol* 1970;29:333–47.
31. Meldrum BS, Balzano E, Wada JA, Vuillon-Cacciuttolo G. Effects of L-tryptophan, L-3,4,dihydroxyphenylalanine and tranylcypromine on the electroencephalogram and on photically induced epilepsy in the baboon Papio papio. *Physiol Behav* 1972;9:615–21.
32. Meldrum B, Braestrup C. GABA and the anticonvulsant action of benzodiazepines and related drugs. In: Bowery N, ed. *Actions and interactions of GABA and benzodiazepines.* New York: Raven Press, 1983:
32a. Meldrum B, Brailowsky S, and Naquet R, Approche pharmacologique de l'epilepsie photosensible de *Papio-papio-* In: *Actualites Pharmacologiques* (30° Serie), Paris: Masson, 1978:81–99.
33. Meldrum BS, Croucher MJ. (1982). Anticonvulsant action of clobazam and desmethylclobazam in reflex epilepsy in rodents and baboons. *Drug Development Research.* 1982;2(Suppl):33–38.
34. Meldrum BS, Croucher MJ, Badman G, Collins JF. Antiepileptic action of excitatory amino acid antagonists in the photosensitive baboon, Papio papio. *Neurosci Lett* 1983;39:101–4.
35. Meldrum BS, Evans MC, Braestrup C. Anticonvulsant action in the photosensitive baboon. Papio papio, of a novel β-carboline derivative, ZK 91296. *Eur J Pharmacol* 1983;91:255–9.
36. Meldrum BS, Horton RW. (1974). Neuronal inhibition mediated by GABA, and patterns of

convulsions in photosensitive baboons with epilepsy (Papio papio). In: Harris P, Mawdsley C, eds. *The natural history and management of epilepsy.* London: Churchill Livingstone, 1974:55–64.

37. Meldrum B, Horton R. Blockade of epileptic responses in the photosensitive baboon, Papio papio, by two irreversible inhibitors of GABA-transaminase, γ-acetylenic GABA (4-amino-hex-5-ynoic acid) and γ-vinyl GABA (4-amino-hex-5-enoic acid). *Psychopharmacology* 1978;69:47–50.
38. Meldrum BS, Horton RW. Anticonvulsant activity in photosensitive baboons. Papio papio, of two new 1,5 benzodiazepines. *Psychopharmacology* 1979;60:277–80.
39. Meldrum BS, Horton RW. Anticonvulsant action of YG 19–256 in baboons with photosensitive epilepsy. *Experientia* 1979;35:796.
40. Meldrum B, Horton R. Effects of the bicyclic GABA agonist, THIP, on myoclonic and seizure responses in mice and baboons with reflex epilepsy. *Eur J Pharmacol* 1980;61:231–7.
41. Meldrum BS, Horton RW, Toseland PA. A primate model for testing anticonvulsant drugs. *Arch Neurol* 1975;32:289–94.
42. Meldrum B, Menini C. Effect of morphine, enkephalins, β-endorphin, and related compounds on seizures thresholds. In: Morselli PL, Lloyd KG, Löscher W, Meldrum B, Reynolds EH, eds. *Neurotransmitters seizures and epilepsy.* New York: Raven Press, 1981:185–94.
43. Meldrum BS, Menini C, Naquet R, Riche D, Silva-Comte C. Absence of seizure activity following focal cerebral injection of enkephalins in a primate. *Regul Pept* 1981;2:383–90.
44. Meldrum BS, Naquet R. Effects of psilocybin, dimethyltryptamine, mescaline and various lysergic derivatives on the EEG and on photically induced epilepsy in the baboon (Papio papio). *Electroencephalogr Clin Neurophysiol* 1971;31:563–72.
45. Meldrum BS, Naquet R, Balzano E. Effects of atropine and eserine on the electroencephalogram on behaviour and on light-induced epilepsy in the adolescent baboon (Papio papio). *Electroencephalogr Clin Neurophysiol* 1970;28:449–58.
46. Meldrum BS, Wilkins AJ. Photosensitive epilepsy in man and the baboon. In: Schwartzkroin P, Wheal HA, eds. *Electrophysiology of Epilepsy,* London: Academic Press, 1983:51–77.
47. Menini Ch. Role du cortex frontal dans l'epilepsie photosensible du singe Papio papio. *J Physiol (Paris)* 1976;72:5–44.
48. Menini Ch, Laurent H. Decharges paroxystiques EEG et EMG induites par la stimulation lumineuse intermittente chez le Papio papio photosensible. *Rev Electroencephalogr Neurophysiol Clin* 1976;6:502–5.
49. Menini Ch, Naquet R. Generalized photosensitive epilepsy in the senegalese baboon (Papio papio). In: Canger R, Angeleri F, Penry K, eds. *Advances in epileptology.* New York: Raven Press, 1980:265–72.
50. Menini Ch, Silva-Barrat C. Cortical visual evoked potentials in the photosensitive epilepsy of Papio papio. *Electroencephalogr Clin Neurophysiol* 1983 (in press).
51. Menini Ch, Silva-Comte C, Stutzmann JM, Dimov S. Cortical unit discharges during photic intermittent stimulation in the Papio papio. Relationships with paroxysmal fronto-rolandic activity. *Electroencephalogr Clin Neurophysiol* 1981;52:42–9.
52. Menini Ch, Silva-Comte C, Valin A, Bryere P, Naquet R. Physiopathogenic mechanisms responsible for two types of myoclonus in the baboon Papio papio. In: Neurophysiological mechanisms of epilepsy. New York: Raven Press, 1983: (in press).
53. Menini Ch, Stutzmann JM, Laurent H, Naquet R. Paroxysmal visual evoked potentials (PVEP) in the Papio papio. I: Morphological and topographical characteristics. Comparison with paroxysmal discharges (PD). *Electroencephalogr Clin Neurophysiol* 1980;50:356–64.
54. Menini Ch, Stutzmann JM, Laurent H, Valin A. Les crises induites—ou non—par la stimulation lumineuse intermittente chez le Papio papio apres injection d'allylglycine. *Rev Electroencephalogr Neurophysiol Clin* 1977;7:232–8.
55. Morrell F, Naquet R, Menini Ch. Microphysiology of cortical single neurons in Papio papio. *Electroencephalogr Clin Neurophysiol* 1969;27:708–9.
56. Naquet R. Conditionnement des decharges hypersynchrones epileptiques chez l'homme et l'animal. In: Fessard A, Gerard RW, Konorski J, eds. Brain mechanisms and learning. Oxford: Blackwell, 1961:625–39.
57. Naquet R. (1973). Contribution of experimental epilepsy to understanding some particular forms in man. In: Brazier MAB, ed. *Epilepsy, its phenomena in man.* New York: Academic Press, 1973:37–65.

58. Naquet R. L'epilepsie photosenible du Papio papio. Un modele de l'epilepsie photosensible de l'homme. *Arch Ital Biol* 1973;111:516–26.
59. Naquet R. L'epilepsie photosensible, donnees humaines et experimentales. *Neurobiol Recife* 1977;40:145–80.
60. Naquet R, Meldrum BS. Photogenic seizures in Baboon. In: Purpura DP, Penry JK, Tower DB, Woodbury DM, Walter RD, eds. *Experimental models of epilepsy.* New York: Raven Press, 1972:373–406.
61. Naquet R, Menini Ch. La photosensibilite excessive du Papio papio: approches neurophysiologique et pharmacologique de ses mecanismes. *Electroencephalogr Clin Neurophysiol* 1972;31:13–26.
62. Naquet R, Menini Ch. New data on the physiopathogeny of experimental generalized epilepsies. *Electroencephalogr Clin Neurophysiol* 1978;34(Suppl):277–84.
63. Naquet R, Menini Ch, Catier J. Photically induced epilepsy in Papio papio. The initiation of discharges and the role of the frontal cortex and of the corpus callosum. In: Petsche H, Brazier MAB, eds. Synchronization of the EEG in the epilepsies. Vienna: Springer Verlag, 1972:347–67.
64. Naquet R, Menini Ch, Cepeda C. Mechanism of appearance of paroxysmal responses induced by intermittent light stimulation. In: Akimoto H, Kazamatsuri H, Seino M, Ward AA Jr, eds. The XIIIth International Epilepsy Symposium. New York: Raven Press, 1982:249–53. (Advances in epileptology).
65. Naquet R, Poncet-Ramade M. Paroxysmal discharges induced by intermittent light stimulation. In: Henri Gastaut and the Marseilles School's Contribution to the Neurosciences. *EEG* 1982;35(Suppl):333–344.
66. Naquet R, Silva-Comte C, Menini Ch. Implication of the frontal cortex in paroxysmal manifestations (EEG and EMG) induced by light stimulation in the Papio papio. In: Speckmann EJ, Elger CE, eds. *Epilepsy and motor system.* Munich: Urban and Schwarzenberg, 1983:220–37.
67. Pedley TA, Horton RW, Meldrum BS. Electroencephalographic and behavioural effects of a GABA agonist (Muscimol) on photosensitive epilepsy in the baboon, Papio papio. *Epilepsia* 1979;20:409–16.
68. Peroutka SJ, Lebovitz RM, Snyder SH. Two distinct central serotonin receptors with different physiological functions. *Science* 1981;212:827–9.
69. Quesney LF, Andermann F, Lal S, Prelevic S. Transient abolition of generalized photosensitive epileptic discharge in humans by apomorphine, a dopamine-receptor agonist. *Neurology* 1980;30:1169–74.
70. Riche D. Afferents to the frontal and occipital lobes in the baboon studied with horseradish peroxidase transport. *Neurosci Lett* 1980;5(Suppl):S198.
71. Riche D, Behzadi G, Calderazzo LS, Guillon R. Cortical and subcortical connections of the parietal area 7 in the baboon, using horseradish peroxidase (HRP) transport. *Neurosci Lett* 1982;10(Suppl):409–10.
72. Silva-Barrat C, Menini Ch. The influence of light stimulation on potentials evoked by single flashes in photosensitive and non-photosensitive Papio papio. *Electroencephalogr Clin Neurophysiol* 1983;(submitted for publication).
73. Silva-Comte C, Velluti J, Menini Ch. Characteristics and origin of frontal paroxysmal responses induced by light stimulation in the Papio papio under allylglycine. *Electroencephalogr Clin Neurophysiol* 1982;53:479–90.
74. Sloper JJ, Powell TPS. An experimental electron microscopic study of afferent connections to the primate motor and somatic sensory cortices. *Philos Trans R Soc Lond [Biol]* 1979;285:199–226.
75. Somogyi P, Freund TF, Wu J-Y, Smith AD. The section-Golgi impregnation procedure. 2. Immunocytochemical demonstration of glutamate decarboxylase in Golgi-impregnated neurons and in their afferent synaptic boutons in the visual cortex of the cat. *Neuroscience* 1983;9:475–90.
76. Somogi P, Nunzi MG, Gorio A, Smith AD. A new type of specific interneuron in the monkey hippocampus forming synapses exclusively with the axon initial segments of pyramidal cells. *Brain Res* 1983;259:137–42.
77. Stutzmann JM, Laurent H, Valin A, Menini Ch. Paroxysmal visual evoked potentials (PVEP) in the Papio papio. II: Evidence for a facilitatory effect of photic intermittent stimulation. *Electroencephalogr Clin Neurophysiol* 1980;50:365–74.
78. Valin A, Cepeda C, Rey E, Naquet R. Opposite effects of lorazepam on two kinds of myoclonus in the photosensitive Papio papio. *Electroencephalogr Clin Neurophysiol* 1981;52:647–51.

79. Valin A, Dodd RH, Liston DR, Potier P, Rossier J. Methyl-β-carboline-induced convulsions are antagonised by Ro 15–1788 and by propyl-β-carboline. *Eur J Pharmacol* 1982;85:93–7.
80. Valin A, Kaijima M, Bryere P, Naquet R. Differential effect of the benzodiazepine antagonist Ro15–1788 on two types of myoclonus in baboon Papio papio. *Neurosci Lett* 1983;38:79–84.
81. Velluti J, Silva-Comte C, Menini Ch. Modifications de l'excitabilité corticale (fronto-rolandique et occipitale par des trains d'éclairs chez le singe Papio papio. *Rev Neurophysiol Electroencephalogr Clin* 1981;11:309–16.
82. Vuillon-Cacciuttolo G, Meldrum BS, Balzano E. Electroretinogram and afferent visual transmission in the epileptic baboon, Papio papio; effects of drugs influencing monoaminergic systems. *Epilepsia* 1973;14:213–21.
83. Wada JA, Balzano E, Meldrum BS, Naquet R. Behavioural and electrographic effects of L-5-hydroxytryptophan and D,L parachlorophenylalanine on epileptic Senegalese baboon (Papio papio). *Electroencephalogr Clin Neurophysiol* 1972;33:520–6.
84. Wada JA, Catier J, Charmasson G, Menini Ch, Naquet R. Further examination of neural mechanisms underlying photosensitivity in the epileptic Senegalese baboon Papio papio. *Electroencephalogr Clin Neurophysiol* 1973;34:786.
85. Wada JA, Terao A, Booker HE. Longitudinal correlative analysis of epileptic baboon Papio papio. *Neurology* 1972;22:1272–85.
86. Walter S, Balzano E, Vuillon-Cacciuttolo G, Naquet R. Effets comportementaux et électrographiques du diéthylamide de l'acide D-lysergique (LSD 25) sur le Papio papio photosensible. *Electroencephalogr Clin Neurophysiol* 1971;30:294–305.
87. Walter WG, Walter V, Gastaut J, Gastaut Y. Une forme electroencephalographique nouvelle de l'epilepsie: L'epilepsie photogenique. *Rev Neurol (Paris)* 1948;80:613–4.

Advances in Neurology, Vol. 43: Myoclonus,
edited by S. Fahn et al. Raven Press,
New York © 1986.

Mechanism of Action of Clonazepam in Myoclonus in Relation to Effects on GABA and 5-HT

P. Jenner, J. A. Pratt, and C. D. Marsden

University Department of Neurology, Institute of Psychiatry and King's College Hospital Medical School, London SE5, United Kingdom

Clonazepam is a 1,4-benzodiazepine, structurally related to diazepam and nitrazepam, that possesses potent anticonvulsant actions (2,33). Clonazepam is employed to control many forms of epilepsy but particularly absence and myoclonic seizures (6). It has become the drug of choice in controlling some forms of myoclonus (4,8,9,20).

The potent anticonvulsant activity of clonazepam is demonstrated by its ability to inhibit pentylenetetrazole-induced seizures in animals (Table 1), in which the drug is more potent than diazepam (26). Like benzodiazepines in general, clonazepam is only weakly effective in blocking maximal electroshock-induced seizures and is less active than diazepam in this model (26). The main action of clonazepam is its ability to interact with benzodiazepine receptors in the brain that facilitate GABAergic transmission (32). Clonazepam potently displaces ligands such as [³H]diazepam or [³H]flunitrazepam from their specific binding sites to benzodiazepine receptors (31), and its ability to do so correlates with its potent anticonvulsant actions. Indeed, there is a good relationship between the ability of benzodiazepines in general both to displace tritiated ligands from the benzodiazepine receptor and to protect against pentylenetetrazole-induced seizures (Table 1) and their potency in conflict tests detecting anxiolytic activity.

The widespread distribution of the GABA receptor complex in the brain (5) enables all benzodiazepines to manipulate the function of a number of neurotransmitter systems, including dopamine, norepinephrine, 5-hydroxytryptamine (5-HT), and acetylcholine (14,25). Interest in clonazepam in myoclonus initially was concentrated on its interaction with brain 5-HT function because of its ability to suppress some forms of postanoxic action myoclonus (8). Postanoxic action myoclonus is associated with low CSF 5-hydroxyindoleacetic acid (5-HIAA) levels and may respond to the administration of the 5-HT precursors L-5-hydroxytryptophan (L-5-HTP), and tryptophan combined with a monoamine oxidase inhibitor (MAOI) (4,8,9). The clinical benefit of clonazepam is associated with a return of CSF 5-HIAA levels to or toward normal. The ability of clonazepam to suppress action myoclonus contrasts with the relative lack of efficacy of diazepam and

TABLE 1. *Comparison of the ability of a range of benzodiazepine drugs to displace [³H]diazepam and to inhibit pentylenetetrazole-induced or maximal electroshock-induced seizures*[a]

Drug	IC_{50} [³H]diazepam (nM)[b]	ED_{50} pentylenetetrazole-induced seizures[c] (mg/kg, i.p.)	ED_{50} maximal electroshock-induced seizures[d] (mg/kg, i.p.)
Clonazepam	2.1	0.009	92.7
Diazepam	8.9	0.165	19.1
Nitrazepam	9.1	0.087	18.1
Flurazepam	16	0.473	47.1
Oxazepam	20	0.360	81.3
Chlordiazepoxide	310	1.61	29.3

[a]Data from Krall et al., ref. 26, and Mohler and Richards, ref. 31.
[b]The ability of benzodiazepine to displace [³H]diazepam was determined using rat cerebral cortex preparations (30).
[c]Pentylenetetrazole (85 mg/kg, s.c.) was administered to mice. This produced seizures in approximately 97% of normal mice. Absence of a single 5-sec episode of clonic spasms (a threshold seizure) was defined as protection (37).
[d]Maximal electroshock seizures were elicited by a 60-Hz alternating current of 50 mA (five to seven times that necessary to elicit minimal seizures) delivered for 0.2 sec via corneal electrodes. Maximal seizures were produced in all normal mice. The maximal seizure typically consists of a short period of initial tonic flexion and a prolonged period of tonic extension (especially of the hindlimbs) followed by terminal clonus. Failure to extend the hindlimbs to an angle with the trunk of greater than 90° is defined as protection (36).

chlordiazepoxide and of nonbenzodiazepine anticonvulsants such as phenobarbital or diphenylhydantoin in this condition (40). The efficacy of newer benzodiazepines such as clobazam or flunitrazepam remains unknown.

ELECTROPHYSIOLOGICAL EVIDENCE FOR ACTION OF BENZODIAZEPINES ON RAPHE CELL FIRING

The cell bodies in the dorsal raphe nucleus of 5-HT projections to the forebrain have 5-HT, GABA, and glycine receptors on their surface, all of which act independently of one another (1,18,42). 5-HT, GABA, and glycine, on microiontophoretic application, inhibit the firing of dorsal raphe neurons. In anesthetized male rats, intravenous administration or the iontophoretic application of diazepam, chlordiazepoxide, or flurazepam by themselves have no effect on the firing rate of dorsal raphe cells, although LSD totally inhibits cell firing (17). However, the inhibition of raphe cell firing produced by a submaximal dose of GABA applied iontophoretically is potentiated by benzodiazepines (17) (Fig. 1). This effect is blocked by the GABA antagonist picrotoxin. Benzodiazepines have no effect on the inhibition of cell firing produced by glycine or 5-HT.

The conclusion reached from these studies is that benzodiazepines do not interact directly with any of the receptors on 5-HT cell bodies, but their actions are mediated via the GABA receptor complex. The failure to observe effects of benzodiazepines

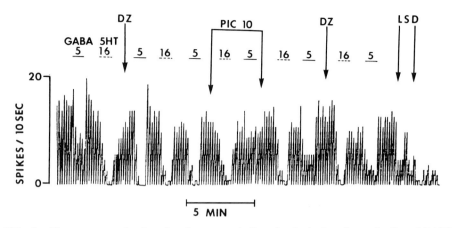

FIG. 1. The response of a dorsal raphe neuron to the microiontophoretic application of GABA and 5-HT. GABA was ejected with a 5-nA current for 60 sec (—); 5-HT was injected with a 16-nA current for 60 sec (---). Immediately following a 1-mg/kg, i.v., dose of diazepam (DZ), a potentiated response to GABA (5 nA) but not to 5-HT (16 nA) was observed. The ejection of picrotoxin (PIC) with a 10-nA current almost completely blocked the response to GABA but did not affect the 5-HT response. An additional 1-mg/kg, i.v., dose of diazepam potentiated the recovering GABA response. The cell was subsequently inhibited by LSD (5 + 5 µg/kg, i.v.). Ordinate spikes/10 sec, scale, 0–20; time marker, 5 min. (From Gallager, ref. 17, with permission.)

in their own right was attributed to low intrinsic GABAergic inhibitory tone. Pretreatment of animals with aminooxyacetic acid, to cause an accumulation of GABA, results in inhibition of raphe cell firing when benzodiazepines alone are administered (17). How benzodiazepines act to potentiate the effects of GABA has not been determined, but the results suggest the presence of a GABA interneuron within the raphe nuclear complex.

The conclusion that ongoing GABA transmission is necessary for the effects of benzodiazepines to be seen has been confirmed by a study of raphe unit activity in freely moving cats (38). Chlordiazepoxide and diazepam produce a dose-dependent decrease in the discharge rate of 5-HT–containing neurons in the dorsal raphe nucleus. Interestingly, doses of benzodiazepines commonly used to produce anxiolytic effects in the cat produce no significant change in the activity of 5-HT raphe neurons. Therapeutic doses of benzodiazepines may not affect the central 5-HT system. Doses of benzodiazepines that do decrease raphe unit activity also produce profound ataxia. This suggests that benzodiazepine-induced suppression of raphe unit activity may be more closely related to general motor behavior and side effects than to the anxiolytic properties of the drugs.

BIOCHEMICAL ACTIONS OF CLONAZEPAM AND OTHER ANTICONVULSANT DRUGS ON BRAIN 5-HT SYSTEMS

A number of investigations have centered on the ability of benzodiazepines and other anticonvulsant drugs to alter cerebral 5-HT metabolism. These arose from evidence suggesting that brain 5-HT may be involved in the control of seizure threshold (3), as well as punishment responding (39). In the photosensitive baboon, compounds that elevate brain 5-HT concentrations such as 5-HTP, or L-tryptophan in conjunction with an MAOI, provide protection against seizures, apparently by modulating the intensity of the provocative visual stimulus (28,41). The threshold for chemically or electrically induced fits in rodents is elevated by raising cerebral 5-HT concentrations, whereas depletion of 5-HT by the use of reserpine or p-chlorophenylalanine (PCPA) lowers the threshold (11,24). A series of anticonvulsant drugs have been shown to elevate brain 5-HT concentrations and that of 5-HT's metabolite, 5-HIAA (3,23).

In this respect, clonazepam is not different from other anticonvulsant drugs. A number of investigators have reported changes in 5-HT parameters in brain following clonazepam administration (Table 2). Some differences exist in the results obtained from the various studies. For example, Fenessey and Lee (16) reported an increase in 5-HT levels in mouse brain but no change in 5-HIAA. Our own studies in mice showed that changes occurred in tryptophan, 5-HT, and 5-HIAA concentrations (7,23,34). Weiner and colleagues (43) also found an increase in brain 5-HT concentrations following clonazepam, but Chung Hwang and van Woert (12) were unable to show any change in brain tryptophan, 5-HT, or 5-HIAA levels following administration to rats. It is not clear why these differences in effect are observed, but we have found that different mouse strains respond differently to clonazepam.

Overall, there is general agreement that some change in 5-HT biochemical parameters is produced by the administration of clonazepam to rodents. However, none of the studies so far described has thrown any light on the mechanism by which clonazepam might alter 5-HT parameters in brain. Recently we carried out a detailed investigation of the alterations in 5-HT function produced by clonazepam looking at the effects of the drug on 5-HT synthesis, utilization, and turnover and on the egress of 5-HT's metabolite, 5-HIAA, from the brain (34).

The acute administration of clonazepam (0.5–8.0 mg/kg, i.p.) to mice resulted in a dose-dependent increase in brain 5-HT, 5-HIAA, and tryptophan levels, as previously reported. The maximal elevations of 5-HT, 5-HIAA, and tryptophan observed were 119, 228, and 158% of control levels, respectively. Since the dose

TABLE 2. *Summary of investigations into the effects of clonazepam on brain 5-HT and 5-HIAA concentrations*

Species	Dose (mg/kg)	Effect of 5-HT	Effect of 5-HIAA	Ref.
Mice	2.5	Increase	No change	16
Mice	0.5–8.0	Increase	Increase	23
Guinea pig	5–20	Increase	—	44
Mice	1–8	Increase	Increase	9
Rat	2	No change	No change	12
Mice	0.5–8.0	Increase	Increase	34

of clonazepam used caused a dramatic fall in body temperature of animals (from $37.2 \pm 0.2°C$ to $33.8 \pm 1.0°C$) after clonazepam (4 mg/kg, i.p.), it could be argued that the changes observed were due to the nonspecific effect of hypothermia. However, in animals housed at a constant environmental temperature of 33°C, which maintained normal body temperature of $36.6 \pm 0.2°C$, identical changes in 5-HT parameters were observed. It would appear that the effects of clonazepam on cerebral 5-HT parameters is a real phenomenon.

Chase and colleagues (10) previously had reported that the administration of diazepam led to an inhibition of the efflux of 5-HIAA from the brain. To determine whether the effects of clonazepam in elevating 5-HIAA levels were due to this mechanism, we studied the effects of clonazepam on 5-HT parameters following inhibition of the breakdown of 5-HT by MAO, using pargyline or tranylcypromine (Fig. 2). The MAOIs themselves elevated brain 5-HT and decreased 5-HIAA. Clonazepam administered in conjunction with the MAOIs elevated brain 5-HT above the levels observed in the presence of the MAOI alone. But despite the large doses of MAOIs administered, clonazepam decreased the reduction of brain 5-HIAA observed in the presence of pargyline or tranylcypromine alone. This finding suggests that clonazepam can inhibit egress of 5-HIAA from brain in agreement with the previous findings for diazepam by Chase et al. (10).

Since clonazepam may impede the egress of 5-HIAA from the brain, the changes in 5-HIAA observed following administration of clonazepam alone might be due entirely to this effect of the drug. So we investigated the ability of clonazepam to

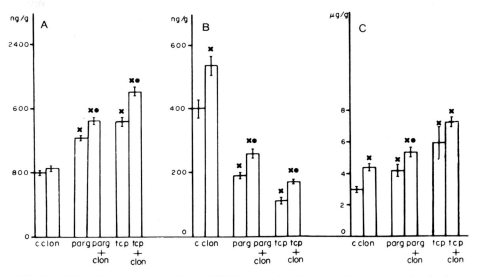

FIG. 2. Effect of pretreatment with the MAOI's pargyline (parg) and tranylcypromine (tcp) on clonazepam (clon)-induced changes in whole brain 5-HT **(A)**, 5-HIAA **(B)**, and tryptophan **(C)**. x, values significantly different from saline-treated controls (c) ($p<0.01$); ●, values significantly different from MAOI-treated animals ($p<0.01$). Statistical analysis by Student's t-test. (From Pratt et al., ref. 34, with permission.)

elevate brain 5-HIAA concentrations following blockade of transport mechanisms by the administration of probenecid (200 mg/kg, i.p., 4 hr and 1 hr prior to death) (Fig. 3). Probenecid induced the expected marked elevation of whole brain 5-HIAA levels, but clonazepam (4 mg/kg, i.p.) induced a further elevation of 5-HIAA concentrations. This suggests that at least some of the change in 5-HIAA was due to an action of clonazepam on 5-HT synthesis or utilization.

We then turned our attention to the possibility that clonazepam alters 5-HT synthesis. We assessed the effects of clonazepam (4 mg/kg) by looking at the accumulation of 5-HTP occurring following blockade of brain aromatic amino acid decarboxylase using the enzyme inhibitor NSD 1034 (Table 3). The decarboxylase inhibitor alone caused a marked increase in whole-brain 5-HTP levels. Clonazepam alone had no effect on 5-HTP concentrations. Similarly, the administration of clonazepam to animals pretreated with NSD 1034 did not alter the 5-HTP content of the brain. This suggests that clonazepam does not alter 5-HT synthesis. This finding was surprising, since previously the acute administration of clonazepam was associated with an increase in brain tryptophan concentrations (Fig. 2). It follows that the elevation of brain tryptophan produced by clonazepam is not likely to be of functional significance, at least in terms of provoking 5-HT synthesis.

Since clonazepam does not increase cerebral 5-HT levels by altering transmitter synthesis, a change in 5-HT utilization might explain the present data. To investigate this, we looked at the rate of decrease of brain 5-HT content following inhibition of tryptophan hydroxylase produced by administration of PCPA (Fig. 4). Pretreatment with PCPA for 3 days caused a marked depletion of whole-brain 5-HT.

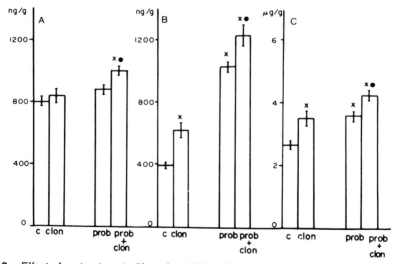

FIG. 3. Effect of pretreatment with probenecid (prob) (200 mg/kg, i.p., 4 hr and 1 hr prior to death) on clonazepam (clon)-induced changes in whole-brain 5-HT **(A)**, 5-HIAA **(B)**, and tryptophan **(C)**. x, values significantly different from saline-treated controls (c) ($p<0.05$); ●, values significantly different from probenecid-treated controls ($p<0.05$). Statistical analysis by Student's t-test. (From Pratt et al., ref. 34, with permission.)

TABLE 3. *Effect of clonazepam on the accumulation of 5-HTP induced by NSD 1034 in whole mouse brain[a]*

Treatment[b]	No. of observations[a]	Whole brain 5-HTP concentrations (ng/g)
Saline controls	9	85 ± 14
NSD 1034	7	257 ± 17[d]
Clonazepam	7	73 ± 24
NSD 1034 + clonazepam	7	280 ± 24[d]

[a]From Pratt et al., ref. 34.
[b]NSD 1034 was administered intraperitoneally 30 min before and 1.5 hr after clonazepam (4 mg/kg, i.p.).
[c]Each observation represents the result obtained from a pool of 10 whole mouse brains.
[d]$p < 0.001$ compared with controls using Student's *t*-test. Data presented as mean ± SEM.

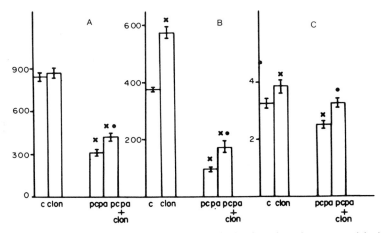

FIG. 4. Effect of pretreatment with p-chlorophenylalanine (pcpa) on clonazepam (clon)-induced changes in whole-brain 5-HT (ng/g) **(A)**, 5-HIAA (ng/g) **(B)**, and tryptophan (μg/g) **(C)**. x, values significantly different from saline-treated controls (c) ($p<0.05$); ●, values significantly different from PCPA alone ($p<0.05$). Statistical analysis by Student's *t*-test. (From Pratt et al., ref. 34, with permission.)

Administration of clonazepam (4 mg/kg) to animals pretreated with PCPA reduced the 5-HT depletion. The ability of clonazepam to decrease the disappearance of 5-HT following synthesis blockade suggests that the rate of utilization of 5-HT is slowed. The changes in cerebral 5-HT and 5-HIAA content produced by clonazepam thus might result from intraneuronal accumulation of 5-HT and its subsequent breakdown resulting from a decrease in transmitter utilization.

One of the problems associated with the previous experiments is that the pharmacological manipulations required to investigate changes in 5-HT function may have altered the dynamics of the system. In an attempt to overcome this we utilized pulse labeling techniques to confirm the actions of clonazepam on brain 5-HT function. We administered L-[G-³H]tryptophan to animals 0.5 hr prior to death to assess incorporation of labeled tryptophan into the 5-HT pool, and at 2.0 hr prior to death when incorporation of labeled tryptophan into 5-HT was complete and this pool was then decreasing due to utilization. We found that administration of clonazepam did not alter the specific activity of 5-HT in the brain during incorporation into the 5-HT pool, confirming the drug to be without effect on brain 5-HT synthesis (Table 4). However, clonazepam increased the brain content of labeled 5-HT and specific activity, compared to control animals, at later time intervals when the labeled pool was decreasing due to utilization. This provides further support to the hypothesis that clonazepam reduces 5-HT utilization.

In summary, the major findings of this study and their implications were as follows. The ability of clonazepam in the presence of an MAOI to elevate 5-HIAA levels, compared to animals receiving MAOI alone, suggests that at least part of the increase in 5-HIAA levels is due to the blockade of the egress of this metabolite from the brain. The ability of clonazepam to further elevate 5-HIAA levels in the presence of probenecid may reflect an increased breakdown of interneuronal 5-HT as a result of a decrease in utilization. Decreased 5-HT utilization is suggested by the pulse-labeling and PCPA experiments. Such a decrease in 5-HT utilization apparently occurs without any change in 5-HT synthesis. The increase in brain 5-HT produced by clonazepam after MAO inhibition may be due to an increase in intraneuronal storage of 5-HT due to normal synthesis but decreased release.

The finding of decreased 5-HT utilization is in accord with evidence of decreased 5-HT neuronal activity in the presence of other benzodiazepine drugs. Indeed, the similar effects on punishment processes produced by the administration of benzodiazepines or by reduction of cerebral 5-HT function (by lesions or PCPA administration) (40) suggests such changes may be of functional significance.

How clonazepam decreases 5-HT utilization remains unclear. In midbrain raphe slices, benzodiazepines act to enhance both spontaneous and potassium-evoked release of [³H]5-HT, an action inhibited by picrotoxin (13). Such an action may be of functional significance, for local injection of chlordiazepoxide into the dorsal raphe in chronically implanted awake rats attenuated the inhibition of lever pressing for food elicited by a signal of punishment (37). This effect, which was abolished by destruction of 5-HT neurons using 5,7-dihydroxytryptamine, could be mimicked or potentiated by the intraraphe administration of 5-HT. Again, chlordiazepoxide or diazepam facilitated the potassium-evoked release of [³H]serotonin from rat midbrain slices. A high density of [³H]flunitrazepam binding sites was found in the dorsal and the median raphe nucleus; the number and affinity of these sites being unaltered by 5,7-dihydroxytryptamine lesions of the raphe system.

There is considerable evidence, therefore, to suggest that clonazepam can interact with brain 5-HT neuronal systems. However, this is not a specific effect of clonazepam, for other benzodiazepines and other anticonvulsant drugs can produce similar changes in 5-HT utilization. In a recent study, we compared the effects of clonazepam, diazepam, chlordiazepoxide, flurazepam, diphenylhydantoin, carbamazepine, and phenobarbital in altering 5-HT utilization as judged by changes in

TABLE 4. Effect of a pulse injection of L-[G-³H]-tryptophan on the specific activity and counts per gram of whole-brain tryptophan and 5-HT in clonazepam-treated mice[a]

Treatment[b]	5-HT		Tryptophan	
	Specific activity DPM/ng 5HT	DPM/g wet weight	Specific activity DPM/ng tryptophan	DPM/g wet weight
0.5 hr after				
L-[G-³H]Tryptophan	6.893 ± 0.533 N = 8	3270 ± 157 N = 8	11.466 ± 0.646 N = 8	2921 ± 193 N = 8
L-[G-³H]Tryptophan + clonazepam	7.130 ± 0.581 N = 8	3758 ± 250 N = 8	15.337[d] ± 1.098 N = 8	4914[d] ± 489 N = 8
2.0 hr after				
L-[G-³H]Tryptophan + clonazepam	3.563 ± 0.166 N = 9	2109 ± 0.88 N = 9	6.419 ± 802 N = 9	6419 ± 802 N = 10
L-[G-³H]Tryptophan + clonazepam	4.849[d] ± 0.444 N = 9	2759[d] ± 277 N = 9	5.910 ± 0.66 N = 9	9309[d] ± 1099 N = 10

[a]From Pratt et al., ref. 34.
[b]L-[G-³H]Tryptophan (25 µCi, s.c.) was administered 30 min and 2 hr before death. Animals were sacrificed 3 hr after clonazepam administration (4 mg/kg, i.p.).
[c]N, number of observations.
[d]$p < 0.05$ compared with L-[G-³H]tryptophan alone as assessed using Student's t-test. Data presented as mean ± SEM.

the brain content of [³H]5-HT following pulse labeling with L-[G-³H]tryptophan (unpublished observations). Although none of the drugs influenced the synthesis of [³H]5-HT from L-[G-³H]tryptophan, clonazepam, diazepam, chlordiazepoxide, and diphenylhydantoin, all decreased 5-HT utilization (Fig. 5). Flurazepam, carbamazepine, and phenobarbital produced no significant change.

RELATIONSHIP OF THE ABILITY OF CLONAZEPAM TO ALTER BRAIN 5-HT FUNCTION TO ITS ACTIONS IN 5-HT–SENSITIVE ACTION MYOCLONUS

The interpretation of the action of clonazepam on 5-HT pathways in rodents is difficult to reconcile with the beneficial effects of the drug in the treatment of postanoxic action myoclonus in humans. Myoclonus in this disease responds to the administration of precursors of 5-HT such as 5-HTP and tryptophan plus an MAOI (8). The myoclonus also responds to clonazepam, and since the actions of clonazepam are accompanied by an increase in CSF 5-HIAA levels, a 5-HT agonist

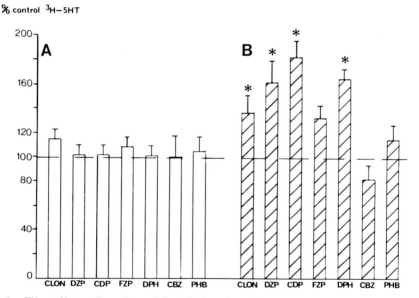

FIG. 5. Effect of benzodiazepines, diphenylhydantoin, carbamazepine, or phenobarbital on the synthesis **(A)** and utilization **(B)** of 5-HT in whole mouse brain following a pulse injection of L-[G-³H]tryptophan 0.5 hr and 2 hr previously (unpublished observations). Animals were administered L-[G-³H]tryptophan (25μCi, s.c.) alone or in combination with clonazepam (clon) (4 mg/kg, i.p., 3 hr prior to death), diazepam (dzp) (32 mg/kg, i.p., 3 hr prior to death), chlordiazepoxide (cdp) (40 mg/kg, i.p., 2 hr prior to death), flurazepam (fzp) (40 mg/kg, i.p., 2 hr prior to death), diphenylhydantoin (dph) (40 mg/kg, i.p., 1.5 hr prior to death), carbamazepine (cbz) (50 mg/kg, i.p., 1 hr prior to death), or phenobarbital (phb) (80 mg/kg, i.p., 2 hr prior to death). *Open columns*, animals receiving L-[G-³H]tryptophan 30min previously; *hatched columns*, animals receiving L-[G-³H]tryptophan 2 hr previously. The data are presented as percentage of [³H]5-HT found in control animals receiving L-[G-³H]tryptophan and vehicle only. Each column represents the mean result ± 1 SEM for at least five estimations. (*), $p < 0.05$ compared to control values using Student's t-test.

action has been proposed (8). Such a hypothesis contrasts with the results obtained from the electrophysiological and biochemical experiments described above, all of which suggest the exact opposite, namely, that clonazepam decreases 5-HT utilization. One explanation for this paradox is that clonazepam might act directly on postsynaptic 5-HT receptors, leading to a feedback inhibition of 5-HT neuronal action. However, clonazepam has no ability to displace tritiated ligands from 5-HT receptors in binding assays (12), and benzodiazepines do not change the actions of 5-HT applied iontophoretically onto raphe neurons (17).

The alterations of 5-HT function caused by clonazepam, however, can result in 5-HT action. Benzodiazepines, including clonazepam, can induce head twitching in mice, a 5-HT–mediated behavior (9). However, this effect is markedly enhanced by pretreatment with MAOIs, so is likely to result from a "spillover" phenomenon from presynaptic accumulations of 5-HT as previously described by Grahame-Smith (22).

Indeed, clonazepam also may exert actions on the uptake and release of [^{3}H]5-HT neuronal terminals. Chung Hwang and Van Woert (12) found clonazepam to inhibit whole-brain synaptosomal [^{3}H]5-HT uptake and to increase [^{3}H]5-HT release in the mouse, although peripheral administration of clonazepam had no effect on these parameters. Similarly, diazepam enhanced spontaneous and potassium-evoked release of [^{3}H]5-HT in rat raphe slices (13). In contrast, however, others have found little effect of diazepam on potassium-evoked release of [^{3}H]5-HT from rat cortical slices (15).

Although clonazepam can alter 5-HT function in the rat, there is no evidence to prove that this is the mechanism by which it is active in depressing some forms of action myoclonus. Weiner and colleagues (43) found clonazepam to induce a moderate elevation of whole-brain 5-HT, but they also found that the drug did not potentiate, or inhibit, 5-HTP–induced myoclonus occurring in guinea pigs. From these results, they suggested that, despite the drug's influencing 5-HT function, it did not have any effect on the physiological activity of 5-HT and might not exert its activity by influencing 5-HT neurons in the brain. Indeed, there is no necessity that the actions of clonazepam should be on 5-HT systems directly.

Benzodiazepines, as discussed above, are capable of modulating GABAergic activity controlling many neurotransmitter systems. It is quite conceivable that the GABA system acted on by clonazepam may lie downstream from 5-HT neurons and that the resulting changes in 5-HT neuronal function observed are the result of a feedback mechanism occurring as a consequence of downstream action. The apparent difference in the effects of clonazepam and those of the 5-HT precursors might be reconciled by such an effect. Also in support of a non–5-HT action of clonazepam is the fact that the doses of clonazepam that need to be administered to animals to produce changes in 5-HT utilization are far greater than those that are required for anticonvulsant action. They also are likely to be in excess of those utilized in humans for the control of myoclonus. The changes in 5-HIAA concentrations in CSF observed in humans following clonazepam administration could be related solely to the ability of the drug to prevent the egress of this metabolite from CSF.

Finally, one must answer the question as to why clonazepam, of all benzodiazepines and of all anticonvulsant drugs, appears to be of such benefit in the treatment of action myoclonus, although the actions of newer, more potent benzodiazepines, such as flunitrazepam or clobazam, remain to be investigated. Diazepam, flurazepam, and chlordiazepoxide, together with diphenylhydantoin and phenobarbital, appear to be of little or no benefit. Certainly, clonazepam is more potent than many of the other benzodiazepine compounds assessed in action myoclonus. However, this alone cannot provide the answer. Potency is only a question of increasing the dose to obtain the same effect. Indeed, in a recent study, Garratini and his colleagues (29) showed that a range of benzodiazepine drugs given in ED_{50} doses for the inhibition of pentylenetetrazole-induced seizures all displaced the *in vivo* binding of [³H]diazepam to rat brain by approximately 50%. There appears to be no evidence whatsoever that the manner in which a range of benzodiazepine drugs interacts with the benzodiazepine receptor or the manner in which this is linked to GABA receptors differs. Subtypes of benzodiazepine receptors have been reported (19), but there is no information that suggests that clonazepam may differentially affect these populations. It is possible that clonazepam shows a differential distribution within the brain that differs from that of other benzodiazepines, but for such lipid-soluble drugs, this would appear unlikely. There is no evidence to support such a hypothesis, so there is no clear explanation for the superiority of clonazepam over other benzodiazepine compounds.

One explanation may lie in the duration of action of the antimyoclonic action of benzodiazepine compounds. From a pharmacokinetic standpoint, in humans it is difficult to differentiate between many of these compounds, since they are all relatively well absorbed, show peak drug concentrations at approximately the same time, and have relatively long plasma half-lives (21) (Table 5). Clinically, however, it is apparent that the antimyoclonic action of diazepam lasts for a much shorter time than the plasma half-life might suggest, whereas that of clonazepam is prolonged. The reasons for this are unclear, but as oral medication, diazepam is not satisfactory for the control of seizures. Meldrum and his colleagues (27) showed

TABLE 5. *Comparison of the pharmacokinetic characteristics of some benzodiazepine drugs in humans*

Drug	% Oral availability	$T_{1/2}$ (hr)	Effective concentration (ng/ml)
Clonazepam	98	39	5–70
Diazepam	100	20–90	>600
Flunitrazepam	85	15	—
Nitrazepam	78	29	—
Chlordiazepoxide	100	10	>700

that in photosensitive baboons, *Papio papio*, treated with a subconvulsant dose of L-allylglycine, diazepam blocked myoclonic responses for only 0.5 to 2.5 hr., the short duration of action apparently being related to the rapid clearance of the drug. Antiepileptic action was evident only while plasma levels remained above 0.5 μg/ml. Clonazepam, however, was more potent, and its antimyoclonic action was prolonged for a considerable period of time. It may be, therefore, that the advantages of clonazepam lie not in a difference in the pharmacological interaction of the drug with benzodiazepine receptors in the brain but rather in some aspect of its pharmacokinetic profile coupled to its potent actions on benzodiazepine receptors.

SUMMARY

Clonazepam is a potent anticonvulsant 1,4-benzodiazepine that controls some types of myoclonus. Its primary mode of action is to facilitate GABAergic transmission in the brain by a direct effect on benzodiazepine receptors.

GABA receptors lie on the cell bodies of dorsal raphe neurons, and GABA acts to inhibit raphe cell firing, an action potentiated by benzodiazepines. Clonazepam does not alter 5-HT synthesis but decreases 5-HT utilization in brain and blocks the egress of 5-HIAA from the brain.

It is not known whether the actions of clonazepam in altering 5-HT function are responsible for its antimyoclonic action, since these are observed only after large doses. Also, the effects of clonazepam are the exact opposite of those predicted from the beneficial effects of 5-HTP in human myoclonic disorders. Finally, why clonazepam, more than other benzodiazepines, is of benefit in the treatment of myoclonus is not clear. This may be due to some pharmacokinetic feature of the drug in conjunction with its potency at benzodiazepine receptors.

ACKNOWLEDGMENTS

This study was supported by the Research Funds of the Bethlem Royal and Maudsley Hospital and King's College Hospital and the Medical Research Council.

REFERENCES

1. Aghajanian G, Haigler H, Bloom F. Lysergic acid diethylamide and serotonin: direct actions in serotonin-containing neurons. *Life Sci* 1972;11:615–22.
2. Blum JE, Haefely W, Jalfre M, Polc P, Scharer K. Pharmakologie und Toxikologie der Antiepiletikums Clonazepam. *Arzneimittelforsch* 1973;23:377–89.
3. Bonnycastle DD, Giarman NJ, Paasonen MK. Anticonvulsant compounds and 5-hydroxytryptamine in rat brain. *Br J Pharmacol* 1957;12:228–31.
4. Boudouresques J, Roger J, Khalil R, Vigouroux RA, Gossett A, Pellisier JF, Tassinari CA. A propos de 2 observations de syndrome de Lance et Adams. Effect therapeutique du Ro-05-4023. *Rev Neurol (Paris)* 1971;125:306–9.
5. Braestrup C, Nielsen M. Benzodiazepine receptors. *Arzneimittelforsch* 1980;30:858–61.
6. Browne TR. Clonazepam: a review of new anticonvulsant drug. *Arch Neurol* 1976;33:326–32.
7. Chadwick D, Gorrod JW, Jenner P, Marsden CD, Reynolds EH. Functional changes in cerebral 5-hydroxytryptamine metabolism in the mouse induced by anticonvulsant drugs. *Br J Pharmacol* 1978;62:115–24.
8. Chadwick D, Hallett M, Harris R, Jenner P, Reynolds EH, Marsden CD. Clinical, biochemical

and physiological features distinguishing myoclonus responsive to 5-hydroxytryptophan, trypto-phan with a monoamine oxidase inhibitor and clonazepam. *Brain* 1977;100:455–87.

9. Chadwick D, Harris R, Jenner P, Reynolds EH, Marsden CD. Manipulation of brain serotonin in the treatment of myoclonus. *Lancet* 1975;2:434–5.

10. Chase TN, Katz RI, Kopin IJ. Effect of diazepam on the fate of intercisternally injected serotonin -^{14}C. *Neuropharmacology* 1970;9:103–8.

11. Chen G, Ensor CR, Bohner BA. A facilitation action of reserpine on the central nervous system. *Proc Soc Exp Biol Med* 1954;86:507–10.

12. Chung Hwang E, Van Woert MH. Antimyoclonic action of clonazepam: the role of serotonin. *Eur J Pharmacol* 1979;60:31–40.

13. Collinge J, Pycock C. Differential actions of diazepam on the release of ^{3}H-5-hydroxytryptamine from cortical midbrain raphe slices in the rat. *Eur J Pharmacol* 1982;85:9–14.

14. Costa E. Benzodiazepines and neurotransmitters *Arzneimittelforsch* 1980;30:858–61.

15. de Boer TH, Stoof JC, van Duijn H. The effects of convulsant drugs on the release of radiolabelled GABA, glutamate, noradrenaline, serotonin and acetylcholine from rat cortical slices. *Brain Res* 1982;253:153–60.

16. Fennessy MR, Lee JR. The effect of benzodiazepines on brain amines of the mouse. *Arch Int Pharmacodyn Ther* 1972;197:37–44.

17. Gallager DW. Benzodiazepines: potentiation of a GABA inhibitory response in the dorsal raphe nucleus. *Eur J Pharmacol* 1978;49:133–43.

18. Gallager DW, Aghajanian GK. Effect of antipsychotic drugs on the firing of dorsal raphe cells. II. Reversal by picrotoxin. *Eur J Pharmacol* 1976;39:357–64.

19. Gee KW, Yamamura HI. Benzodiazepine receptor heterogeneity: a consequence of multiple conformational sites of a single receptor or multiple populations of structurally distinct macro-molecules. In: Usdin E, Skolnick P, Tallman JF Jr, Greenblatt D, Paul SM, eds. Pharmacology of benzodiazepines. London: Macmillan, 1982:93–108.

20. Goldberg MA, Dorman JD. Intention myoclonus: successful treatment with clonazepam. *Neurology* 1976;26:24–6.

21. Goodman Gilman A, Goodman LS, Gilman A, eds. Goodman & Gilman's. The pharmacological basis of therapeutics. 6th ed. New York: Macmillan, 1980:

22. Grahame-Smith DG. Studies *in vivo* on the relationship between brain tryptophan, brain 5HT synthesis and hyperactivity in rats treated with a monoamine oxidase inhibitor and L-tryptophan. *J Neurochem* 1971;18:1052–66.

23. Jenner P, Chadwick D, Reynolds EH, Marsden CD. Altered 5HT metabolism with clonazepam, diazepam and diphenylhydantoin. *J Pharm Pharmacol* 1975;27:707–10.

24. Killian M, Frey HH. Central monoamines and convulsive thresholds in mice and rats. *Neuropharmacology* 1973;12:681–92.

25. Koe K. Biochemical effects of antianxiety drugs on brain monoamines. In: Fielding S, Lal H, eds. Anxiolytics. Mount Kisco, New York: Future, 1979:173–95.

26. Krall RL, Penry JK, White BG, Kupferberg HJ, Swinyard EA. Antiepileptic drug development: II Anticonvulsant drug screening. *Epilepsia* 1978;19:409–28.

27. Meldrum BS, Anlezark G, Balzano E, Horton RW, Trimble M. Photically induced epilepsy in Papio papio as a model for drug studies. In: Meldrum BS, Marsden CD, eds. Primate models of neurological disorders. New York: Raven Press, 1975:1199–28. (Advances in neurology; Vol. 10)

28. Meldrum BS, Balzano E, Wada JA, Vuillon-Caccuittolo G. Effects of L-tryptophan L-3,4,dihydroxyphenylalanine and tranylcypromine on the electroencephalogram and on photically induced epilepsy in the baboon, Papio papio. *Physiol Behav* 1972;9:615–21.

29. Mennini T, Cotecchia S, Caccia S, Garattini S. Benzodiazepines: relationship between pharma-cological activity in the rat and *in vivo* receptor binding. *Pharmacol Biochem Behav* 1982;16:529–32.

30. Mohler H, Okada T. Demonstration of benzodiazepine receptors in the central nervous system. *Science* 1977;198:849–51.

31. Mohler H, Richards JG. Receptors for anxiolytic drugs. In: Malik JB, Enna SJ, Yamamura HI, eds. Anxiolytics: neurochemical, behavioural and clinical perspectives. New York: Raven Press, 1983:15–40.

32. Pieri L, Haefely W. The effect of diphenylhydantoin, diazepam and clonazepam on the activity of Purkinje cells in the rat cerebellum. *Naunyn Schmiedebergs Arch Pharmacol* 1976;296:1–4.

33. Pinder RM, Brogden RN, Speight TM, AVery GS. Clonazepam: a review of its pharmacolgical properties and therapeutic efficacy in epilepsy. *Drugs* 1976;12:321–61.
34. Pratt J, Jenner P, Reynolds EH, Marsden CD. Clonazepam induces decreased serotonergic activity in the mouse brain. *Neuropharmacology* 1979;18:791–9.
35. Swinyard EA. Assay of antiepileptic drug activity in experimental animals: standard tests. In: Mercier J, ed. Anticonvulsant drugs, international encyclopedia of pharmacology and therapeutics. sec 19. New York: Pergamon Press, 1972:47–65.
36. Swinyard EA, Brown WC, Goodman LS. Comparative assays of antiepileptic drugs in mice and rats. *J Pharmacol Exp Ther* 1952;106:319–30.
37. Thiebot M-H, Hamon M, Soubrie P. Attenuation of induced-anxiety in rats by chlordiazepoxide: role of raphe dorsalis, benzodiazepine binding sites and serotonergic neurones. *Neuroscience* 1982;7:2287–94.
38. Trulson ME, Preussler DW, Howell GA, Fredrickson CJ. Raphe unit activity in freely moving cats: effects of benzodiazepines. *Neuropharmacology* 1982;21:1045–50.
39. Tye NC, Everitt BJ, Iversen SD. 5-Hydroxytryptamine and punishment. *Nature* 1977;268:741–3.
40. Van Woert MH, Chung Hwang E. Biochemistry and pharmacology of myoclonus. In: Klawans HL, ed. Clinical neuropharmacology. New York: Raven Press, 1978;3:167–84.
41. Wada JA, Balzamo E, Meldrum BS, Naquet R. Behavioural and electrographic effects of L-5-hydroxytryptophan and D,L-para-chlorophenylalanine on epileptic Senegalese baboon (Papio papio). Electroencephalogr Clin Neurophysiol 1972;33:520–6.
42. Wang RY, Aghajanian GK. Physiological evidence for habenula as a major link between forebrain and midbrain raphe. *Science* 1977;197:89–91.
43. Weiner WJ. Goetz C, Nausieda PA, Klawans HL. Clonazepam and 5-hydroxytryptophan-induced myoclonic stereotypy. *Eur J Pharmacol* 1977;46:21–4.

Advances in Neurology, Vol. 43: Myoclonus,
edited by S. Fahn et al. Raven Press,
New York © 1986.

Clonazepam-Induced Up-Regulation of Serotonin₁ and Serotonin₂ Binding Sites in Rat Frontal Cortex

*H. Ryan Wagner, †Avinoam Reches, †Elena Yablonskaya, and †Stanley Fahn

*Departments of *Pharmacology and *†Neurology, Columbia University,
New York, New York 10032*

Cerebrospinal fluid (CSF) levels of the serotonin (5-HT) metabolite 5-hydroxyindoleacetic acid (5-HIAA) are decreased in posthypoxic action myoclonus, and clinical improvement is often associated with recovery of CSF 5-HIAA levels (4). The benzodiazepine clonazepam is one drug of choice in the management of action myoclonus (2). We have investigated the possibility that the antimyoclonic action of clonazepam is mediated through its effect on brain 5-HT receptors. Brain 5-HT₁ and 5-HT₂ binding sites were assessed following chronic *in vivo* exposure of rats to clonazepam. We observed increases in the density of both binding sites in frontal cortex membranes following chronic clonazepam treatment. Increases in receptor density did not reflect direct antagonism of 5-HT binding sites by clonazepam. Although we failed to note clonazepam-induced changes in brain 5-HIAA levels, we cannot exclude transsynaptic receptor up-regulation as a mechanism.

MATERIALS AND METHODS

Animals

Male Sprague-Dawley rats (150–175 g) were injected daily with clonazepam (5 mg/kg, i.p.) (courtesy of Hoffman-La Roche Inc., Nutley, NJ) or vehicle for 10 days unless otherwise specified. Forty-eight hours after the final injection, rats were sacrificed and brains were removed and dissected over ice. Tissue was frozen in aluminum foil on dry ice and stored at $-70°C$ until assayed.

Binding Assays

For receptor-binding assays, frozen tissue samples were homogenized in 50 mMTRIS HCl buffer (pH 7.6) by polytron (Brinkman; setting 4 for 10 sec). Homogenates were centrifuged at $40,000 \times G$ for 10 min and resuspended. Tissue was preincubated for 10 min at 37°C to degrade endogenous 5-HT, then recentrifuged, and the final pellet was resuspended in assay buffer (8) containing 50 mM

TRIS HCl, 4mM $CaCl_2$, 10 μM pargyline, and 0.1% ascorbate (pH 7.6). Final tissue concentrations were 400 μg protein per sample. 5-HT_1 binding sites were assayed using [^{3}H]5-HT (SA, 25–30 Ci/mmol; New England Nuclear). Specific binding was defined as the difference in [^{3}H]5-HT bound in the presence and absence of 10 μM unlabeled 5-HT (Sigma Chemical Co., St. Louis). 5-HT_2 binding sites were assayed with [^{3}H]spiperone (SPIP) (SA, 23–32 Ci/mmol; New England Nuclear). Specific binding was defined as the difference in total binding in the presence and absence of 1 μM unlabeled spiperone (courtesy of Janssen Pharmaceutical Co., New Brunswick). For both assays, drugs and ligands were combined with membrane suspensions to a final volume of 1 ml. Incubations were for 30 min at 23°C. Following incubation, bound and free ligand were separated by vacuum filtration over glass-fiber filters (Whatman GF/B) and washed with 10 ml of assay buffer. After drying, filters were suspended in a commercial fluor (Aquasol; New England Nuclear) and counted by using standard liquid scintillation spectroscopy techniques.

High-Performance Liquid Chromatography Procedures

Measurements of 5-HT and 5-HIAA were made using high-performance liquid chromatography (HPLC) with electrochemical detection (10). Frozen tissue samples were sonicated (Kontes Microultrasonic Cell Disrupter) in approximately 5 vol iced perchloric acid (0.1 M) containing 10 μl/ml $NaHSO_3$ (0.1 M) and Na_2 ethylenediaminotetraacetate (EDTA) (2 mM). After centrifugation (15,600×G for 5 min), 20 to 100 μl of supernatant was injected directly into the HPLC (C18 ODS column, DuPont) and an LC-4A amperometric detector coupled to a TL-5 glassy carbon electrode (Bioanalytical Systems) at 0.7 V. The mobile phase contained sodium acetate buffer (0.1 M), Na_2 EDTA (2 mM) and 4% (vol/vol) methanol (pH 4.7); the flow rate was 1.25 ml/min, and at 23°C retention times for 5-HT and 5-HIAA were 7.72 and 10.83 min, respectively. Signals were assessed on a Spectra-Physics graphic integrator (SP 4100). Proteins were measured by the Lowry (7) procedure, using bovine serum albumin as a standard.

RESULTS

Specific binding of both ligands was rapid, reversible, and saturable. Scatchard (11) analysis of [^{3}H]5-HT binding was linear over a concentration range of 0.5 to 15.0 nM. Unlabeled 5-HT (K_I, 4.0 nM) was considerably more potent in displacing specifically bound [^{3}H5-HT than was the serotonin antagonist cyproheptadine (K_I, 3.3 μM) as is characteristic of 5-HT_1 binding sites (8). Scatchard analysis of [^{3}H]SPIP binding was linear over a range of 0.05 to 3.5 nM; unlabeled cyproheptadine (K_I, 4.2 nM) was considerably more potent in displacing specifically bound [^{3}H]SPIP than unlabeled 5-HT (K_I 2.1) μM) as expected of a 5HT_2 binding site (8).

Binding of both radioligands to frontal cortex membranes, as determined in single point analysis, was significantly increased by chronic clonazepam exposure (Fig. 1A and B). Regional specificity was apparent, since binding in brainstem

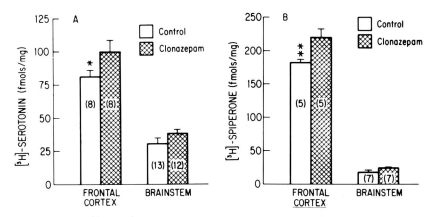

FIG. 1. Specific binding of [³H]5-HT **(A)** and [³H]SPIP **(B)** to rat brain membranes. Rats were injected daily with clonazepam (5 mg/kg) or vehicle for 10 days and killed 48 hr after the final injection. Binding was assayed at a single ligand concentration ([³H]5-HT, 4 nM; [³H]SPIP, 0.3 nM). (*) $p \leqslant 0.05$, (**) $p < 0.001$, as determined by Student's t-test for mean differences. Bars represent one SEM.

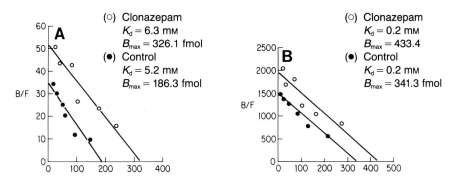

FIG. 2. Analysis of [³H]5-HT **(A)** and [³H]SPIP **(B)** specific binding in rat frontal cortex membranes. Rats were injected daily with clonazepam (5 mg/kg) or vehicle for 10 days and killed 48 hr after the final injection. Membranes were pooled and binding was assayed at ligand concentrations of 1.0 to 20 nM for [³H]5-HT and 0.05 to 2.0 nM for [³H]SPIP.

membranes was not significantly increased by clonazepam (Fig. 1A and B). As determined by Scatchard (11) analyses, increases in frontal cortex membrane binding reflected increases in the maximum densities of binding sites (B_{max}) with no change in ligand affinities (K_D) (Fig. 2A and B).

Effects of clonazepam on binding were dose dependent. Specific binding of [³H]5-HT and [³H]SPIP were significantly increased in rats treated daily for 10 days with 5 mg/kg clonazepam (Fig. 3). Binding of [³H]SPIP was also significantly increased in rats receiving 2.5 mg/kg but not 1.0 mg/kg doses. [³H]5-HT was increased only at the highest (5.0 mg/kg) dose. No effect was seen at lower (1.0 or 2.5 mg/kg) doses. Daily injections of the benzodiazepine diazepam (30 mg/kg)

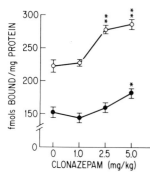

FIG. 3. Specific binding of [³H]5-HT (●) and [³H]SPIP (○) to rat frontal cortex membranes. Rats were injected for 10 days with clonazepam at the specified doses or vehicle and killed 48 hr after the final injection. Binding was assayed at a single ligand concentration ([³H]5-HT, 4 nM; [³H]SPIP, 0.3 nM). (*) $p < 0.05$, (**), $p < 0.01$, from control as determined by analysis of variance with *post hoc* comparison (Duncan). Bars represent one SEM. *N*, 9 per group.

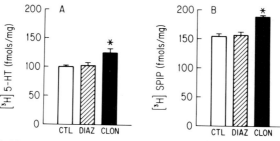

FIG. 4. Specific binding of [³H]5-HT **(A)** and [³H]SPIP **(B)** to rat frontal cortex membranes. Rats were injected with diazepam (DIAZ) (30 mg/kg), clonazepam (CLON) (5 mg/kg), or vehicle (CTL) for 10 days and killed 48 hr after the final injection. Binding was assayed at a single ligand concentration ([³H]5-HT, 4 nM; [³H]SPIP, 0.3 nM). (*), $p < 0.05$ from control as determined by analysis of variance with *post hoc* comparison (Duncan). Bars represent one SEM. *N*, 5 per group.

FIG. 5. Specific binding as percent control of [³H]5-HT and [³H]SPIP to rat frontal cortex membranes. Rats were injected with clonazepam (5 mg/kg) or vehicle for the specified periods of time and killed 48 hr after the final injection. Binding was assayed at a single ligand concentration ([³H]5-HT (●), 4 nM; [³H]SPIP (○), 0.3 nM). (*), $p < 0.05$, as determined by Student's *t*-tests for mean differences. Bars represent one SEM. *N*, 9 per group.

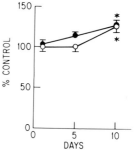

for 10 days failed to induce up-regulation of either binding site (Fig. 4A and B). Higher diazepam doses were not explored.

Increased binding apparently required continued drug exposure, since specific binding of [³H]5-HT and [³H]SPIP did not differ significantly from vehicle-treated controls in animals injected with clonazepam (5 mg/kg/day) for 1 or 5-day intervals (Fig. 5).

Clonazepam-induced changes in binding site densities were not mediated through the direct antagonism of clonazepam at serotonin receptors. Clonazepam failed to displace specifically bound [³H]5-HT in competitive binding studies at doses of up to 100 μM (Fig. 6A). Slight displacement of specifically bound [³H]SPIP was noted only at high (100 μM) clonazepam concentrations (Fig. 6B).

Frontal cortex levels of 5-HT and 5-HIAA in clonazepam-treated rats (5 mg/kg/ day for 10 days) did not differ from control levels (Table 1). Failure to observe a difference may have reflected the long (48-hr) post-drug interval. Accordingly, 5-HT and 5-HIAA were measured in a second set of experiments 2 hr after the final drug injection. Despite pronounced behavioral effects (sedation, ataxia, and shakes) at this shorter interval, 5-HT and 5-HIAA levels remained unaffected (Table 1).

DISCUSSION

We have observed a significant increase in the density of 5-HT and 5-HT$_2$ binding sites in rat frontal cortex membranes following chronic *in vivo* clonazepam administration. Increases in binding site density occurred after prolonged exposure to high levels of drug. Effects were regional in that changes were found in membranes from frontal cortex but not brainstem. Drug specificity also was apparent, since a second benzodiazepine, diazepam (30 mg/kg), failed to induce binding changes. 5-

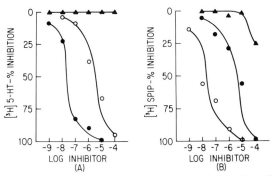

FIG. 6. Competition binding experiments in rat frontal cortex showing displacement of specifically bound [³H]5-HT **(A)** and specifically bound [³H]SPIP **(B)** by various concentrations of unlabeled serotonin (5-HT) (●), cyproheptadine (○), or clonazepam (▲).

TABLE 1. *Concentrations of 5-HT and 5-HIAA in frontal cortex after chronic clonazepam administration*[a]

Post-drug interval	No. of animals	5-HT		5-HIAA	
		Control (ng/mg ± SEM)	Clonazepam (ng/mg ± SEM)	Control (ng/mg ± SEM)	Clonazepam (ng/mg ± SEM)
2 hr	8	0.11 ± 0.2	0.11 ± 0.1	0.07 ± 0.01	0.06 ± 0.01
48 hr	10	0.33 ± 0.1	0.43 ± 0.1	0.06 ± 0.01	0.09 ± 0.02

[a]Rats were injected daily with clonazepam (5 mg/kg) or vehicle for 10 days. Two or 48 hr after the final injection, rats were killed and frontal cortices were assayed for 5-HT and 5-HIAA (see Materials and Methods).

HT_2 binding increased at slightly lower doses of clonazepam but otherwise drug effects on the two 5-HT receptors were similar.

The mechanism underlying clonazepam-induced up-regulation of binding sites is unclear. In competitive binding experiments, clonazepam showed no direct affinity for either binding site even at high concentrations (100 μM). Similar findings have been reported for clonazepam displacement of [³H]5-HT binding in mouse brain (5). Failure to observe clonazepam-induced changes in frontal cortex levels of 5-HT or 5-HIAA levels suggests that presynaptic nerve activity was unaffected by clonazepam and that receptor changes do not reflect transynaptic regulatory events. However, this conclusion may be premature. Acute clonazepam administration in mice elevates brain levels of 5-HT (1,3,6,9) and 5-HIAA (1,6,9). Effects of clonazepam on brain 5-HIAA levels apparently reflect a drug-induced reduction in the clearance of 5-HIAA from the CSF. Clonazepam does not affect 5-HT synthesis (5,9), leading to the suggestion that clonazepam-induced increases in brain 5-HT levels reflect decreased utilization of 5-HT (9). Failure to observe increases in frontal cortex 5-HT and 5-HIAA levels in our study may reflect an attenuation of the drug effect with chronic administration (1). The latter data do not preclude a compensatory up-regulation of serotonin binding sites in response to drug-induced decreases in 5-HT release during the initial stages of drug exposure. Dose-response data are consistent with this explanation, since clonazepam-induced increases in 5-HT levels and receptor binding occur at similar dose ranges (3,6,9,12); ataxia and sedation are common at these doses. The relevance of clonazepam-induced changes in brain 5-HT function to its antimyoclonic actions remains to be established, since clinical drug responses occur in a much lower dose range.

SUMMARY

Chronic administration of the benzodiazepine clonazepam increased the number of [³H]5-HT (5-HT$_1$) and [³H]SPIP (5-HT$_2$) binding sites in rat frontal cortex. In each instance, binding changes reflected increases in the maximum densities of binding sites (B_{max}) with no change in ligand affinities (K_D). Increases in binding required continued clonazepam exposure (10 days) at high doses. [³H]5-HT binding was significantly elevated at daily dose levels (i.p.) of 5.0 mg/kg but not 2.5 mg/kg. [³H]SPIP binding was significantly increased at drug doses of 2.5 mg/kg but not 1.0 mg/kg. Binding changes were regional in that they occurred in membranes from frontal cortex but not brainstem. A second benzodiazepine, diazepam, did not affect either binding site at daily doses of 30 mg/kg. These data suggest that serotonin receptor changes seen after chronic clonazepam may occur as a compensatory response to decreases in the presynaptic release of serotonin.

ACKNOWLEDGMENTS

This research was supported by a grant from the Myoclonus Research Foundation. We wish to express our appreciation to Ms. Donna Johnson, Mr. James Fahn, and Ms. Maddy Moshel for administrative and secretarial assistance.

REFERENCES

1. Chadwick D, Gorrod JW, Jenner P, Marsden CD, Reynolds EH. Functional changes in cerebral 5-hydroxytryptamine metabolism in the mouse induced by anticonvulsant drug. *Br J Pharmacol* 1978;62:115–24.
2. Fahn S. Posthypoxic action myoclonus: review of the literature and report of two cases with response to valproate and estrogen. In: Fahn S, Davis JN, Rowland LP, eds. *Advances in neurology; vol. 26. Cerebral hypoxia and its consequences*, New York: Raven Press, 1979 49–84.
3. Fennessy MR, Lee JR. The effects of benzodiazepines on brain amines of the mouse. *Arch Int Pharmacodyn Ther* 1972;197:37–44.
4. Guilleminault C, Tharp BR, Cousin D. HVA and 5-HIAA CSF measurements and 5-HTP trials in some patients with involuntary movements. *J Neurol Sci* 1973;18:435–41.
5. Hwang EC, Van Woert MH. Antimyoclonic action of clonazepam: the role of serotonin. *Eur J Pharmacol* 1979;60:31–40.
6. Jenner P, Chadwick D, Reynolds EH, Marsden CD. Altered 5-HT metabolism with clonazepam, diazepam and diphenylhydantoin. *J Pharm Pharmacol* 1975;27:707–10.
7. Lowry OH, Rosebrough NJ, Farr AL, Randall RJ. Protein measurement with the folin phenol reagent. *J Biol Chem* 1951;193:265–75.
8. Peroutka SJ, Snyder SH. Multiple serotonin receptors. differential binding of [^{3}H]5-hydroxytryptamine, [^{3}H]lysergic acid diethylamide and [^{3}H]spiroperidol. *Mol Pharmacol* 1979;16:687–99.
9. Pratt J, Jenner P, Reynolds EH. Clonazepam induces decreased serotoninergic activity in the mouse brain. *Neuropharmacology* 1979;18:791–9.
10. Reinhard JF, Maskowitz MA, Sved AE, Fernstrom JD. A simple, sensitive and reliable assay for serotonin and 5-HIAA in brain tissue using liquid chromatography with electrochemical detector. *Life Sci* 1980;27:435–41.
11. Scatchard G. The attractions of proteins for small molecules and ions. *Ann NY Acad Sci* 1949;51:660–72.
12. Weiner WJ, Goetz C, Nausieda PG, Klawans HL. Clonazepam and 5-hydroxytryptophan-induced myoclonic stereotypy. *Eur J Pharmacol* 1977;46:21–4.

Advances in Neurology, Vol. 43: Myoclonus,
edited by S. Fahn et al. Raven Press,
New York © 1986.

Possible Mechanisms of Action of Valproic Acid in Myoclonus

Melvin H. Van Woert and Eunyong Chung

*Departments of Neurology and Pharmacology, Mount Sinai School of Medicine,
New York, New York 10029*

Valproic acid (2-*n*-propyl-pentanoic acid, *n*-dipropyl-acetic acid) (DPA) is an anticonvulsant that is particularly effective treatment for absence seizures, generalized tonic-clonic seizures, and progressive myoclonus epilepsy (1,20,34). The myoclonus associated with postanoxic encephalopathy also may occasionally respond to therapy with DPA (14). DPA has several pharmacological actions in the central nervous system. The possible relevance of DPA's pharmacological effects to antimyoclonic action will be reviewed in this paper.

Several investigators have demonstrated that DPA increases the concentration of the inhibitory neurotransmitter γ-aminobutyric acid (GABA) in the central nervous system (12,15,18,19,30). The increase in brain GABA levels after DPA administration is due predominantly to the drug's inhibition of GABA catabolism. DPA is a weak inhibitor of GABA-transaminase and a more potent inhibitor of succinic semialdehyde dehydrogenase (3,16,17). Inhibition of succinic semialdehyde dehydrogenase also elevates GABA concentration because the increased succinic semialdehyde is converted back to GABA by the reverse reaction of GABA transaminase (33). Succinic semialdehyde also inhibits the degradation of GABA by GABA-transaminase (33). DPA-induced increase in brain GABA may also be due, in part, to an activation *in vivo* of the glutamic acid decarboxylase, the enzyme responsible for converting glutamate to GABA (21). Simlar et al. (30) reported a correlation between the increase in brain GABA levels produced by DPA and the protection against audiogenic seizures in genetically sensitive mice. Electrophysiological evidence also suggests that DPA may enhance neuronal inhibition by GABA (4,22). However, other studies have questioned the clinical relevance of DPA-induced changes in brain GABA. For example, the doses of DPA necessary to increase GABA levels in rat brain are much greater than those used in clinical treatment (3,27,32). Further, the concentration of DPA required to inhibit succinic semialdehyde dehydrogenase is higher than anticonvulsant levels (3,33). Recently, it has been shown that DPA has a much longer anticonvulsant action than would be expected based on its relative short half-life, suggesting that a metabolite might be the active agent (29). This also suggests that the effect of large doses of DPA on GABA metabolism may not be relevant to its therapeutic action. Thus, the evidence that the therapeutic effect of DPA is due to an increase in brain GABA is not totally convincing.

What is the evidence for a role of GABA in the pathogenesis of myoclonus? Tarsy et al. (31) reported that unilateral injections of the GABA antagonists picrotoxin and bicuculline into the caudate nucleus of the rat produced focal myoclonus consisting of rhythmic jerking movements of the contralateral limbs. Intracaudate injection of GABA inhibits the myoclonus produced by intracaudate injection of GABA antagonists. The authors compared this animal model to the clinical myoclonus syndrome seen in certain neurological disorders such as Creutzfeldt–Jakob disease, subacute sclerosing panencephalitis, and epilepsia partialis continua. There is evidence that cerebral GABA metabolism also may be abnormal in patients with certain types of myoclonus. We found that the concentration of GABA in the CSF was decreased in seven patients with postanoxic intention myoclonus and three patients with progressive myoclonus epilepsy (13). Whole-blood GABA levels were normal in these myoclonic patients. Recently, Airaksinen and Leino (2) also observed low CSF GABA levels in patients with progressive myoclonus epilepsy.

We have examined the effects of various GABA agonists on a stimulus-sensitive serotonin (5-HT)-responsive animal model of myoclonus produced by intragastric injection of DDT [1,1,1-trichloro-2,2-bis(p-chlorophenyl)ethane] in mice. The direct GABA agonist muscimol, GABA transaminase inhibitors, acetylenic GABA, aminooxyacetic acid, as well as DPA, had no significant effect on myoclonic activity (Table 1).

We previously reported that drugs that increase the action of 5-HT in the brain —L-5-hydroxytryptophan (L-5HTP), quipazine, 5-HT uptake blockers (chlorimipramine, fluoxetine, Org 6582) and the 5-HT releaser H75/12—decreased DDT-induced myoclonic movements, and drugs that block 5-HT receptors (methysergide,

TABLE 1. Effects of GABA and 5-HT agents on DDT-induced myoclonus in mice

Drug	Dosage (mg/kg)	Counts/5 min		% Change from control	Paired t-test
		Control[a]	After therapy[a]		
Muscimol	1	382 ± 24	420 ± 43	+10	NS
Muscimol	5	414 ± 30	425 ± 63	+3	NS
Acetylenic GABA	100	434 ± 54	465 ± 74	+7	NS
Acetylenic GABA	200	450 ± 24	506 ± 15	+12	NS
Aminooxyacetic acid	25	331 ± 29	397 ± 80	+19	NS
DPA	400	379 ± 31	324 ± 31	−12	NS
L-5-HTP	100	410 ± 19	345 ± 39	−14	NS
Chlorimipramine	10	405 ± 26	367 ± 17	−9	NS
Chlorimipramine + L-5-HTP	10 + 100	432 ± 47	120 ± 16	−72	p < 0.001
Chlorimipramine + DPA	10 + 400	418 ± 40	139 ± 31	−68	p < 0.001

[a]Each value is the mean ± SE of five or six observations. Details on the evaluation of myoclonic activity have been described (8).

metergoline, cinanserin) increased the intensity of DDT-induced myoclonus in mice and rats (7). Chlorimipramine and L-5-HTP, in doses that have no effect when given separately, produce a 72% decrease in myoclonic activity when given concomitantly (Table 1). Although DPA has little effect when given alone, in combination with chlorimipramine it produces a 68% decrease in myoclonus. Potentiation of the antimyoclonic action of L-5-HTP and DPA by the 5-HT uptake blocker chlorimipramine suggests that DPA, like L-5-HTP, may increase intrasynaptic 5-HT. This observation is consistent with the clinical finding that certain forms of myoclonus, such as progressive myoclonus epilepsy and postanoxic intention myoclonus, are responsive to drugs that enhance serotonergic neurotransmission.

Thus, the effect of DPA on 5-HT metabolism may be relevant to its therapeutic action. Horton et al. (18) reported that DPA (400–600 mg/kg, i.p.) produced a maximum increase in brain 5-hydroxyindoleacetic acid (5-HIAA) of 134% in mice. They postulated that DPA increased brain 5-HIAA by inhibiting the active transport system for removing acidic metabolites from the brain. Kukino and Deguchi also found that DPA increased 5-HIAA concentrations in the brain as well as elevating brain tryptophan levels (19). We have investigated further the effect of DPA in 5-HT metabolism in mice and rats (8). Serum and brain tryptophan analyses were carried out according to the method of Denckla and Dewey (11) as modified by Bloxam and Warren (5), and brain 5-HT and 5-HIAA according to the method of Curzon and Green (10). Table 2 shows the effect of acute and chronic treatment with DPA on serum free and total tryptophan and brain tryptophan, 5-HT, and 5-HIAA in rats. Total serum tryptophan decreased by 66% after one injection and by 73% after seven daily injections of DPA. DPA readily binds to serum protein and displaces tryptophan, which is normally bound to albumin, thus lowering total serum tryptophan and increasing the level of free tryptophan. Free serum tryptophan was increased 77% and 87% after a single dose and seven daily doses of DPA, respectively. The unbound tryptophan in the serum readily crosses the blood–

TABLE 2. *Effects of single and seven daily injections of DPA (400 mg/kg, i.p.) on rat free and total serum tryptophan and brain tryptophan 30 min after the last injection*

Treatment	Serum tryptophan[a] (μg/ml)		Brain concentration (μg/g)		
	Free	Total	Tryptophan	5-HT	5-HIAA
Saline	0.75 ± 0.03	30.98 ± 1.76	2.32 ± 0.02	0.40 ± 0.02	0.30 ± 0.02
DPA (single dose)	1.33 ± 0.08^d	10.63 ± 1.45^d	3.54 ± 0.16^d	0.41 ± 0.02	0.37 ± 0.03^d
DPA (7 days)	1.40 ± 0.26^c	8.34 ± 0.88^d	3.07 ± 0.02^d	0.37 ± 0.02	0.37 ± 0.02^c

[a]Serum tryptophan values are the mean $\pm$ SEM of five determinations, and the remaining results are the mean $\pm$ SEM of 10 determinations.
[b]$p < 0.05$ vs. saline control.
[c]$p < 0.01$ vs. saline control.
[d]$p < 0.001$ vs. saline control.

brain barrier and increases brain tryptophan levels, which are converted to 5-HT and then to its metabolite 5-HIAA (Table 2).

In order to determine whether the DPA-induced increase in brain 5-HT metabolism occurred diffusely throughout the brain or only in selected regions, the effect of a single injection of DPA (400 mg/kg, i.p.) on tryptophan, 5-HIAA, and 5-HT turnover rate were determined in seven regional areas of the rat brain (Table 3). DPA produced a significant increase in the concentration of tryptophan (32% in striatum to 65% in medulla) and 5-HIAA (11% in midbrain to 46% in hippocampus) in all seven regional areas examined. However, DPA did not significantly increase 5-HT synthesis in all regional brain areas (Table 3). Minimal changes in the small functional pool of 5-HT, which is readily released by nerve impulses, may not always be reflected by measurement of brain 5-HT accumulation after monoamine oxidase inhibition. In summary, it would appear that DPA elevated freely diffusible serum tryptophan that is not bound to serum albumin, which in turn raises brain tryptophan levels. Since tryptophan hydroxylase is normally not saturated with its substrate, elevated brain tryptophan concentration results in an increase in 5-HT synthesis. This may be reflected by the increase in brain 5-HIAA, the major metabolite of 5-HT. However, the DPA-induced increase in 5-HT synthesis appears marginal, since it was not evident in 5-HT turnover estimations employing mono-

TABLE 3. *Effect of a single DPA injection (400 mg/kg, i.p.) on rat brain tryptophan, 5-HIAA, and 5-HT synthesis, 30 min later*

Region	Treatment	Tryptophan[a] (μg/g)	5-HIAA[a] (μg/g)	Rate of 5-HT synthesis[a] (μg/g/hr)
Cerebellum	Saline	2.63 ± 0.07	0.06 ± 0.01	0.01
	DPA	3.96 ± 0.13[d]	0.08 ± 0.01[c]	0.02
Medulla	Saline	1.96 ± 0.05	0.51 ± 0.02	0.13
	DPA	3.23 ± 0.10[d]	0.70 ± 0.02[c]	0.21
Hypothalamus	Saline	2.96 ± 0.26	0.44 ± 0.02	0.20
	DPA	4.35 ± 0.34[c]	0.61 ± 0.04[c]	0.31
Striatum	Saline	2.91 ± 0.13	0.49 ± 0.02	0.08
	DPA	3.85 ± 0.22[c]	0.62 ± 0.04[c]	0.17
Midbrain	Saline	2.21 ± 0.13	0.80 ± 0.02	0.14
	DPA	3.13 ± 0.20[c]	0.89 ± 0.02[c]	0.35
Hippocampus	Saline	2.31 ± 0.16	0.28 ± 0.01	0.21
	DPA	3.52 ± 0.26[c]	0.41 ± 0.02[c]	0.16
Cortex	Saline	2.88 ± 0.07	0.17 ± 0.01	0.16
	DPA	3.73 ± 0.25[c]	0.23 ± 0.01[b]	0.17

[a]Each value is the mean ± SEM of four to six determinations. Rate of 5-HT synthesis was determined by measuring 5-HT accumulation 1 hr after inhibition of monoamine oxidase by pargyline (75 mg/kg, i.p.). Pargyline was given 30 min after DPA. Regional areas from 3 rats were pooled for each determination. Control rats were injected with the same volume of saline (0.1 ml), i.p.
[b]$p < 0.05$ vs. control.
[c]$p < 0.01$ vs. control.
[d]$p < 0.001$ vs. control.

amine oxidase inhibition. The increase in brain 5-HIAA also may partially be due to interference with the active transport process that removes 5-HIAA from the brain as suggested by Horton et al. (18) and MacMillan (23).

The mechanism of antimyoclonic action of DPA can not be satisfactorily explained by its minimal effects on GABA or 5-HT metabolism. More recently, DPA has been found to alter two putative amino acid neurotransmitters, aspartate and glycine. DPA decreases the excitatory amino acid aspartate in the central nervous system (6,19), and there is a temporal correlation between the reduction in brain aspartate concentrations and anticonvulsant activity (28). It has been argued that a reduction in excitatory amino acids, like aspartate, could be associated with a decreased excitatory state in the central nervous system. The possible role of aspartate in myoclonic disorders has not been investigated.

Kukino and Deguchi (19) suggested that DPA might affect pyridoxal phosphate-dependent enzymes, such as aspartate aminotransferase and certain enzymes in the tricarboxylic acid cycle. This hypothesis was based on their observations that DPA suppressed oxygen consumption in rat brain slices and that this suppression was counteracted by adding 1 mM pyridoxal phosphate to the incubation mixture. Further, DPA inhibited the catabolism of aspartate in brain slices. Pyridoxal is converted to the active cofactor pyridoxal phosphate by the enzyme pyridoxal kinase. Therefore, we examined the effect of DPA on rat brain pyridoxal kinase activity *in vivo* and *in vitro*. As seen in Table 4, DPA had no effect on pyridoxal kinase activity. Semicarbazide and isoniazid, known inhibitors of pyridoxal kinase, significantly reduced pyridoxal kinase activity under these assay conditions.

Glycine is an inhibitory neurotransmitter which, like GABA, may modulate neuronal excitability and seizure threshold. Seizures can be induced by systemic administration of the glycine receptor antagonist strychnine. We observed that strychnine produced myoclonic movements when injected directly into the medul-

TABLE 4. *Effect of DPA on pyridoxal kinase activity*

Treatment	Pyridoxal kinase activity[a] pyridoxal phosphate (μmol/g/hr)
Control	257.8 ± 9.8
DPA (400 mg/kg i.p.)	261.8 ± 9.0
10^{-5} M DPA	265.8 ± 14.7
10^{-4} M DPA	259.8 ± 11.3
10^{-3} M DPA	256.3 ± 10.3
10^{-5} M Semicarbazide	188.8 ± 5.2[b]
10^{-4} M Isoniazide	87.8 ± 3.5[c]
10^{-5} M Isoniazide	160.0 ± 6.6[b]

[a]Each value is mean $\pm$ SE of four to six determinations. Whole brain excluding medulla was used for the assay. Pyridoxal kinase activity was measured according to the method of Nearly and Niven (25).
[b]$p < 0.002$ vs. control.
[c]$p < 0.00005$ vs. control.

TABLE 5. *Effect of DPA on glycine levels*

Region	Glycine (μg/mg protein)[a]	
	Saline	DPA
Pons	1.42 ± 0.07	1.26 ± 0.25
Trapezoid	2.01 ± 0.21	1.82 ± 0.25
Lower medulla	2.07 ± 0.10	2.37 ± 0.12
Spinal cord	1.10 ± 0.08	1.16 ± 0.13

[a]Each value is the mean ± SE of six rats. Glycine levels were determined according to the method of Sardesai and Provido (26).

lary reticular formation of the rat (9). Further, urea, in concentrations that produce myoclonus in rats, interferes with glycine receptor binding (E. Chung and M. H. Van Woert, *this volume*). Hayashi and Negishi (17) have shown that iontophoretically applied DPA augments the inhibitory effects of glycine, as well as GABA on retinal ganglion cells *in vitro*. In addition, it was reported that DPA increases plasma and urinary glycine by inhibiting hepatic glycine cleavage enzymes (24), but has no effect on whole-brain (19) or cortical glycine levels (6). Since glycine acts as an inhibitory neurotransmitter predominantly in the pons, medulla, and spinal cord, we measured the concentration of glycine in these areas 30 min after an intraperitoneal injection of 400 mg/kg of DPA. Table 5 shows that DPA treatment had no effect on pons, trapezoid, lower medulla, or spinal cord glycine levels in rats. Thus, there is no evidence to suggest that the antimyoclonic action of DPA is related to central nervous system glycine.

In summary, DPA has multiple biochemical and physiological effects in the brain, but the mechanism of antimyoclonic action remains elusive.

ACKNOWLEDGMENTS

The authors thank M. Dvorozniak for his technical assistance. This work was supported by USPHS grant NS 12341.

REFERENCES

1. Adams DJ, Luders H, Pipenger C. Sodium valproate in the treatment of intractable seizure disorders: a clinical and electroencephalographic study. *Neurology* 1978;28:152–7.
2. Airaksinen EM, Leino E. Decrease of GABA in the cerebrospinal fluid of patients with progressive myoclonus epilepsy and its correlation with the decrease of 5-HIAA and HVA. *Acta Neurol Scand* 1982;66:666–72.
3. Anlezark GM, Horton RW, Meldrum BS, Sawaya MCB. Anticonvulsant action of ethanolamine-o-sulphate and di-n-propylacetate and the metabolism of γ-aminobutyric acid (GABA) in mice with audiogenic seizures. *Biochem Pharmacol* 1976;25:413–6.
4. Baldino F, Geller HM. Sodium valproate enhancement of γ-aminobutyric acid (GABA) inhibition: electrophysiological evidence for anticonvulsant activity. *J Pharm Exp Ther* 1981;217:445–50.
5. Bloxam DL, Warren WH. Error in the determination of tryptophan by Denckla and Dewey. A revised procedure.*Anal Biochem* 1974;60:621–5.

6. Chapman AG, Riley K, Evans MC, Meldrum BS. Acute effects of sodium valproate and γ-vinyl GABA on regional amino acid metabolism in the rat brain. *Neurochem Res* 1982;7:1089–1105.

7. Chung Hwang E, Van Woert MH. p,p'-DDT-induced neurotoxic syndrome: experimental myoclonus. *Neurology* 1978;28:1020–5.

8. Chung Hwang E, Van Woert MH. Effect of valproic acid on serotonin metabolism. *Neuropharmacology* 1979;18:391–7.

9. Chung E, Van Woert MH. DDT myoclonus: sites and mechanism of action. *Exp Neurol* 1984;85:273–82.

10. Curzon G, Green AR. Rapid method for the determination of 5-hydroxytryptamine and 5-hydroxyindoleacetic acid in small regions of rat brain. *Br J Pharmacol* 1970;39:653–5.

11. Denckla WD, Dewey HH. The determination of tryptophan in plasma, liver and urine. *J Lab Clin Med* 1967;69:160–9.

12. Emson PC. Effects of chronic treatment with amino-oxyacetic or sodium n-dipropylacetate on brain GABA levels and the development and regression of cobalt epileptic foci in rats. *J Neurochem* 1976;27:1489–94.

13. Enna SJ, Ferkany JW, Van Woert M, Butler IJ. Measurement of GABA in biological fluids: effect of GABA transaminase inhibitors. *Adv Neurol* 1979;23:741–50.

14. Fahn S. Post-anoxic action myoclonus: improvement with valproic acid. *N Eng J Med* 1978;299:313–4.

15. Godin Y, Heinler HL, Mark J, Mandel P. Effect of dipropylacetate, an anticonvulsant compound, on GABA metabolism. *J Neurochem* 1969;16:869–73.

16. Harvey PKP, Bradford HF, Davison AN. The inhibitory effect of sodium-n-dipropyl acetate on the degradative enzymes of the GABA shunt. *FEBS Lett* 1975;52:251.

17. Hayashi T, Negishi K. Suppression of retinal spike discharge by dipropylacetate (depakene); a possible involvement of GABA. *Brain Res* 1979;175:271–8.

18. Horton RW, Anlezark GM, Sawaya MCB, Meldrum BS. Monoamine and GABA metabolism and the anticonvulsant action of di-n-propylacetate and ethanolamine-o-sulfate. *Eur J Pharmacol* 1977;41:387–97.

19. Kukino K, Deguchi T. Effects of sodium dipropylacetate on γ-aminobutyric acid and biogenic amines in rat brain. *Chem Pharm Bull (Tokyo)* 1977;25:2257–62.

20. Lance JW, Anthony M. Sodium valproate and clonazepam in the treatment of intractable epilepsy. *Arch Neurol* 1977;34:14–7.

21. Loscher W, Frey HH. On the mechanism of action of valproic acid in mice. Arzneimittel-forsch 1977;27:1081–2.

22. Macdonald RL, Bergey GK. Valproic acid augments GABA-mediated postsynaptic inhibition in cultured mammalian neurons. *Brain Res* 1979;170:558–62.

23. MacMillan V. The effects of the anticonvulsant valproic acid on cerebral indole amine metabolism. *Can J Physiol Pharmacol* 1979;57:843–7.

24. Mortensen PB, Kolvraa S, Christensen E. Inhibition of the glycine cleavage system: hyperglycinemia and hyperglycinuria caused by valproic acid. *Epilepsia* 1980;21:563–9.

25. Nearly JT, Diven WF. Purification, properties and a possible mechanism for pyridoxal kinase from bovine brain. *J Biol Chem* 1970;245:5585–93.

26. Sardesai VM, Provido HS. The determination of glycine in biological fluids. *Clin Chim Acta* 1970;29:67–71.

27. Sawaya MCB, Horton RW, Meldrum BS. Effects of anticonvulsant drugs on the central enzymes metabolizing GABA. *Epilepsia* 1975;16:649–52.

28. Schecter PJ, Trainer Y, Grove J. Effect of n-dipropylacetate on amino acid concentrations in mouse brain: correlation with anticonvulsant activity. *J Neurochem* 1978;31:1325–7.

29. Schobben F, Vree TB, van der Kleijn E, Claessens R, Reiner WO. Metabolism of valproic acid in monkey and man. In : Johnnnessen SI, Svein I, Morselli PL, Pippinger CE, Richens A, Schmitt D, Meinardi H, eds. Advances in drug monitoring. New York: Raven Press; 1980:91–102.

30. Simler S, Ciesielski L, Maitre M, Rondrianisoa H, Mandel P. Effects of sodium n-dipropylacetate on audiogenic seizures and brain gamma aminobutyric acid level. *Biochem Pharmacol* 1973;22:1701–8.

31. Tarsy D, Pycock CJ, Meldrum BS, Marsden CD. Focal contralateral myoclonus produced by inhibition of GABA action in the caudate nucleus of rats. *Brain* 1978;101:143–62.

32. Turner AJ, Whittle SR. Sodium valproate, GABA and epilepsy. *Trends Pharmacol Sci* 1980;1:257–60.

33. van der Loan JW, DeBoer T, Bruinvals J. Di-n-propylacetate and GABA degradations. Preferential inhibition of succinic-semialdehyde dehydrogenase and indirect inhibition of GABA transaminase. *J Neurochem* 1979;32:1769–80.
34. Wilder BJ, Bruni J. Seizure disorders: a pharmacological approach to treatment. New York: Raven Press, 1981: ch 7.

Advances in Neurology, Vol. 43: Myoclonus,
edited by S. Fahn et al. Raven Press,
New York © 1986.

Valproate and Myoclonus

Astrid G. Chapman

*Department of Neurology, Institute of Psychiatry, Rayne Institute,
London, SE5 9NU, United Kingdom*

Valproate, or dipropyl acetic acid, is a broad-spectrum anticonvulsant that offers potent protection against a wide range of clinical and experimental forms of epilepsy (8,11,13,32,44,46,56,68,76). It is also effective against different types of clinical myoclonus. Progressive myoclonus epilepsy is well controlled by valproate alone or in combination with clonazepam or phenobarbital (36). Valproate alone also protects against myoclonic jerks in children and adolescents (37), and some cases of posthypoxic myoclonus are well controlled by valproate alone or in combination with clonazepam (24; S. Fahn, *this volume*; J. W. Lance, *this volume*).

Among the drugs that are therapeutically beneficial against different forms of myoclonus are several classical antiepileptic drugs. The benzodiazepine clonazepam is, in addition to valproate, the drug most commonly used for posthypoxic myoclonus (28,78; S. Fahn, *this volume*; P. Jenner et al., *this volume*). Other anticonvulsants, such as phenytoin and barbiturates, have also, to a lesser extent, shown antimyoclonic activity (24).

Myoclonus, in contrast to most forms of epilepsy, also responds to treatment with drugs designed to enhance serotonergic activity, such as the serotonin precursor 5-hydroxytryptophan (5-HTP) in combination with a peripheral aromatic amino acid decarboxylase inhibitor carbidopa (24,78). In order to reduce the adverse side effects of the high doses of serotonin or serotonin precursors required for protection, lower doses are currently administered in combination with the serotonin uptake inhibitor fluoxetine (M. Van Woert et al., *this volume*).

An understanding of the mechanism of action of valproate would provide a rational basis for the design of new drugs with an even more potent antimyoclonic action than valproate. Valproate administration has been shown to affect a number of neurotransmission systems, including the γ-aminobutyric acid (GABA), glycine, serotonin, and excitatory amino acid systems (13,32,40), but the causal relationship between these effects and the anticonvulsant and antimyoclonic activity of valproate remains to be established.

The aim of the present chapter is to describe the effects of valproate on different neurotransmitter systems and, whenever possible, examine how these effects relate to the anticonvulsant action of valproate.

VALPROATE AND ANIMAL MODELS OF MYOCLONUS

The difficulties encountered in developing animal models for sustained myoclonus without a significant accompanying contribution from either clonic seizures or tremors are discussed elsewhere in this volume. Table 1 lists a number of animal models in which the drug treatment or stimulus produces a response that consists predominantly (at least transiently) of myoclonic jerks. The efficacy of valproate or benzodiazepines in suppressing these myoclonic seizures is also shown in the table.

DDT, when given intragastrically (600 mg/kg), produces myoclonic movements in mice (16; J. A. Pratt et al., *this volume*). Valproate alone (400 mg/kg, i.p.) has only a slight protective effect against myoclonus, but it potentiates the protective effect of chlorimipramine (17). Clonazepam (2 mg/kg) also protects against DDT-induced myoclonic activity in mice (18).

5-HTP (100–150 mg/kg, i.p., or 30–60 mg/kg in combination with carbidopa) produces myoclonus in guinea pigs (42) that is inhibited by some of the serotonin receptor blockers (10,80). Clonazepam administration does not modify the myoclonic activity in this model (G. Luscombe et al., *this volume*).

Intravenous urea infusion produces sustained myoclonus accompanied by spike-and-wave discharges in the reticular formation in cats (83) and transient myoclonus developing into seizures in rats (S. Muscatt et al., *this volume*). Very high doses of clonazepam (10–20 mg/kg) causes a slight but significant delay of the onset of

TABLE 1. *Animal models for seizures with prominent myoclonic features:*
effects of valproate and benzodiazepines

Animal model	Effect of valproate	Effect of benzodiazepines	Ref.
DDT, mice	Slight protection	Clonazepam: protection	17,18; Pratt et al. (*this volume*)
Morphine, rats	Acute administration: no effect Pretreatment: protection	—	Shohami et al. (*this volume*)
Urea, rats	—	Clonazepam: protection	Muscatt et al. (*this volume*)
5-HTP, guinea pigs	—	Clonazepam: no effect	Luscombe et al. (*this volume*)
High-pressure neurological syndrome (mice)	Protection	Flurazepam: protection	6
Lorazepam, baboons	Protection	—	9
Photic stimulation (baboons)	Protection	Diazepam, clonazepam clobazam: protection	12,59,63,66
GABA agonists, rats (muscimol, THIP)	Potentiation	Clonazepam: protection	25

urea-induced myoclonus in rats (S. Muscatt et al., *this volume*). The effect of valproate has not been tested in this model (S. Muscatt et al., *this volume*).

Morphine, when administered intraventricularly (77) or intrathecally (E. Shohami et al., *this volume*) has been shown to produce myoclonic movements in rats. Acute valproate (300 mg/kg) administration does not block morphine-induced myoclonus, whereas 3 days of valproate pretreatment (300 mg/kg/day) protects against this type of myoclonus (E. Shohami et al., *this volume*). The effect of valproate has not been tested.

Exposure of mice to elevated pressure (above 70–90 atmospheres) produces myoclonus and subsequently clonic seizures in mice (31,64). Valproate (400 mg/kg) significantly elevates the threshold for myoclonus, as does flurazepam (10 mg/kg) (6).

Some benzodiazepines, though potently anticonvulsant in most seizure models (60) can induce myoclonus in baboons *(Papio papio)* that is not accompanied by paroxysmal discharges (9). Lorazepam (1 mg/kg)-induced myoclonus in baboons is strongly inhibited by valproate (200 mg/kg) (9).

A high percentage of Senegalese baboons has a genetic defect that makes them sensitive to photically induced seizures (41). These seizures can develop into full clonic-tonic seizures, but often they consist of myoclonic jerks of facial muscles, trunk, and limbs. Valproate (22-130 mg/kg) protects against photically induced myoclonus in baboons (66). Different benzodiazepines, including diazepam (1 mg/kg) (63), clonazepam (0.11–0.18 mg/kg) (59), and clobazam (2–6 mg/kg) (12) also suppress photically induced myoclonus in baboons.

GABA agonists have anticonvulsant activity in different seizure models (57,58); however, at high concentrations muscimol (0.25–1.0 mg/kg) and 4,5,6,7-tetrahydroisoxazolo-[5,4-c]pyridin-3ol(THIP) (8 mg/kg) produce myoclonus in rodents and baboons (62,67). Valproate (200 mg/kg) potentiates and clonazepam (1 mg/kg) protects against THIP-induced myoclonus in rats (25).

VALPROATE AND GABA

It is well established that a number of anticonvulsants act by enhancing GABA-mediated inhibition (55,57,58). Benzodiazepines and barbiturates interact with the GABA-receptor complex and have been shown in electrophysiological studies to augment the inhibitory action of GABA (30,52). In addition, specific GABAergic compounds such as GABA transaminase (GABA-T) inhibitors (γ-vinyl GABA, aminooxyacetic acid, gabaculine, or ethanolamine-*O*-sulfate) or certain GABA uptake inhibitors (*cis*-4-OH-nipecotic methyl ester and 4,5,6,7-tetrahydroisoxazolo[4,5-c]pyridin-3-ol)(THPO) exhibit anticonvulsant activity in a number of animal models of epilepsy (57,58).

Most studies of valproate-induced cerebral metabolic changes in animals have been carried out following the acute administration of anticonvulsant doses of valproate. Higher doses of valproate (150–400 mg/kg) are required in rodents to achieve anticonvulsant protection than in humans (5–60 mg/kg/day) (13). During the period of maximal protection against pentylenetetrazol seizures in mice following the acute administration of valproate, the drug levels are approximately 400 µg/ml in plasma and 150 µg/g (or approximately 1 mM) in the brain (45).

The ability of anticonvulsant doses of valproate to elevate cortical or whole-brain levels of the inhibitory transmitter GABA has been recognized since the early studies of Godin et al. (27) and has been confirmed by numerous studies in different animal models (13). The rise in GABA concentration is observed throughout the period of valproate-induced protection (Fig. 1). However, the anticonvulsant effect of valproate is not absolutely dependent on a cerebral GABA elevation since valproate exhibits anticonvulsant action against sound-induced seizures in DBA/2 mice at doses insufficient to raise brain GABA levels (200 mg/kg, i.p.) (1) and since the protection against electroshock-induced convulsions is established (at 2 min) before the GABA level has increased (39). The valproate-induced GABA increase is observed in most brain regions in mice (74,75). In rats, following the acute administration of anticonvulsant doses of valproate, the GABA levels increase in the cortex, substantia nigra, and colliculus (35), with no changes in the GABA levels in the hippocampus, striatum and cerebellum (15). When valproate is administered intracerebroventrically (i.c.v.), there is a dose-dependent increase in GABA concentration in the forebrain of mice, which correlates with the anticonvulsant potency of valproate (Fig. 2). The cerebellar GABA level is less affected by valproate administration (Chapman, Croucher, and Meldrum, *unpublished observations*).

A number of structural analogs of valproate (short branched-chain fatty acids) have anticonvulsant activity against pentylenetetrazol seizures (72) and sound-induced seizures (14) in mice, that is of similar potency to that of valproate. The four most potent anticonvulsant analogs, 2-ethylhexanoic acid, 2-butylhexanoic acid, 2-propylhexanoic acid, and 2-propylheptanoic acid, all elevate brain GABA levels (Fig. 3), whereas most of the less potent anticonvulsant analogs (with the exception of pentanoic acid and 2-ethylpentanoic acid) have little effect on the brain GABA levels.

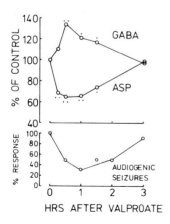

FIG. 1. **(Bottom):** Sound-induced seizures in audiogenic mice (DBA/2) following the administration of valproate (400 mg/kg, i.p.; 15 min to 3 hr). **(Top):** Valproate-induced changes in whole-brain GABA and aspartate (ASP) levels in audiogenic mice during the period of valproate protection. (*),$p < 0.05$; (**),$p < 0.01$. (Data from Schechter et al., ref. 70.)

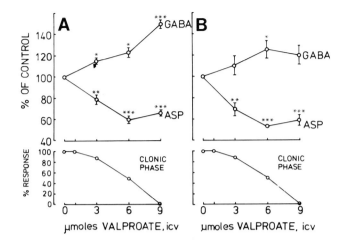

FIG. 2. Protection against sound-induced seizures in audiogenic (DBA/2) mice following the intracerebroventricular injection of valproate (30 min) **(bottom)** and the concomitant changes in forebrain and cerebellar GABA and aspartate (ASP) levels **(top)**. Control levels (μmol/g brain, mean $\pm$ SEM) were as follows: in forebrain, aspartate, 2.70 ± 0.10; GABA, 1.98 ± 0.11; in cerebellum, aspartate, 2.94 ± 0.18; GABA, 1.63 ± 0.12. (*),$p < 0.05$, (**)$p < 0.01$; (***)$p < 0.001$ (Student's *t*-test). (Chapman, Croucher, and Meldrum, *unpublished results*.)

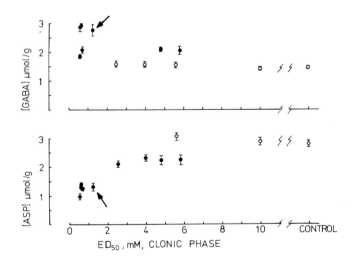

FIG. 3. GABA and aspartate (ASP) levels in forebrain of audiogenic DBA/2 mice following the administration of valproate *(arrows)* or valproate analogs (2 mmol/kg, i.p., 30 min) versus the potency of these analogs to protect against sound-induced seizures (ED_{50}, clonic phase). ($\bullet$), Levels significantly different from control values. (From Chapman et al., ref. 14, with permission.)

Measurement of GABA in the CSF obtained via lumbar puncture indicate, when corrected for rostrocaudal concentration gradients (29) and postsampling GABA increases (49), a correlation between the levels of GABA in the brain and in cisternal CSF (7,29). Decreased GABA levels have been reported in the CSF of children with febrile convulsions (50). It has also been shown that valproate administration increases the level of GABA in human plasma (51) and dog CSF (47).

GABA is synthesized by the decarboxylation of glutamate. This reaction is catalyzed by glutamate decarboxylase (GAD) (EC, 4.1.1.15). The sequential metabolism of GABA to succinic semialdehyde and succinate is catalyzed by the enzymes GABA-T (EC, 2.6.1.19) and succinic semialdehyde dehydrogenase (SSADH) (EC. 1.2.1.16), respectively. High valproate concentration inhibits the reversible GABA-T reaction *in vitro* (K_I, 10–100 mM) (13), whereas the subsequent GABA metabolizing enzyme SSADH is much more sensitive to valproate inhibition *in vitro* (K_I, 0.5-4.8 mM) (13), allowing for a cumulative inhibition of GABA metabolism by valproate. This mechanism may explain the observed valproate-induced increase in GABA levels, but the relationship to the anticonvulsant action of GABA is not known.

When GABA turnover is studied *in vivo* in rodents by either (a) determining the rate of GABA accumulation following the blocking of further GABA metabolism with potent GABA-T inhibitors (4,5) or (b) by determining the rate of ^{14}C-labeling of glutamate and GABA following the *in vivo* administration of ^{14}C-labeled precursors (15,19), it is found that valproate inhibits the rate of GABA turnover.

In contrast to GABAergic action of other anticonvulsants, such as benzodiazepines or barbiturates, there is no evidence for the interaction of valproate with the GABA receptor complex (48), nor is there any effect of valproate on the uptake and release of GABA (2,48,69).

The most compelling evidence for GABA-mediated valproate action comes from electrophysiological studies. Iontophoretic application of valproate potentiates the inhibitory action of GABA on neuronal activity *in vivo* in several brain areas, such as the cortex (3,38,71), spinal cord (53) and reticular formation (26). Reticular formation and cerebellum have been implicated in myoclonic activity (78,79) Figure 4 shows the effects of valproate on the responses of reticular neurons to GABA and glycine. Valproate potentiates the response to GABA, but not the response to glycine (26). The local concentration of valproate following iontophoretic application *in vivo* cannot be estimated. When the effect of valproate is studied using isolated neurons in bathing solution, quite high valproate concentrations (3–10 mM) are required in order to enhance the GABA-mediated inhibition of neuronal firing (33).

VALPROATE AND GLYCINE

Glycine is an inhibitory transmitter in the spinal cord (21), and some myoclonic activity has been shown to have a spinal cord origin (78). A loss of glycine neurons

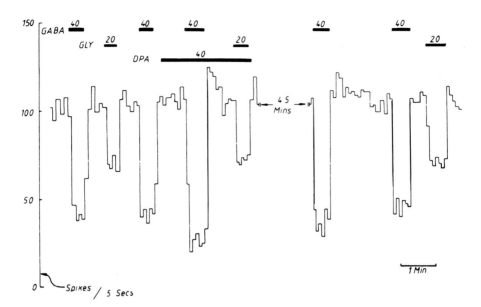

FIG. 4. The effects of valproate (DPA) on the responses of reticular neurons to GABA and glycine (GLY). Drugs were applied microiontophoretically during the periods indicated by the bars (currents are shown above in nanoamperes). *Ordinate*, the firing rate in successive 5-sec epochs. Valproate potentiates the responses to GABA but not to glycine. The recovery from the valproate effect took approximately 6.5 min. (From Gent and Phillips, ref. 26, with permission.)

in the spinal cord has been reported in cats following transient ischemia (23), which could be related to posthypoxic myoclonus deficits.

The levels of glycine are elevated in the plasma and urine of patients receiving valproate (65,73) and in rats given chronic anticonvulsant doses of valproate. The mechanism for the elevated glycine levels appears to be the valproate-mediated inhibition of the glycine cleavage system in liver, which is the major route for glycine metabolism (65). Despite the elevated plasma glycine levels, there are no changes in the brain glycine levels following acute or chronic valproate administration in rodents (15,27,43). The effect of valproate administration on spinal cord glycine levels has not been established.

VALPROATE AND SEROTONIN

Photically induced myoclonus in baboons and intention myoclonus in humans can be blocked by 5-HTP and other drugs acting on serotonergic transmission (78,81). Valproate has potent antimyoclonic activity in both forms of reflex epilepsy, indicating a possible direct or indirect serotonin-mediated action of valproate (24,66; S. Fahn, this volume).

Following the acute administration of valproate, there is a large increase in the plasma concentration of free tryptophan due to the displacement by valproate of protein-bound tryptophan (17,54). This leads to an increased influx of the serotonin precursor tryptophan into the brains of rodents, with resulting increases in the brain levels of tryptophan, serotonin, and the serotonin metabolite 5-hydroxyindoleacetic acid (17,34,54). However, the anticonvulsant action of valproate does not depend on this elevation in the brain levels of serotonin precursors and metabolites, since valproate has undiminished anticonvulsant activity against sound-induced seizures in DBA/2 mice that have been pretreated with *p*-chlorophenylalanine in order to block serotonin synthesis and thus deplete the serotonin and 5-hydroxyindoleacetic acid levels in the brain (34). The anticonvulsant potency of valproate in control and *p*-chlorophenylalanine–pretreated audiogenic mice is shown in Fig. 5 along with the valproate-induced changes in brain levels of GABA, serotonin, and 5-hydroxyindoleacetic acid in the presence and absence of *p*-chlorophenylalanine pretreatment.

VALPROATE AND EXCITATORY AMINO ACIDS

It has recently been shown that antagonists of excitatory amino acid transmission (compounds that specifically antagonize excitation induced by *N*-methyl-D-aspartic acid) exhibit potent anticonvulsant and antimyoclonic activity in a number of animal models. The most potent of these antagonists is 2-amino-7-phosphonoheptanoic acid (2-APH). Photically induced myoclonus in baboons (61) and myoclonus in-

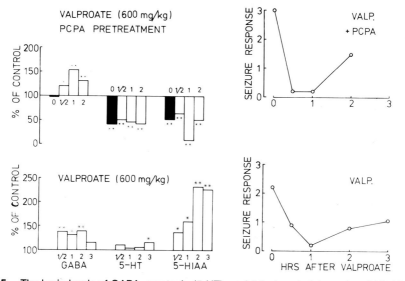

FIG. 5. The brain levels of GABA, serotonin (5-HT), and 5-hydroxyindoleacetic acid (5-HIAA) **(left)** and sound-induced seizure response **(right)** in DBA/2 mice following the administration of valproate (600 mg/kg, i.p., 30 min) with **(top)** and without **(bottom)** pretreatment of the mice with *p*-chlorophenylalanine (PCPA) to block 5-HT synthesis. Filled bars **(top left)** indicate the metabolite levels in the PCPA-pretreated mice before the valproate administration; open bars indicate the same metabolite levels 30 min and 1, 2, and 3 hr after valproate administration. (*),$p < 0.05$; (**),$p < 0.01$. Seizure response is scored: 1, wild running; 2, clonic seizures; 3, tonic seizures. (Data from Horton et al. ref. 34.)

duced by high pressures (above 70–90 atmospheres) in mice (64) are strongly suppressed by anticonvulsant doses of 2-APH (0.3–1.0 mmol/kg). In addition, sound-induced seizures in DBA/2 mice (20) and several types of chemically induced seizures in Swiss mice (22) are inhibited by 2-APH and other excitatory amino acid antagonists. Regional aspartate levels in fasted rats and mice are decreased following 2-APH administration (82).

Relatively little is known about the effect of valproate on the excitatory amino acid neurotransmitter system (presumed transmitters aspartate and glutamate). The administration of acute anticonvulsant doses of valproate leads to a simultaneous increase in the level of the inhibitory transmitter GABA and a decrease in the level of the excitatory transmitter aspartate (70). The aspartate decrease is observed in most brain regions in rats (15). The time course for the valproate-induced aspartate decrease in mouse brain coincides with the period of valproate protection (Fig. 1). There is also a dose-dependent decrease in aspartate levels in mouse forebrain and cerebellum following i.c.v. administration of anticonvulsant doses of valproate (Fig. 2), and finally, there is a very good correlation between the anticonvulsant potency against sound-induced seizures in mice of a number of valproate structural analogs and the ability of these analogs to depress brain aspartate levels (Fig. 3). Therefore, there exists a time-dependent, a dose-dependent, and an anticonvulsant potency-dependent correlation between brain aspartate levels and the administration of valproate or valproate analogs. The brain level of glutamate is less affected by the administration of valproate (15).

It remains to be established whether valproate has any effect on endogenous aspartate transmission or turnover, aspartate release, or aspartate synthesis or metabolism.

CONCLUSIONS

Valproate offers protection against several forms of clinical myoclonus and has antimyoclonic activity in several animal models. Several neurotransmitter systems are affected directly or indirectly by valproate administration, but the mechanism of valproate action remains unknown. The widely held belief that valproate enhances GABAergic transmission by making more GABA available for synaptic release (analogous to the mechanism of action of the anticonvulsant GABA-T inhibitors such as γ-vinyl-GABA) is not supported by the observed effects of valproate on GABA turnover and release. A postsynaptic action, mimicking or enhancing the effect of synaptically released GABA, is more consistent with the metabolic and electrophysiological effects of valproate. However, the recent findings of a close correlation between valproate action and aspartate response suggest that an action of valproate on excitatory aspartergic transmission could play an important part in the anticonvulsant or antimyoclonic action. A valproate-induced reduced activity at excitatory neurons converging on GABAergic inhibitory neurons might also be related to the decreased GABA turnover. This potential aspartergic component of valproate action merits further consideration, especially in light of the recently observed potent anticonvulsant and antimyoclonic activity of drugs antagonizing excitatory amino acid transmission.

SUMMARY

Valproate exhibits potent antiepileptic and antimyoclonic activity in a number of clinical and experimental syndromes. The mechanism of action of valproate remains unknown, but several neurotransmitter systems are affected directly or indirectly by valproate administration.

The levels of the serotonin precursor and the principal serotonin metabolite, tryptophan and 5-hydroxyindoleacetic acid, respectively, are elevated in rodent brain following the administration of anticonvulsant doses of valproate. However, the anticonvulsant action of valproate is preserved in mice pretreated with *p*-chlorophenylalanine, which depletes the brain levels of serotonin and serotonin metabolites.

Valproate administration elevates the level of the inhibitory transmitter glycine in the urine and plasma of patients and experimental animals, and the hepatic glycine cleavage enzyme is inhibited by valproate. The cerebral glycine levels in rodents are not affected by valproate administration, and the inhibitory action of glycine on reticular neuron firing is not affected by iontophoretically applied valproate.

Valproate exerts multiple effects on the inhibitory GABA transmitter system. Elevation in brain GABA level occurs in parallel with the anticonvulsant activity observed following valproate administration, and high levels of valproate inhibit the GABA-metabolizing enzymes GABA-T and SSADH and cause a reduction in the rate of GABA turnover. Valproate has no effect on GABA uptake, release, or binding to the GABA receptor complex. Iontophoretically applied valproate augments the inhibitory action of GABA on neuronal firing in a number of brain regions including the reticular formation.

Excitatory amino acid antagonists have recently been shown to possess anticonvulsant and antimyoclonic activity in a number of animal models. The ability of these compounds to decrease the brain level of the excitatory transmitter aspartate is shared by valproate. The valproate-induced decrease in aspartate level is dose dependent and coincides with the period of anticonvulsant protection. There is also a strong correlation between the anticonvulsant potency of a number of valproate analogs and their ability to reduce cerebral aspartate levels.

REFERENCES

1. Anlezark G, Horton RW, Meldrum BS, Sawaya MCB. Anticonvulsant action of ethanolamine-o-sulphate and di-n-propylacetate and the metabolism of γ-aminobutyric acid (GABA) in mice with audiogenic seizures. *Biochem Pharmacol* 1976;25:413–7.
2. Balcar VJ, Mandel P. Inhibition of high affinity uptake of GABA by branched fatty acids. *Experientia* 1976;32:906–8.
3. Baldino F, Geller HM. Sodium valproate enhancement of γ-aminobutyric acid (GABA) inhibition: electrophysiological evidence for anticonvulsant activity. *J Pharmacol Exp Ther* 1981;217:445–50.

4. Bernasconi R, Maitre L, Martin P, Raschdorf F. The use of inhibitors of GABA-transaminase for the determination of GABA turnover in mouse brain regions: an evaluation of amino-oxyacetic acid and gabaculine. *J Neurochem* 1982;38:57–66.
5. Bernasconi R, Schmutz M, Martin P, Hauser K. The GABA hypothesis of the mechanism of action of antiepileptic drugs: its usefulness and limitation. In: Fariello RG, Morselli PL, Engel J, eds. Neurotransmitters, seizures and epilepsy. New York: Raven Press, 1983.
6. Bichard AR, Little HJ. Drugs that increase γ-aminobutyric acid transmission protect against the high pressure neurological syndrome. *Br J Pharmacol* 1982;76:447–52.
7. Böhlen P, Huot S, Palfreyman MG. The relationship between GABA concentrations in brain and cerebrospinal fluid. *Brain Res* 1979;167:297–305.
8. Bruni J, Wilder BJ. Valproic acid: review of a new antiepileptic drug. *Arch Neurol* 1979;36:393–8.
9. Cepeda C, Valin A, Calderazzo L, Stutzman JM, Naquet R. Myoclonies induites par certaines benzodiazepines chez le Papio papio. Comparison avec les myoclonies induites par la stimulation lumineuse intermittente. *Rev EEG Neurophysiol Clin* 1982;12:32–7.
10. Chadwick D, Hallett M, Jenner P, Marsden CD. 5-Hydroxytryptophan-induced myoclonus in guinea pigs. A physiological and pharmacological investigation. *J Neurol Sci* 1978;35:157–65.
11. Chapman AG. The effect of valproate on cerebral amino acid metabolism and its relationship to anticonvulsant effects. In: Rose FC, ed. Research progress in epilepsy. London: Pitman Press, 1982:371–83.
12. Chapman AG, Horton RW, Meldrum BS. Anticonvulsant action of a 1,5-benzodiazepine, clobazam, in reflex epilepsy. *Epilepsia* 1978;19:293–9.
13. Chapman A, Keane PE, Meldrum BS, Simiand J, Vernieres JC. Mechanism of anticonvulsant action of valproate. *Prog Neurobiol* 1982;19:315–59.
14. Chapman AG, Meldrum BS, Mendes E. Acute anticonvulsant activity of structural analogues of valproic acid and changes in brain GABA and aspartate content. *Life Sci* 1983;32:2023–31.
15. Chapman AG, Riley K, Evans MC, Meldrum BS. Acute effects of sodium valproate and γ-vinyl GABA on regional amino acid metabolism in the rat brain: incorporation of 2-(^{14}C) glucose into amino acids. *Neurochem Res* 1982;7:1089–1105.
16. Chung Hwang E, Van Woert MH. p,p'-DDT-induced neurotoxic syndrome: Experimental myoclonus. *Neurology* 1978;28:1020–5.
17. Chung Hwang E, Van Woert MH. Effect of valproic acid on serotonin metabolism. *Neuropharmacology* 1979;18:391–7.
18. Chung Hwang E, Van Woert MH. Role of prostaglandins in the antimyoclonic action of clonazepam. *Eur J Pharmacol* 1981;71:161–4.
19. Cremer JE, Sarna GS, Teal HM, Cunningham VJ. Amino acid precursors: their transport into brain and initial metabolism. In: Fonnum F, ed. Amino acids as transmitters. New York, London: Plenum Press, 1978:669–89.
20. Croucher MJ, Collins JF, Meldrum BS. Anticonvulsant action of excitatory amino acid antagonists. *Science* 1982;216:899–901.
21. Curtis DR, Hösli L, Johnston GAR, Johnston IH. Glycine and spinal inhibition. *Brain Res* 1967;5:112–4.
22. Czuczwar SJ, Meldrum BS. Protection against chemically-induced seizures by 2-amino-7-phosphonoheptanoic acid. *Eur J Pharmacol* 1982;83:335–8.
23. Davidoff RA, Graham LT, Shank RP, Werman R, Aprison MH. Changes in amino acid concentrations associated with loss of spinal interneurons. *J Neurochem* 1967;14:1025–31.
24. Fahn S. Posthypoxic action myoclonus: review of the literature and report of two new cases with response to valproate and estrogen. In: Fahn S, Davis JN, Rowland LP, eds. Cerebral hypoxia and its consequences. New York: Raven Press, 1979:49–84. (Advances in neurology; vol. 26).
25. Fariello RG, Golden GT. The epileptogenic action of some direct GABA agonists. Effects of manipulation of the GABA and glutamate systems. In: Fariello RG, Morselli PL, Engel J, eds. Neurotransmitters, seizures and epilepsy. New York: Raven Press, 1983: in press.
26. Gent JP, Phillips NI. Sodium di-n-propylacetate (valproate) potentiates responses to GABA and muscimol on single central neurones. *Brain Res* 1980;197:275–8.
27. Godin Y, Heiner L, Mark J, Mandel P. Effects of di-n-propylacetate, an anticonvulsant compound, on GABA metabolism. *J Neurochem* 1969;16:869–73.
28. Goldberg MA, Dorman JD. Intention myoclonus: successful treatment with clonazepam. *Neurology* 1976;26:24–6.

29. Grove J, Schechter PJ, Hanke NFJ, de Smet Y, Agid Y, Tell G, Koch-Weser J. Concentration gradients of free and total γ-aminobutyric acid and homocarnosine in human CSF: comparison of suboccipital and lumbar sampling. *J Neurochem* 1982;39:1618–22.

30. Haefely W, Pieri L, Polc P, Schaffner R. General pharmacology and neuropharmacology of benzodiazepine derivatives. In: Hoffmeister F, Stille G, eds. Handbook of experimental pharmacology. Berlin: Springer Verlag, 1981:13–262 (55/II).

31. Halsey MJ. Effects of high pressure on the central nervous system. *Physiol Rev* 1982;62:1342–77.

32. Hammond EJ, Wilder BJ, Bruni J. Central actions of valproic acid in man and in experimental models of epilepsy. *Life Sci* 1981;29:2561–74.

33. Harrison NL, Simmonds MA. Sodium valproate enhances responses to GABA receptor activation only at high concentrations. *Brain Res* 1982;250:201–4.

34. Horton RW, Anlezark GM, Sawaya MCB, Meldrum BS. Monoamine and GABA metabolism and the anticonvulsant action of di-n-propylacetate and ethanolamine-O-sulphate. *Eur J Pharmacol* 1977;41:387–97.

35. Iadarola MJ, Raines A, Gale K. Differential effects of n-dipropylacetate and amino-oxyacetic acid on γ-aminobutyric acid levels in discrete areas of rat brain. *J Neurochem* 1979;33:1119–23.

36. Iivanainen M, Himberg J-J. Valproate and clonazepam in the treatment of severe progressive myoclonus epilepsy. *Arch Neurol* 1979;39:236–8.

37. Jeavons PM, Clark JE, Maheshwari MC. Treatment of generalised epilepsies of childhood and adolescence with sodium valproate ("Epilim"). *Dev Med Child Neurol* 1977;19:9–25.

38. Kerwin RW, Olpe HR. The effect of sodium valproate on single unit activity in the rat brain. *Br J Pharmacol* 1980;70:76P.

39. Kerwin RW, Olpe HR, Schmutz M. The effect of sodium-n-dipropylacetate on γ-aminobutyric acid dependent inhibition in the rat cortex and substantia nigra in relation to its anticonvulsant activity. *Br J Pharmacol* 1980;71:545–51.

40. Kerwin RW, Taberner PV. The mechanism of action of sodium valproate. *Gen Pharmacol* 1981;12:71–5.

41. Killam KF, Naquet R, Bert J. Paroxysmal responses to intermittent light stimulation in a population of baboons (Papio papio). *Epilepsia* 1966;7:215–9.

42. Klawans HL, Goetz BA, Weiner WJ. 5-Hydroxytryptophan-induced myoclonus in guinea pigs and the possible role of serotonin in infantile myoclonus. *Neurology* 1973;23:1234–40.

43. Kukino K, Deguchi T. Effects of sodium dipropylacetate on γ-aminobutyric acid and biogenic amines in rat brain. *Chem Pharm Bull (Tokyo)* 1977;25:2257–62.

44. Kupferberg HJ. Sodium valproate. In: Glaser GH, Penry JK, Woodbury DM, eds. Antiepileptic drugs: mechanisms of action. New York; Raven Press, 1980:643–54.

45. Lacolle JY, Ferrandes B, Eymard P. Profile of anticonvulsant activity of sodium valproate. Role of GABA. In: Meinardi H, Rowan AJ, eds. Advances in epileptology—1977. Amsterdam; Swets & Zeitlinger, 1978;162–7.

46. Lance JW, Anthony M. Sodium valproate and clonazepam in the treatment of intractable epilepsy. *Arch Neurol* 1977;34:14–17.

47. Löscher W. GABA in plasma and cerebrospinal fluid of different species. Effects of γ-acetylenic GABA,γ-vinyl GABA and sodium valproate. *J Neurochem* 1979;32:1587–91.

48. Löscher W. Effect of inhibitors of GABA transmission on the synthesis, binding, uptake and metabolism of GABA. *J Neurochem* 1980;34:1603–8.

49. Löscher W, Ahnfelt-Rønne I. EDTA inhibits in vitro increases in the GABA content of human CSF. *J Neurochem* 1982;39:251–4.

50. Löscher W, Rating D, Siemes H. GABA in cerebrospinal fluid of children with febrile convulsions. *Epilepsia* 1981;22:697–702.

51. Löscher W, Schmidt D. Increase of human plasma GABA by sodium valproate. *Epilepsia* 1980;21:611–5.

52. Macdonald RL, Barker JL. Enhancement of GABA-mediated postsynaptic inhibition in cultured mammalian spinal cord neurons: a common mode of anticonvulsant action. *Brain Res* 1979;167:323–36.

53. Macdonald RL, Bergey GK. Valproic acid augments GABA-mediated postsynaptic inhibition in cultured mammalian neurons. *Brain Res* 1979;170:558–62.

54. MacMillan V. The effects of the anticonvulsant valproic acid on cerebral indole amine metabolism. *Can J Physiol Pharmacol* 1979;57:843–7.

55. Meldrum BS. Epilepsy and GABA-mediated inhibition. *Int Rev Neurobiol* 1975;17:1–36.
56. Meldrum BS. Mechanism of action of valproate. *Brain Res Bull* 1980;5(suppl. 2):579–84.
57. Meldrum BS. Anticonvulsant drugs and GABA-mediated inhibition. In: Sandler M, ed. *Psychopharmacology of anticonvulsant drugs*, Oxford University Press, 1982:62–78.
58. Meldrum BS. Pharmacology of GABA. *Clin Neuropharmacol* 1982;5:293–316.
59. Meldrum BS, Anlezark G, Balzamo E, Horton RW, Trimble M. Photically induced epilepsy in Papio papio as a model for drug studies. In: Meldrum BS, Marsden CD, eds. Primate models for neurological disorders. New York: Raven Press, 1975:119–28.
60. Meldrum B, Braestrup C. GABA and the anticonvulsant action of benzodiazepines and related drugs. In: Bowery N, ed. Actions and interactions of GABA and benzodiazepines. New York: Raven Press, 1983: in press.
61. Meldrum BS, Croucher MJ, Badman G, Collins JF. Antiepileptic action of excitatory amino acid antagonists in the photosensitive baboon, Papio papio. *Neurosci Lett* 1983;39:101–4.
62. Meldrum B, Horton R. Effects of the bicyclic GABA agonist, THIP, on myoclonic and seizure responses in mice and baboons with reflex epilepsy. *Eur J Pharmacol* 1980;61:231–7.
63. Meldrum BS, Horton RW, Toseland PA. A primate model for testing anticonvulsant drugs. *Arch Neurol* 1975;32:289–94.
64. Meldrum B, Wardley-Smith B, Halsey M, Rostain J-C. 2-Amino-phosphonoheptanoic acid protects against the high pressure neurological syndrome. *Eur J Pharmacol* 1983;87:501–2.
65. Mortensen PB, Kølvraa S, Christensen E. Inhibition of the glycine cleavage system: hyperglycinemia and hyperglycinuria caused by valproic acid. *Epilepsia* 1980;21:563–9.
66. Patry G, Naguet R. Action de l'acide dipropylacetique chez le Papio papio photosensible. *Can J Physiol Pharmacol* 1971;49:568–72.
67. Pedley TA, Horton RW, Meldrum BS. Electroencephalographic and behavioural effects of a GABA agonist (muscimol) on photosensitive epilepsy in the baboon, Papio papio. *Epilepsia* 1979;20:409–16.
68. Pinder RM, Brogden RN, Speight TM, Avery GS. Sodium valproate: a review of its pharmacological properties and therapeutic efficacy in epilepsy. *Drugs* 1977;13:81–123.
69. Ross SM, Craig CR. Studies on γ-aminobutyric acid transport in cobalt experimental epilepsy in the rat. *J Neurochem* 1981;36:1006–11.
70. Schechter PJ, Tranier Y, Grove J. Effect of n-dipropylacetate on amino acid concentrations in mouse brain: correlation with anticonvulsant activity. *J Neurochem* 1978;31:1325–7.
71. Schmutz M, Olpe HR, Koella WP. Central actions of valproate sodium. *J Pharm Pharmacol* 1979;31:413–4.
72. Keane PE, Simiand J, Mendes E, Santucci V, Morre M. The effects of analogues of valproic acid on seizures induced by pentylenetetrazol and GABA content in brain of mice. *Neuropharmacol* 1983;22:875–9.
73. Simila S, Von Wendt L, Linnaa SI. Dipropylacetate and aminoaciduria. *J Neurol Sci* 1980;45:83–6.
74. Simler S, Gensburger C, Ciesielski L, Mandel P. Effets du n-dipropylacetate de sodium sur le taux de GABA de certaines zones du cerveau de la souris. *Comp Rend Soc Biol* 1976;170:1285–8.
75. Simler S, Gensburger C, Ciesielski L, Mandel P. Time course of the increase in GABA level in different mice brain regions following n-dipropylacetate treatment. *Commun Psychopharmacol* 1978;2:123–30.
76. Simon D, Penry JK. Sodium di-N-propylacetate (DPA) in the treatment of epilepsy. A review. *Epilepsia* 1975;16:549–73.
77. Urca G, Frenk H, Liebeskind JC, Taylor AN. Morphine and enkephalin: analgesic and epileptic properties. *Science* 1977;197:83–6.
78. Van Woert MH, Chung Hwang E. Biochemistry and pharmacology of myoclonus. In: Klawans HL, ed. Clin Neuropharmacol 1978;3:167–84.
79. Van Woert MH, Chung E. Stimulus-sensitive myoclonus: Hyperexcitable medullary reticular neurons. In: Fariello RG, Morselli PL, Engel J, eds. Neurotransmitters, seizure and epilepsy. New York: Raven Press, 1983: in press.
80. Volkman PH, Lorens SA, Kindel GH, Ginos JZ. 5-Hydroxytryptophan-induced myoclonus in guinea pigs: a model for the study of central serotonin-dopamine interactions. *Neuropharmacology* 1978;17:947–55.
81. Wada JA, Balzano E, Meldrum BS, Naquet R. Behavioural and electrographic effects of L-5-

hydroxytryptophan and D,L parachlorophenylalanine on epileptic Senegalese baboon (Papio papio). *Electroencephalogr Clin Neurophysiol* 1972;33:520–6.

82. Westerberg E, Chapman AG, Meldrum BS. The effect of 2-amino-7-phosphonoheptanoic acid administration on regional brain amino acid levels in fed and fasted rodents. *J Neurochem* 1983;41:1755–60.

83. Zuckermann EG, Glaser GH. Urea-induced myoclonic seizures. An experimental study of site of action and mechanism. *Arch Neurol* 1972;27:14–28.

Advances in Neurology, Vol. 43: Myoclonus,
edited by S. Fahn et al. Raven Press,
New York © 1986.

Piracetam: Physiological Disposition and Mechanism of Action

Maria T. Tacconi and Richard J. Wurtman

*Laboratory of Neuroendocrine Regulation, Department of Nutrition and Food Science,
Massachusetts Institute of Technology, Cambridge, Massachusetts 02139*

Piracetam (2-oxo-1-pyrrolidine acetamide; Nootropil®) has been proposed (13) as the prototype of a new class of psychoactive drugs, the "nootropic" drugs, which allegedly "selectively improve the efficiency of high telencephalic integrative activities" (Fig. 1). Properties reportedly associated with piracetam include the "enhancement of learning acquisition, the conferring of resistance to agents that impair acquisition, the facilitation of interhemispheric transfer, and the absence of other psychological or general pharmacological effects" (18).

Piracetam apparently is virtually nontoxic: its lethal dose (LD) is higher than 8 to 10 g/kg in mice, rats, and dogs (19). Rats treated chronically with 100 to 1,000 mg/kg orally for 6 months and dogs treated with as much as 10 g/kg orally for 1 year did not show any toxic effect. No teratogenic effects were found, nor was behavioral tolerance noted (14).

Piracetam administration to experimental animals has been described as affecting learning acquisition (34) when studied using Y-maze and drinking tests (56), habituation (11), retrieval (45), hypoxia-induced amnesia (15), electroconvulsive-shock–induced amnesia (44), barbiturate intoxication (29), and alcohol withdrawal (46). Studies on human subjects have investigated piracetam's effects on aging, alcohol withdrawal, postelectroconvulsive cognitive deficiency, and schizophrenia. Results in geriatric patients are controversial: Stegink (48) and Macchione et al. (28) found significant improvement in several symptoms (asthenia, disordered alertness, psychomotor agitation) in geriatric patients with "senile involution" (48) or the "cerebral psycho-organic syndrome" (28), using daily doses of 2.4 and 4.8 g, respectively. Bente et al. (5) found positive effects on communicative behavior and cognitive functions, which were correlated with EEG changes suggestive of increased vigilance (dose: 4.8 g daily for 8–13 months). However, in other studies, piracetam did not significantly affect behavior in people with memory impairment (1), or organic dementia (23).

Denker et al. (9) compared the effects of piracetam (4.8 g daily) or chlormethiazole in patients with an alcohol-withdrawal syndrome and found that piracetam was as effective as chlormethiazole in reducing abstinence symptoms. However, its lack of sedative effects meant that other drugs also had to be used to treat patients with sleep disturbances. Psychotic patients reportedly showed improvement in drug-

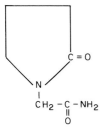

FIG. 1. Chemical structure of piracetam: 2-oxo-1-pyrrolidine aceta-mide.

resistant depression and schizophrenia after piracetam (2.4 g daily) (27). No effect of piracetam was noted in recovery rates of patients with postelectroconvulsive-treatment cognitive deficiency, in a double-blind trial (3).

PHYSIOLOGIC DISPOSITION

Rat

Piracetam given orally to rats is quickly absorbed through the stomach, and distributed in all tissues (19), concentrating in the brain (41). In an attempt to identify the central nervous system (CNS) locus at which piracetam exerts its behavioral actions, we studied the drug's kinetics and distribution in rat plasma and brain. Animals received piracetam by gavage (doses ranging from 1 to 1,000 mg/kg), with or without addition of [^{3}H]piracetam as a tracer, and were killed after various intervals. Serum and brain piracetam levels were measured using a gas chromatographic method (26) after protein precipitation with formic acid acetone. Extracts were evaporated to dryness, resuspended in water, and submitted to further purification before injection into the gas chromatograph, i.e., washing with hexane and separation by thin-layer chromatography (TLC) in order to eliminate some interfering peaks. Figure 2 shows data from experiments in which [^{3}H]piracetam (100 mg/kg, containing 1 μCi/kg) was given to starved rats, which were killed after 30 min to 36 hr. Drug absorption was very quick, peak serum levels being attained between 30 and 60 min; levels then dropped exponentially (half-life, 2 hr) for 8 hr, after which the rate of elimination from serum decreased (half-life, 3.5 hr). Brain concentrations equilibrated with those in serum after about 4 hr; there-after, brain levels were approximately double those in serum. The two exponential curves obtained by plotting our data suggested the presence of two metabolic compartments, one including plasma and tissues that offer no diffusion barrier to piracetam, and the other including tissues with a slow diffusion rate. The brain may be part of this second compartment; the compound is very polar and might be expected to cross the blood–brain barrier with difficulty.

Although the high doses of piracetam required to produce behavioral effects might suggest that the drug works via an active metabolite, virtually no metabolism of piracetam could be detected by identifying ^{3}H-labeled compound in urine, feces, blood, liver, or brain of animals given [^{3}H]piracetam (19). Moreover, in the ranges studied, excretion of unchanged [^{3}H]piracetam was not affected by dosage or by

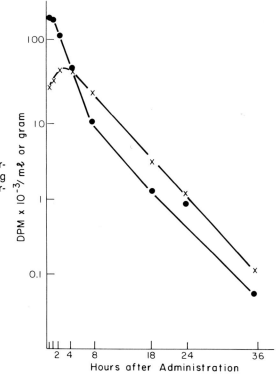

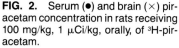

FIG. 2. Serum (●) and brain (×) piracetam concentration in rats receiving 100 mg/kg, 1 μCi/kg, orally, of ³H-piracetam.

chronic administration (6 weeks in humans) of the drug. Our studies confirmed these earlier results: 98% of the radioactivity found in serum and brain extracts of rats given [³H]piracetam (100 μCi/kg) orally 4 hr earlier co-migrated with the unlabeled piracetam added as reference standard. In related studies on the possible metabolism of piracetam *in vitro*, [³H]piracetam (5×10^{-5} M, SA, 1 μCi/μmole) was incubated with a liver homogenate (5% wt/vol in 0.05 M TRIS buffer pH 8.8) with or without 10^{-4} M S-adenosine methionine (SAM) for 60 min at 37°C. Control incubations (at 0°C) were run in parallel. The incubation was stopped by the addition of formic acid in acetone, and the samples were extracted as described above. Aliquots of the acetone phase, water phase, and hexane phase, after washing, were taken for the radioactivity measure. Thereafter, aliquots were run on TLC, after which the silica gel of the plate was divided into six fractions, which were scraped and extracted with methanol; the radioactivity in all fractions was counted. No difference was found in the amount of piracetam before and after incubation, and in the presence or absence of SAM (Table 2).

We investigated the regional distribution of piracetam in rat brain after a single oral dose (500 mg/kg) given 4 hr earlier (Table 1). Pons and medulla showed piracetam level 30 to 40% lower than those of olfactory bulb, cortex, and colliculi. These data are in agreement with those of Ostrowsky et al. (39), who observed

TABLE 1. *Regional distribution of oral piracetam in rat brain*[a]

Region	Piracetam (μg/g $\pm$ SE)	Region	Piracetam (μg/g $\pm$ SE)
Olfactory bulb	56.8 $\pm$ 1.3	Striatum	46.7 $\pm$ 0.3
Colliculi	54.2 $\pm$ 1.3	Cerebellum	42.0 $\pm$ 2.4
Cortex	52.0 $\pm$ 5.0	Thalamus	39.8 $\pm$ 2.0
Hypothalamus	51.2 $\pm$ 1.5	Medulla	36.1 $\pm$ 1.1
Hippocampus	49.4 $\pm$ 0.5	Pons	31.1 $\pm$ 4.0

[a]Animals were killed 4 hr after receiving piracetam (500 mg/kg) by gavage.

higher concentrations of piracetam radioactivity in cortical areas, using autoradiography.

The subcellular distributions of [^{3}H]piracetam in brain were examined in rats treated with various piracetam doses: 1 and 100 mg/kg, containing [^{3}H]piracetam, 100 μCi/kg (Table 3). The [^{3}H]piracetam in aliquots of total brain homogenate was present in the cytosol, regardless of the piracetam dose given or the extent of isotope dilution. The remaining radioactivity was distributed in the various particulate fractions. (When [^{3}H]piracetam was added to the homogenate *in vitro*, no drug was found in the particulate fractions.)

Humans

Oral piracetam is rapidly absorbed in humans, peak plasma levels (after an 800-mg dose) being attained after 30 min (20) (Fig. 3). Thereafter, concentrations decrease rapidly for 1 hr and subsequently fall exponentially with a half-life of 5.2 hr, similar to that observed after intravenous injection of piracetam. Piracetam is excreted without metabolic modification via the urine; only 1 to 2% of a dose is found in feces. The drug recovery is almost complete within 30 hr in humans, as in rats and dogs (19). The renal clearance was found to be 86 ml/min in humans.

POSSIBLE MECHANISMS OF ACTION

Biochemical Effects

Piracetam administration can reportedly affect brain neurotransmitter levels, but these effects are, in general, small. In spite of its resemblance to γ-aminobutyric acid (GABA), piracetam does not elicit specific GABAergic effects (17), nor does it modify GABA levels in the brain (51). Dopamine levels in the brain (36) and striatum (41) also are unaffected by piracetam, but a slight decrease in homovanillic acid (HVA) levels (35–45%) was found at very high dosages [5 g/kg, i.p., for 90 min (36); 1 g/kg, i.p. (41)], respectively.

Valzelli et al. (50) studied the levels and turnover of brain serotonin (5-HT) in young and old mice given 1 g/kg of piracetam, i.p., daily for 7 days. No differences in 5-HT levels were noted: 5-hydroxyindole acetic acid (5-HIAA) was slightly

TABLE 2. *Effect of added S-adenosylmethionine on piracetam metabolism of rat liver homogenate[a]*

Piracetam	SAM	Time of incubation (min)	[³H]Piracetam DPM/mg liver ± SE									
			Initial	After acetone	After washing		After TLC					
					Hexane	H₂O	1	2	3	4	5	6
+	−	0	11,500	10,400 ± 230	50 ± 7	10,000 ± 360	18	12	18	81	10,950	43
+	−	60	11,500	10,600 ± 300	75 ± 7	8,100 ± 390	12	12	20	129	10,856	92
+	+	0	11,700	10,100 ± 80	61 ± 6	10,700 ± 340	11	11	15	89	9,904	68
+	+	60	11,700	10,700 ± 80	60 ± 5	10,700 ± 230	14	11	16	103	10,114	93

[a]Piracetam (5×10^{-5} M; SA, 1 μCi/μmole) was incubated for 60 min at 37°C with a 5% liver homogenate, in TRIS buffer (pH 8,8), with or without S-adenosylmethionine (SAM) (10^{-4} M). The incubation was stopped by addition of 15% formic acid in acetone, and the piracetam in it was washed with hexane prior to thin-layer chromatography (TLC) of the aqueous phase. After TLC, the silica gel of the plate was divided into six fractions; these were extracted with methanol and their radioactivity then measured.

TABLE 3. *Subcellular distribution of oral piracetam in rat brain[a]*

Dose (mg/kg)	Disintegrations per minute as % of total homogenate					
	Nuclei	Mitochondria	Microsomes	Synaptosomes	Myelin	Cytosol
1	3.5 ± 0.5	2.2 ± 0.3	1.7 ± 0.1	2.7 ± 0.3	2.3 ± 0.3	87.6 ± 0.8
100	3.3 ± 0.4	3.1 ± 0.1	1.6 ± 0.1	2.8 ± 0.2	1.8 ± 0.2	87.3 ± 0.5
Added to homogenate	3.9	0.001	0.77	0.002	0.007	95.3

[a]Animals were killed 2 hr after receiving piracetam (1 or 100 mg/kg; 100 μCi) by gavage. As a control, piracetam (10 μg, 0.1 μCi/ml) was added to brain homogenates and its subcellular distribution determined.

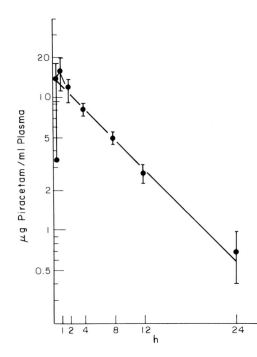

FIG. 3. Plasma piracetam concentrations in subjects receiving 800 mg piracetam orally. (From Gobert and Baltes, ref. 21, with permission.)

increased in both the young and the old groups; and brain tryptophan was elevated by piracetam in old mice. File and Hyde (12) observed an increase in cortical 5-HT, a decrease in 5-HIAA, and no changes in norepinephrine (NA) and dopamine in brains of rats killed 30 min after receiving piracetam (100 mg/kg, i.p.).

Wurtman et al. (57) found that piracetam (300 mg/kg, i.p.) decreased acetylcholine levels by 32% in the hippocampus of naive rats. Similarly, Bartus et al. (4) found a slight decrease (19%) in hippocampal acetylcholine in aged rats receiving 100 mg/kg of piracetam in drinking water for 14 days, and a higher increase of hippocampal choline (88%). When choline was given together with piracetam, no further significant changes in choline and acetylcholine levels were observed in comparison to the choline-treated animals, but the choline-induced improvement of the passive-avoidance learning test was potentiated.

Preliminary studies by Gobert and Temmerman (22) presented evidence that piracetam caused a substantial increase in energy-rich adenosine nucleotides in the brain; Nickolson and Wolthuis (33) were unable to detect changes in adenine nucleotide contents, but did find stimulation of adenylate cyclase. Woelk and Peiler-Ichikawa (55) investigated the effect of piracetam on electron transport system in the neuronal and glial microsomes, measuring the formation of ethanolamine plasmalogen from the corresponding ether lipid, a step that is dependent on cytochrome b_5. Piracetam (60–100 mg/kg daily, i.p., for 10 days) increases formation of the ethanolamine plasmalogen in neuronal cells. Moreover, evidence obtained by adding a specific antibody against cytochrome b_5 to the reaction mixture suggested that piracetam effect is mediated by an increase in the synthesis or turnover of cytochrome b_5.

Burnotte et al. (6) showed that piracetam (100 mg/kg, i.p., for 4 days) increased the ratio of polyribosomes to free ribosomes, a marker for protein synthesis, in brains of old rats. Platt et al. (40) found that piracetam (100 mg/kg daily for 8 days) increased the *in vivo* leucine incorporation into cerebral proteins in young and old rats. Nickolson and Wolthuis (33) confirmed that piracetam (10 mM) increased leucine uptake into rat cortical slices, but incorporation of the leucine into the brain proteins was unaffected even after 180 min of incubation. Similarly, no effect of piracetam was observed on the *in vivo* incorporation of [^{3}H]leucine into rat cortical proteins. No increase in the synthesis of labeled proteins was found in brain slices incubated with labeled glucose in the presence of piracetam (10).

Several authors reported that piracetam increased the incorporation of ^{32}P into brain phospholipids. Rochus and Reuse (43) found that piracetam (600 mg/kg daily for 10 days, i.p.) had this effect only when the synthesis was depressed by chloropromazine. Woelk (53) described increased incorporation of ^{32}P (given intracisternally) into neuronal phosphatidyl inositol (PI) and phosphatidyl choline (PC) among rabbits receiving piracetam (100 mg/kg, i.p., daily) for 3 weeks. Woelk also studied the effect of piracetam on phospholipase A_2 activity in rat neurons and synaptosomes. The hydrolysis of different glycerophosphatides *in vitro* was increased by 40 to 50% among animals receiving piracetam (100 mg/kg daily, i.p.) for 10 days (54).

Nikolov et al. (35) found that piracetam restored the resistance to hypoxia impaired by prostaglandin $F_{2\alpha}$ ($PGF_{2\alpha}$) but no direct interaction between piracetam and $PGF_{2\alpha}$ or PGE_2 could be shown *in vivo* or *in vitro*. In rats subjected to immobilization stress, piracetam was shown to decrease free fatty acid (FFA) levels in both plasma and brain (32,47). Domenskaja-Janik and Zalewska (10) studied the effect of piracetam on glucose metabolism in brain slices: a 500 μg/ml concentration increased O_2 consumption and lactate and CO_2 production when the media were normally oxygenated; the drug had no effect in high-potassium or anoxic media. Henry et al. (24) found that piracetam (5–50 mM) reduced adenosine diphosphate (ADP) and NA-induced platelet aggregation in a dose-dependent manner. Piracetam also reportedly increased erythrocyte deformability (1–5 mM) in normal and sickle erythrocytes (2,30,31).

Vlahov et al. (52) reported a small effect of piracetam on cerebral blood flow (increases of 15–25%) in anesthetized cats receiving 100 mg/kg of piracetam. Reuse-Blom (42) found that giving piracetam i.v. (0.02–2 mg/kg) to rabbits caused a dose-dependent dilation of the pial arterioles *in situ* and restored previously contracted arterioles to normal diameter.

Physiological Effects

Few data are available on electrophysiological effects of piracetam. Giurgea and Moyersoon (16) showed an increase in transcallosal evoked potentials in cats receiving piracetam (10–500 mg/kg) intravenously. Olpe and Steinman (38) studied the discharge rate of noradrenergic neurons of the locus ceruleus, using single-cell recording techniques. Piracetam elicited a 30 to 40% increase in firing rate at doses of 300 to 1,000 mg/kg. He also examined the effect of piracetam on the electrical responses of rat hippocampal slices studied *in vitro* (37). Piracetam increased the amplitude of the population–spike response of pyramidal neurons that was evoked by stimulation of the afferent Schaeffer–commissural fibers. (This effect resembled that of opiate compounds such as enkephalin and morphine.)

CLINICAL CORRELATIONS

Clinical studies provide few correlations with the biochemical and metabolic changes reportedly produced by giving piracetam to experimental animals. Herrschaft (25) found a slight increase in cerebral blood flow after piracetam, or a tendency to normalization in ischemic regions, whereas others (23) found no effect.

Lactate levels in blood and cerebrospinal fluid were studied in patients with head injuries (7); among piracetam-treated patients (4–8 g, i.v.), a correlation was shown between the decrease of lactate levels and clinical improvement.

Kabés et al. (27) found a positive correlation between clinical improvement and ratio of ADP to adenosine triphosphate (ATP) in red blood cells of psychotic patients receiving continuous psychotropic medication treated with piracetam (2 g daily).

On the basis of its hypothesized effect on energy metabolism, piracetam has been tested in two cases of postanoxic intention myoclonus (8,49) and was found effective.

CONCLUSIONS

That piracetam can benefit some patients with cognitive deficits seems likely, if for no other reason than its widespread continued use for this purpose. However, the mechanism by which it and other nootropic drugs produce their therapeutic effects remains obscure. High doses apparently are needed, suggesting that it might enter the brain with great difficulty, or work via an active metabolite; however, pharmacokinetic and metabolic studies show that piracetam does enter the brain well (so that brain levels exceed those in plasma several hours after its administration) and that it is metabolized only to an unmeasurably small extent. The agent does concentrate better in some brain areas (e.g., olfactory bulb, colliculi, and cortex) than in others (e.g., brainstem). However, differences are only on the order of 50 to 60%; it does not concentrate to a major extent within any subcellular fraction that might suggest a specific biochemical function. Piracetam administration has been claimed to produce a variety of biochemical effects in experimental animals; however, few of these effects have repeatedly been confirmed in several laboratories. Perhaps the most promising biochemical leads now available concern piracetam's possible effects on energy metabolism (e.g., increased synthesis and turnover of cytochrome b_5) and its ability to enhance acetylcholine release from certain brain neurons; however, evidence supporting either of these effects is only fragmentary. Piracetam has been tried in a very few cases in the treatment of myoclonus; evidence for its utility in this disorder is not compelling. The enormous current interest in the treatment of Alzheimer's disease and especially in the development of nootropic drugs promises a rapid increase in our understanding of how and when piracetam works.

SUMMARY

Piracetam, the prototype of nootropic drugs, is claimed to have therapeutic value in some patients suffering from cognitive deficits, especially when hypoxia may be a factor in the deficits. The drug lacks sedative or stimulatory effects and apparently does not influence behavior in normal people. The site of action and the mechanism by which piracetam exerts its beneficial effects are not well established. This review has summarized experimental and clinical data on its absorption, distribution, and excretion, and described the biochemical data available that bear on its mechanism of action.

REFERENCES

1. Abuzzahab FS, Merwin GE, Zimmerman RL, Sherman MC. A double blind investigation of piracetam (Nootropil) vs placebo in geriatric memory. *Pharmakopsychiatry* 1977;10:49–56.
2. Asakura T, Ohnishi ST, Adachi K, Ozguc M, Hashimoto K, Devlin MT, Schwartz E. Effect of piracetam on sickle erythrocytes and sickle haemoglobin. Biochim Biophys Acta 1981;668:397–405.
3. Bagadia VM, Gada MT, Mundra VK, Simon S, Doshi JM. A double blind trial of piracetam in cases of post ECT-cognitive deficiency. *J Postgrad Med* 1980;26:116–20.
4. Bartus RT, Dean RL, Sherman KA, Friedman E, Beer B. Profound effect of combining choline and piracetam in memory enhancement and cholinergic functions in aged rats. *Neurobiol Aging* 1981;2:105–11.
5. Bente D, Glatthaar G, Ulrich G, Lewinsky M. Piracetam und Vigilanz. Elektroenzephalographische und klinische Ergebnisse einer Langzeitmedikationen bei gerontopsychiatrischen Patienten. *Arzneimittelforsch/Drug Res* 1978;28:1529–30.
6. Burnotte RE, Gobert JG, Temmerman JJ. Piracetam induced modifications of the brain polyribosome pattern in ageing rats. *Biochem Pharmacol* 1973;22:811–14.
7. Calliauw L, Marchau M. Clinical trial of piracetam in disorders of consciousness due to head injury. *Acta Anaesthesiol Belg* 1975;26:51–60.

8. Cremieux C, Serratrice A. Myoclonus d'intention postanoxique. Amélioration par le piracetam. *Nouv Presse Med* 1979;8:3357—8.

9. Dencker SJ, Wihelmsson F, Carlsson E, Bereen FJ. Piracetam and cloromethiazole in acute alcohol withdrawal. A controlled clinical trial. *J Int Med Res* 1978;6:395–400.

10. Domenskaja-Janik K, Zalewska M. The action of piracetam on ^{14}C glucose metabolism in normal and posthypoxic rat cerebral cortex slices. *Pol J Pharmacol Pharm* 1977;29:111–6.

11. File SE, Hyde JRC. The effect of piracetam on acquisition and retention of habituation. *Br J Pharmacol* 1977;61:475P.

12. File SE, Hyde JRC. Evidence that piracetam has an anxiolytic effect. *J Affective Disord* 1979;1:227–36.

13. Giurgea C. Vers une pharmacologie de l'activité intégrative du cerveau. Tentative du concept nootrope en psychopharmacologie. *Actual Pharmacol (Paris)* 1972;115–56.

14. Giurgea M. Piracetam toxicity and reproduction studies. *Il Farmaco* 1977;32:47–52.

15. Giurgea C, Lefevre D, Lescrenier C, David-Remacle M. Pharmacological protection against hypoxia-induced amnesia. *Psychopharmacology* (Berlin) 1971;20:160–8.

16. Giurgea D, Moyersoon F. Differential pharmacological reactivity of three types of cortical evoked potential. *Arch Int Pharmacodyn Ther* 1970;188:401–4.

17. Giurgea C, Moyersoon F, Evraerd AC. A GABA-related hypothesis on the mechanism of action of the antimotion-sickness drugs. *Arch Int Pharmacodyn Ther* 1967;166:238–51.

18. Giurgea C, Salama M. Nootropic drugs. *Prog Neuropsychopharmacol Biol Psychiatry* 1977;1:235–47.

19. Gobert JG. Genèse d'un medicament: le piracetam. Métabolisation et recherche biochimique. *J Pharm Belg* 1972;27:281–304.

20. Gobert JG. Availability and plasma clearance of piracetam in man. *Il Farmaco* 1977;32:84–91.

21. Gobert JG, Baltes EL. *Il Farmaco* 1977;32:84–91.

22. Gobert JG, Temmerman J. Piracetam-induced increase of the rat brain energetic metabolism and polyribosome/ribosome ratio in old rats. *Int Soc Neurochemistry*, Tokyo, 1973; Japan 8:23–31.

23. Gustafson L, Risberg J, Johanson M, Fransson M. Effect of piracetam in regional blood flow and mental functions in patient with organic dementia. *Psychopharmacology (Berlin)* 1978;56:115–7.

24. Henry RL, Nabaldian RM, Herman GE, Ho T. Release of PF_4 and βTG from platelets and inhibition by piracetam. *Blood* 1978;52(suppl I):163.

25. Herrschaft H. Die Wirkung von Piracetam auf die Gehirndurchblutung des Menschen. Quantitative regionale Hindurchblutung messungen bei der akuten zerebralen Ischaemie. *Med Klin* 1978;73:195–202.

26. Hesse C, Schulz M. Gas-chromatographische Bestimmung von Piracetam in Serum und biologischen Material. *Chromatographie* 1979;12:12–16.

27. Kabés J, Erban L, Hanzliček V, Skondia V. Biological correlates of piracetam clinical effects in psychotic patients. *J Int Med Res* 1979;7:277–84.

28. Macchione C, Molaschi M, Fabris F, Feruglio FS. Results with piracetam in the management of senile psychoorganic syndromes. *Acta Ther* 1976;213:261–9.

29. Moyersoon F, Giurgea C. Protective effect of piracetam in experimental barbiturate intoxication. EEG and behavioural studies. *Arch Int Pharmacodyn Ther* 1974;210:38–48.

30. Nalbaldian RJ, Blood RL. Desickling mechanism of piracetam. *Blood* 1979;54:56a.

31. Nalbaldian RJ, Henry RL. Molecular reactions useful in sickle-cell disease. *Blood* 1978;52:116.

32. Navratil J, Sklenowsky A, Chmela Z, Rypka M. Effect of piracetam on free fatty acids in the plasma during immobilisation stress. *Acta Nerv Super* 1981;23:222–4.

33. Nickolson VJ, Wolthuis OL. Protein metabolism in the rat cerebral cortex in vivo and in vitro as affected by the acquisition-enhancing drug piracetam. *Biochem Pharmacol* 1976;25:2237–41.

34. Nickolson VJ, Wolthuis OL. Effect of acquisition enhancing drug piracetam on rat cerebral energy metabolism. *Biochem Pharmacol* 1976;25:2241–4.

35. Nikolov R, Rakovska A, Dushkova R, Dimitrova L, Pavlidu A. Study of PG antagonistic activity of Aligeron and piracetam. *Methods Find Exp Clin Pharmacol* 1982;4:397–402.

36. Nybäck CK, Wiesel FA, Skett P. Effect of piracetam on brain monoamines metabolism and serum prolactine levels in the rat. *Psychopharmacology (Berlin)* 1979;61:235–8.

37. Olpe HR, Lynch GS. The action of piracetam on the electrical activity of the hippocampal slice preparation: a field potential analysis. *Eur J Pharmacol* 1982;80:415–9.

38. Olpe HR, Steinman MW. The activating action of vincamine, piracetam and hydergine on the activity of the noradrenergic neurons of the locus coeruleus. *Behav Neural Biol* 1981;33:249–51.
39. Ostrowki J, Keil M, Schraven E. Autoradiographische Untersuchungen zur Verteilung von Piracetam ^{14}C bei Ratte und Hund. *Arzneimittelforsch/Drug Res* 1975;25:589–96.
40. Platt D, Hering H, Hering F. Messungen Lysosomaler Enzyme-Activitaten sowie von Leuzin Inkorporationraten im Gehirn Yunger and alter Ratten nach Gabe von Piracetam. *Arzneimittelforsch/Drug Res* 1974;24:1588–92.
41. Rägo LK, Allikmets LH, Zarkowsky, AM. Effect of piracetam on the central dopaminergic transmission. *Naunyn Schmiedebergs Arch Pharmacol* 1981;318:36–7.
42. Reuse-Blom S. Effect of piracetam on pial vasculature in the rabbit. In: Betz E, Grote J, Heuser D, eds. Pathophysiol Pharmacother Disord, Sat Symp 2nd 1980;413–415. (Baden-Baden).
43. Rochus L, Reuse JJ. Chlorpromazine and phospholipids metabolism in the rat hypothalamus. Effect of pretreatment with piracetam. *Arch Int Physiol Biochim* 1974;82:1010–1.
44. Sara SJ, David-Remacle M. Recovery from electroconvulsive shock-induced amnesia by exposure to the training environment. Pharmacological enhancement by piracetam. *Psychopharmacologia (Berlin)* 1974;36:59–66.
45. Sara SJ, David-Remacle M, Levander S. Piracetam facilitates retrieval but does not impair extinction of bar-pressing in the rat. *Psychopharmocologia (Berlin)* 1979;61:71–5.
46. Serby M, Segarnick DJ, Mandio Cordasco D, Rotrosen J. Piracetam reduces alcohol withdrawal in mice without potentiating alcohol sedative effects. *Alcoholism: Clin Exp Res* 1982;6:520–2.
47. Sklenowsky A, Chmela Z. Effect of piracetam on FFA in the brain during immobilisation stress. *Acta Nerv Super* 1981;23:221–2.
48. Stegink AJ. The clinical use of piracetam, a new nootropic drug. The treatment of senile involution. Arzneimittelforsch/Drug Res 1972;22:975–7.
49. Terwinghe G, Daumerie J, Nicaise C, Nichaise CE, Rosillon O. Effet thérapeutique du piracetam dans un cas de myoclonus d'action post-anoxique. *Acta Neurol Belg* 1978;78:30–6.
50. Valzelli L, Bernasconi S, Sala A. Piracetam activity may differ according to the age of the recipient mouse. *Int Pharmacopsychiatry* 1980;15:150–6.
51. Vial H, Claustre Y, Pacheco H. Effets de substances stimulantes, sedatives, et hypnotiques sur le taux d'amino-acides cérébrales libres chez le rat. *J Pharmacol* 1974;5:461–78.
52. Vlahov V, Nikolova M, Nikolov R. The effect of piracetam on the local cortical blood flow in cats. *Arch Int Pharmacodyn Ther* 1980;243:103–10.
53. Woelk H. Effect of piracetam on the incorporation of ^{32}P into the phospholipids of neural and glial cells isolated from rabbit cerebral cortex. *Pharmacopsychiatry* 1979;12:251–6.
54. Woelk H. On the influence of piracetam upon neuronal and synaptosomal A phospholipase activity. *Arzneimittelforsch/Drug Res* 1979;29:615–8.
55. Woelk H, Peiler-Ichikawa K. The action of piracetam on the formation of ethanolamine plasmalogen by neuronal microsomes of the developing rat brain. *Arzneimittelforsch/Drug Res* 1978;28:1752–6.
56. Wolthuis OL. Experiments with UCB 6215, a drug which enhances acquisition in rats: its effects compared with those of methamphetamine. *Eur J Pharmacol* 1971;16:283–97.
57. Wurtman RJ, Magil SG, Reinstein DK. Piracetam diminishes hippocampal acetylcholine levels in rats. *Life Sci* 1981;1091–3.

Advances in Neurology, Vol. 43: Myoclonus,
edited by S. Fahn et al. Raven Press,
New York © 1986.

Drugs Acting on Amino Acid Neurotransmitters

B. S. Meldrum

Department of Neurology, Institute of Psychiatry, London, SE 5 8AF, United Kingdom

Amino acids are the most universal neurotransmitters, in terms of the number of neurons or terminals that release them in the mammalian nervous system. They are also the most consistent in their postsynaptic effects. Thus, the neutral amino acids, glycine and γ-aminobutyric acid GABA, are universally inhibitory (56a), and the dicarboxylic amino acids, aspartate and glutamate, are universally excitatory (21,95). By contrast the monoamines, norepinephrine, dopamine, and serotonin occur in a very restricted number of neurons, and their postsynaptic effects vary with the site and with coincident excitatory or inhibitory inputs (69,70).

Burst firing of neurons in the cortex, striatum, hippocampus, or brainstem can be induced either by impaired inhibitory synaptic action or by enhanced excitatory input (68,83). Either abnormality could thus provide the basis for myoclonic or epileptic activity. Evidently, two therapeutic approaches are suggested: pharmacological enhancement of inhibitory transmission and impairment of excitatory transmission.

This chapter reviews both of these approaches. Enhancement of GABA-mediated inhibition is thought to contribute to the mechanism of action of benzodiazepines and valproic acid (11,34,63). Recent experiments utilizing potent and selective antagonists of certain types of excitatory amino acid transmitters suggest that particular types of receptors play a special role in the induction of myoclonus. This provides a novel and as yet unexploited approach to the therapy of myoclonus.

POSSIBLE INVOLVEMENT OF INHIBITORY AND EXCITATORY INTERNEURONS IN POSTHYPOXIC MYOCLONUS

Inhibitory GABAergic interneurons can be identified at the light- and electron-microscopic level by immunocytochemical methods utilizing antibodies to the enzyme glutamic acid decarboxylase (74,82). Such neurons are particularly vulnerable to hypoxic injury. Thus, in infant monkeys, following 30 min of moderate hypoxia, there is a loss of the aspinous stellate neurons in the lamina IV of the neocortex that provide symmetric synapses to the cell bodies of pyramidal neurons (87). Forebrain ischemia in the rat leads to a loss of GABAergic interneurons in the striatum (30,31). GABAergic interneurons in the hippocampus (the hilar polymorphic neurons) are particularly vulnerable to abnormally sustained neuronal activity or drug-induced limbic system status epilepticus (56,88,89).

Studies of enzyme activities in postmortem human brain show that glutamic acid decarboxylase activity is decreased in the cortex and deep brain nuclei when death is preceded by a significant period of impaired cerebral oxygenation, e.g., in death from bronchopneumonia (5). Loss of GABAergic interneurons in human cortex, basal ganglia, or brainstem following hypoxic ischemia has not yet been demonstrated by immunocytochemical means.

It is evident that loss of the recurrent inhibition provided by output neurons activating intrinsic GABAergic neurons could permit the sustained burst discharges that produce myoclonus (68,83).

There is also evidence that ischemia of the spinal cord selectively damages interneurons. In an experimental study in cats, occlusion of the thoracic aorta for 15 to 60 min led to a reduction in the number of interneurons in the spinal gray matter, with a corresponding reduction in the content of both glycine and aspartate (25). This is consistent with electrophysiological data showing that glycine is an inhibitory transmitter in the spinal cord (21) and that aspartate is probably the transmitter for excitatory interneurons responsible for polysynaptic reflex responses (27,77). This type of ischemic lesion at the spinal level is associated with spasticity and myoclonus. It is possible that loss of aspartergic interneurons leads to supersensitivity of postsynaptic N-methyl-D-aspartate (NMDA) receptors, and thus contributes to the myoclonic phenomena.

In the hippocampus, pyramidal neurons in the Sommer sector and end folium are particularly vulnerable to hypoxia/ischemia and to epileptic brain damage (56). These are excitatory neurons liberating glutamate or aspartate. Secondary synaptic changes (both pre- and postsynaptic) have been identified in the hippocampus (17,71) and are presumably a feature of similar neuronal loss at other sites, including the neocortex, striatum, and brainstem.

GLYCINERGIC INHIBITION

Glycine is a major inhibitory transmitter in the spinal cord and brainstem, providing reciprocal inhibition via Ia afferents and interneurons, and recurrent inhibition on motoneurons via Renshaw cells (21). A selective loss of glycinergic interneurons following spinal ischemia is thought to contribute to the spasticity characteristic of this syndrome and may contribute to spinal myoclonus.

Strychnine relatively specifically blocks glycinergic inhibition, producing a syndrome initially characterized by enhanced polysynaptic reflexes and subsequently by intermittent or sustained tonic extension (24).

There are no definitively established mechanisms for enhancing glycinergic inhibition. It has been proposed that some central myorelaxant compounds may do this because they depress polysynaptic reflexes. However, it is more probable that their principal action is to impair the release or postsynaptic action of excitatory transmitters, such as aspartate (see below).

TABLE 1. *Mechanisms for pharmacological enhancement of GABA-mediated inhibition*

GABA agonist
    e.g., muscimol, THIP, imidazoleacetic acid
GABA prodrug
    e.g., cetyl-GABA, benzoyl-GABA, progabide
Facilitating GABA release from terminals
    e.g., baclofen (?), γ-acetylenic GABA (?)
GABA-transaminase inhibition
    e.g., γ-vinyl-GABA, ethanolamine-*O*-sulphate
Allosteric enhancement of affinity (or efficacy) of GABA recognition site
    e.g., benzodiazepines, triazolopyridazines, β-carbolines
Action on chloride ionophore or related site
    e.g., barbiturate, valproate (?)
Inhibition of GABA reuptake
    e.g., nipecotic acid, ethylnipecotate

GABAERGIC INHIBITION

GABA is the principal inhibitory transmitter substance in the brain. GABAergic terminals surround the soma of output neurons in cortex, thalamus, cerebellum, hippocampus, etc., mediating feedback and feedforward inhibition (68). Any treatment that significantly impairs the function of this system will induce focal or generalized seizure activity (51,53). Furthermore, partial impairment, as by a subconvulsant dose of a drug that inhibits the enzyme synthesizing GABA (glutamic acid decarboxylase), induces a condition in which sensory stimulation readily provokes myoclonic responses (53,66).

Thus, pharmacological enhancement of GABA-mediated inhibition is a rational approach to therapy of myoclonus and may be the basis of the two most effective drugs currently available (clonazepam and valproate). Curiously, there is also evidence that GABAergic agents can induce myoclonus (see below).

PHARMACOLOGICAL ENHANCEMENT OF GABAERGIC INHIBITION

Possible mechanisms for pharmacological enhancement of GABA-mediated inhibition have been reviewed previously (55). They are listed in Table 1.

Evidently, the drugs that have been shown to be effective against myoclonus in humans act primarily on a site or sites interacting with the GABA recognition site to enhance the affinity of the site for GABA or the efficacy of GABA at the site. The biochemistry and electrophysiology of this interaction between benzodiazepines and the GABA recognition site have been extensively reviewed (33,58,75). Benzodiazepines increase the number of chloride channels opened in response to a given quantity of GABA (91). This effect is seen *in vitro* with benzodiazepine concentrations similar to those effective against myoclonus *in vivo*.

Valproate also can enhance the inhibitory effects of locally applied GABA in *in vitro* preparations but only at concentrations substantially in excess of those likely to be found in the brain or spinal cord during chronic treatment with valproate (36,45).

A new class of agents acting on the same site as benzodiazepines has recently been identified. These are β-carbolines, which can have either convulsant or anticonvulsant actions (58,61). One such compound, ZK 91296, potently suppresses photically induced myoclonus in the baboon, *Papio papio* (61), suggesting that this or related compounds might be effective in human myoclonic syndromes.

The specific irreversible inhibitor of GABA-transaminase, γ-vinyl-GABA is currently undergoing trials as an antiepileptic agent. This has previously been shown to produce a sustained suppression of myoclonic responses in the photosensitive baboon (63) and thus merits trial in patients with myoclonus.

It is possibly significant that the GABAergic agents that are apparently most efficacious against myoclonic syndromes are the compounds that also appear to modify excitatory amino acid transmission (13). This has been discussed by Chapman (11; *this volume*). Benzodiazepines have been shown to decrease stimulated release of excitatory amino acid transmitters in *in vitro* test systems (2,16), and the inverse agonist at the benzodiazepine site, 6,7-dimethoxy-4-ethyl-β-carboline-3-carboxylate (DMCM) enhances the release of [^{3}H]D-aspartate (40).

SITE OF ANTIMYOCLONIC ACTION OF GABAERGIC AGENTS

There is strong evidence that clonazepam, given intravenously in experimental animals at doses corresponding to those having antimyoclonic activity, enhances the intrinsic inhibition due to GABAergic interneurons in the cortex. Thus, in the cat, clonazepam 0.1 mg/kg, i.v., inhibits the recovery cycle for cortical responses to paired cortical surface stimuli (an effect attributed to enhanced intracortical inhibition) (98). That a similar phenomenon occurs in humans can be concluded on the basis of the enhanced giant somatosensory evoked potential recorded in a patient with cortical myoclonus, after clonazepam (Obeso et al., *this volume*). The increase in the amplitude of the P 25 wave is due to enhanced hyperpolarization of the soma of pyramidal neurons, due to augmentation of the effect of the intrinsic GABAergic inputs (see Fig. 11.1 in ref. 54).

Enhancement of the inhibitory action of GABA applied iontophoretically to cortical neurons has been demonstrated with local application of valproate (41). Action at the cortical level is indicated by biochemical studies in the rat showing changes in cortical GABA and aspartate concentration (14; A. Chapman, *this volume*).

An important antiepileptic action of GABAergic agents at the level of the substantia nigra has been proposed on the basis of suppression of tonic seizures induced by electroshock or pentylenetetrazol in rats (39). This action may, however, be more important for preventing the evolution to the tonic phase of seizure activity rather than as a specific antimyoclonic activity.

In the brainstem of the rat, the inhibitory responses of reticular neurons to iontophoretically applied GABA or muscimol are enhanced by the simultaneous application of valproate (33) in the rat. Intravenous administration of clonazepam, 0.1 to 0.2 mg/kg, reverses the antagonism of GABA-induced inhibition produced

TABLE 2. *GABAergic agents producing myoclonus*

Agent	Afferent type
GABA agonists Muscimol, THIP	Cortical (diffuse)
Benzodiazepines Lorazepam (baboons)	Reticular (generalized)
Barbiturates Etomidate	Cortical and reticular

by iontophoretically applied bicuculline in the rat brainstem (6). There is evidence that the serotonergic neurons of the raphe nuclei are under GABAergic inhibitory control and that intravenous benzodiazepines can potentiate the inhibitory action (32). This effect would explain the decrease in serotonin turnover produced by clonazepam (81). However effects on serotonergic activity do not appear to contribute to the antimyoclonic or antiepileptic activity of clonazepam or valproate (38,81).

In contrast, it is possible that altered function of the serotonergic system is responsible for the head jerks induced in mice by clonazepam (72) and the reticular myoclonus induced in baboons by lorazepam (8). The syndrome in mice is blocked by cyproheptadine and that in baboons by L-5-hydroxytryptophan (8,72). Benzodiazepines probably differ in their relative activity at different levels of the nervous system (43,58). In general, their antimyoclonic actions overcome their myoclonic effects, but differences in relative potencies of benzodiazepines at different sites, or species, or individual differences in the proportions of benzodiazepine receptor subtypes may permit the emergence of myoclonic phenomena (see next section).

MYOCLONIC SYNDROMES INDUCED BY GABAERGIC AGENTS

Paradoxically, several GABAergic agents can induce myoclonic syndromes (Table 2). A diffuse distal myoclonus is seen in baboons and humans after the potent GABA agonist muscimol (15,76) and in baboons after moderately high doses of the bicyclic GABA agonist tetrahydroisooxazolopyridineol (THIP) (65). The mechanism for this is not clear but some possibilities are listed in Table 3. A depolarizing action of the agonists on dendritic or axonal sites at the cortical level is most probable. The mechanism is not the same as for the benzodiazepines that induce myoclonus, e.g. lorazepam and diazepam in baboons (8,93). This latter myoclonus appears to be reticular in origin. It is not associated with any paroxysmal cortical activity and involves the limbs and trunk simultaneously. It is exacerbated by L-allylglycine (an inhibitor of glutamic acid decarboxylase) and is prevented by valproate and by L-5-hydroxytryptophan. A somewhat similar myoclonus has been reported in humans after etomidate, a short-acting, barbiturate-like compound that acts on the GABA receptor complex to enhance GABAergic inhibition (50).

TABLE 3. *GABA agonists—possible mechanism for induction of myoclonus*

Action at GABA$_A$ sites
Postsynaptic, hyperpolarizing action
Desensitization (effect of endogenous GABA limited to hippocampus)
Diffuse activation (interferes with temporospatial patterning of recurrent inhibition)
Postsynaptic, depolarizing action
Dendrites and axons
Presynaptic
Decreasing GABA release
Enhancing glutamate release
Action at GABA$_B$ site
Inhibiting NA, DA, 5-HT release

FUTURE USE OF GABAERGIC AGENTS IN HUMAN MYOCLONIC SYNDROMES

Enhancement of GABA-mediated inhibition as by clonazepam and valproate is currently the most successful pharmacological approach to the therapy of myoclonus. What are the possibilities for improved therapy exploiting this approach? The particular advantage of the benzodiazepines appears to be that they enhance the physiological effect of synaptically released GABA and thus preserve required temporospatial patterning of inhibition in relation to normal and abnormal output from the cortex or elsewhere. Agents acting on the benzodiazepine receptor differ in terms of their behavioral pharmacological actions and in terms of their binding characteristics to membranes prepared from different brain regions (e.g., hippocampus and cerebellum) (58). Such differences are small when the traditional 1,4-benzodiazepines are studied but are marked, for example, with β-carbolines. Experimental studies have shown that 1,5-benzodiazepines, such as clobazam, may have antimyoclonic activity similar to 1,4-benzodiazepines (12,64) but may produce less sedation or impairment of complex motor performance.

The other significant therapeutic approach that provides a GABAergic effect is inhibition of GABA-transaminase by γ-vinyl GABA or similar agents. Trials of such agents would provide information of great theoretical value and might identify an important sole or adjunctive therapy.

EXCITATORY AMINO ACIDS

Figure 1A illustrates the molecular formulas of the amino acids found in the mammalian brain that have a direct excitatory action on single cells when applied iontophoretically in the spinal cord or brain (21,90,95).

A neurotransmitter role is highly probable for both glutamate and aspartate in many brain regions. Evidence relating to the sulfinic and sulfonic amino acids is much less conclusive.

Two or more ionic mechanisms underlie the excitatory action of glutamate and aspartate. An increase in G_{Na} provides direct depolarization and may be associated with an increase in G_{Ca} that is either primary or secondary to the depolarization

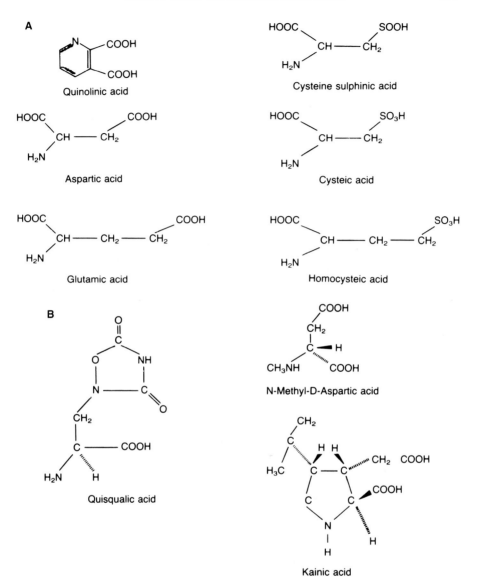

FIG. 1. Molecular formulas of **(A)** acidic amino acids found in the brain that have potent excitatory actions on single units when applied iontophoretically, and **(B)** three analogs of the naturally occurring compounds that act preferentially on distinct receptors to produce differing patterns of excitation.

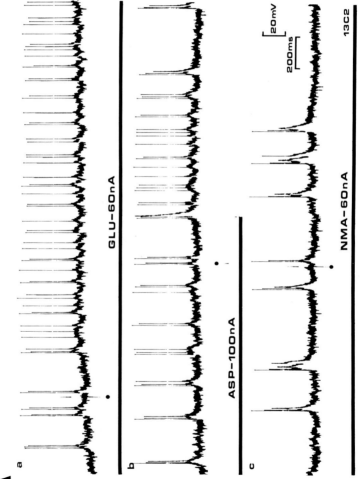

FIG. 2. Differing excitatory actions of various dicarboxylic amino acids as shown by intracellular records from neurons in the head of the caudate nucleus in the cat. **(A):** Extracellular iontophoretic application of glutamate, aspartate or N-methyl-DL-aspartate (as indicated by the horizontal bars). Note that in this cell N-methyl-DL-aspartate induced only burst firing and that relatively more burst firing is induced by aspartate than by glutamate. **(B):** Iontophoresis of quisqualate induced repetitive firing without depolarization plateaus or burst firing. In the same cell, N-methyl-DL-aspartate and quinolinic acid induce depolarization plateaus and burst firing. (From Herrling et al., ref. 37, with permission.)

B

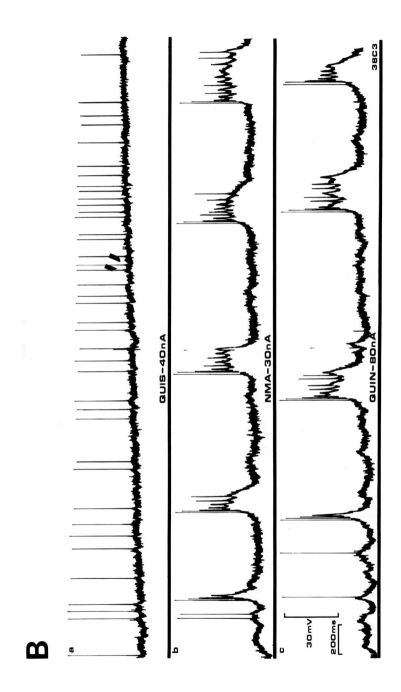

QUIS-40nA

NMA-30nA

QUIN-80nA

30mV

200ms

38C3

produced by the increase in G_{Na}. There is a further effect, which was initially described in spinal neurons with iontophoresis of homocysteic acid but is also seen in *in vitro* spinal neuron preparations with administration of aspartate or other amino acids (29,42,48). This appears as a decrease in membrane conductance, probably due to diminished G_K. However, it may also be interpreted in terms of induction of a region of negative slope in the current–voltage relationship (47).

The membrane receptor sites can be classified into three or four types according to the preferred agonists (95). Studies on amphibian or rodent spinal cord give a classification into receptors preferring (a) NMDA, (b) quisqualic acid, and (c) kainic acid (Fig. 1B).

Studies utilizing Na^+ release from brain slices give a broadly similar classification but suggest a fourth type of glutamate-preferring receptor (44,92). Not only do these receptors show preferential responses to specific agonists, which can be differentially blocked by selective antagonists, but they also seem to be coupled to different membrane ionic channels. Thus the pattern of firing, induced by activation of the different types of receptor, is distinctive. NMDA produces repetitive burst firing when applied to spinal interneurons (46) or to striatal neurons (37) (Fig. 2). This pattern of firing is dependent on a paroxysmal membrane potential shift similar to that associated with myoclonus or epileptic activity (83). Quisqualate does not produce this burst pattern of firing but rapidly enhances firing rate to a plateau. In contrast, kainic acid produces a slow progressive enhancement of firing frequency (53). The endogenous agents acting on these receptors are not yet definitively identified. Among those found in the brain, aspartic acid is most effective at NMDA-preferring receptors and can induce burst firing. Glutamate is the strongest candidate for the endogenous agent acting at the quisqualic acid–preferring receptor. There is no clear candidate for the kainic acid receptor. It remains possible that the sulfinic and sulfonic acid analogs of glutamate and aspartate or various di- or tripeptide derivatives are significantly involved in excitatory transmission.

In the spinal cord, "monosynaptic" excitation of anterior horn cells (from stretch or Ia afferents) utilizes quisqualate-preferring receptors, whereas polysynaptic excitation of anterior horn cells (that mediates, for example, crossed extensor reflexes) utilizes NMDA-preferring receptors (27,77). The latter appear to be activated principally by aspartergic interneurons. Relative overactivity in this system could result from impaired concurrent inhibition, from a faulty pattern of activation of spinal interneurons through corticospinal or reticulospinal inputs, or from supersensitive postsynaptic receptors (arising from "deafferentation"). Thus, the pattern of neuronal activation illustrated in Fig. 2 can be seen as the *final common pathophysiology of myoclonus*, for spinal and for reticular and cortical myoclonus. It can explain how a brief volley in the corticospinal tract can be translated into a more sustained "myoclonic" discharge of anterior horn cells. It does not explain asterixis or "negative myoclonus."

However, burst firing can also be induced in spinal interneurons, and shows somewhat different properties from that in motoneurons. It is readily evoked by

TABLE 4. *Antimyoclonic action by impairment of excitatory transmission*

Decrease maximal rates of synthesis of glutamate, aspartate, etc.
Decrease synaptic release (selectively)
  Glutamate autoreceptors
  Other presynaptic receptors, e.g., baclofen
  Ca^{2+} calmodulin-dependent protein kinase
Decrease postsynaptic action
  Selective antagonists (*not* receptors on inhibitory interneurons)
  Down-regulation of receptors

---

iontophoresis of glutamate (an effect not seen in motoneurons) (73). Thus, negative myoclonus could arise as a result of abnormal inputs to spinal interneurons and motoneurons, as a specific result of burst firing in inhibitory interneurons, or as a result of supersensitivity of motoneurons to glycine.

There is also evidence for aspartergic synapses within the brainstem and cerebellum (97). The best documented pathway is the eighth nerve relay in the cochlear nucleus (49,96).

In the neocortex, there is evidence for glutamatergic and aspartergic transmission, providing the output from a proportion of the pyramidal neurons, including some that project intracortically and some that act at the thalamic level (including the lateral geniculate) (3).

IMPAIRMENT OF EXCITATORY TRANSMISSION

It is evident that agents that impair excitatory transmission might reduce myoclonic activity by actions at almost every level of the central nervous system, including (most obviously) afferent and efferent pathways but also cortical and brainstem relay systems. Mechanisms for such impairment are listed in Table 4. It is possible that valproate acts on the synthesis of aspartate and on long-term regulation of membrane receptor numbers (11) and that benzodiazepines and barbiturates diminish synaptic release of excitatory amino acids (58,86).

However, we shall consider in detail postsynaptic antagonists of excitatory amino acids, as we have recently identified a potent and specific action of NMDA antagonists against myoclonus in a wide range of animal models.

ANTAGONISTS OF EXCITATORY AMINO ACIDS

Many natural and synthetic analogs of dicarboxylic amino acids have now been shown to block excitation induced by glutamate or aspartate but not to alter excitation induced by, for example, acetylcholine or substance P. Table 5 lists some of these and indicates their relative specificity for the different types of excitatory amino acid receptor. Whereas several compounds are highly potent and selective for NMDA, comparably selective agents are not available for the other receptor types.

Administered focally *in vivo*, these antagonists block physiologically evoked activity in particular pathways. Thus, NMDA antagonists block reflexly evoked

TABLE 5. *Antagonists of excitatory amino acids[a]*

	Potency against[b] NMDA	Quisqualate	Kainic acid
Glutamic acid diethylester	0	+ +	0
γ-D-Glutamylglycine	+ + +	+	+ +
2-Amino-5-phosphonopentanoic acid	+ + +	0	0
2-Amino-7-phosphonoheptanoic acid	+ + +	0	0
cis-2,3-Piperidine decarboxylic acid	+ +	+	+ +
D-α-aminoadipic acid	+ +	0	+
3-Amino-1-hydroxy-2-pyrrolidone	+	0	0

[a]Data from Peet et al., ref. 77, and Watkins and Evans, ref. 95.
[b]Relative potency against excitation induced in the spinal cord by selective agonists represented on a three-point scale.

polysynaptic excitatory activity on dorsal horn interneurons (22,27). Monosynaptic excitation is not blocked by specific NMDA antagonists but is blocked by *cis*-2,3-piperidine dicarboxylate (which impairs excitation at quisqualate and kainic acid receptors as well as NMDA receptors) (27).

ANTIMYOCLONIC ACTION OF EXCITATORY AMINO ACID ANTAGONISTS

We have tested a wide range of antagonists of excitatory amino acids as potential antimyoclonic or antiepileptic agents in the animal models listed in Table 6.

Because these antagonists are highly polar compounds and might therefore have difficulty penetrating the blood–brain barrier, we began by evaluating them by intracerebroventricular injection in DBA/2 mice (that show a sound-stimulus–induced sequence of wild running, clonus, and tonus) (10) (Table 7). This preliminary study established that antagonists that potently block excitation induced by NMDA are effective anti-epileptic agents (19). In particular, the straight-chain

TABLE 6. *Protection against myoclonus by systemic administration of amino acid antagonists*

Animal model	Protection	mmol/kg	Ref.
DBA/2 mice	2-APH	0.04–0.33	19
Sound-induced seizures	cis-2,3-PDA	0.33–1.0	20
Swiss S mice	2-APH	0.33	23
Chemically induced seizures			
Rats			
High-pressure neurological syndrome	2-APH	0.8	67
	cis-2,3-PDA	2.0	1
Papio papio			
Photically induced myoclonus	2-APH	1.00	59
	2-APV	3.0	
	cis-2,3-PDA	1.0–3.3	

TABLE 7. *Protection against clonic seizure phase following sound stimulation in DBA/2 mice by intracerebroventricular injection of antagonists of excitation due to NMDA (and of diazepam and valproate)[a]*

Antagonist	ED_{50} (μmole)
γ-D-Glutamyl glycine	0.046
2-Amino-5-phosphonopentanoic acid	0.022
2-Amino-6-phosphonohexanoic acid	0.14
2-Amino-7-phosphonoheptanoic acid	0.0018
cis-2,3-Piperidine dicarboxylic acid	0.017
Diazepam	0.011
Valproate	6.00

[a]Data from Chapman et al., ref. 10, and Croucher et al., refs. 19, 20.

phosphono higher analogs of glutamate and aspartate, such as 2 amino-5-phosphonopentanoic acid (2-APP) and 2-amino-7-phosphonoheptanoic acid (2-APH) (which have minimal activity against quisqualic acid– or kainic acid–induced excitation) were very potent. Indeed, they were more active when administered by this route in DBA/2 mice than any established anticonvulsants, including benzodiazepines (10) (Table 7) (Fig. 3). We have subsequently established, using ³H-labeled 2-APH that 2-APH does enter the brain when administered systemically (9) and is effective when given intraperitoneally or intravenously against the different myoclonic models listed in Table 6.

The activity against chemically induced seizures is of particular interest (Table 8). Convulsant compounds that were effectively antagonized by 2-APH pretreatment

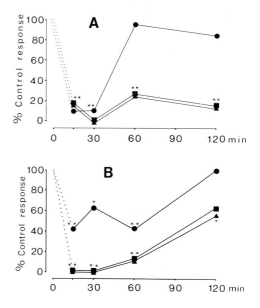

FIG. 3. Time course of antiepileptic action following the intracerebroventricular injection of **(A)** 2-amino-5-phosphonovaleric acid, 0.033 μmol, and **(B)** 2-amino-phosphonoheptanoic acid, 0.0033 μmol, in DBA/2 mice, age 20 to 27 days. Mice were exposed to a white sound (109 dB) at the indicated times after the injection and the incidence of wild running (●) (WR), clonic jerking (▲), and tonic extension (■) recorded. (*N*, 10 for each time point). (*)$p < 0.05$; (**)$p < 0.01$. (From Croucher, De Sarro, and Meldrum, *unpublished data.*)

TABLE 8. *Protection against clonus by pretreatment with 2-amino-7-phosphonoheptanoic acid (0.33 mmol/kg) on seizures in Swiss S mice*[a]

Convulsant	ED_{50} (mmol/kg, i.p.) for clonic convulsions	
	Control	After 2-APH
N-Methyl-DL-aspartate	1.38	2.32
Kainic acid	0.38	0.35
Quinolinic acid	7.00	6.40
3-Mercaptopropionic acid	0.33	0.48
Thiosemicarbazide	0.11	0.28
Bicuculline	0.012	0.013
Picrotoxin	0.0087	0.0156
Methyl-6,7-dimethoxy-4-ethyl-β-Carboline-3-carboxylate	0.035	0.23

[a]From Czuczwar and Meldrum, ref. 23.

included 3-mercaptopropionic acid, thiosemicarbazide, and 6,7-dimethoxy-4-ethyl-β-carboline-3-carboxylate. These compounds greatly enhance the stimulated release of preloaded [^{3}H]D-aspartate from rat cortical minislices (40,84,86). Thus, the clonus and the tonic seizures induced by these convulsants may be a direct consequence of the excessive release of aspartate, or some other transmitter acting on the NMDA receptor. The protective effect of 2-APH presumably results from direct competition at this site.

Tremor and clonus are a characteristic feature of the *high-pressure neurological syndrome* seen in experimental animals at pressures above 40 atmospheres absolute (35). Substantial protection against this syndrome is provided by 2-APH and by *cis*-2,3-piperidine dicarboxylic acid (36,67). Interestingly, other drugs offering protection include valproate and benzodiazepines (4).

Of all animal models of stimulus-induced myoclonus, photically induced myoclonic activity in the Senegalese baboon, *Papio papio* shows the closest correspondence to posthypoxic action myoclonus in terms of its pharmacological responsiveness (see Naquet and Meldrum, *this volume*). Thus, it is highly sensitive to valproate and clonazepam (52,57,66) and also responds to L-5-hydroxytryptophan (94). This syndrome also responds to the NMDA antagonists when given intravenously. In particular, 2-APH provides complete protection for several hours (59; Naquet and Meldrum, *this volume*).

SITE OF ACTION OF EXCITATORY AMINO ACID ANTAGONISTS

Electrophysiological studies on the cat and rat spinal cord indicate that antagonists such as 2-APH and *cis*-2,3-piperidine dicarboxylic acid have a powerful influence on motoneuron firing. Nevertheless, actions at the brainstem level and in the cortex are likely following systemic administration.

Direct application of 2-APP or of 2-APH to cortical neurons is as effective at blocking excitation due to aspartate or NMDA on cortical neurons as on spinal motoneurons (60,79). Furthermore, intraperitoneal administration of 2-APH in the rat blocks the excitatory effect of quinolinic acid applied iontophoretically to cortical neurons (78). Myoclonic jerks in the rat made epileptic by cobalt implantation in the sensorimotor cortex can be suppressed by superfusing the cortex with 2-APP (18). Focal injection of small quantities of 2-APH into the substantia nigra pars reticulata suppresses tonic extension induced by electroshock (28a).

CENTRALLY ACTING MYORELAXANT DRUGS

Drugs that act at the spinal or brainstem level to reduce spasticity, such as mephenesin and baclofen, have antimyoclonic action in some animal models (7,62) and are occasionally of value in the treatment of myoclonus. Their mechanism of action is not well understood, but *in vitro* studies with brain slices show that baclofen decreases the stimulation-induced release of excitatory amino acids (80). A similar mechanism of action for the novel myorelaxant DS103-282, tizanidine, has been proposed on the basis of single unit responses in the spinal cord (26). However, this compound has been shown to have a relatively selective postsynaptic action against the excitation induced by NMDA (22). It suppresses reflexly induced myoclonus in DBA/2 mice and in photosensitive baboons (28). The potential use of this or related compounds in the therapy of myoclonus merits further study.

IMPAIRMENT OF EXCITATORY TRANSMISSION: FUTURE CLINICAL APPLICATION

None of the potent selective antagonists of excitation due to NMDA has been tested in humans. It is not known whether any of them are suitable for this purpose, as relevant toxicity data are not available. They are highly polar compounds with very much greater activity when given directly into the brain then when given systemically. Thus, the development of prodrugs that release the active moiety in the brain could be useful. Development of variants of valproate and of the benzo-diazepines with greater or more specific actions on excitatory transmission could provide a therapeutic advance.

This pharmacological approach is of great theoretical importance. Experimental studies in humans based on the new understanding of the role of particular types of excitatory receptor in the physiology of the motor system could contribute importantly to our understanding of the different myoclonic syndromes.

SUMMARY

The most potent agents currently available for suppressing myoclonic activity in animals and humans act to enhance GABA-mediated inhibition and/or to diminish amino acid–induced excitation.

Postsynaptic GABA-mediated inhibition plays an important role at the cortical level, diminishing the effect of augmented afferent activity and preventing patho-logically enhanced output. Enhancement of GABAergic inhibition, principally at the cortical level but also at lower levels, by clonazepam and by valproate appears to be a predominant element in their antimyoclonic action. Studies in various animal models, including photically induced myoclonus in the baboon, *P papio*, indicate the value of other approaches to enhancing GABA-mediated inhibition. Among such approaches meriting evaluation in humans are inhibition of GABA-transaminase activity by γ-vinyl GABA and action at some of the benzodiazepine receptors to enhance the action of GABA, as by the novel anticonvulsant β-carbolines.

Excitatory transmission mediated by dicarboxylic amino acids appears to play a role in myoclonus, especially at the spinal level, but also in the brainstem, cerebellum, basal ganglia, and cortex. Among various novel agents that act at the postsynaptic receptor site to antagonize such excitation, those specifically blocking excitation induced by aspartate and/or NMDA prevent myoclonic activity in a wide range of animal models. Further research is required before such agents can be evaluated in humans.

ACKNOWLEDGMENTS

We thank the Wellcome Trust and the Medical Research Council for financial support.

REFERENCES

1. Angel A, Halsey MJ, Little H, Meldrum BS, Ross JAS, Rostain JC, Wardley-Smith B. Specific effects of drugs at pressure: animal investigations. *Proc R Soc Lond [Biol]* 1984;304:85–94.
2. Baba A, Okumura S, Mizuo H, Iwata H. Inhibition by diazepam and γ-aminobutyric acid of depolarisation-induced release of ^{14}C cysteine sulfinate and ^3H-glutamate in rat hippocampal slices. *J Neurochem* 1983;40:280–4.
3. Baughman RW, Gilberg CD. Aspartate and glutamate as possible neurotransmitters of cells in layer 6 of the visual cortex. *Nature* 1980;287:848–50.
4. Bichard AR, Little HJ. Drugs that increase γ-aminobutyric acid transmission protect against the high pressure neurological syndrome. *Br J Pharmacol* 1982;76:447–52.
5. Bowen DM, Smith CB, White P, Davison AN. Neurotransmitter-related enzymes and indices of hypoxia in senile dementia and other abiotrophies. *Brain* 1976;99:459–96.
6. Bowery NG, Dray A. Reversal of the action of amino acid antagonists by barbiturates and other hypnotic drugs. *Br J Pharmacol* 1978;63:197–215.
7. Bowser-Riley F. Mechanistic studies on high-pressure neurological studies. *Phil Trans Soc Lond [Biol]* 1983;304:31–41.
8. Cepeda C, Valin A, Calderazzo L, Stutzmann JM, Naquet R. Myoclonies induites par certaines benzodiazepines chez le *Papio papio*. *Electroencephalogr Clin Neurophysiol* 1981;52:647–51.
9. Chapman AG, Collins JF, Meldrum BS, Westerberg E. Uptake of a novel anticonvulsant compound, 2-amino-7-phosphono (4,5¹-³H-heptanoic acid, into mouse brain. *Neurosci Lett* 1983;37:75–80.
10. Chapman AG, Croucher MJ, Meldrum BS. Evaluation of anticonvulsant drugs in DBA/2 mice with sound-induced seizures. *Arznmittelforsch* 1984;34:1261–4.
11. Chapman A, Keane PE, Meldrum BS, Simiand J, Vernieres JC. Mechanism of anticonvulsant of valproate. *Prog Neurobiol* 1982;19:315–59.
12. Chapman AG, Horton RW, Meldrum BS. Anticonvulsant action of a 1,2-benzodiazepine, clobazam, in reflex epilepsy. *Epilepsia* 1978;19:293–9.
13. Chapman AG, Meldrum BS, Mendes E. Acute anticonvulsant activity of structural analogues of valproic acid and changes in brain GABA and aspartate content. *Life Sci* 1983;32:2023–31.

14. Chapman AG, Riley K, Evans MC, Meldrum BS. Acute effects of sodium valproate and γ-vinyl GABA on regional amino acid metabolism in the rat brain. *Neurochem Res* 1982;7:1089–1105.
15. Chase TN, Taminga CA. GABA system participation in human motor, cognitive and endocrine function. In: Krogsgaard-Larsen P, Scheel-Kruger J, Kofod H, eds. GABA-neurotransmitters. Copenhagen: Munksgaard, 1979;283–94.
16. Collins GGS. The effects of chlordiazepoxide on synaptic transmission and amino acid neuro-transmitter release in slices of rat olfactory cortex. *Brain Res* 1981;224:389–404.
17. Cotman CW, Nadler JV. Reactive synaptogenesis in the hippocampus. In: Cotman CW, ed. Neuronal plasticity. New York: Raven Press, 1978;227–71.
18. Coutinho-Netto J, Abdul-GHani AS, Collins JF, Bradford, HF. Is glutamate a trigger factor in epileptic hyperactivity? *Epilepsia* 1981;22:289–96.
19. Croucher MJ, Collins JF, Meldrum BS. Anticonvulsant action of excitatory amino acid antagonists. *Science* 1982;216:899–901.
20. Croucher MJ, Meldrum BS, Collins JF. Anticonvulsant and proconvulsant properties of a series of structural isomers of piperidine dicarboxylic acid. *Neuropharmacology* 1984;23:476–72.
21. Curtis DR, Johnston GAR. Amino acid transmitters in the mammalian central nervous system. *Ergeb Physiol Biol Chem Exp Pharmacol* 1974;69:97–188.
22. Curtis DR, Leah JD, Peet MJ. Spinal interneurone depression by DS 103-282. *Br J Pharmacol* 1983;79:9–11.
23. Czuczwar SJ, Meldrum B. Protection against chemically induced seizures by 2-amino-7-phos-phonoheptanoic acid. *Eur J Pharmacol* 1982;83:335–8.
24. Davidoff RA. Studies of neurotransmitter actions, GABA, glycine and convulsants. In: Ward AA, Penry JK, Purpura D, eds. Epilepsy. New York: Raven Press, 1983:53–85.
25. Davidoff RA, Graham LT, Shank RP, Werman R, Aprison MH. Changes in amino acid concen-trations associated with loss of spinal interneurons. *J Neurochem* 1967;14:1025–1031.
26. Davies J. Selective depression of synaptic transmission of spinal neurones in the cat by a new centrally acting muscle relaxant, 5-chloro-4-(2-imidazolin-2-yl-amino)-2,1,3-benzothiodazole (DS 103-282). *Br J Pharmacol* 1983;76:473–81.
27. Davies J, Watkins JC. Role of excitatory amino acid receptors in mono- and polysynaptic excitation in the cat spinal cord. *Brain Res* 1983;266:83–95.
28. De Sarro CB, Croucher MJ, Meldrum BS. Anticonvulsant actions of DS 103-282: Pharmacological studies in rodents and the baboon, *Papio papio*. *Neuropharmacology* 1984;23:525–30.
28a. De Sarro, G, Meldrum BS, Reavill C. Anticonvulsant action of 2-amino-7-phosphonoheptanoic acid in the substantia nigra. *Eur J Pharmacol* 1984;106:175–9.
29. Engberg I, Flatman JA, Lambert JDC. The actions of excitatory amino acids on motoneurons in the feline spinal cord. *J Physiol (Lond)* 1979;288:227–61.
30. Francis A, Pulsinelli W. Response of GABAergic and cholinergic neurons to transient cerebral ischemia. *Brain Res* 1982;243:271–8.
31. Francis A, Pulsinelli W. Increased binding of ³H-GABA to striatal membranes following ischaemia. *J Neurochem* 1983;40:1497–9.
32. Gallager DW. Benzodiazepines: potentiation of a GABA inhibitory response in the dorsal raphe nucleus. *Eur J Pharmacol* 1978;49:133–43.
33. Gent JP, Phillips NI. Sodium di-n-propylacetate (valproate) potentiates responses to GABA and muscimol on single central neurones. *Brain Res* 1980;197:275–8.
34. Haefely W, Pieri L, Polc P, Schaffner R. General pharmacology and neuropharmacology of benzodiazepine derivatives. In: Hoffmeister F, Stille G, eds. Handbook of experimental phar-macology 55/11, pp. 13–262, Berlin: Springer-Verlag, 1981.
35. Halsey MJ. Effects of high pressure on the central nervous system. *Phys Rev* 1982;62:1342–77.
36. Harrison NL, Simmonds MA. Sodium valproate enhances responses to GABA receptor activation only at high concentrations. *Brain Res* 1982;250:201–4.
37. Herrling PL, Morris R, Salt TE. Effects of excitatory amino acids and their antagonists on membrane and action potentials of cat caudate neurones. *J Physiol (Lond)* 1983;339:207–22.
38. Horton RW, Anlezark GM, Sawaya MCB, Meldrum BS. Monoamine and GABA metabolism and the anticonvulsant action of di-n-propylacetate and ethanolamine-O-sulphate. *Eur J Pharmacol* 1977;41:387–97.
39. Iadarola MJ, Gale K. Substantia nigra: site of anticonvulsant activity mediated by γ-aminobutyric acid. *Science* 1982;218:1237–40.

40. Kerwin RW, Meldrum BS. Effect on cerebral ³H-D-aspartate release of 3-mercaptopropionic acid and methyl 6,7-dimethoxy-4-ethyl-β-carboline-3-carboxylate. *Eur J Pharmacol* 1983;89:265–9.
41. Kerwin RW, Olpe HR, Schmutz M. The effect of sodium-n-dipropyl-acetate on γ-aminobutyric acid-dependent inhibition in the rat cortex and substantia nigra in relation to its anticonvulsant activity. *Br J Pharmacol* 1980;71:545–51.
42. Lambert JDC, Flatman JA, Engberg I. Actions of excitatory amino acids on memrane conductance and potential in motoneurones. In: Di Chiara G, Gessa GL, eds. Glutamate as a neurotransmitter. New York: Raven Press; 1981:205–16.
43. Laurent JP, Mangold M, Humbel U, Haefely W. Reduction by two benzodiazepines and pentobarbitone of the multiunit activity in substantia nigra, hippocampus, nucleus locus coeruleus and nucleus raphe dorsalis of encephale isole rats. *Neuropharmacology* 1983;22:501–11.
44. Luini A, Goldberg O, Teichberg VI. Distinct pharmacological properties of excitatory amino acid receptors in the rat striatum: A study by Na⁺ efflux assay. *Proc Natl Acad Sci USA* 1981;78:3250–4.
45. MacDonald RL, Bergey GK. Valproic acid augments GABA-mediated postsynaptic inhibition in cultured mammalian neurons. *Brain Res* 1979;170:558–62.
46. MacDonald JF, Nistri A. A comparison of the action of glutamate, ibotenate, and other related amino acids on feline spinal interneurones. *J Physiol (Lond)* 1978;275:449–65.
47. MacDonald JF, Porietis AV, Wojtowicz JM. L-aspartic acid induces a region of negative slope conductance in the current-voltage relationship of cultured spinal cord neurones. *Brain Res* 1982;237:248–53.
48. MacDonald JF, Wojtowicz JM. The effects of L-glutamate and its analogues upon the membrane conductance of central murine neurones in culture. *Can J Physiol Pharmacol* 1982;60:282–96.
49. Martin MR. The effects of iontophoretically applied antagonists on auditory nerve and amino acid evoked excitation of anteroventral cochlear nucleus neurons. *Neuropharmacology* 1980;19:519–28.
50. Meink HM, Mohlenhof O, Kettler D. Neurophysiological effects of etomidate, a new short acting hypnotic. *Electroencephalogr Clin Neurophysiol* 1980;50:515–22.
51. Meldrum BS. Epilepsy and GABA-mediated inhibition. *Int Rev Neurobiol* 1975;17:1–36.
52. Meldrum BS. Photosensitive epilepsy in Papio papio as a model for drug studies. In: Cobb WA, van Duijn H, eds. Contemp Clin Neurophys Supp. 34, Electroenceph Clin Neurophysiol. Amsterdam: Elsevier, 317–322, 1978.
53. Meldrum B. Convulsant drugs, anticonvulsants and GABA-mediated neuronal inhibition. In: *GABA-Neurotransmitters*, Krogsgaard-Larsen P, Scheel-Kruger J, Kofod H, eds. Copenhagen: Munksgaard, 1979;390–405.
54. Meldrum B. Epilepsy. In: Davidson AN, Thompson RHS, eds. The molecular basis of neuropathology. London: Edward Arnold, 1981;265–301.
55. Meldrum B. Pharmacology of GABA. *Clin Neuropharmacol* 1982;5:293–316.
56. Meldrum BS. Metabolic factors during prolonged seizures and their relation to nerve cell death. In: Delgado-Escueta AV, Wasterlain CG, Treiman DM, Porter RJ, eds. Status epilepticus. New York: Raven Press, 1983;261–75. (Advances in Neurology, vol. 34).
56a. Meldrum BS. GABA and other amino acids. In: Frey HH, Janz D, eds. Antiepileptic drugs. Berlin: Springer-Verlag, 1985:153–188.
57. Meldrum BS, Anlezark G, Balzano E, Horton RW, Trimble M. Photically induced epilepsy in Papio papio as a model for drug studies. In: Meldrum BS, Marsden CD, eds. Primate models of neurological disorders. New York: Raven Press, 1975;119–28. (Advances in Neurology, vol. 10).
58. Meldrum BS, Braestrup C. GABA and the anticonvulsant action of benzodiazepines and related drugs. In: Bowery N, ed. Actions and interactions of GABA and benzodiazepines. New York: Raven Press.
59. Meldrum BS, Croucher MJ, Badman G, Collins JF. Antiepileptic action of excitatory amino acid antagonists in the photosensitive baboon, Papio papio. *Neurosci Lett* 1983;39:101–4.
60. Meldrum BS, Croucher MJ, Czuczwar SJ, Collins JF, Curry K, Joseph M, Stone TW. A comparison of the anticonvulsant potency of (±) 2-amino-5-phosphonopentanoic acid and (±) 2-amino-7-phosphonoheptanoic acid. *Neuroscience* 1983;9:925–30.
61. Meldrum BS, Evans MC, Braestrup C. Anticonvulsant action in the photosensitive baboon, Papio papio, of a novel β-carboline derivative, ZK 91296. *Eur J Pharmacol* 1983;91:255–9.
62. Meldrum BS, Horton RW. Neuronal inhibition mediated by GABA, and patterns of convulsions

in photosensitive baboons with epilepsy *(Papio papio)*. In: Harris P, Mawdsley-Churchill C, eds. The natural history and management of epilepsy. Edinburgh: Livingstone, 1974;55–64.

63. Meldrum B, Horton R. Blockade of epileptic responses in the photosensitive baboon, Papio papio, by two irreversible inhibitors of GABA-transaminase, γ-acetylenic GABA (4-amino-hex-5-enoic acid) and γ-vinyl GABA (4-amino-hex-5-enoic acid) *Psychopharmacology* 1978;69:47–50.

64. Meldrum BS, Horton RW. Anticonvulsant activity in photosensitive baboons, *Papio papio*, of two new 1,5-benzodiazepines. *Psychopharmacology* 1979;60:277–80.

65. Meldrum B, Horton R. Effects of the bicyclic GABA agonist, THIP, on myoclonic and seizure responses in mice and baboons with reflex epilepsy. *Eur J Pharmacol* 1980;61:231–37.

66. Meldrum BS, Horton RW, Toseland PA. A primate model for testing anticonvulsant drugs. *Arch Neurol* 1975;32:289–94.

67. Meldrum B, Wardley-Smith B, Halsey H, Rostain J-C. 2-Amino-phosphonoheptanoic acid protects against the high pressure neurological syndrome. *Eur J Pharmacol* 1983;87:501–2.

68. Meldrum BS, Wilkins AJ. Photosensitive epilepsy. In: Schwartzkroin PA, Wheal HV, eds. Electrophysiology of epilepsy. London: Academic Press, 1983:51–77.

69. Moore RY, Bloom FE. Central catecholamine neuron systems: anatomy and physiology of the dopamine system. *Annu Rev Neurosci* 1978;1:129–69.

70. Moore RY, Bloom FE. Central catecholamine neuron systems: anatomy and physiology of the norepinephrine and epinephrine systems. *Annu Rev Neurosci* 1979;2:113–68.

71. Nadler JV, Perry BW, Cotman CW. Selective reinnervation of hippocampal area CA$_1$ and the fascia dentata after destruction of CA$_3$-CA$_4$ afferents with kainic acid. *Brain Res* 1980;182:1–9.

72. Nakamura M, Fukushima H. Head twitches induced by benzodiazepines and the role of biogenic amines. *Psychopharmacology* 1976;49:259–61.

73. Nistri A, Arenson MS. Differential sensitivity of spinal neurones to amino acids: an intracellular study on the frog spinal cord. *Neuroscience* 1983;8:115–22.

74. Oertel WH, Schmechel DE, Mugnaini E, Tappaz ML, Kopin IJ. Immunocytochemical localization of glutamate decarboxylase in rat cerebellum with a new antiserum. *Neuroscience* 1981;6:2715–35.

75. Olsen RW. GABA benzodiazepine-barbiturate receptor interactions. *J Neurochem* 1981;37:1–17.

76. Pedley TA, Horton RW, Meldrum BS. Electroencephalographic and behavioural effects of a GABA agonist (muscimol) on photosensitive epilepsy in the baboon, Papio papio. *Epilepsia* 1979;20:409–16.

77. Peet MJ, Leah JD, Curtis DR. Antagonists of synaptic and amino acid excitation of neurones in the cat spinal cord. *Brain Res* 1983;266:83–95.

78. Perkins MN, Stone TW. On the interaction of 2-amino-7-phosphonoheptanoic acid and quinolinic acid in mice. *Eur J Pharmacol* 1983;89:297–300.

79. Perkins MN, Stone TW, Collins JF, Curry K. Phosphonate analogues of carboxylic acids as aminoacid antagonists on rat cortical neurons. *Neurosci Lett* 1981;23:333–6.

80. Potashner SJ. Baclofen: effects on amino acid release and metabolism in slices of guinea pig cerebral cortex. *J Neurochem* 1979;32:103–9.

81. Pratt J, Jenner P, Reynolds EH, Marsden CD. Clonazepam induced decreased serotoninergic activity in the mouse brain. *Neuropharmacology* 1979;18:791–9.

82. Ribak CE, Vaughn JE, Saito K. Immunocytochemical localization of glutamic acid decarboxylase in neuronal somata following colchicine inhibition of axonal transport. *Brain Res* 1978;140:315–22.

83. Schwartzkroin PA, Wyler AR. Mechanisms underlying epileptiform burst discharge. *Ann Neurol* 1980;7:95–107.

84. Skerritt JH, Johnston GAR. Enhancement of excitant amino acid release from rat brain slices by the convulsant 3-mercapto-propionic acid. *Brain Res* 1983;258:165–9.

85. Skerritt JH, Johnston GAR. Enhancement of GABA binding by benzodiazepines and related anxiolytics. *Eur J Pharmacol* 1983;89:193–8.

86. Skerritt JH, Johnston GAR. Modulation of excitant amino acid release by convulsant and anticonvulsant drugs. In: Fariello RG, et al., eds. Neurotransmitters, seizures and epilepsy II. New York: Raven Press, 1983;215–26.

87. Sloper JJ, Johnson P, Powell TRS. Selective degeneration of interneurons in the motor cortex of infant monkeys following controlled hypoxia: a possible cause of epilepsy. *Brain Res* 1980;198:204–9.

88. Sloviter RS. "Epileptic" brain damage in rats induced by sustained electrical stimulation of the

perforant path. I. Acute electrophysiological and light microscopic studies. *Brain Res Bull* 1983;10:675–97.

89. Sloviter RS, Damiano BP. Sustained electrical stimulation of the perforant path duplicates kainate-induced electrophysiological effects and hippocampal damage in rats. *Neurosci Lett* 1981;24:279–84.

90. Stone TW, Perkins MN. Quinolinic acid: a potent endogenous exitant at amino acid receptors. *Eur J Pharmacol* 1981;72:411–2.

91. Study RE, Barker JL. Diazepam and (−)pentobarbital: fluctuation analysis reveals different mechanisms for potentiation of GABA responses in cultured central neurons. *Proc Natl Acad Sci USA* 1981;78:7180–4.

92. Tal N, Goldberg O, Luini A, Teichberg VI. An evaluation of glutamyl dipeptide derivatives as antagonists of amino acid-induced Na^+ fluxes in rat striatum slices. *J Neurochem* 1982;39:574–6.

93. Valin A, Cepeda C, Rey E, Naquet R. Opposite effects of lorazepam on two kinds of myoclonus in photosensitive Papio papio. *Electroencephalogr Clin Neurophysiol* 1981;52:647–51.

94. Wada JA, Balzano E, Meldrum BS, Naquet R. Behavioural and electrographic effects of L-5-hydroxytryptophan and D,L-parachlorphenylalanine on epileptic Senegalese baboon Papio papio. *Electroencephalogr Clin Neurophysiol* 1972;33:520–6.

95. Watkins JC, Evans RH. Excitatory amino acid transmitters. *Annu Rev Pharmacol Toxicol* 1981;21:165–204.

96. Wenthold RJ. Release of endogenous glutamic acid, aspartic acid and GABA from cochlear nucleus slices. *Brain Res* 1979;162:338–43.

97. Wiklund L, Toggenburger G, Cuenod M. Aspartate: possible neurotransmitter in cerebellar climbing fibres. *Science* 1982;216:78–80.

98. Zakusov VV, Ostrovskaya RU, Kozhechkin SN, Markovich VV, Molodavkin GM, Voronina TA. Further evidence for GABA-ergic mechanisms in the action of benzodiazepines. *Arch Int Pharmacodyn Ther* 1977;229:313–26.

Advances in Neurology, Vol. 43: Myoclonus,
edited by S. Fahn et al. Raven Press,
New York © 1986.

Concluding Remarks

James W. Lance

*Department of Neurology, The Prince Henry Hospital, Little Bay,
New South Wales, 2036, Australia*

Myoclonus is a brief involuntary muscle contraction of abrupt onset. At the meeting on which this volume is based, an attempt was made to define myoclonus more precisely but met with semantic difficulties. Myoclonus must clearly be differentiated from tremor, and it was generally agreed that rhythmic repetitive movements such as "palatal myoclonus" belong in a separate category. Perhaps this interesting condition could be called "palatal tremor," or the original term, "palatal nystagmus," could be revived. Similarly, the symmetrical limb movements seen in advanced cerebral disease such as subacute sclerosing panencephalitis were considered to be a repetitive dystonia distinct from myoclonus. The slow semipurposive movements of sleep were also thought to be a distinct entity and should therefore not be called nocturnal myoclonus. On the other hand, "night starts" and the startle response were considered to fall under the descriptive heading of myoclonus.

Myoclonus can be subdivided or classified on clinical grounds by the frequency, regularity, and duration of movements, the muscles or muscle groups involved, the precipitation of movement by action or sensory stimulation, and the association in some cases with epilepsy or with degenerative diseases of the nervous system. There are no clinical grounds for separating Ramsay Hunt syndrome from Unverricht–Lundborg disease among the progressive myoclonic epilepsies. Myoclonus may tentatively be classified on physiological grounds as being of cortical, reticular, or spinal origin and, on pharmacological grounds, by response to various forms of therapy. A more complete and satisfying classification will have to await the acquisition of knowledge about the excitatory and inhibitory mechanisms involved and the cellular and molecular basis of the disorders that produce them.

Myoclonus is frequently associated with transient involuntary cessation of muscular contraction during attempts at sustained movement, signaled by a "silent period" in the electromyogram, which interrupts the maintenance of posture and may cause an affected limb to drop or the patient to fall to the ground. The myoclonic jerk can be regarded as a positive physiological phenomenon and the silent period as a related negative phenomenon.

There is no pathological change that can be demonstrated consistently in all types of myoclonus studied. Degeneration of the cerebellum and its dentatorubral projection, the basal ganglia, thalamus, optic and auditory pathways, motoneurons, and muscle fibers have all been described in conjunction with progressive myoclonic epilepsy. No single site has been implicated as the source of posthypoxic action myoclonus, but three of the four reported autopsies have shown changes in the lower midbrain in an area corresponding to the nucleus raphe dorsalis, which is a serotonergic nucleus in animals. The demonstration of defects in the respiratory chain in mitochondrial myopathy associated with progressive myoclonic epilepsy may point to a more extensive change in mitochondria within the central nervous system. Further understanding of storage diseases may enable some forms of myoclonus to be understood in terms of the enzymatic defects involved, although the site of storage may be more important in the production of myoclonus than the nature of the substance stored.

Observations in humans and ingenious experimental models in animals (Table 1) suggest that neurotransmission mediated by serotonin [and possibly γ-aminobutyric acid (GABA)] may be disordered, leading to excessive excitation, diminished inhibition, or both processes in the brainstem and possibly other levels in the motor pathways. The systemic injection of 5-hydroxytryptophan in the guinea pig may inhibit cortical function and permit the reticular formation of the brainstem to discharge spontaneously as well as in response to afferent stimuli. Experiments with DDT and urea suggest that the nucleus gigantocellularis may be an important generator of myoclonus. The catechol model involves a complex pattern of excitation and inhibition with resulting hyperactivity of reticular and thalamic transmission. Intrathecal opiates may induce spinal myoclonus.

Many questions have been raised during the productive workshop on which this volume is based. Why is adrenocorticotropic hormone (ACTH) effective in infantile myoclonic encephalopathy and some cases with an underlying neuroblastoma? Can an autoimmune process be demonstrated in these patients? How do female hormones alter myoclonus? Some patients with myoclonus apparently improve during pregnancy or other causes of amenorrhoea, and others may improve with estrogen

TABLE 1. *Animal models of myoclonus*

Model	Spontaneous	5-HTP[a]	DDT	Urea	Catechol	Opiate
Animal	*Papio papio*	Guinea pig	Rat	Rat	Rat	Rat
Myoclonus						
Rhythmic		+				
Stimulus-sensitive	+	?	+ (Sound)	+	+	+
Generator						
Cortical	+	−				
Thalamic					+	
Reticular		+	+	+	+	
Spinal						+
Drugs						
Improve	Anticonvulsants	Methysergide	5-HTP MAOI[b]	Clonazepam	Atropine	
Worsen					5-HTP	

[a]5-HTP, 5-hydroxytryptophan.
[b]MAOI, monoamine oxidase inhibitor.

therapy. Why do some posthypoxic patients develop action myoclonus and others not? Comparative neuropathology with immunofluorescent studies of serotonin-containing neurons in the raphe nuclei may give us an answer here. Studies of GABA transmission in the cortex (which Brian Meldrum showed is affected by hypoxia) are obviously important. Why do some patients with system degenerations—cerebellar atrophy, for example—develop myoclonus and others (even in the same family) with a similar neurological deficit remain free of myoclonic jerking? How applicable to human disease are the various animal models studied so far? Nucleus reticularis gigantocellularis certainly requires further investigation. There are enough questions here to keep us all busy for a while.

In the meantime, we can be thankful that such enormous advances have been made in the treatment of this devastating condition. The introduction of serotonin precursors, clonazepam, and sodium valproate have completely changed the outlook for patients afflicted by myoclonus.

Subject Index